The Handbook of Fashion Studies

THE HAND FASHION

BOOK OF STUDIES

Edited by

Sandy Black, Amy de la Haye,
Joanne Entwistle, Agnès Rocamora,
Regina A. Root and Helen Thomas

Bloomsbury Academic
An imprint of Bloomsbury Publishing Plc
BLOOMSBURY
LONDON • OXFORD • NEW YORK • NEW DELHI • SYDNEY

Bloomsbury Academic
An imprint of Bloomsbury Publishing Plc

50 Bedford Square
London
WC1B 3DP
UK

1385 Broadway
New York
NY 10018
USA

www.bloomsbury.com

First published 2013
Reprinted 2014
Paperback edition first published 2017

British Library Cataloguing-in-Publication Data
A catalogue record for this book is available from the British Library.

ISBN: HB: 978-0-8578-5194-9
PB: 978-1-3500-2986-6
ePub: 978-1-4725-7743-6
ePDF: 978-1-4725-7744-3

Library of Congress Cataloging-in-Publication Data
The handbook of fashion studies : international perspectives / [edited by]
Amy de la Haye... [et al.]. – First edition.
pages cm
Includes bibliographical references and index.
ISBN 978-0-85785-194-9 (hardback)
1. Fashion–Handbooks, manuals, etc. 2. Clothing and dress–Handbooks, manuals, etc.
3. Clothing trade–Handbooks, manuals, etc. I. De La Haye, Amy.
TT507.H178 2013
746.9'2–dc23
2013024031

Typeset by Apex CoVantage, LLC, Madison, WI, USA.
Printed and bound in Great Britain

CONTENTS

SECTION II: FASHION, IDENTITY, AND DIFFERENCE

SECTION III: SPACES OF FASHION

SECTION IV: FASHION AND MATERIALITY

SECTION V: FASHION, AGENCY, AND POLICY

SECTION VI: SCIENCE, TECHNOLOGY, AND NEW FASHION

SECTION VII: SUSTAINABLE FASHION IN A GLOBALIZED WORLD

LIST OF ILLUSTRATIONS

FIGURES

TABLES

ACKNOWLEDGMENTS

This *Handbook* has been an incredible journey spanning years, continents, and cyberspace. The generosity of many people shaped its pages and ideas from inception to finish. The editors look forward to the many conversations that this handbook will surely inspire.

Early on in the process, the editorial team at Berg Publishers (now Bloomsbury) demonstrated a kind professionalism that is not easily matched. Kathryn Earle and Hannah Shakespeare brought together the international team of editors who ultimately engaged this project. Tristan Palmer and Julia Hall were most thoughtful professionals throughout the early and middle stages of this project. Emily Roessler and Anna Wright provided helpful support and information as we brought this text together. At the University of the Arts and London College of Fashion, Marie Stanley and Laura Thornley both played seminal roles in managing this project. The editors are especially grateful to Laura for the meticulous and thoughtful care with which she approached this project during its final stages and through to submission. Benjamin Whyman also provided much-needed support.

Throughout the process, anonymous reviewers provided important feedback and ideas that ultimately made for a stronger handbook. We are very grateful for their insights. The editors also have pleasure in offering immense thanks to the contributing authors in this volume. Their erudite texts will have lasting influence on the multidisciplinary interpretations of our subject. Our respective institutions have offered us all great support, without which such a far-flung collaboration would not have been possible.

We all have incurred debts along the way. Our families, our friends, our colleagues with whom we have had meaningful conversations along the way, all deserve our heartfelt thanks.

CONTRIBUTORS

Katherine Appleford completed her PhD at the London College of Fashion, University of the Arts London, in 2011. Her research examines the relationship between fashion and class in contemporary British women's dress and explores class distinctions in fashion tastes and fashion practice. Her work highlights important relationships between fashion, class, gender, and space and also emphasizes the important role that mothers play in cultivating classed practices and attitudes in relation to fashion. She teaches sociology at Kingston University London and cultural and historical studies at the London College of Fashion, University of the Arts London. She is currently pursuing further research into class, fashion and public performance, and fashion and body image.

Patrik Aspers is professor and chair of sociology in the Department of Sociology at Uppsala University and professor of fashion management at the Swedish School of Textiles, University of Borås. He is the author of numerous articles and several books, including *Orderly Fashion: A Sociology of Markets* (Princeton University Press, 2010), *Markets* (Polity Press, 2011, translated into Swedish in 2013), *The Worth of Goods* (edited with Jens Beckert; Oxford University Press, 2011), and *Markets in Fashion: A Phenomenological Approach* (City University Press, 2001; 2nd ed., Routledge, 2006). The book *Etnografiska Metoder* (Liber, 2007; 2nd ed., 2011) was published in Swedish. He has worked at the Max Planck Institute for the Study of Societies in Cologne for several years and has been a visiting scholar at the London School of Economics, Harvard University, Columbia University, and Sciences Po. His main fields of research are economic sociology and sociological theory.

Donatella Barbieri is senior research fellow in design for performance, jointly at the Victoria and Albert Museum and London College of Fashion. From 2007 to 2010 she was the London College of Fashion's graduate school director of programs (design cluster). She had previously led the London College of Fashion undergraduate courses in design for performance and established the theater design course at Rose Bruford

College. Her research interests are focused around design for performance, the dress and performance, and the relationship between archived objects and the here and now. As a designer, performance maker, and visual artist she has presented work nationally and internationally. Her projects travel between theory and practice; *Encounters in the Archive,* for example, is a filmed exploration of interaction between the archived object and artist. She is coauthoring *Costume in Performance* (Bloomsbury, 2014) with Melissa Trimingham and has written and presented on methodologies of embodiment and dress in papers such as "Costume Re-Considered" ("Endyesthai": To Dress: Conference, Athens, 2010) and "The Embodied Researcher: Effecting Change through the Body, Creative Processes Material and Interaction" (with Melissa Trimingham, public lecture at the Barbican, 2012). She is curator of costume events at World Stage Design in 2013.

Joanna Berzowska is assistant professor of design and computation arts at Concordia University and a member of the Hexagram Research Institute in Montreal. She is the founder and research director of XS Labs, where her team develops innovative methods and applications in electronic textiles and responsive garments. She lectures internationally about the field of electronic textiles and related social, cultural, aesthetic, and political issues. She received her master's of science from MIT for her work titled Computational Expressionism and subsequently worked with the Tangible Media Group of the MIT Media Lab and cofounded International Fashion Machines in Boston. She holds a BA in pure math and a BFA in design arts. Her art and design work has been shown in the Cooper-Hewitt Design Museum and Art Directors Club in New York, the Victoria & Albert Museum in London, the Millenium Museum in Beijing, various SIGGRAPH Art Galleries, ISEA, the Australian Museum in Sydney, NTT ICC in Tokyo, and Ars Electronica Center in Linz among others.

Sandy Black is professor of fashion and textile design and technology at London College of Fashion, University of the Arts London, and a key researcher within the university's Centre for Sustainable Fashion based at the London College of Fashion. Her focus is interdisciplinary research including design for textiles and fashion, technology, science and mathematics, and the important role of design in sustainable futures. She teaches at the graduate level and supervises a number of PhD candidates in practice-led interdisciplinary research in fashion and textiles. She developed the Interrogating Fashion research network in 2005 (a Designing for the 21st Century initiative funded by the Engineering and Physical Sciences Research Council/Arts and Humanities Research Council), and she founded and coedits the journal *Fashion Practice: The Journal of Design, Creative Process and the Fashion Industry* (Berg). She is principal investigator for the collaborative project Considerate Design for Personalised Fashion Products and in 2013 of the Fashion, Innovation Research and Enterprise (FIREup) project. She has lectured and published widely on the interfaces of design, technology, and sustainability in knitwear, fashion, and textiles. Key books she has written include *The Sustainable Fashion Handbook* (Thames and Hudson, 2012), *Knitting: Fashion, Industry, Craft* (V&A Publishing, 2012), *Eco Chic: The Fashion Paradox* (Black Dog, 2008; 2nd ed., 2011),

Fashioning Fabrics: Contemporary Textiles in Fashion (Black Dog, 2006), and *Knitwear in Fashion* (Thames and Hudson, 2002). Her published chapters include "Nanotechnologies: Their Role in Sustainable Textiles" in *Sustainable Textiles* (ed. R. Blackburn, Woodhead, 2009) and "Trends in Smart Textiles" in *Smart Textiles for Medicine and Healthcare* (ed. L. van Langenhove, Woodhead, 2007).

Regina Lee Blaszczyk is professor of history and chair in the history of business and society at the University of Leeds in the United Kingdom and an associate editor of the *Journal of Design History.* Her work focuses on the history of design and innovation for the consumer culture. She has published eight books, including *The Color Revolution* (MIT Press, 2012), *American Consumer Society, 1865–2005: From Hearth to HDTV* (Harlan Davidson, 2009), *Rohm and Haas: A Century of Innovation* (University of Pennsylvania Press, 2009), *Producing Fashion: Commerce, Culture, and Consumers* (University of Pennsylvania Press, 2008), *Major Problems in American Business History* (Houghton Mifflin, 2005), and *Imagining Consumers: Design and Innovation from Wedgwood to Corning* (Johns Hopkins University Press, 2000). In 2011, together with Richard Coopey of Aberystwyth University, she cofounded FAB, the Fashion and Business History Project. Her new work focuses on three areas: the role of synthetic fiber companies in fashion and interior design, high-street retailing, and the transatlantic fashion business.

Simonetta Carbonaro holds a third-cycle postgraduate degree in consumer psychology and is an expert in strategic marketing and design management. She carries out research in consumer ethos and behavior, forecasting the directions in which consumer culture is moving. For the last fifteen years, Carbonaro has been working as a senior strategic advisor for major retail and manufacturing companies. She is a partner at REALISE, a business consulting firm based in Germany, where she is actively involved in values branding, strategic design, and innovation management. She is professor of design management and humanistic marketing at the Swedish School of Textiles at the University of Borås and a visiting professor at the London College of Fashion.

Jennifer Craik has a bachelor of arts with honors in sociology from the Australian National University and a doctorate in social and political sciences from the University of Cambridge. She is research professor of fashion and textiles at the Royal Melbourne Institute of Technology University. She also lectures in the bachelor of design (fashion) at the Canberra Institute of Technology, Australia. Her research interests are primarily in the culture of fashion and dress, and arts and cultural policy. As a member of the International Scientific Committee for Cultural Policy Research, she is co-organizer of biennial conferences on international cultural policy research. She has published in the areas of tourism, media policy, cultural policy, and fashion theory. Her books include *Resorting to Tourism: Cultural Policies for Tourist Development in Australia* (Allen & Unwin, 1989), *The Face of Fashion* (Routledge, 1994), *Uniforms Exposed* (Berg, 2005), *Re-visioning Arts and Cultural Policy* (ANU e-Press, 2007), and *Fashion: The Key Concepts* (Berg, 2009). Currently, she is completing (with Dr. Sharon Peoples) *The Fashion Studies Book* (Routledge).

Greer Crawley is a senior lecturer in the bachelor's and master's programs in spatial design at Buckinghamshire New University, United Kingdom, and is visiting lecturer at the Institute of Art History, University of Zurich, and in the master's program in spatial design at the University of the Arts, Zurich. A practicing designer and researcher, she received a master's of advanced studies in scenography from the Institute of Design and Technology, the University of the Arts, Zurich, and a PhD from the Institute for Theatre, Film and Media Studies, University of Vienna. She is an associate of the Museums Association and member of the Thinking through Performance Research Group, London College of Fashion, University of the Arts London. She is the editor of *Blue Pages,* the quarterly journal of the Society of British Theatre Designers, and member of the exhibition coordination committee and editor for the exhibition catalog *Transformation & Revelation: UK Design for Performance 2007–2011.* She is coauthor of the Victoria and Albert Museum publication *Gormley to Gaga: UK Design for Performance* (2012), UK commissioner for OISTAT Publications commission, editorial leader for World Stage Design in 2013, and co-curator for Scenofest Architecture World Stage Design.

Amy de la Haye is Rootstein Hopkins Chair of Dress History and Curatorship at London College of Fashion. Her publications on London couture 'Material Evidence' in *The Golden Age of Couture: Pairs and London 1947–57* (ed. Claire Wilcox, V&A Publishing, 2007), *Lucile* (with Valerie D. Mendes, V&A Publishing, 2009), *Britain's Women's Land Army* (The Royal Pavilion & Museums, Brighton & Hove, 2010), and *Chanel* (V&A Publishing, 2012) and her children's book *Clara Button and the Magical Hat Day* (V&A, 2012) are object-led narratives. Her curated exhibitions include Fashion and Fancy Dress: The Messel Family Dress Collection 1865–2005 (with Lou Taylor and Eleanor Thompson, Brighton Museum, 2005) and Cinderellas of the Soil: The Women's Land Army (Brighton Museum, 2010). From 2007 to 2011 she was joint course director, with Professor Judith Clark, of the London College of Fashion's master's course in fashion curation. From 1991 to 1999 she was curator of twentieth-century dress at the Victoria and Albert Museum, where she curated Streetstyle: From Sidewalk to Catwalk (1994) and The Cutting Edge: 50 Years of British Fashion (1997), along with smaller shows including One Woman's Wardrobe (1998).

Marsha A. Dickson is professor and chairperson in the Department of Fashion and Apparel Studies at the University of Delaware. She is lead author of the book *Social Responsibility in the Global Apparel Industry.* She has published in journals such as *Business and Society, Journal of Business Ethics,* and *Journal of Fashion Marketing and Management* and is internationally known for her research and teaching on social responsibility. Dickson is president of Educators for Socially Responsible Apparel Business. She is also a member of the board of directors of the Fair Labor Association, a nongovernmental organization originally formed by President Clinton to improve working conditions in factories around the world. In 2009 Dickson was recognized for her academic contributions with the All Star Award from *Apparel Magazine.* In 2011 Dickson was named Distinguished Scholar of the International Textile and Apparel Association.

Joanne Entwistle is senior lecturer in culture, media, and creative industries at King's College, London. She has previously worked at the University of the Arts, London, and the University of Essex. She holds a doctorate in sociology from Goldsmiths College and has published widely on fashion and dress, cultural and economic value, the body, and gender. Her most recent publications include *Fashioning Models: Image, Text, Industry* (Berg, 2011), *The Aesthetic Economy of Fashion: Markets and Value in Clothing and Modelling* (Berg, 2009), and *The Fashioned Body: Fashion, Dress and Modern Social Theory* (Polity, 2000).

Sarah Fee holds degrees in anthropology and African studies from Oxford University and the Institut National des Langues et Civilisations, Paris. For over twenty years she has been carrying out field research on textiles and dress in Madagascar, as art forms, gifts, and objects of action for their female makers. In recent years her research has broadened to the textile trades of the western Indian Ocean rim. She has edited a volume on gender in Madagascar, coauthored a dictionary of the Tandroy dialect, and is author of numerous articles and chapters on the textile arts of Madagascar and beyond.

Kate Fletcher's work is rooted in nature's principles and engaged with the cultural and creative forces of fashion and design. Over the last fifteen years, her original thinking and progressive outlook have shaped the field of fashion, textiles, and sustainability and come to define it. Fletcher is one of the founders of the "slow fashion" movement and instigator of directional sustainability projects, including Local Wisdom, which has engaged thousands of people worldwide with the "craft of use" and "postgrowth" fashion. She has over fifty scholarly and popular publications in the field. She is author of *Sustainable Fashion and Textiles: Design Journeys* (Earthscan, 2008) and coauthor of *Fashion and Sustainability: Design for Change* (Laurence King, 2012). She is reader in sustainable fashion at the Centre for Sustainable Fashion, London College of Fashion, where she has a remit spanning enterprise, education, and research. Her strategic leadership permeates the center's activities, including its role as co-secretariat to the All Party Parliamentary Group on Ethics and Sustainability in Fashion at the House of Lords.

Judy Frater is the cofounder and project coordinator for the Kala Raksha Trust, a 1,000-person artisan group in Bhuj, Kutch, India. As coordinator she has guided the enterprise since 1993, culminating in the establishment of the first design school in India specifically for traditional artisans. In recognition of her accomplishments, Frater was awarded an Asoka Fellowship for social entrepreneurship, the 2009 Sir Misha Black Medal for Distinguished Services to Design Education, and the Crafts Council of India Kamala Award. Frater is author of *Threads of Identity: Embroidery and Adornment of the Nomadic Rabaris,* for which she received the Costume Society of America's Milla Davenport award. Prior to her residence in India, Frater served as associate curator of the Eastern Hemisphere Collections at the Textile Museum in Washington, D.C. She lectures widely and serves as a consultant to museums with South Asian collections throughout the world.

David Goldsmith is a PhD candidate at the Swedish School of Textiles at the University of Borås, Sweden, and an adjunct professor at Parsons the New School for Design in New York City. He is a practicing textile designer whose doctoral research centers on developing a model for holistically assessing the value of small-scale and local textile production in relationship to long-term sustainability and new concepts of prosperity. His current primary fieldwork is with WomenWeave Charitable Trust in Maheshwar, Madhya Pradesh, India. Additionally, he has extensive managerial experience in the field of contemporary art and teaching English as a second language in many locations around the world.

Karen Tranberg Hansen is professor emerita of anthropology at Northwestern University. As an urban and economic anthropologist, she has conducted extensive research in Zambia. She has published on urban life in Zambia, gender, housing, the informal economy, and work and consumption, including *Salaula: The World of Secondhand Clothing and Zambia* (University of Chicago Press, 2000) and essays on secondhand clothing, dress practices, fashion, and consumption. Together with D. Soyini Madison she is coeditor of *African Dress: Fashion, Agency, Power* (Bloomsbury, 2013).

Robyn Healy is an associate professor in the School of Fashion and Textiles at Royal Melbourne Institute of Technology University. She is the deputy head of research and innovation. In 2009 she completed her PhD thesis, entitled *Striptease: An Investigation of Curatorial Practices for Fashion in the Museum.* Healy was formerly senior curator of fashion and textiles at the National Gallery of Victoria, Melbourne, and the inaugural curator of international fashion at the National Gallery of Australia in Canberra. Her exhibitions have included Gianni Versace: The Retrospective 1982–1997 (National Gallery of Victoria, 2000), Housemix: Highlights of the International Fashion and Textiles Collection (National Gallery of Victoria, 2003), Noble Rot: An Alternate View of Fashion (National Trust of Australia, Melbourne, 2006), Nomadic Archive (Craft Victoria, Melbourne, 2008), and The Endless Garment: The New Craft of Machine Knitting (RMIT Gallery, Melbourne, 2010).

Paul Jobling is senior lecturer in the School of Humanities at the University of Brighton. He has research interests in gender and queer theory, the intertextuality of material culture and visual culture, and the ways in which objects of design are translated into words and images. Among his publications are *Man Appeal: Advertising Menswear and Modernism* (Berg, 2005) and *Fashion Spreads: Word and Image in Fashion Photography since 1980* (Berg, 1999). His forthcoming book, *Advertising Menswear,* deals with print, television, and cinema publicity for men's clothing in Britain between 1945 and 2000 and elaborates the complex interface between advertising and gender theory, and design issues and consumer habits. Further details about his current research projects can be found at http://arts/brighton.ac.uk/research/academic/jobling.

Jennifer M. Jones is associate professor of history at Rutgers University, New Brunswick. She holds a PhD in history from Princeton University. Her research specialties are gender history and eighteenth-century France. She is author of several articles on early modern fashion and commercial culture in journals such as *French Historical Studies* and *Yale French Studies.* Her first book, *Sexing La Mode: Gender, Fashion and Commercial Culture in Old Regime France* (Berg, 2004) explores the history of the gendering of the production and consumption of clothing and fashion in early modern France, with a focus on Paris. She is currently writing a book titled *Therese's Enlightenment: Women in the Shadows of the Public Sphere in Old Regime France,* which examines the life of Jean-Jacques Rousseau's mistress, Thérèse Levasseur, to explore the relationship of nonelite women to the social and cultural projects of the Enlightenment.

Vicki Karaminas is associate professor of fashion studies and associate head of the School of Design at the University of Technology, Sydney, Australia. She is the president of the Popular Culture Association of Australia and New Zealand (2012–2015) and the chair of fashion and the chair for subcultural style and identity for the Popular Culture Association/American Culture Association. Her book publications include *The Men's Fashion Reader* (Berg, 2009), *Fashion in Fiction: Text and Clothing in Literature, Film and Television* (Intellect, 2009), *Fashion and Art* (Bloomsbury, 2013), *Queer Style* (Bloomsbury, 2013), *Shanghai Street Style* (Intellect, 2013), and *Fashion in Popular Culture: Literature, Media and Contemporary Studies* (Intellect, 2013). She is the coeditor of the *Australasian Journal of Popular Culture* and is on the editorial boards of *Fashion Theory: The Journal of Dress, Body and Culture*; *The International Journal of Fashion Studies, Film, Fashion and Consumption*; *Critical Studies in Men's Fashion*; and *Fashion, Style and Popular Culture.*

Mary A. Littrell is research associate at the Museum of International Folk Art in Santa Fe, New Mexico, and is professor and department head emeritus in design and merchandising at Colorado State University. Littrell's research addresses multiple facets of business social responsibility, with special focus on artisan enterprises, fair trade, and nongovernmental organizations. Across her work, she has examined how artisan textile enterprises achieve sustainability in the increasingly competitive global market for artisan products. Her books with coauthor Marsha Dickson include *Social Responsibility in the Global Market: Fair Trade of Cultural Products* and *Artisans and Fair Trade: Crafting Development.* In recognition of their research, the coauthors were named Rockefeller Center Scholars in Bellagio, Italy. Littrell is a fellow of the International Textile and Apparel Association and of the Society for Applied Anthropology.

Margaret Maynard is an associate professor in the School of English, Media Studies and Art History and honorary research consultant at the University of Queensland. Her special research interests are dress, identity, and consumption with particular focus on Australian clothing including indigenous dress. Her publications include "Clothing: Art Clothes or Wearable Art?" in *Fashion and Art* (ed. Adam Geczy and Vicki Karaminas, Bloomsbury, 2013), "What Is Australian Fashion Photography? A Dilemma" (*Fashion Theory* 13 [4], 2009), "The Fashion Photograph: An Ecology," in *Fashion Photography: Thinking Critically about Fashion Photography* (ed. Eugenie Shinkle, I. B. Tauris, 2007), "Where Do Flappers Fit In? The Photography of Modern Fashion in Australia" (*Australian*

Cultural History 25, 2006), *Fashioned from Penury: Dress as Cultural Practice in Colonial Australia* (Cambridge University Press, 1994), *Out of Line: Australian Women and Style* (University of New South Wales Press, 2001), and *Dress and Globalisation* (Manchester University Press, 2004). She edited volume 7, *Australia, New Zealand and the Pacific Islands,* for the *Berg Encyclopedia of World Dress and Fashion* (Berg, 2010).

Marie O'Mahony is an academic and consultant. She is professor of advanced fashion and textiles at Ontario College of Art and Design (OCAD) University, Toronto, and visiting professor at University of the Arts, London. She is also a textile and technology consultant, author, and curator. Her books include *TechnoTextiles 2* (2005), *TechnoTextiles* (1998), *Cyborg: The Man Machine* (2002), and *Sportstech* (2002), all published by Thames and Hudson with the most recent, *Advanced Textiles for Wellness and Health,* published in October 2011. Exhibitions she has curated include Cyborg for the Stedelijk Museum in Amsterdam; The Fabric of Fashion, an international touring exhibition for the British Council; and TechnoThreads for Science Gallery, Trinity College, Dublin. Her clients include Zaha M. Hadid, Seymour Powell, Ove Arup and Partners, Nike, and Hussein Chalayan. She has also served on the Australian government's Textile, Clothing and Footwear (TCF) Industries Innovation Council from 2009 to 2011.

Alexandra Palmer is the Nora E. Vaughan Senior Curator, Textiles and Costume, at the Royal Ontario Museum (ROM), associate professor in the Department of Fine Art at the University of Toronto, and adjunct professor in York University's graduate program in art history. She has curated many exhibitions and has published extensively on postwar fashion; her book *Couture and Commerce: The Transatlantic Fashion Trade in the 1950s* (UBC Press with Royal Ontario Museum, 2001) won a Clio Award for Ontario history. She is exhibition editor for the journal *Fashion Theory.*

Bradley Quinn is a British author and consultant with expertise in fashion, technology, textiles, and design. His books include *Techno Fashion, The Fashion of Architecture, Textile Designers at the Cutting Edge, UltraMaterials, Textile Futures, Design Futures, Fashion Futures,* and the recently published *Textile Visionaries.* As his trend forecasts and publications chart new ways of thinking about products and materials, Quinn explores the furthermost boundaries of what today's generation of designers can achieve.

Agnès Rocamora is a reader in social and cultural studies at the London College of Fashion, University of the Arts London. She is the author of *Fashioning the City: Paris, Fashion and the Media* (I. B. Tauris, 2009). Her writing on the field of fashion, fashion media, and fashion blogging has appeared in various journals, including *Fashion Theory, Sociology,* and the *Journal of Consumer Culture.* She is a coeditor of *Thinking Through Fashion: A Guide to Key Thinkers* (I. B. Tauris, forthcoming in 2014) and *Fashion Media: Past and Present* (Bloomsbury, 2013), and a contributor to *Fashion's World Cities* (Berg, 2006) and *Fashion as Photograph* (I. B. Tauris, 2008). She is currently developing her work on fashion and digital media.

Regina A. Root, associate professor of Hispanic studies, environmental science and policy, and global studies at the College of William and Mary, has published numerous works on fashion and cultural production. Her award-winning *Couture and Consensus: Fashion and Politics in Postcolonial Argentina* (University of Minnesota Press, 2010) and *The Latin American Fashion Reader* (Berg, 2005) have been touted by reviewers as pioneering work in the area of Latin American material culture. Root's work on sustainable design practices—which includes a volume on ecofashion (special issue of *Fashion Theory*, 2008) and contributions as president *ad honorem* of the scientific committee of Ixel Moda, Latin America's fashion congress, and as a consultant for various design and industry initiatives—has focused on opening new areas of research with links to cultural policy. Her recent work includes the coedited volumes *Pasado de moda: Expresiones culturales y consumo en la Argentina* (with Susan Hallstead, Edhasa, 2014) and "Latin American Fashion Now" (a special issue of *Fashion Theory*, with Rita Andrade, 2014). She serves on the editorial board of *Fashion Theory*, *d[O]bras*, and *IARA, Revista de Moda, Cultura e Arte*.

Philip Sams's background is in industrial chemistry, with a long career as a research scientist and "research entrepreneur" at Unilever PLC. Now a research consultant, his reputation is as a catalyst for and champion of new design/science collaborations with a mission to help industry make inspirational use of new science and technology by engaging designer and fashion thinkers into dialogue with industry. His credits include many design and fashion/science projects, academic papers, and more than 30 patents. He received academic recognition for his collaborative work with an honorary doctorate from London College of Fashion, University of the Arts London. Sams is a visiting professor in the Faculty of Art and Design at Northumbria University.

Philip A. Sykas is currently a research associate within the Manchester Institute for Research and Innovation in Art and Design at Manchester Metropolitan University. With a background in textile conservation and curatorship, he brings to his research an interest in the material and technical makeup of historical dress and the ways in which this evidence reveals cultural meaning. His past work has included a study of constructional sewing and sewing threads, but his current work is focused on printed textiles: cloth grounds, engraving for calico printing, and the technical evolution of printing for dress. He has particularly studied the evidence found in manufacturers' pattern books, looking at the influence of technology on pattern design, and the development of British merchanting practice within the international trade in printed textiles.

Lou Taylor is professor of dress and textile history at the University of Brighton and author of *Mourning Dress: A Costume and Social History* (1983, republished by Routledge in 2010) and *The Study of Dress History* (2002) and *Establishing Dress History* (2004), both published by Manchester University Press.

José Teunissen holds a professorship of fashion theory and research at ArtEZ Institute of the Arts, Arnhem, the Netherlands, and works as an independent fashion curator. In addition, she is a chair member of Premsela, the Institute for Fashion and Design. Teunissen studied Dutch language and literature and film and television science. From

1998 to 2007 she was curator of fashion and costumes at the Centraal Museum in Utrecht. Her research interests focus on fashion as performance, identity, and presentation. Among her publications are *Mode in Beweging* (NFM, 1990), *De Nieuwe Kleren* (Balie, 1992), *Droog & Dutch Design* (Centraal Museum, 2000), *The Ideal Woman* (SUN, 2004), *Global Fashion, Local Tradition* (Terra, 2005), *Mode in Nederland* (Terra, 2006), *The Power of Fashion* (Terra and ArtEZ Press, 2006), *Fashion and Accessories* (Terra and ArtEZ Press, 2007), *Fashion and Imagination* (ArtEZ Press and d'jonge Hond, 2009), *the New Man* (ArtEZ Press and d'jonge Hond, 2010).

Helen Thomas is a professor and director of doctoral programs at the University of the Arts London. From 2004 to 2010 she was director of research at London College of Fashion. Before that, she was professor of sociology of dance and culture and director of the Interdisciplinary Research Centre for the Body and Performance at Goldsmiths University of London. Her research interests center on sociology of the body and dance in culture and performance; cultural theories; and methodologies. She mostly works with PhD students whose work centers on dance and fashion, fashion curation, and costume and performance. Recent publications include "Mapping Embodiment: Methodologies for Representing Pain and Injury" (with Jen Tarr, *Qualitative Research* 11 [2], 2011); "Dancers Perceptions of Pain and Injury: Positive and Negative Effects" (with Tarr, *Journal of Dance Medicine and Science* 13 [2], 2009); *The Body, Dance and Cultural Theory* (Palgrave Macmillan, 2003); *Cultural Bodies: Ethnography and Theory* (coedited with Jamilah Ahmed, Polity, 2004); and *The Body and Everyday Life* (Routledge, 2013).

Julia Twigg is professor of social policy and sociology at the University of Kent in the United Kingdom. She is currently engaged in a series of interconnected projects exploring the role of clothing and dress in the changing constitution of age. She recently completed an Economic and Social Research Council (ESRC)–funded study of dress in later life, drawing on the views and experiences of older women and the responses of the media and the fashion industry, published by Bloomsbury in 2013 as *Fashion and Age: Dress, the Body and Later Life.* She is currently working on an ESRC-funded project on dementia and dress, exploring issues of embodied personhood and the role of clothing in its expression. She is coediting the *Routledge Handbook of Cultural Gerontology,* which aims to be a position statement for this emerging field. Her earlier work focused on embodiment, particularly on the role of bodywork in care, and in 2006 she published *The Body in Health and Social Care.* Twigg's original degree was in history, and she is interested in the historical dimension of these topics of research.

Introduction

SANDY BLACK, AMY DE LA HAYE, JOANNE ENTWISTLE, AGNÈS ROCAMORA, REGINA A. ROOT, AND HELEN THOMAS

Most published collections on fashion tend to be organized on the basis of disciplinary frameworks. Such an approach to the field of fashion studies limits all too quickly the scope and diversity of the scholarly contributions that ground this field and move it forward. With *The Handbook of Fashion Studies,* the editors have aimed to offer a unique, thematically based approach to map the field of historical and contemporary fashion theory and history. This volume highlights new collaborations and international connections that ground the current study of fashion, while also pointing to the very real potential of fashion research that is interdisciplinary and pan-disciplinary in nature. In so doing, *The Handbook of Fashion Studies* overcomes the limits of approaches that have often described fashion in somewhat binary terms: as the site of tension between theory and practice, production and consumption, high art and popular culture. While such analysis can indeed be useful, it risks overlooking the complexity of key strands and concepts guiding fashion studies research. Furthermore, there are issues relevant to fashion theory and history—from the archival process to creative agency to the quest for sustainable design—that have been virtually unaddressed by previous volumes.

The Handbook of Fashion Studies defines the key areas generally addressed as specific subjects and integral to the study of fashion, such as identity, materiality, dress history, technology, and globalization, among others. The themes of production and consumption, designers and design practices, and the body are woven into the fabric of the collection as opposed to being set out as individual themes, and they function as core strands in each of the *Handbook*'s sections. The methodological issues that arise in relation to these core strands are also embedded in the chapters.

Each section carefully situates the *Handbook* within the contemporary context of an expanding "fashion studies." Early chapters lay the groundwork for working definitions of key terms such as *fashion, dress,* and *clothing* to ensure consistency of terminology.

Readers will also find the multidisciplinary and interdisciplinary nature of fashion studies reflected in the *Handbook* with sections organized thematically to identify key concepts and issues. The themes that are developed cover multiple aspects of the study of fashion: its relationship with time, identity and difference, space, materiality, policy and agency, science and technology, and not least sustainability, all in the context of a significant global economic reach whether in terms of production, consumption, or communication.

While the coeditors have ensured breadth of coverage with the methodological range covered across sections, from historical methods to contemporary social and cultural theory, and from theory to praxis, it is also evident that the field continues to expand. A critical questioning of the definitions guiding the field, the recovery of fashion histories traditionally overlooked by scholars, and the need for research to engage the communities it represents are vibrant new connections for fashion studies. Readers will note the parallel treatment of theory and practice throughout the *Handbook*; the editors believed it was important to show these not as separate, autonomous entities but as scholarly perspectives that inform and reflect on each other. Such an approach thereby alters the traditional analysis of fashion that has often privileged theory over and above practice. For the editors, theory and practice are intimately connected and offer important counterpoints for fashion studies analysis.

One of this volume's contributions represents an internationalization process underway in fashion studies research. As indicated in chapter 1, change in the study of dress and fashion has been slow to occur in part because of cultural values that have not ordinarily taken into account fashion's seriousness as a subject of study. In addition, linguistic barriers and geographic distances have made it difficult to bring the field together more cohesively. However, with its ten volumes representing scholars from across the globe, the *Berg Encyclopedia of World Dress and Fashion* (Eicher 2010) represented an important first step in bridging this divide. Further publications have started to appear that address a new wave of emerging (non-Western) fashion designers, such as works by Juanjuan Wu (2009, 2012) and Christine Tsui (2010) on Chinese designers. Linguistic barriers continue to present an important obstacle in assessing the field in its entirety, something of which the editors of this volume were very aware. While contributors to this handbook are largely English speaking, those who are multilingual aimed to integrate scholarly work published in languages other than English to provide the most holistic view of the field through the key strands identified.

As is to be expected, any coedited handbook is the result of collaborative connections. In many ways, this project has been an experiment across institutions and the expanse of topics within our field. To capture the diversity of subjects that comprise fashion studies, we sought the input of diverse contributors and received generous feedback from numerous reviewers and scholars, with the expectation that a rigorous approach to the field's ideas and assertions was the only way to push individual and collective work forward. While many of us still experiment with new research models to engage the meaning of dress and fashion to produce new knowledge, it remains clear that a wide range of approaches exist. This *Handbook* therefore highlights some of the best practices available to scholars, with a methodological focus that will undoubtedly help to expand the realm of fashion studies.

Section I, entitled "Fashion/Dress and Time," edited by Helen Thomas, seeks to map out interdisciplinary approaches to "dress" and "fashion" within the contexts of particular time frames: "historical," "contemporary," and "new times." The concern with history and changing times is central to the four chapters in this section as they relate to shifts in discourse on dress and fashion that have had, or will have, an impact on the increasingly interdisciplinary studies on fashion and dress. It brings together scholars with a keen interest in dress and fashion whose main disciplinary bases are in dress history and curation, design for performance, sociology, and social gerontology, which in turn evidences the interest in fashion and dress in other areas of study.

Although the words *dress* and *fashion* are generally considered to have emerged out of different disciplinary bases, they are often used interchangeably (Entwistle 2000). The former, as indicated in regard to section IV in this *Handbook,* has by and large been studied within an art historical approach in relation to the interpretation of dress in the context of museums and within anthropology. The latter is usually associated with the rise of modernity in the West, with its accompanying rapid social and political change and a quickening of time, although this viewpoint has been criticized for privileging fashion as a Western construct (Craik 1993).

In chapter 1, Lou Taylor, a historian and curator of dress whose work has had a considerable impact on the field, notes that definitions of *dress* and *fashion* are often contested within the literature. Taylor analyzes the major developments in recent research and critical theory on fashion and dress and the emergence of fashion studies (also a contested term), beginning with an examination of the material culture approach. Taylor's chapter provides an impressive historical map of the impact of theories and frameworks from other disciplines on the field in the context of a burgeoning fashion studies. From a design-for-performance perspective, Greer Crawley and Donatella Barbieri examine the ways in which the absent body in historical dress in certain innovative contemporary curatorial practices may be seen to challenge traditional curatorial approaches to the "object of dress." This has resulted in a paradigmatic shift through the incorporation of postmodern "performative" strategies and narratives, with a focus on "exhibition making" (that is to say, curation as practice or in practice), opening up the possibility of a dialogue between historical dress and the spectator. These new approaches to exhibition making, as the authors show, draw on contemporary theoretical and often interdisciplinary frames such as postmodernist, narrative, and psychoanalytic theories.

In her chapter "New Fashion Times," Agnès Rocamora, a sociologist whose research focuses on fashion and culture (and who is the editor of section III in this volume), addresses the ways in which fashion and time are related in contemporary culture. She considers the ways in which the concept of time has accelerated exponentially since the latter half of the twentieth century through the advances in new technologies that heralded a new phase of modernity. By drawing on a range of social and cultural theorists Rocamora examines how time and space are increasingly collapsed into the immediacy of the "now" of real time, suggesting we may need to think about "instant fashion" rather than "fast fashion."

Julia Twigg's chapter, "Fashion, the Body, and Age," focuses on the function that dress has played historically in the construction of age. Twigg is a social gerontologist whose recent research has focused on the relationship between dress, the body (particularly women's bodies), and age. The chapter addresses and assesses the ways in which the sociohistorical construction of age has changed with the increasing rise of consumer culture since the latter half of the twentieth century, to the extent that the old patterns of age ordering are no longer applicable. This chapter forms a link to the next section, which addresses the issues of identity and difference.

Dress has long been associated with categories of social difference, marking out class, gender, race, ethnicity, sexualities (gay, lesbian, and transgender), and subcultural affiliations. Section II, entitled "Fashion, Identity, and Difference," edited by Joanne Entwistle, discusses some of these issues, and specifically how fashion—as an industry and a discursive practice—has "played" with, exaggerated, and marked out differences. Within the field of fashion studies, issues concerning identity have been widely analyzed. This was a preoccupation from the earliest sociological and anthropological work in the late nineteenth and early twentieth centuries, which set out to examine the ways in which dress shapes social and individual expressions of self. More recent expositions of subjectivities have sought to address the increasing proliferation of identities that has come to the fore in late modernity (Blumer 1969; Crane 2000; Entwistle 2000, 2001; Tseëlon 1997). This section takes on some of these issues through an examination of recent historiographical work on eighteenth-century femininity and fashion (Jennifer M. Jones), analysis of class and identity (Katherine Appleford), and a consideration of the ways in which lesbian identities have been articulated in recent years, from "butch" and "femme" to "lesbian chic" (Vicki Karaminas).

Historical and contemporary examples demonstrate the ways fashion is influential in constructing important social distinctions. Katherine Appleford highlights the pivotal role that class has traditionally played in understanding British fashion consumption and, more important, demonstrates its continuing significance for an understanding of mainstream fashion practices and discourses in Britain today. Looking at historical precedents, Jennifer M. Jones discusses how in the course of the eighteenth century fashion became female. This new association of fashion with femininity was connected to new forms of production, new forms of consumption, and new fashion styles themselves. The transformation in the meaning of fashion and practices of dressing is placed within a broader context of changes in gender and political ideologies and economic and social practices in increasingly commercial and urban societies. Complementing this is a discussion on fashion, identity, and gender, as Vicki Karaminas addresses the stereotypical view of lesbian sartorial style as simply the adoption of masculine attire and explores the diverse mix of cultural forms and multiethnic styles in "lesbian chic" since the early twentieth century.

The section cannot hope to cover all the many varied aspects of fashion and identity, but in taking on some of the key elements—class, gender, sexuality—it demonstrates the diversity of work in this area. Discussions of race and ethnicity are not included here, but we acknowledge that work in this area continues to expand (Black 2009; Eicher, Evenson, and Lutz 2008; Kondo 1997).

As both a symbolic and a material form, fashion evolves at the intersection of a varied constituency of spaces and places that shape, as they are shaped by, practices of fashion. Section III, "Spaces of Fashion," edited by Agnès Rocamora, focuses on these often complex spaces of fashion. Some of these spaces are mentioned in other sections, for example, in Jennifer Craik's chapter "Fashion, Tourism, and Global Culture." Section III, however, takes space as its central focus of interest. It brings together academics from different disciplines: Paul Jobling, a historical and critical studies scholar; Regina Lee Blaszczyk, a business historian; José Teunissen, a fashion curator; and Patrik Aspers, a sociologist. While Jobling focuses on the relation between fashion on and off the cinema screen, Blaszczyk looks at the hidden spaces of fashion, where it is made and negotiated behind the scenes before it reaches the scrutinizing eye of the consumer. In contrast, Teunissen looks at some of the spaces where fashion is displayed for scrutiny, fueling the economy of desire that is the essence of fashion: the catwalks, galleries, and stores where it is displayed, the distinction between the realm of commerce and that of art being made ever more tenuous. Finally, in his discussion of the fashion market in its various incarnations, Aspers interrogates the notion of the market as a space for the constitution of fashion.

Although informed by the tradition of the discipline each belongs to, the authors' approach to the topic of space and fashion is premised on a shared understanding of the concept of space as that which makes and is made by fashion. It shows that fashion in space has to be thought of in the plural—spaces rather than a space of fashion—and that these spaces are all intrinsic to the production, circulation, and consumption of fashion. These are also spaces that are historically determined, which draws attention to their fluid and constantly changing nature.

Although various authors have attended to some aspects of the spatiality of fashion, concentrating on one or another of its dimensions—the three-dimensional space of the city as in the work of Rebecca Arnold (2008) or Christopher Breward (2004), or the two-dimensional space of print magazines or film screens as in the work of Stella Bruzzi (1997), Paul Jobling (1999), Jane Gaines and Charlotte Herzog (1990), or Agnès Rocamora (2009), for instance—the varied and complex nature of the spatiality of fashion is still largely left unexplored. Except maybe for John Potvin's 2009 *The Places and Spaces of Fashion, 1800–2007,* there is still a dearth of systematic and in-depth explorations of the various genres and manifestations of fashion spaces, as well as of the processes whereby fashion is made through space, pointing to a real opportunity for further research.

At a time when the forces of globalization are continually renewing the geography of fashion, and with the proliferation of new digital platforms such as websites and apps that take fashion through virtual spaces and on the move almost instantly, it is more important than ever to interrogate the complex and differentiated spatiality of fashion, its many places, sites, and modalities.

Recent developments in the manner, place, and times in which historical fashion is experienced are evidenced by the purposeful opening up of museums and public institutions to wider audiences, seeking to encourage new audience demographics. In tandem with the "always-on" connectedness of much of contemporary networked society, many significant city-based institutions opened their doors to new types of activities such as late-night openings and themed events, becoming a greater part of the urban entertainment and leisure culture. Fashion exhibitions and related events have continued to play a significant role in attracting larger numbers of visitors to museums and expanding engagement with the materiality and sometimes performativity of fashion and clothing.

Section IV of the *Handbook,* "Fashion and Materiality," edited by Amy de la Haye, explores various methodologies involved in object-led analysis of fashion clothing, research typically conducted in museums and archives. Here we provide an overview of the intersection of core disciplines, direct the reader to key sources, and argue for the methodological specificity of materiality.

Within academia, the term *materiality* is allied closely with material culture studies, which has its roots in anthropology and sociology and has been developed within the university sector since the 1970s in studies of semiotics, modernity, and consumption. Its chronology corresponds with the burgeoning of the field of fashion studies, within which fashion history has a much longer genealogy, and the inclusion, presentation, and interpretation of fashionable dress within the context of the museum. These have been paralleled by the growth of related academic interests in life histories, gender, and ethnicity.

Lou Taylor's erudite books *The Study of Dress History* (2002) and *Establishing Dress History* (2004) document respectively the history and historiography of dress history—including fashionable dress—within texts and exhibitions. Another key source that has explored and extended the debates on object-led fashion research is the journal *Fashion Theory* (launched by Valerie Steele in 1997): special issues titled "Methodologies" (Steele 1998), "Exhibitionism" (Steele 2008), and "Fashion Curation" (O'Neill 2008) are especially pertinent.

Material culture researchers have generally interpreted objects (items that have been made or modified by humans, also referred to as *artifacts*) as markers that shape the culture from which they have emerged. And, in turn, they have explored how objects can inform our understanding of that culture, placing special emphasis on people-object relationships across time and space. For a now seminal formulation of material culture analysis we direct the reader to Jules Prown's *Art as Evidence: Writings on Art and*

Material Culture (2001) and, for a historiography and expansion of recent debate, to Ian Woodward's *Understanding Material Culture* (2007).

It was not until the mid-2000s that material culturalists engaged actively with dress and the fabric from which it is made. The work of Daniel Miller has been hugely instrumental within material culture studies, and his engagement with dress has been important for the purposes of this *Handbook.* His core texts include *Clothing as Material Culture,* coedited with Susanne Küchler (2005), and, more recently, an examination of world fashion, *Global Denim,* coedited with Sophie Woodward, which investigates denim as a case study (2010). To date, material culture studies on fashion are rare (see, for example, Sophie Woodward's 2007 *Why Women Wear What They Wear*), and their central tenet is the meaning, rather than the object specificity, of fashion clothing.

Within section IV, de la Haye's concerns extend the study of the social biography and social life of objects (Appadurai 1986; Kopytoff 1986)—in this case fashion clothing—beyond the world of consumption and consumption-based identity to the point at which they expose meanings and values as "objects." She argues that materiality is a research process that is still underutilized. One of the reasons underlying this might be that "objects are harder to access than text, both physically and intellectually," as one of the contributors to this section, Alexandra Palmer, argues in chapter 13. Philip A. Sykas, in his chapter "Investigative Methodologies: Understanding the Fabric of Fashion," stresses that

> materiality is directed to the values and meanings attached to objects. The qualities that give rise to these are inextricably bundled together, such as color, drape, indicators of maker and origin, contributing alongside form and substance. Thus the materiality approach shifts attention toward a holistic account of fashion, integrating maker and making (and re-making), wearers and wearing, along with cultural values—values that are interpreted in full cognizance of their mutable meanings.

In 2012, de la Haye argues, while the detailed object-centeredness of materiality as a fashion studies methodology is entirely complementary to and influenced by material culture studies, it remains distinctive.

In order to understand fully the complexities of dress, the body, and culture, scholars have also begun to address the dynamics of creative agency, demonstrating how fashion as expression asserts power, imitates and emerges as hybrid form, challenges authority, and enacts change. The essays in section V, "Fashion, Agency, and Policy," edited by Regina A. Root, examine the creation, production, sale, and consumption of dress and fashion within select world culture regions.

Recognizing the multivalent nature of fashion studies, the essays in this section challenge the hegemony of Western fashion constructs as much as they decenter the field through a critical questioning of the workings of culture and power. To understand "fashion" as a globalized phenomenon, scholars have engaged in a long-term recovery project to unlock fashion studies and create a more inclusive field in the process. Global fashion studies have registered the complexities of self-fashioning and style appropriations, competing discourses and pockets of resistance, crises and disruptions, among other sociocultural issues. The scholars represented in this section delve into topics as diverse as the proliferation of fashion weeks around the globe and the rise of fashion tourism as the twenty-first century's version of consumer citizenship (Jennifer Craik, chapter 16), the complex issues faced by Indian artisans struggling to maintain their cultural heritage within the globalized marketplace (Mary A. Littrell and Judy Frater, chapter 17), efforts underway to map Latin American fashion (Regina A. Root, chapter 18), and the complex dynamics of secondhand clothing in Africa (Karen Tranberg Hansen, chapter 19). While it would be difficult to capture the diversity of global fashion studies in but one section of a handbook, these contributions reveal the unfinished nature of the fashion canon and point us toward important new directions that will expand the field.

The impact of the total fashion system on global society and the environment is such that "business as usual" is no longer an option. The inclusion of both sustainability and technology among the *Handbook*'s themes marks a point of change in academic studies of fashion. The relationship between science, technology, design, and fashion has until recent decades been little acknowledged in the academic literature, although there is a burgeoning list of books now being published (see below). The fundamental importance of textiles in the Industrial Revolution sets the context in which these disciplines are normally delineated, with clearly defined but polarized perspectives of practice and theory: for example, fiber and textile technology, design theory, analysis of historical dress and fashion, and contemporary design. Viewing fashion and clothing as an embodied and experiential practice, and giving importance to design and the material culture of fashion (Entwistle 2000; Evans 2003), is central to current and emerging research approaches that take a more holistic standpoint. As Caroline Evans puts it, this more empirical integrated approach is a methodology that does not "eclipse fashion with theory" (2003: 3).

Section VI of the *Handbook,* "Science, Technology, and New Fashion," edited by Sandy Black, examines recent developments in fashion studies that straddle traditional disciplines. Late twentieth-century developments in technology and science (not least the electronic and digital revolution that has enabled rapid convergence of previously unrelated areas) have blurred boundaries and created new experimental nodes of knowledge and practice, in which design is fundamental and fashion plays an increasing role. The fertile territories for research have been visionary academic organizations and research labs, which have sought to seed and cross-fertilize new concepts through multidisciplinary teams and agendas. After small beginnings in the 1980s with pioneers such as the Xerox research lab in Palo Alto, California, and the MIT Media Lab in Boston, Massachusetts, cross-disciplinary research is flourishing in academia, bringing together normally divergent sectors such as fashion design, computing, engineering, and polymer science. The potential has increasingly been recognized in funding initiatives across the United Kingdom, Europe, and Canada, for example, whether involving the better use of raw materials, efficient energy use, or the development of smart cities. Designers may have previously used concepts in science and technology as inspiration, but through the insightful (and occasionally serendipitous) forging of new collaborations, experimental research is increasingly taking place, creating new hybrid practices and propositional prototypes that would not have come into existence through individual endeavor. A number of these are discussed in chapters 20 to 23, exemplifying the concepts of practice as research and research through practice (Frayling 1993). A simple taxonomy for collaborations between fashion, science, and technology is proposed by industrial research scientist Philip Sams and design practitioner/researcher Sandy Black (chapter 23).

New territories have been mapped out for fashion that harness pure science and technology to practical applications, often originating in research for the space sector or for military or medical purposes. Gradually, this research spread from specialist commercial products for protective clothing to mainstream design and fashion. In the 1990s several fashion designers and artists were inspired by the technical qualities of such textiles, often in the context of dystopian urban visions of the future (Bolton 2002). Similar scenarios have continued to be explored as fashion and functionality become increasingly merged.

The fashion industry has traditionally had a very low capacity for research and development, due to its complex structure of multiple suppliers and producers, together with the speed of its product cycles and constraints of specific price points. The industry has therefore relied on external organizations to provide new research concepts, especially in technology. For example, the Netherlands-based consumer electronics giant Philips catalyzed new thinking by engaging textile and fashion designers with industrial designers and engineers in the mid-1990s. More recently, as the global reach of sportswear brands such as Nike has increased, research and development to provide elite athletes' clothing with optimum performance have stimulated the expectation of enhanced functionalities in everyday clothing. Fashion and clothing research has become more collaborative between science and technology providers and academic institutions. The acknowledgment of "design thinking" as a new approach for business stems from the specific nature of design and designers, which Tim Brown of the creative agency IDEO styles as being "T-shaped" (Brown 2005; Guest 1991). That is, a designer is able to empathize and work broadly across disciplinary boundaries and a wide scope but maintains in-depth knowledge that can be applied to specific problems (Cross 2011; Rowe 1987). Furthermore, in chapter 23, Sams and Black make the case for "fashion thinking" as a distinctive complement to and subset of design thinking (see also Nixon and Blakley 2012).

Fashion is harnessing emerging technology to enhance both the functional and emotional experience of clothing, creating new scenarios and altering the relationship of individuals to their clothing. In this section, chapters by the writer Bradley Quinn and practitioner/researcher Joanna Berzowska trace the development of the field of wearable technology from the relatively crude distribution of hardware around the body to the ongoing development of embedded electronics and other sensing capability in the textiles from which clothing is fabricated. The impact and consequences (both positive and negative) of revealing traces of touch and other sensory communication are explored through the mechanism of experimental prototyping and testing scenarios.

The role of the creative imagination in research is explored by author Marie O'Mahony in chapter 22, discussing the remarkable synergy and mutual inspiration between science fiction in film and literature and "science fact"—the realization of new textile and fashion functionality and experiences. Textiles are fundamental to the progression of fashion, yet in certain cases traditional methods can now be bypassed by technological developments such as three-dimensional printing, heralded as the next revolution in production, set to be as influential as two-dimensional desktop printing. Collaborative cross-disciplinary research has been instrumental in developing remarkable new paradigms for the creation of textiles, for example, the growing and harvesting of bacterial cellulose as textile (the BioCouture project) or the creation of fabric-in-a-can from Fabrican (both discussed in chapter 23). The rate at which such experimental projects are being generated has continued to increase, evidenced by the growing number of survey publications produced by observers, curators, and practitioners (see, for example, Braddock Clarke and O'Mahony 2005; Lee 2005; Quinn 2002; Seymour 2008). The experimental methods and interdisciplinary dialogues discussed in the "Science, Technology, and New Fashion" section represent a maturing of imaginative practice-led research in the fashion and clothing context. These research directions clearly signal future potential to create and experience fashion in new ways that could provide lasting delight while addressing some of the major environmental concerns facing society.

The complex issue of sustainability—environmental, social, and economic—is discussed further in the final section of the *Handbook,* "Sustainable Fashion in a Globalized World," coedited by Sandy Black and Regina A. Root. Given the trajectory spanned by fashion in the previous century, fueled by technological developments and scientific discoveries, we can only speculate about the future. However, the current business paradigms for fashion are no longer sustainable (as discussed in chapters 26 and 27), and visionary developments for a sustainable future are necessary.

While *The Handbook of Fashion Studies* approaches sustainability and globalization throughout fashion theory and history, especially as related to practice, this concluding section highlights the cultural shifts that are already informing and challenging everyday fashion practices around the globe. It considers the fast-changing practices within fashion production and consumption, precipitated by the global environmental and economic imperatives that have impacted fashion since the Industrial Revolution and through to the early twenty-first century. Both practical and cultural shifts have resulted, and are still emerging, due to increased awareness of issues endemic to the complex fashion system of global manufacturing and the pressing need for enhanced sustainability. The section discusses issues from a range of perspectives and indicates future directions for the practice of fashion.

In recent decades, the democratization of fashion (from the diffusion of luxury brands to the "fast fashion" phenomenon of the mass market) has made fashion accessible to an ever wider public. But there has been a severe human and environmental cost to the rapid expansion of low-priced fashion, creating pressures felt most keenly by manufacturers and garment workers in developing countries and subsistence farmers who grow fibers such as cotton or cashmere. Media coverage and high-profile campaigns exposing malpractices raised the bar in the 1990s; a major shift has seen increasing consumer demand for transparency and traceability in the production of clothing, following the lead of similar successful campaigns around food production. An uncompromising global agenda has been set, and the "greening" of the fashion industry has become an imperative. Margaret Maynard in chapter 25 examines how far the industry has traveled and identifies issues and directions, whereas Marsha A. Dickson shines the spotlight on the human rights agenda in fashion production and its integration into and impact on company policies via the adoption of clear strategies for corporate social responsibility.

Different forms of fashion work at a different pace: limited-edition handcrafted pieces may become future heirlooms; conceptual fashion pieces have a life beyond the catwalk in the art gallery or museum and in the academic record; designer fashions continue to inspire and stimulate mainstream fashion, one of the most significant global industries. Fashion provides livelihoods, and sustainable fashion must continue to meet both personal and symbolic needs, while addressing the problems associated with the fashion system. Sustainable fashion does not imply the end of fashion; it can instead become a catalyst for change and empowerment. Kate Fletcher's contribution (chapter 26) to the debate on sustainability in the fashion context strongly advocates the potential for design thinking and design practice to catalyze change at three levels within the sector: the fashion and textile product, service, and system. She also distinguishes between the concepts of green design, ecodesign, and design for sustainability. Simonetta Carbonaro and David Goldsmith, however, look to new synergies between business, culture, and sustainable practices to effect long-term change. It may still be too early to assess the efficacy of design as a response to sustainability, as scholars and practitioners are engaged in a process that is still beginning; this is an exciting time to initiate this conversation in multiple languages, across cultures, with an awareness of all that preservation and innovation can mean. While the precepts of sustainable fashion have yet to fully transform bodies, objects, and behavior, the scholars of this section ultimately concur that sustainable fashion has the potential to reposition the fashion system and imagine alternatives for the future.

CONCLUSION

Through the connections within our scholarly work the editors of *The Handbook of Fashion Studies* have intended to provide an integrated, holistic view of the current state of and possible futures for the field of fashion studies. While we sought to map the field for professionals, scholars, and practitioners alike, we also look forward to the conversation that we hope this *Handbook* inspires.

BIBLIOGRAPHY

Appadurai, Arjun. 1986. "Introduction: Commodities and the Politics of Value." In Arjun Appadurai (ed.), *The Social Life of Things: Commodities in Cultural Perspective.* Melbourne: Cambridge University Press.

Arnold, Rebecca. 2008. *The American Look.* London: I. B. Tauris.

Black, Daniel. 2009. "Wearing Out Racial Discourse: Tokyo Street Fashion and Race as Style." *Journal of Popular Culture* 42 (2): 239–56.

Blumer, Hebert. 1969. "Fashion: From Class Differentiation to Collective Selection." *Sociological Quarterly* 10: 275.

Bolton, Andrew. 2002. *The Supermodern Wardrobe.* London: V&A Publishing.

Braddock Clarke, Sarah E., and Marie O'Mahony. 2005. *TechnoTextiles 2.* London: Thames and Hudson.

Breward, Christopher. 2004. *Fashioning London.* Oxford: Berg.

Brown, Tim. 2005. "Strategy by Design." *Fast Company,* June 1. http://www.fastcompany.com/52795/strategy-design (accessed January 9, 2012).

Bruzzi, Stella. 1997. *Undressing Cinema: Clothing and Identity in the Movies.* London: Routledge.

Craik, Jennifer. 1993. *The Face of Fashion.* London: Routledge.

Crane, Diane. 2000. *Fashion and Its Social Agendas: Class, Gender, and Identity in Clothing.* Chicago: University of Chicago Press.

Cross, Nigel. 2011. *Design Thinking.* Oxford: Berg.

Eicher, Joanne B. (ed.). 2010. *Berg Encyclopedia of World Dress and Fashion.* 10 vols. Oxford: Berg.

Eicher, Joanne B., Sandra Lee Evenson, and Hazel A. Lutz. 2008. *The Visible Self: Global Perspectives on Dress, Culture, and Society.* Oxford: Berg.

Entwistle, Joanne. 2000. *The Fashioned Body: Fashion, Dress and Modern Social Theory.* Cambridge, UK: Polity.

Entwistle, Joanne. 2001. "Fashioning of the Career Woman: Power Dressing as a Strategy of Consumption." In Mary R. Talbot and Mary Margaret Andrews (eds.), *All the World and Her Husband: Women and Consumption in the Twentieth Century,* 224–38. London: Cassell.

Evans, Caroline. 2003. *Fashion at the Edge: Spectacle, Modernity and Deathliness.* New Haven, CT: Yale University Press.

Frayling, Christopher. 1993. "Research in Art and Design." RCA Research Papers 1 (1). London: Royal College of Art.

Gaines, Jane, and Charlotte Herzog (eds.). 1990. *Fabrications: Costume and the Female Body.* London: Routledge.

Guest, David. 1991. "The Hunt Is on for the Renaissance Man of Computing." *The Independent* (London), September 17.

Jobling, Paul. 1999. *Fashion Spreads: Word and Image in Fashion Photography since 1980.* Oxford: Berg.

Kondo, Dorine. 1997. *About Face: Performing Race in Fashion and Theater.* New York: Routledge.

Kopytoff, Igor. 1986. "The Cultural Biography of Things: Commodities in Cultural Perspective." In Arjun Appadurai (ed.), *The Social Life of Things: Commodities in Cultural Perspective.* Melbourne: Cambridge University Press.
Lee, Suzanne. 2005. *Fashioning the Future: Tomorrow's Wardrobe.* London: Thames and Hudson.
Miller, Daniel, and Susanne Küchler (eds.). 2005. *Clothing as Material Culture.* Oxford: Berg.
Miller, Daniel, and Sophie Woodward (eds.). 2010. *Global Denim.* Oxford: Berg.
Nixon, Nathalie, and Johanna Blakley. 2012. "Fashion Thinking: Towards an Actionable Methodology." *Fashion Practice: The Journal of Design, Creative Process and the Fashion Industry* 4 (2): 153–75.
O'Neil, Alistair (ed.). 2008. "Fashion Curation." Special issue, *Fashion Theory* 12 (2).
Potvin, John (ed.). 2009. *The Places and Spaces of Fashion, 1800–2007.* London: Routledge.
Prown, Jules David. 2001. *Art as Evidence: Writings on Art and Material Culture.* New Haven, CT: Yale University Press.
Quinn, Bradley. 2002. *Techno Fashion.* Oxford: Berg.
Rocamora, Agnès. 2009. *Fashioning the City: Paris, Fashion and the Media.* London: I. B. Tauris.
Rowe, Peter G. 1987. *Design Thinking.* Cambridge, MA: MIT Press.
Seymour, Sabine. 2008. *Fashionable Technology: The Intersection of Design, Fashion, Science and Technology.* Vienna: Springer.
Steele, Valerie (ed.). 1998. "Methodologies." Special issue, *Fashion Theory* 2 (4).
Steele, Valerie (ed.). 2008. "Exhibitionism." Special issue, *Fashion Theory* 12 (1).
Taylor, Lou. 2002. *The Study of Dress History.* Manchester: Manchester University Press.
Taylor, Lou. 2004. *Establishing Dress History.* Manchester: Manchester University Press.
Tseëlon, Efrat. 1997. *The Masque of Femininity.* London: Sage.
Tsui, Christine. 2010. *China Fashion: Conversations with Designers.* Oxford: Berg.
Woodward, Ian. 2007. *Understanding Material Culture.* Los Angeles: Sage.
Woodward, Sophie. 2007. *Why Women Wear What They Wear.* Oxford: Berg.
Wu, Juanjuan. 2009. *Chinese Fashion from Mao to Now.* Oxford: Berg.
Wu, Juanjuan (ed.). 2012. "Contemporary Chinese Fashion." Special issue, *Fashion Practice: The Journal of Design, Creative Process and the Fashion Industry* 4 (1).

SECTION I

Fashion/Dress and Time

Introduction

HELEN THOMAS

This first section of *The Handbook of Fashion Studies* considers research on fashion and dress through the lens of various approaches to "time": historical, museological, new, and biographical. Rather than simply focusing on the history of fashion and dress in terms of past times, the approach adopted for this section takes on various "time"-related foci. In so doing, the four chapters address respectively the following concerns:

- the theoretical and methodological issues confronting the analysis of fashion and dress history in the context of current theoretical shifts and the cultural flows with which these are associated (Taylor);
- the challenges to curatorial practice in locating past fashion and dress, which was "modern" in its day, within the context of the museum (of art) in contemporary culture, where the essential ingredient of the wearing of clothes, the lived body, is absent (Crawley and Barbieri);
- the potential democratization or shift from professional to lay approaches to fashion criticism and journalism made possible through the global interconnectedness of the new social media and the meteoric rise of fashion blogging today (Rocamora); and
- the ways in which fashion, with its ever-increasing close association with youth, contributes to "age ordering" throughout the life course, where the requirement to "act your age" (Laz 1998) that accompanies it may increase rather than decrease the invisibility and denigration of older or different bodies (Twigg).

Lou Taylor is a renowned dress historian and curator whose approach to dress history, as she readily acknowledges in chapter 1, has been grounded in "close assessment of the actualities of garments themselves." For Taylor, it is from the garments that the (hi)stories emerge. However, she is aware that the object-based approach she advocates is not shared by a number of academics whose interest, like hers, is in fashion and dress. In this first chapter, "Fashion and Dress History," Taylor's wide-ranging discussion sets out and assesses the mushrooming of academic interest in fashion from a range of disciplines, which in turn has generated new methodologies over the past fifteen or so years.

The chapter begins with a discussion of what she has called the old "great divide" (Taylor 2002) between academic fashion, curatorial research, and fashion history research, which remained resolutely separate from each other. To a large extent, as Taylor notes, this divide has begun to fray at the edges with students and researchers moving toward a position of recognizing value in other approaches. The newest kid on the block, as Taylor notes, is *fashion studies,* and as she indicates, distinctions between fashion studies and fashion/dress history are not clear-cut, and definitions may vary from one academic to another. Defining terms such as *fashion, dress, clothes, costume,* and so on has been a key topic for specialists in different areas for a number of years, as Joanne Entwistle (2000) has also noted. Entwistle points out that the terminology used is generally related to the particular field of study that a scholar is rooted in. So, for example, sociologists whose area of study is their own culture tend to focus on "fashion," seen as a feature of modernity, which is characterized by its rapidly shifting industrial, social, and economic configuration.

Taylor sets out the major developments in recent research and critical theory beginning with an examination of the material culture approach to clothing and dress, which then broadens out to encompass approaches to, for example, "social and economic history," "dress and ethnography," "uses of literature in dress history research," "oral history and oral testimony as a source for dress history and fashion studies," and so on. Taylor acknowledges the contribution that the burgeoning area of fashion studies and the criss-crossing of disciplines has made to the field, including the loosening of the old "great divide" and the generation of international research developments, not restricted to the West. Nonetheless, she remains attached to the importance of "touching, looking, listening, and reflecting," which entails taking time to "research, reflect on, and then interpret objects of clothing in their specific and yet interdisciplinary historical gendered, class, or ethnic context."

While Taylor does engage with curatorial practices and policies briefly, in chapter 2, "Dress, Time, and Space," Donatella Barbieri and Greer Crawley consider the ways that "the perception, interpretation, and representation of time have acquired a new significance" in a number of "contemporary exhibitions of historical dress." They argue that by drawing on postmodernist frames of reference on "temporality, memory, and narrative" there have been significant "curatorial attempts" to play with "temporality, spatiality, materiality, and performativity" to rupture the dominant perception of historical dress as being fixed or locked in times past.

The "curated and conserved dress, as museum object," references the absent body, which at the same time is brought into play by what the authors term the "curatorial intervention." Here the authors draw on John L. Austin's notion of the "performative" in language, which he suggests is a "doing" word rather than simply describing something. For example, in voicing the words, "I name this ship Queen Elizabeth," or saying, "I do," in a wedding ceremony, we are not simply making a statement, according to Austin (1962: 222); rather we are *doing* something: we are performing an action. From this viewpoint, words act and enact what they name. Following along these lines, Barbieri and Crawley are concerned to reveal the "doing" in exhibition making's imaginative processes. They draw on Elizabeth Wilson's (1985) notion of the "uncanny" experience of looking at items of clothing in museums that once adorned a body that is no longer there but is invoked by the presentation of the dress. They consider that the "something only half understood" has been an issue for "contemporary curators of dress," and the chapter sets out to examine how this challenge has been met by particular contemporary exhibition makers.

The authors first explain the ways in which Andy Warhol's curation of objects from the costume collection for the Museum of Art of the Rhode Island School of Design in 1969 challenged conventional hierarchical approaches to displaying objects and itemizing them in the catalog accordingly. Rather, Warhol insisted that all the shoes in the collection, together with "parasols as costume accessories," were displayed in a cabinet the visitors could open and close, opening up possibilities for audience engagement and participation. Warhol's radical experimental approach was highly influential and led to other experiments in the presentation of museum objects, including dress. Barbieri and Crawley discuss the impact of later exhibitions that were influenced by this approach, looking at, for example, other curatorial interventions by Peter Wollen, Claire Wilcox, and Judith Clark that had an impact on the field. The authors show how, for example, Wilcox and Clark were searching for new, experimental ways to exhibit historical dress within the museum context, which drew on other artists and curators who were not involved in dress curation. Clark's Malign Muses: When Fashion Turns Back exhibition for MoMu Museum in 2004, which was retitled Spectres: When Fashion Turns Back when the exhibition transferred to the Victoria and Albert Museum in 2005, was viewed by Valerie Steele as "paradigm shifting." Barbieri and Crawley show how Clark drew on "experimental methods of display, based on a dialogue between dress, space, and ideas" that privileged a "conceptual approach" that employed performative strategies, rather than the more conventional "instructive" approach to dress display that is rooted in a chronological time line. In so doing, the authors argue that curators like Wilcox and Clark in particular deepen the "the complex relationship between dress and culture."

In chapter 3, Agnès Rocamora takes the discussion away from fashion and dress history to address "New Fashion Times," as her chapter is titled. In this chapter, Rocamora argues that where fashion time was once neatly paced by the biannual collections, by the spring/summer takeover of the autumn/winter collections, and by the monthly publications of glossies, now fashion time has accelerated and fragmented into a series of moments that have shattered its orderly pace. She points to the fact that pre-collection, pre-fall, cruise, and resort collections are all new moments in this restructured fashion time, a time ruled by the imperative of immediacy John Tomlinson (2007) has identified as constitutive of today's "culture of speed." The recent creation and rapid proliferation of new digital media such as fashion blogs has supported, and been supported by, this culture of "immediacy" (Bolter and Grusin 2000). Based on an analysis of the development of digital fashion media, Rocamora interrogates the notion of time, drawing on a variety of theoretical approaches from Karl Marx to Gilles Deleuze and Félix Guattari to situate the shifts in modernity from old to new times.

The chapter begins by contextualizing the development of fashion within the context of the rise of modernity, which was characterized by industrialization and the associated values of "progress, rationality, and rapid change." As modernity went full speed ahead in the nineteenth century, with the expansion of new communication systems such as the railways and the need to "synchronize" the mass labor force, time, as Rocamora shows, became perceived as a "scarce resource" and a "central dimension of capitalism," which gave rise to important theoretical analyses of the consequences of its formation. As the speed of change accelerated into the late twentieth century, theorists began to speak of an "information society," that is, a society that is no longer founded on the production of goods and materials but rather on the "creation and circulation of information," due to the rapid expansion of "new information technologies." Modernity's former strict adherence to "clock time" has given way to "timeless time" (Castells 2000) in a society that is constantly networked via new technologies such as the Internet and the mobile phone. It is in this sense that time and space are compressed into one, characterized by "a culture of speed" (Tomlinson 2007).

Rocamora discusses the acceleration of the speed of time in relation to fashion and the recent developments in "fast fashion," where new or emergent fashion trends and styles are copied and made up for purchase in retail outlets as soon as they have appeared on the catwalk, challenging the exclusivity of the haute couture model of fashion. Rocamora cites, among others, the global high street retail company Zara, which produces 30,000 different designs a year, as a leader in the fast fashion trend of providing almost instant access to new fashion styles. She notes that the speeding up of fashion has been accompanied by "an increasingly rapid flow of immaterial fashion" in the guise of fashion websites, which have become "key platforms for the circulation of fashion discourse." Rocamora points to the trajectory of the first fashion websites, which began to appear from the mid-1990s, such as UK Vogue.com, followed by others like WGSN, Net-a-porter.com, and SHOWstudio, to mention but a few. However, she sees that a "key moment in the history of digital fashion" came into being in the early twenty-first century with the introduction of fashion blogs, which were first created by "nonprofessional" independent individuals and were subsequently taken up by different fashion organizations as a means of "further disseminating their visions and values" to a potentially global audience, contributing to the acceleration of fashion. Rocamora argues that the increasing rapidity of material and symbolic fashion have supported what has become "a defining trait of contemporary society," "acceleration," and a collapsing of time and space.

In chapter 4, Julia Twigg addresses yet another notion of time through a consideration of the relationship between fashion, the body, and age. Twigg's discussion takes its starting point from the idea that "clothes lie at the interface between the body and its social presentation," and following Entwistle (2000) she considers that dress should be understood as a "situated body practice." There are cultural norms associated with dressing, and one of these norms is in relation to age, the central topic of her chapter. Here, the author carefully addresses the ways in which fashion and dress relate to notions of "age" and "aging" in contemporary Western cultures. The popular images of age in contemporary popular culture, shored up by the dominant biomedical master narrative, tend to categorize age as a consequence of physiology, as "something rooted in the processes of bodily decline." Twigg argues that aging needs to be considered as a social and cultural construct as research on aging has clearly demonstrated that "many of the key features of later life are determined as much by social as physiological processes."

She mobilizes current themes of embodiment to explore the intersections between forms of dress and changes in the body as people age in the context of the cultural assumptions that attach to these. The discussion of the issues surrounding age and dress is predominantly centered on women. The author locates the shifts in perceptions of aging historically, noting that in Western cultures the entry into what is called old age has been largely defined in terms of retirement, although it is important to note that what counts as old may vary from culture to culture and within cultural contexts. The analysis demonstrates that the boundaries of what counts as "old" in contemporary Western culture are not as rigid as they were before, which is highlighted by the oft-heralded slogan in the media that "sixty is the new forty," or what Twigg calls "moving younger." The triumph of youth culture and the growth of consumer culture that accompanied the 1960s revolution is often considered to have contributed to a more relaxed or perhaps less moralistic approach to notions of what form of dress is appropriate for individuals at different stages of the life course. By drawing on the presentation of fashion and age in the fashion industry, the media, fashion magazines, and a UK project on clothing and age funded by the Economic and Social Research Council (see Twigg 2013), the chapter considers the subtle ways that dress plays a key role in "age ordering" within contemporary culture. This, it might be argued, contributes further to the technologies of the aging (bodily) self as opposed to a freedom from previous social constraints and negative conceptions of older people. The social enhancement to be gained from looking ten years younger, as Twigg notes, "has its limits." Wearing clothes designed for a much younger market in order to look younger can point up the aging body. Moreover, "moving younger" has become "a central cultural ideal," which is part and parcel of what Higgs and colleagues (2009) call the "'will to health' in later life."

The author concludes that fashion studies have largely ignored age, just as studies of age have paid scant attention to the "areas of consumption, performance, and identity." Twigg indicates that recent developments in the field have sought to attend to this gap. As such, this chapter may be seen to form a bridge between this section on time and the following one, which focuses on identity and difference.

BIBLIOGRAPHY

Austin, John L. 1962. *How to Do Things with Words: The William James Lectures Delivered at Harvard 1955.* London: Clarendon.

Bolter, Jay David, and Richard Grusin. 2000. *Remediation.* Cambridge, MA: MIT Press.

Castells, Manuel. 2000. *The Rise of the Network Society.* Oxford: Blackwell.

Entwistle, Joanne. 2000. *The Fashioned Body: Fashion, Dress and Modern Social Theory.* Cambridge, UK: Polity.

Higgs, Paul, Miranda Leontowitsch, Fiona Stevenson, and Ian R. Jones. 2009. "Not Just Old and Sick—the 'Will to Health' in Later Life." *Ageing & Society* 29 (5): 687–707.

Laz, Cheryl. 1998. "Act Your Age." *Sociological Forum* 13 (1): 85–95.

Taylor, Lou. 2002. *The Study of Dress History.* Manchester: Manchester University Press.

Tomlinson, John. 2007. *The Culture of Speed.* London: Sage.

Twigg, Julia. 2013. *Fashion and Age: Dress, the Body and Later Life.* London: Bloomsbury.

Wilson, Elizabeth. 1985. *Adorned in Dreams: Fashion and Modernity.* London: Virago.

1

Fashion and Dress History: Theoretical and Methodological Approaches

LOU TAYLOR

INTRODUCTION

This chapter discusses approaches to and developments in researching and theorizing dress and fashion history. After a lifetime involved in this field it would seem straightforward enough to write such an introductory chapter in a scholarly handbook. After one has been a fashion design student in the early 1960s, worked as a museum dress curator from the mid-1960s to the early 1980s, and taught dress history in art schools/polytechnics and universities for a lifetime, such a task would seem unproblematic. Yet this has proved far from easy, because over the last fifteen years our field has broken its banks and flooded into a fertile plain of new approaches and methodologies. Each of these is as exciting and valid as the others, and each has developed its own methodologies and specific interests. Now, as well as the "old" base of art and social history, we have academic texts about clothing from the specialisms of design history; ethnography; gender, feminist, film, and photography studies; and media studies as well as business and economic history, performance studies, geography, urban studies, colonial and postcolonial studies, literature studies, and on it goes.

One outcome of all this has been a clear escalation of interdisciplinary research, a theme that will run through this chapter. No one can possibly be skilled in every one of these academic fields, each of which has its own sets of specific critical approaches, interests, and standpoints, so where does this leave the bewildered incoming student? What critical stances does the drowning researcher leave in, without overconfusing the story, and what can she/he leave out without compromising it?

The central interest of my own dress history research has always been based around close assessment of the actualities of garments themselves—from the stories they offer us and from the critical possibilities inherent within those stories (Taylor [1983] 2009, 2002, 2004). While it is a fact that many scholars are now working from clothing "things," many more are not and will not do so. Fundamental questions recently asked by colleagues, seemingly unconvinced by this approach, have included: "Why do you need to look at clothes in the museum?" or "How you can tell anything by just looking?" These questions have reminded me that object-based material culture analysis undertaken through examination of surviving clothing has yet to convince a good few academics who nevertheless share this driving interest in *dress/fashion/clothes/costume* but approach these from quite different starting points. This chapter therefore seeks to outline current developments in the fields of dress and fashion history, which sit alongside and are intertwined with those rooted in the field of fashion studies today; the conclusion will point to possible future developments in this area of study.

OLD DIVIDES AND ANCIENT ANTAGONISMS

Today, new generations of students looking for their ideal undergraduate or postgraduate course are confronted by a range of terms and consequential confusions. They can study in a plethora of programs in fashion/dress history and fashion studies from the bachelor's to the doctoral level. Students are surprised to find out that this is a comparatively recent state of affairs, achieved not without struggle. I have named the old divides between the university, museum curatorial research, and the wider fashion history world as a "great divide" (Taylor 2002: 65–71). In 2009 Negley Harte, from his viewpoint as an economic textile historian and a key player in professionalizing dress history studies within the university system, summed up the old situation perfectly:

> Historians were defeated by clothes. Archaeologists fussed about the surviving evidences of their absence; art historians were interested only in the portraited upper classes; social historians were torn between thinking clothes were either too trivial to bother with or too complex to master, and economic historians could not count them and therefore paid no attention. Clothes were dismissed from academic history. Archaeology, art history, social history, economic history, all flourished, as indeed did history—academic conferences and departments and degrees and debates, all booming, but clothes were left to art colleges plus a few enthusiastic eccentrics. (2009: 176)

As Harte notes, such a view has now been eroded by the weight of new first-rate interdisciplinary research and publications.

Daniel Miller, a social anthropologist, has dealt with "ancient antagonisms" of his own, those between students of "textile conservation, design or museum collections" set against students with backgrounds in "cultural studies, sociology or social anthropology with training in semiotics and symbolic analysis and an interest in the 'social life' of clothing." He explains:

> Specialists in textiles may have very little respect for those disciplines they lump together as cultural studies.... In turn, social scientists may denigrate scholars of textile, pattern, form and technology as "positivists," who study such things merely because they have collections. They see such attention to details as emulating the assumptions of objectivity in the natural sciences and thus as a kind of "right wing" failure properly to appreciate the politicized nature of all such research which they have been trained to elicit from the material as what really matters. (2005: 1)

While it would be foolish to believe that all of this tension has dissolved, I have watched with much interest as this "great divide" begins to disintegrate. Now researchers from various of fields of study have realized the fascinating potential of the history and present of the design, making, retailing, and consumption of clothing and now accept that, as Daniel Roche has clarified astutely, "the history of clothing tells us much about civilisations; it reveals their codes" (1987: 5). Specialist academic journals that regularly feature interdisciplinary texts on dress/fashion and use such approaches include *Costume, Cloth and Culture, Textile History,* the *Winterthur Portfolio,* the *Journal of Design and Studies in the Decorative Arts,* the *Material Culture Journal,* and more.

ESTABLISHED AND NEW FIELDS OF STUDY

Today there is an additional new stream flooding into the subject area—fashion studies. Notions of what the differences between fashion studies and fashion/dress history actually are have become a further crisscross of confusion for students and early researchers alike. Definitions are far from clear, differing from one university to the other and one scholar to the other. Some fashion studies programs and texts may build on a foundation of critical dress/fashion theory and social history, while many barely contain elements of historical study at all. Others are based on analysis of today's global fashion industry.

Undergraduate and master's programs in fashion/dress history and fashion studies that include historical and critical approaches can be found in universities in Australia, the United States, Britain, Denmark, Sweden, Canada, and France, for example. Most fashion studies courses lay critical emphasis on analysis of twentieth- and twenty-first-century fashion studies, while dress and fashion history programs are normally rooted in a far wider time span. Both would normally include high levels of critical theory. Francesca Granata suggests that "arguments could be made for fashion studies to develop as a self-standing discipline with its own methodology and departmental structures... or for it to remain a subject to be studied across a range of disciplines from visual culture to sociology" (2012: 75). Fashion studies departments indeed are currently based across departments of art and design history and theory or allied to programs in visual culture, media studies, film studies, gender studies, history, marketing and performance studies, business studies, fashion design, and home economics.

A survey of websites reveals many commonalities, particularly interdisciplinarity. To give a few examples, the University of Stockholm's MA in fashion studies, based in its Faculty of Humanities, "addresses questions concerning fashion as a discourse and the construction of identity with regard to fashion as an industry. The programme also investigates fashion as an aesthetic and material form, including representations of fashion in the visual arts, photography, theatre, film, advertising and marketing."[1] The web page for the MA in fashion studies at Parsons New School, New York, based in their School of Art and Design History and Theory, stated in 2012: "Using an interdisciplinary approach, [students] explore fashion as object, image, text, practice, theory, and concept and develop a critical understanding of fashion and its complex global intersections with identities, histories, and cultures in the contemporary world."[2] The University of Brighton's web page for its BA in fashion and dress history highlights that it emphasizes history and consumption more than many other programs and assesses the "ways in which different social, national, ethnic and gender groups project their identities through their dress."[3] The web page for the BA in fashion history and theory at Central Saint Martins also stresses its interdisciplinarity, considering the "design, manufacture, promotion and consumption of fashion" and their "relation to relevant social, historical and cultural contexts."[4] The web page on the MA in the history of dress at the Courtauld Institute of Art stresses first that "art historical methodologies provide the starting point" but then, similarly, highlights the program's emphasis on "design, manufacture, promotion and consumption of fashion . . . within social, historical and cultural contexts."[5] The web page of the London College of Fashion's MA in fashion curation notes its stress on "specialist practice-based, critical and interpretative skills involved within the discipline of fashion curation."[6] Now undergraduates can study fashion in a university department of "big history," at the University of Warwick. The description of its course Fashion in History: A Global Look, 1300–2000, notes, "Why was fashion so important in the life of millions of people at least since the Middle Ages? What is the relationship between economic change, social and cultural transformation and fashion?"[7]

That there is much overlap across all these courses is evident, and, now that we are functioning in this world of interdisciplinary developments, maintaining real or imagined differences seems futile. What remains is to further enhance the depth and breadth of our field of study by embracing this interdisciplinarity.

DEFINITION OF TERMS

Attempts at defining terms—*dress, fashion, clothing,* and *costume*—have exercised specialists in the fields for many years. Negley Harte has commented that such definitions crucially affect "not just the approach to a topic but to a whole sub-discipline: are we doing the history of dress, of clothing, of costume, or of fashion? For each of these four words contains intrinsic indicators of different approaches, and each of them can be used to describe the field itself" (2009: 176). In her survey of the historiography of dress/fashion history terminology, Fadwa El Guindi's preference was to use the term *dress* as defined in Ruth Barnes and Joanne Eicher's *Dress and Gender* (1992). They proposed a "sociocultural approach comprehensive, cross-cultural, and grounded in ethnography" (El Guindi 1999: 55). Daniel Roche's preference is for the term *clothes* rather than *costume:* "Let us speak of 'clothes' as the best word suited to a social and cultural history of appearances." He defines the term *costume,* a word of Italian origin, as "too ambiguous in its double meaning of custom and or way of dressing" (1994: 4). Suzanne Baizerman, Joanne Eicher, and Catherine Cerny share this view and comment that "to some, the term *costume* contains an inherent bias that differentiates the unfamiliar from the familiar. In English usage the term costume often refers to exceptional dress, dress outside the context of everyday life: Halloween costume, masquerade costume, theatre costume" (1993: 23). Emma Tarlow agrees, noting that "the term 'costume' is more associated with history and theatre than everyday living" (1996: 5).

There is now also further recognition that applying the term *fashion* only to Euro-American and global styles betrays a strong sense of culturally dominating Eurocentricity that is no longer acceptable. Baizerman, Eicher, and Cerny made it clear in 1993 that such "privileged positions" reflected "the predilections of a society that has given precedence to the status and lifestyle of the middle and upper class EuroAmerican, with far less concern shown for dress from the rest of the world." They proposed therefore "nesting the study of EuroAmerican dress conceptually within the broadest topic of world dress. . . . Such a focus recognises that the people of the world interact, have interacted, and will continue to interact with concomitant changes in dress" (1993: 26). They point to Renato Rosaldo's stress on cultural interconnections around the world (Baizerman, Eicher, and Cerny 1993: 19). Rosaldo commented in 1989 that "in the present postcolonial world, the notion of an authentic culture as an autonomous internally coherent universe no longer seems tenable, except perhaps as a 'useful fiction' or a revealing distortion." He stressed that "rapidly increasing global interdependence has made it more and more clear that neither 'we' nor 'they' are as neatly bounded and homogeneous as once seemed to be the case" (1989: 19). Finally, he suggested significantly that in examining colonial or postcolonial themes of cross-cultural consumption, we need to be aware that "all of us inhabit an interdependent late twentieth century world marked by borrowing and lending across porous national and cultural boundaries that are saturated with inequality, power and dominion" (217).

Such fashion and textile bleedings across porous boundaries have been dated back to the fourteenth century when printed cottons were already specifically produced in India for the Egyptian market (Barnes 1997: 8–9). Recent innovative research into cotton chintz's history has exposed similar manufacturing, trade, and fashion interdependencies across the porous cultural, political, and economic boundaries between India and Europe, and, significantly, back again, from the late sixteenth century through to the nineteenth century (Hartkamp-Jonxis 1994; Lemire 2003; Riello and Parthasarathi 2009; Riello and Roy 2009). Elisha Renne researched the introduction of specifically designed cotton prints by the John Holt Company of Liverpool into the Yoruba Kabba-Bunu district of Kogi State in Central Nigeria in the 1930s, noting that this roller-printed cloth was admired not only because it was light in weight and easy to wash but also because, locally, it represented "notions of modern 'civilised behaviour'" (1995: 174).

So we are all aware now that notions of modernity and fashionability are embedded into evolving dress practices the world over, and research has gone from strength to strength. Judith Perani and Norma H. Wolff, for example, have shown us the centrality of fashion on Yoruba terms within the design of *aso-oke* strip-weave fabrics in Nigeria, for example. They note that as well as being the preferred Yoruba choice of "wealthy urbanites as visible symbols of prosperity, status and pride in ethnic heritage" (1999: 171), the cloth is both costly and fashionable. They highlighted the role of the skilled craft handweavers and traders, who "have their fingers on the pulse of fashion through on-going interaction with their elite consumer-patrons" (172). *Aso-oke* has thus become a powerful symbol of Yoruba modernity that pays no allegiance whatsoever to Western fashion roots. Thus, today dress history and fashion studies are now subject areas that embrace the study of dress and textiles from all over the world with equal respect, seeking an equal understanding of their specific forms of tradition, modernity, and fashion.

All the writers and researchers noted here are absorbed by their use of clothing/dress/fashion as a vehicle for all manners of historical and contemporary cultural and social history analysis. The most marginalized field of all was garment reenactment work, but that too, at its best, has become increasingly respected as a lively teaching aid at heritage sites and museums (Poppy 1997). The old divides have collapsed so far that museums such as the Victoria and Albert Museum and the Designmuseum in Copenhagen, for example, employ their own "academic" research staff to help develop exhibitions, and some dress curators around the world are now also university lecturers. Now museums and universities apply for funding grants together as a norm.

KEY DEVELOPMENTS IN RESEARCH APPROACHES AND CRITICAL THEORY

Material Culture Approaches to the Study of Clothing

One of the key factors in these positive developments has been the embracing of material culture approaches and the now widely held acceptance that probing objects, including clothing, can pull out "stories" accessible by no other methods. As Roche has clarified astutely, "Clothing is a good indication of the material culture of a society for it introduces us immediately to consumers' patterns and enables us to consider the social hierarchy of appearances" (1987: 160). While Roche did not examine surviving garments and textiles, the anthropologist Daniel Miller, writing over twenty years later, understands the cultural significances built into the very materiality of garments and appearances. "We are prepared now to see clothes themselves as having agency, as part of what constitutes and forms lives, cosmologies, reasons, causes and effect" (Miller 2005: 2). Miller firmly believes that material culture studies "as they pertain to textiles and clothing... lead to a new respect for scholarship that considers draping, feel, comfort and assemblage... [and that] patterns of value are created not just patterns of style" (16). Leora Auslander argues too that "people's relation to language is not the same as their relation to things; all that they express through their creation and use of material objects is, furthermore, not reducible to words" (2005: 1017). Susan Pearce follows up the same theme, writing, "Objects hang before the eyes of the imagination, continuously representing ourselves to ourselves and telling the stories of our lives in ways which would be impossible otherwise" (1993: 147).

Material culture approaches to the study of dress thus focus on its design, manufacture, retailing, and consumption and on the end life of objects of clothing, in order finally to speculate on themes such as past and present social hierarchies; histories of making, manufacturing, and trading; and the cultural, gendered meanings of specific garments to wearers, to communities, and indeed to nations, past and present. The requirement, however, is to set these exactly in the context of their own period, geographical, and cultural consumption spaces.

This approach places sharp focus on the materiality of surviving items of dress. One key to success is to pay attention to the "trivial" details, such as fabric, sewing, trimmings, and accessories—a viewpoint often derided in the past by social and economic historians, who took no interest in the actuality of garments, failing to understand the nuanced cultural importances embedded in supposedly trivial details. Beatrix Le Wita, examining the material culture of young Parisian bourgeois women in the 1980s in the context of ideas by Fernand Braudel, Pierre Bourdieu, and Claude Levi-Strauss, noted what she deliberately termed the "trivia" of their clothing (the cut of jeans, the similar engagement rings, and silk scarves) "because when these are added together they create 'distinction'" which "enables [man] to mark out a sphere for himself in which he will live with himself and his fellows" (1994: 57). Such trivia can be located by sight, hearing, touch, taste, and smell as well as by text and image. Auslander stresses that

> each provide certain kinds of information, and people create unique (and non-interchangeable) forms in each of these sensorial domains. A symphony cannot be rendered visually; the aroma of roasting coffee cannot be put into words; the feeling of cashmere or burlap cannot be expressed in music. In the particular domain of concern here—material culture—sight and touch are the relevant senses, and objects, words, and images the relevant genres. (2005: 1016)

Kaori O'Connor is also convinced that close study of objects is needed and that the "ubiquity, intimacy, and materiality of cloth and clothing mean that by studying them we can obtain nuanced insights into the dynamism of society on many levels not easily arrived at by other means, if at all" (2005: 41). Amy de la Haye, Lou Taylor, and Eleanor Thompson, researching a collection of the surviving dress of the Messel women from the 1860s on, noted that "the clothes are far more than elegant fashion items. They live on as material fragments through which it is possible to trace the biographies of six generations of women from this exceptional family" (2005: 3). Through examination of hundreds of surviving dresses and accessories, they were also able to highlight for the first time a specific Messel feminine fashion taste—a luxurious but slightly arty-historical, English style developed across four generations of wealthy Messel women from the 1860s. It was a subtle style designed to project a nonworldly elegance based on historical family heritage (though that in truth was of dubious reality). Figure 1.1, for example, shows the front panel of a London couture evening gown made for Maud Messel by Sarah Fullerton Monteith Young, in deep purple velvet, dating from about 1907. This one was personalized, highly unusually, through the addition of an embroidered section cut from a late eighteenth-century man's waistcoat, almost certainly from Maud's own textile collection (de la Haye, Taylor, and Thompson 2005: 59, 740). The authors concluded, "We have sought to demonstrate... that the application of a close garment-focused study of surviving clothes can help us touch the memories, emotions, aspirations

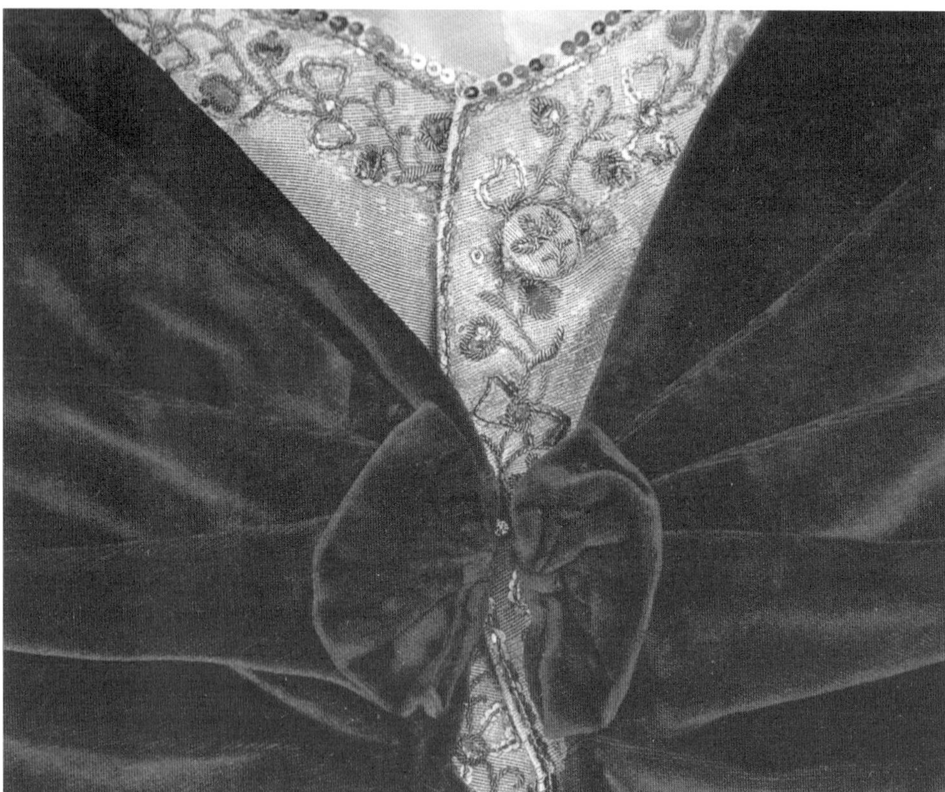

FIGURE 1.1 Center-front panel of evening gown, made from late eighteenth-century waistcoat embroidery, Sarah Fullerton Monteith Young, worn by Maud Messel, about 1907.
Credit: Brighton Museum, CT004015. Courtesy of the Royal Pavilion, Libraries and Museums of Brighton and Hove.

and sensitivities of their owners, characteristics which drive the world along and yet which are so often left out of historical study and museum interpretations" (166–67). Such approaches are now widely accepted. Auslander, among many others, is convinced that objects act "as memory cues . . . or expressions of the psyche, or extensions of the body, as well as sites of aesthetic investment, involving pleasure, distress, or conscious indifference" (2005: 1016).

Social and Economic History

Over the last twenty years, social and economic historians too have come to accept the historical and cultural significances to be drawn from what Janet Andrewes terms "the lived experience of dress" (2005: 310). The pioneer in this approach was Daniel Roche with his seminal books *The People of Paris: An Essay in Popular Culture in the 18th Century* (1981) and *The Culture of Clothing: Dress and Fashion in the Ancien Régime* (1994, first published in 1989). He was clear that assessing historical clothing "is another way of penetrating the heart of social history" (Roche 1994: 5). Both his texts extensively used clothing sources unearthed from eighteenth-century inventories, wills, notarial documents, court reports, and police, witness, and mortuary reports. Roche examined dress from the nobility to the poor in pre-Revolutionary Paris. Choosing not to access surviving clothes of the rich (few clothes of the poor have survived), he produced a masterly account of the clothing of the citizens of Paris nevertheless. To give just one example, using notary listings of shop clothing belonging to the Parisian *fripiers* (dealers selling new and secondhand garments) he was able to demonstrate that two-thirds of the colors chosen across Parisian society in 1789, at the dawn of the French Revolution, were drab—"black, brown, maroon and grey" and usually plain (Roche 1994: 137). His final question noted that pre-Revolutionary hierarchical difference in dress in Paris was "one of the visible manifestations of the coherence of the old world." He asks whether, during the Revolution, its function changed into a more egalitarian stance: "Did it . . . in its social specificity, by its nature, unite the instinct for equalisation within the distinctive hierarchies . . . and the appeal of egalitarian imitation?" (519).

Roche's pioneering studies paved the way for today's interdisciplinary material culture-social and economic history approaches. John Styles and Amanda Vickery, approaching material culture study from just such roots, have usefully discussed the interdisciplinary problems of twinning text with artifact-based research:

> Some have treated material evidence as an adjunct to text-based history; others have argued for the superiority of the material over textual evidence—for studying the illiterate majorities that characterized most historical societies; others again have made a case for according empirical precedence to material evidence over textual evidence. But all those who share a material culture framework share a commitment to thinking about the social and cultural work performed by artefacts. (2006: 21)

Even without surviving examples of their fabrics and clothes, these approaches take us close to understanding social differences, personal memories, aspirations, and even the life regrets of consumers. Vickery identified the moderate character of Mrs. Elizabeth Shackleton, for example, through her care for her clothing. She was the financially secure widow of a textile merchant living on the edges of merchant and gentry class circles in the West Midlands. Through Mrs. Shackleton's diaries, domestic account books from 1762 to 1781, and local regional archives, even without a surviving whole garment, Vickery identified Mrs. Shackleton's reuse of a much-loved fabric. Once her "favourite, pritty, red and white linen gown," in 1773 she used one scrap to make "a working bag" and three years later "made a cover for the dressing drawers of my pritty red and white linnen gown" (Vickery 1993: 183). Vickery notes too that wherever possible "outdated or faded gowns were often unpicked" to the original fabric lengths and that Mrs. Shackleton sent these "to be dyed in Manchester or London" (151). Vickery interpreted all of this as a rebuttal of the stereotypic view of women as spendthrift consumers of frivolous fashion, and thus she seminally challenged historical prejudices against women, characterized as "parasitic and pointless" consumers (274).

Styles makes clear his approach to the use of dress in his well-received *The Dress of the People: Everyday Fashion in Eighteenth-Century England* (2007). "In analysing plebeian fashion *The Dress of the People* has focused on how it was embedded in the practices of everyday life, not on issues of meaning and identity which have so often engaged those who study dress—emphasis is on 'distinction between best and working clothes'" (323). Through this, Styles questions previous assumptions about the low consumption levels of even stylish clothing among working people in England in the eighteenth century. He accessed sources similar to those used by Roche but additionally used more illustrations, including samples of period fabrics, to illustrate the significance of his emphasis on the existence of "best" as well as everyday garments within the "dress of the people."

Dress and Ethnography

Ethnographic approaches to the study of dress examine the lives of world communities, assessing homes, religious practice, social organization, land ownership, agricultural and consumption systems, gender relationships, and domestic and clothing artifacts. Today these methods are applied equally to remote or urban settings, as Le Wita (1994) has shown. All now propose a view of "living cultures" assessed through the eyes of the community who made and wore the clothing. No longer are they examined from colonial and imperial viewpoints. Researchers today, as already noted, are probing issues of cross-cultural design and consumption, and no country is seen as isolated from the global ebb and flow of human exchange and contact. Giorgio Riello and Tirthankar Roy note, just for one example, that as early as the fourteenth century, West Africa exchanged primary products for Asian manufactured goods such as cottons and other fine textiles and that "considerable quantities of Asian textiles also arrived in Congo as luxury cloths designed in rich and colourful ways" (2009: 4).

Portraiture as a Source of Dress History Studies

Renne comments on the inevitable rotting and destruction of cloth and clothing, stating that "unless specially preserved, cloths—like human bodies—eventually disintegrate and disappear" (1995: 9). The survival of complete European garments (apart from clothes preserved in bogs or tombs) dating from before 1550–1700 is rare, hence the long-established use of period portraits, drawings, and engravings within dress history study, a complex and fascinating subject dealt with by Aileen Ribeiro, for one, over a lifetime of pioneering research and scholarship. She has written extensively on eighteenth- and nineteenth-century dress and has explained with care her methodologies. Aware of the view put forward, for example, by Auslander that "objects that are not just seen, but also felt and touched (thereby distinguishing between visual and material culture)" (2005: 1016), Ribeiro offers in her recent book, *Fashion and Fiction: Dress in Art and Literature in Stuart England* (2006), a masterly account of seventeenth-century dress through, yet again, a skillful interdisciplinary fusion of analysis of period portraiture, rare surviving fabrics and garments, and text drawn from period novels and other texts.

Use of Literature in Dress History Research

Ribeiro's emphasis on the use of fiction as a source for the study of fashion/dress history is an indication that this source is now accepted in the field as a means of breathing life, emotion, and movement into our study of historical clothing. Miller has stressed that "the sensual and aesthetic—what cloth feels and looks like—is the source of its capacity to objectify myth, cosmology and also morality, power and values" (2005: 1). Yet how can this be extracted from static clothes on frozen mannequins in dimly lit galleries or stored in boxes? The use of novels, diaries, and travelers' tales has become one answer and is now an established tool for injecting movement into dress history. In the 1980s both Anne Buck (1983) and Daniel Roche (1994) drew insightful ideas from period novels. Roche noted that descriptions of the clothing of characters in late eighteenth-century French novels helped clarify period social hierarchies and that novelists' accounts of clothing of women in the 1770s evoked "dissolute seduction, sexual display and the dangers of city life for virtuous girls but…also [drove] home the importance of social masks, since the fascination of clothes, fashion and the circulation of objects promoted the confusion of *ranks*" (Roche 1994: 413). Clair Hughes has further emphasized that "clothes in fiction are clothes in action, clothes experienced and clothes observed…Dressed in fiction, clothes of the past are warmed into life" (2006: 185).

Travelers' tales also carry precious historical descriptions of all kinds of clothing from those of royalty to the poverty-stricken, all of which have to "read" with extreme care with an eye on the viewpoint of the traveler. Mildred Cable and Francesca French,

Christian missionaries traveling in remote Buddhist Mongolian China, were deeply impressed by the richness of dress of a Kalmuk princess from the Altai Mountains in the 1920s and provide us today with a detailed account of her appearance both in text and visually. They photographed her (Figure 1.2), noting that "her hair hung down in two long glistening plaits, outlining the pure oval of her face, and was gathered into jewelled sheaths, forming part of her regal head-dress . . . Jade, gold and silver ornaments covered her breast and a satin garment of sombre richness fell from her shoulders to her feet" (Cable and French 1927: 28).

Travelers' tales, however, are often rooted in imperialism, colonialism, right- or left-wing politics, gendered prejudices, or sentimentality and can also offer far less neutral views. In 1938 Sacheverell Sitwell published an account of his journey around Romania, where he enjoyed the hospitality of aristocratic circles and villages alike. However, the anti-Semitism embedded in his comments about the Jews of Hotin, a small, poor Jewish town in Romanian Galicia, is clear: "It is the tattered greasy caftans of the Jews to which the greatest horror attaches . . . The Jews of small towns like Hotin are upon

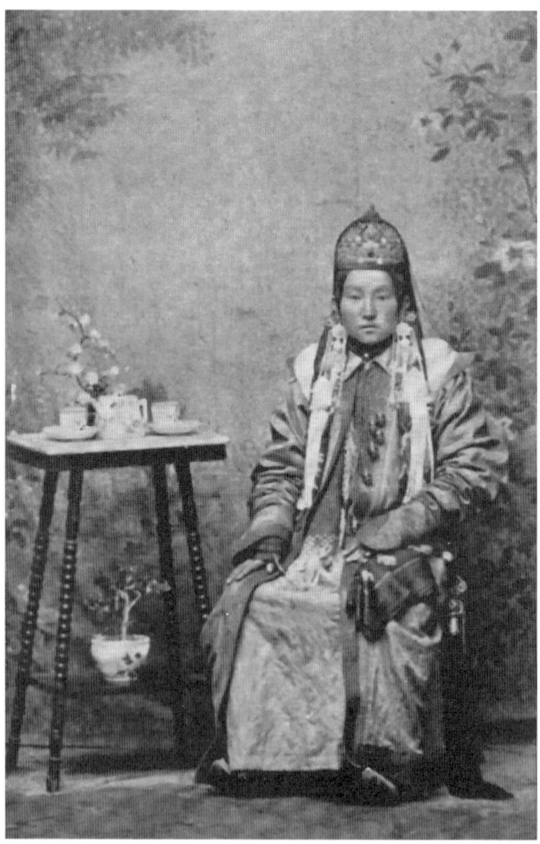

FIGURE 1.2 Kalmuk princess, Chinese Mongolia, about 1925, from Mildred Cable and Francesca French, *Through Jade Gate and Central Asia* (London: Constable, 1917), facing p. 28.
Credit: Photograph by the author.

a lower scale of life, physically, than any other slum population in the world" (Sitwell [1938] 1992: 85). As Taylor notes, Sitwell then endorsed the proposal made that year by Julius Streicher, the Nazi *Gauleiter* of Franconia, that Romanian Jews should be "settled in Madagascar" (Taylor 2004: 238). Reader beware.

Oral History and Oral Testimony as a Source for Dress History and Fashion Studies

Oral history and testimony form another, still underused but now established, tool in dress history and fashion studies. Again, such work needs always to be set in its related interdisciplinary context of social, cultural, and dress history. The preciousness of this method is that it brings the interviewer close to the "personal" aspect of clothing, through memories, most especially those of people once marginalized from "big history." This process requires sensitivity to the interviewee, patience over transcription, and open-mindedness, as the results may be entirely unexpected. Robert Perks and Alistair Thompson's 2006 *Oral History Reader* demonstrates the scope of research, with

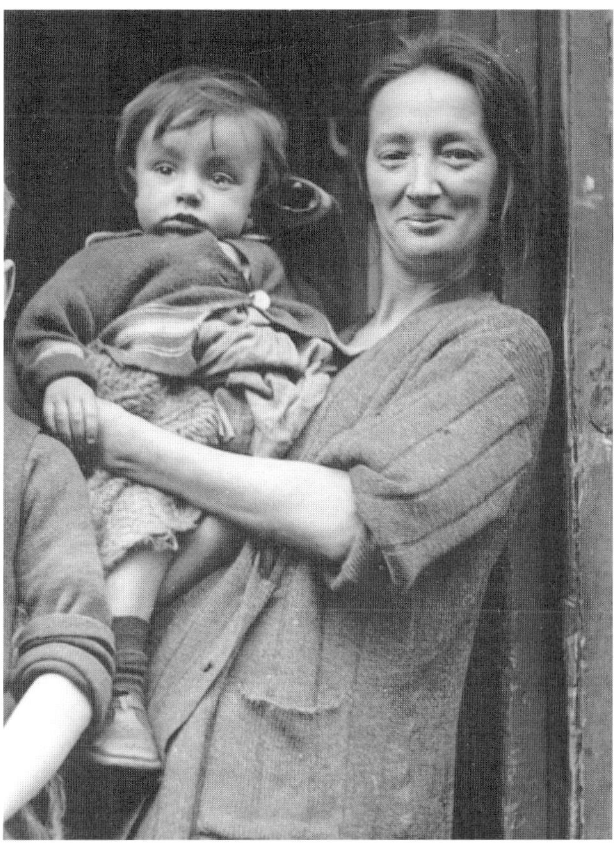

FIGURE 1.3 Edith Tudor Hart, photograph of *Mrs B. Clarendon Street, Paddington,* 1934.
Credit: Pearl Binder Collection. Courtesy of Wolf Suschitzky.

its texts on lesbian history, women's role in the Ku Klux Klan, World War II memories, and so on. Alan Wieder, too, believes "in the power of testimony and the importance of those who are historically invisible having a public voice that adds a deeper human understanding to the historical record" (2004: 23).

Use of Photography and Film in Dress History Studies

There is now a whole academic industry of film fashion studies with its own academic journals, including *Film, Fashion & Consumption.* My personal interest lies in documentary and amateur film and photography. If novels and travelers' tales offer some injection of spirit into the field of dress history, documentary, amateur film, and photographs offer even more. Again, these sources are used by researchers because they offer images of those who might otherwise be left out of dress history—such as Edith Tudor Hart's documentary photograph of a poor but cheery London woman, *Mrs B. Clarendon Street, Paddington,* in a ragged cardigan in 1934 (Figure 1.3).[8]

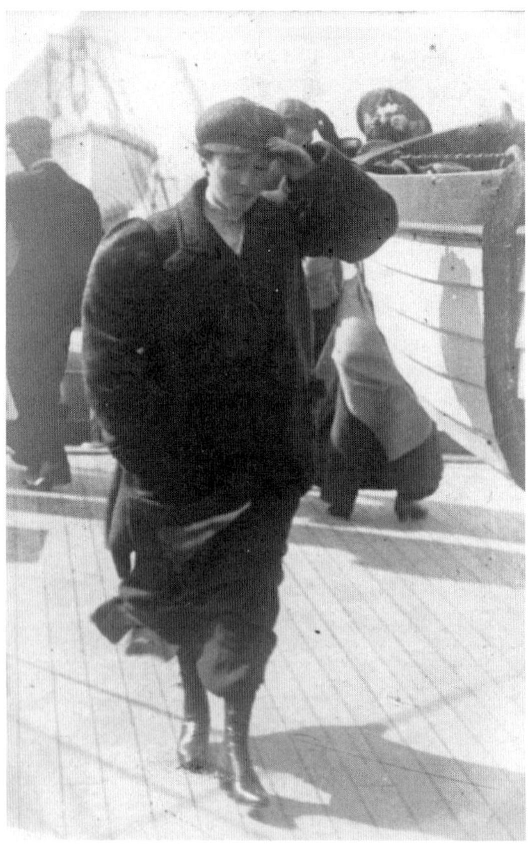

FIGURE 1.4 Unknown woman on the cross-Channel ferry in tweed coat and cap, April 3, 1906, photographed by Linley Sambourne, Maud Messel's father.
Credit: Courtesy of the Royal Borough of Kensington and Chelsea, the Sambourne Family Archives.

Images taken "in action," rather than posed formally in a photographer's studio, again offer missing information on clothing in movement. On April 3, 1906, the *Punch* political cartoonist Linley Sambourne, father of Maud Messel, a keen experimental "street" photographer, traveled in a gale on the cross-Channel ferry. Sambourne photographed a woman traveler struggling against the wind wrapped in a body-concealing, masculine-styled, heavy tweed coat, with her tweed cap rammed inelegantly over her forehead (Figure 1.4). This snatched image of dress in action is a far cry from the posed, static elegance of the decorative feminized outdoor clothing choices seen in the studio photograph of Sambourne's daughter in about 1907–1908. In it Maud has carefully arranged both her large hat with its huge silk bow and her swansdown stole in their precise and fashionably correct positions before permitting the studio photographer in Oxford to take the photograph (Figure 1.5).

The sense of movement to be found in documentary and amateur film also offers useful evidence of clothing in movement. Among the short documentary films made by Sagar Mitchell and James Kenyon is one taken as workers leave the Alfred Butterworth cotton mill, in Hollinwood, Lancashire, in July 1901 (Mitchell and Kenyon 1901). This

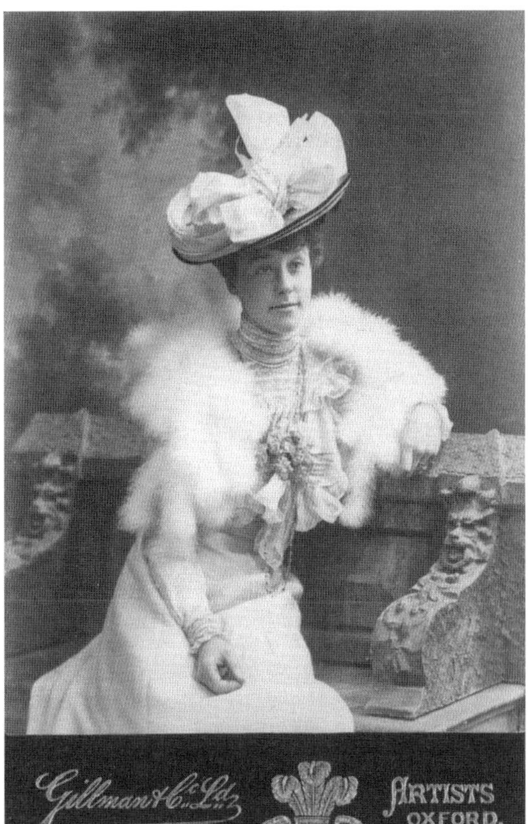

FIGURE 1.5 Studio photograph of Maud Messel, taken by Gillman and Co. in Oxford, about 1907–1908. *Credit*: Courtesy of the Royal Borough of Kensington and Chelsea, the Sambourne Archives.

shows in detail women and girls in clogs, wrapping their heavy shawls around their bodies, with no sign yet of the consumption of the more fashionable ready-made jackets, already available as daily outerwear. Cathy Eck and Hannah Kauffman, using the resources of Screen Archives South East at the University of Brighton, set out to reveal the research value of amateur film for fashion history. Using themes of sport, leisure, work, and travel, related to 1920s and 1930s fashions, they matched garments filmed at public and family events to dress surviving in local museums in the south of England. This fascinating interdisciplinary research tour de force reveals interwar dress both in movement and in its provenanced consumption context.[9] Eck and Kauffman identify the settings as mostly middle class, confirming aptly that these films show "everyday dress within its context rather than separated from it... [allowing us to]... read clothes not just as a static image but with the added associations of body shape, gesture and mannerisms" (2011: 77).

Business and Fashion History

Business history has also finally become a growing field within dress and textile studies. Today's accounts recognize the power of consumer choice and style change as major driving forces in business, past and present. Philip Sykas, for example, has shown how these impacted on business success within the English cotton print trade in the nineteenth century. Through examination of 900 print sample books, he clarified the complex annual business export cycle of printed cottons, noting the fashion-driven seasonality of related designs (2005: 120). The business historian Regina Blaszczyk has made a seminal contribution to this field through her edited book, *Producing Fashion: Commerce, Culture and Consumers* (2008), as has Andrew Godley through his business history research, such as "The Development of the Clothing Industry: Technology and Fashion" (1997). The business history of Dior's haute couture salon has finally also been examined, revealing the salon to be very much more than the most glamorous leading couture house in postwar Paris, as depicted in most fashion history accounts. Examining its huge financial success, Alexandra Palmer emphasizes Dior's direct, energetic involvement in the business success of the company. She clarifies for the first time that by 1953, having opened only in 1947, the House of Dior impressively "grossed more than $7 million a year" and was "by the far the most profitable couture company ever created," with its couture exports "accounting for more than half the total of the Paris couture's export market by 1957" and with flourishing related companies across five continents (Palmer 2009: 98).

DRESS AND COLLECTING

We learn our dress history and build images of the appearance of our past in no small part from displays of historic dress in local and national museums. Today, because of the extraordinary popular fascination with fashion, especially that related to designers and women celebrities, glamorous fashion exhibitions have become a financial and publicity prop for museums all over the world, even at the expense of other, more historically based displays. This in turn has generated much debate at fashion studies conferences, including critical reviews of fashion exhibitions and in-depth analysis of display motivations and theory. The journal *Fashion Theory* produced a special edition, "Exhibitionism," edited by Alexandra Palmer and Valerie Steele (2008), which confronted passionate current exhibition-related debates, noting issues such as the tensions in museum displays between scholarship and contemporary fashion styling and between experimental display and historical artifact, all of which indicate the vibrancy of our field today.

CONCLUSION

For me the crucial, vital processes are touching, looking, listening, and reflecting: touching first (when allowed) and then looking closely at garments—from poor worn-out clothing to perfect couture—and examining stitching, restitching, patching, cutting, and so on. Listening to voices recorded through oral history or voices lying mute in archives is a key element of research. These are thoroughly creative processes. It takes time to research, reflect on, and then interpret objects of clothing in their specific and yet interdisciplinary historical gendered, class, or ethnic context. Figure 1.6 shows a magnificent shawl, handwoven in the hills of Kashmir perhaps in the 1865–1870 period, exported to and worn probably in France or England; it was altered with the highest of tailoring skills into a fashionable and elegant bustle-backed lady's coat in about 1885, finally finding itself locked away in the stores of Worthing Museum, brought out for occasional exhibition (Figure 1.6). Fred Davis asserts significantly that fashion styles and ideas are "the irrepressible out comings of localities, regionalisms and particular-isms of every sort" (1994: 205). This unprovenanced coat raises exactly these issues within the history of European/Indian cross-cultural consumption, colonialism, Euro-American fashion, and orientalism in the 1860–1890 period and in the context of cultures bleeding across Rosaldo's "porous boundaries" (1989: 217). Through all of this, we need to be alert to our own contemporary cultural and historical assumptions. These are often so deeply embedded in our minds that it is hard to even realize their presence, and they can catch us unawares and lead to errors in dating garments or a false decoding of their historical social place and cultural meanings.

Clothes are important. Miller notes that new studies on dress and material culture "seek to convey the experiences of peoples... where cosmology, that is one's understanding of the nature of the universe and one's place within it, is often formulated through the making, wearing, displaying and destruction of fibres" (2005: 10). For me, studying artifacts of surviving dress along the lines and approaches discussed here brings us very close to the breath of the past. The possibilities for future research are many. For example, there is growing interest in examining the design, making, retailing, and

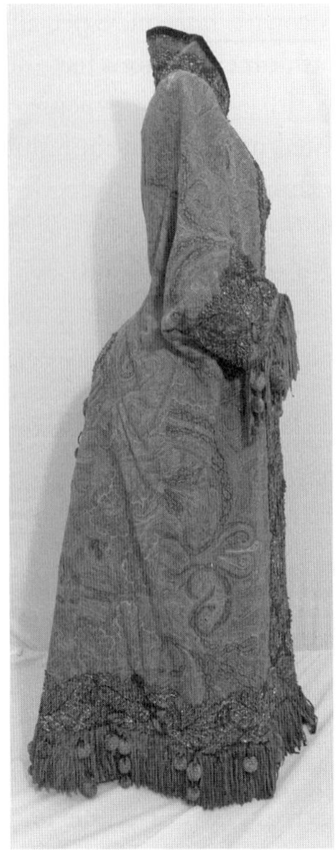

FIGURE 1.6 Woman's coat, about 1885, made from a Kashmir shawl. Worthing Museum, no. 4313. *Credit*: Courtesy of the Leisure and Culture Services, Worthing Borough Council.

consumption of everyday dress across the world, past and present, in its specific global and local contexts. Karen Tranberg Hansen (2000), Lucy Norris (2010), and Hazel Clark and Alexandra Palmer (2005) have triggered new research dealing with the global circulation and local meanings of secondhand and recycled clothing. Analysis of global tourism's cultural, economic, and design impact on textiles and clothing produced in the remotest corners of the world for tourist sale and export is another growing area of interest, opened up by Eric Cohen back in 1989 with his article "The Commercialisation of Ethnic Crafts." In the blossoming fields of dress history and fashion studies these themes point to positive and rapidly growing international research developments. The horizons seem limitless, and there is no end to research possibilities in sight, with much still to be done.

NOTES

1. "Magister Course in Fashion Studies, 60 hp," University of Stockholm, http://sisu.it.su.se/search/info/FS7000/en (accessed September 8, 2012).
2. "Fashion Studies (MA)," Parsons the New School for Design, http://www.newschool.edu/parsons/ma-fashion-studies (accessed September 8, 2012).

3. "Fashion and Dress History BA(Hons)," University of Brighton Faculty of Arts, http://arts.brighton.ac.uk/study/history-art-design/fashion-dress-history-ba (accessed September 8, 2012).
4. "Fashion History and Theory," Central Saint Martins, http://www.csm.arts.ac.uk/courses/ba-fashion/fht/ (accessed September 8, 2012).
5. "Research: History of Dress," The Courtauld Institute of Art, http://www.courtauld.ac.uk/research/sections/historyofdress.shtml (accessed September 8, 2012).
6. "MA Fashion Curation," London College of Fashion, http://www.fashion.arts.ac.uk/courses/graduate-school/ma-fashion-curation/ (accessed September 8, 2012).
7. "Fashion in History: A Global Look, 1300–2000 (HI169)," University of Warwick, http://www2.warwick.ac.uk/fac/arts/history/undergraduate/modules/fashion/ (accessed September 8, 2012).
8. This information is taken from Edith Tudor Hart's notation on the back of the photograph.
9. Screen Search Fashion, http://www.brighton.ac.uk/screenarchive/fashion/ (accessed August 31, 2012).

BIBLIOGRAPHY

Andrewes, Janet. 2005. *Bodyworks: Dress as Cultural Tool; Dress and Demeanour in the South of Senegal.* Leiden: Brill.

Auslander, Leora. 2005. "Beyond Words." *American Historical Review* 110 (4): 1015–45.

Baizerman, Suzanne, Joanne Eicher, and Catherine Cerny. 1993. "Eurocentrism in the Study of Ethnic Dress." *Dress* 20: 19–32.

Barnes, Ruth. 1997. *Indian Block-Printed Textiles in Egypt: The Newberry Collection in the Ashmolean Museum.* Oxford: Clarendon.

Barnes, Ruth, and Joanne Eicher. 1992. *Dress and Gender.* Oxford: Berg.

Blaszczyk, Regina (ed.). 2008. *Producing Fashion: Commerce, Culture and Consumers.* Philadelphia: University of Pennsylvania Press.

Buck, Anne. 1983. "Clothes in Fact and Costume, 1825–1865." *Costume: The Journal of the Costume Society* 17: 89.

Cable, Mildred, and Francesca French. 1927. *Through Jade Gate and Central Asia.* London: Constable.

Clark, Hazel, and Alexandra Palmer. 2005. *Old Clothes, New Looks: Second-Hand Fashion Fashion.* Oxford: Berg.

Cohen, Eric. 1989. "The Commercialisation of Ethnic Crafts." *Journal of Design History* 2 (2–3): 161–68.

Davis, Fred. 1994. *Fashion, Culture and Identity.* Chicago: University of Chicago Press.

de la Haye, Amy, Lou Taylor, and Eleanor Thompson. 2005. *A Family of Fashion: The Messels: Six Generations of Dress.* London: Philip Wilson.

Eck, Carly, and Hannah Kauffman. 2011. "Non-fiction Film in Fashion History." *Costume: The Journal of the Costume Society* 45: 75–84.

El Guindi, Fadwa. 1999. *Veil: Modesty, Privacy and Resistance.* Oxford: Berg.

Godley, Andrew. 1997. "The Development of the Clothing Industry: Technology and Fashion." *Textile History* 28 (1): 3–10.

Granata, Francesca. 2012. "Fashion Studies Inbetween: A Methodological Case Study and an Inquiry into the State of Fashion Studies." *Fashion Theory: The Journal of Dress, Body and Culture* 16 (1): 67–81.

Harte, Negley. 2009. "Review: John Styles, The Dress of the People." *Costume: The Journal of the Costume Society* 43: 176.

Hansen, Karen Tranberg. 2000. *Salaula: The World of Secondhand Clothing and Zambia.* Chicago: University of Chicago Press.

Hartkamp-Jonxis, E. 1994. *Indian Chintzes.* Amsterdam: Rijksmuseum, Waanders.

Hughes, Clair. 2006. *Dressed in Fiction.* Oxford: Berg.

Lemire, Beverly. 2003. "Domesticating the Exotic: Floral Culture and the East India Calico Trade with England, c. 1600–1800." *Textile: The Journal of Cloth and Culture* 1 (1): 65–85.

Le Wita, Beatrix. 1994. *French Bourgeois Culture.* Cambridge: Cambridge University Press.

Miller, Daniel. 2005. "Introduction." In Susanne Küchler and Daniel Miller (eds.), *Clothing as Material Culture,* 1–19. Oxford: Berg.

Mitchell, Sagar, and James Kenyon. 1901. *Alfred Butterworth and Sons, Gleb Mills, Hollinwood (1901).* London: British Film Institute. Documentary film. http://www.youtube.com/watch?v=G3Dw9ZNiqoI (accessed August 31, 2012).

Norris, Lucy. 2010. *Recycling Indian Clothing: Global Contexts of Reuse and Value.* Bloomington: Indiana University Press.

O'Connor, Kaori. 2005. "The Material Culture of New Fibres." In Susanne Küchler and Daniel Miller (eds.), *Clothing as Material Culture*, 22–41. Oxford: Berg.

Palmer, Alexandra. 2009. *Dior.* London: V&A Publishing.

Palmer, Alexandra, and Valerie Steele. 2008. "Exhibitionism." *Fashion Theory: The Journal of Dress, Body and Culture* 12 (1): 7–30.

Pearce, Susan M. 1993. *Museums, Objects and Collection: A Cultural Study.* Leicester: Leicester University Press.

Perani, Judith, and Norma H. Wolff. 1999. *Cloth, Dress, and Art Patronage in Africa.* Oxford: Berg.

Perks, Robert, and Alistair Thompson. 2006. *The Oral History Reader.* 2nd ed. Abingdon, UK: Routledge.

Poppy, P. 1997. "Fancy Dress? Costume for Re-enactment." *Costume: The Journal of the Costume Society* 31: 100–105.

Renne, Elisha P. 1995. *Cloth That Does Not Die: The Meaning of Cloth in Bunu Social Life.* Seattle: University of Washington Press.

Ribeiro, Aileen. 2006. *Fashion and Fiction: Dress in Art and Literature.* New Haven, CT: Yale University Press.

Riello, Giorgio, and Prasannan Parthasarathi (eds.). 2009. *The Spinning World: A Global History of Cotton Textiles.* Oxford: Oxford University Press.

Riello, Giorgio, and Tirthankar Roy (eds.). 2009. *How India Clothed the World: The World of South Asian Textiles, 1500–1850.* Leiden: Brill.

Roche, Daniel. 1987. *The People of Paris: An Essay in Popular Culture in the 18th Century.* Oxford: Berg.

Roche, Daniel. 1994. *The Culture of Clothing: Dress and Fashion in the Ancien Régime.* Cambridge: Cambridge University Press.

Rosaldo, Renato. 1989. *Culture and Truth: The Remaking of Social Analysis.* Boston: Beacon.

Sitwell, Sacheverell. [1938] 1992. *Roumanian Journey.* London: B. T. Batsford.
Styles, John. 2007. *The Dress of the People: Everyday Fashion in Eighteenth-Century England.* New Haven, CT: Yale University Press.
Styles, John, and Amanda Vickery. 2006. *Gender, Taste and Material Culture in Britain and North America.* New Haven, CT: Yale University Press.
Sykas, Philip. 2005. *The Secret Life of Textiles: Six Pattern Book Archives in North West England.* Bolton, UK: Bolton Museums, Art Gallery and Aquarium.
Tarlow, Emma. 1996. *Clothing Matters: Dress and Identity in India.* London: Huest.
Taylor, Lou. [1983] 2009. *Mourning Dress: A Costume and Social History.* Abingdon, UK: Routledge.
Taylor, Lou. 2002. *The Study of Dress History.* Manchester: Manchester University Press.
Taylor, Lou. 2004. *Establishing Dress History.* Manchester: Manchester University Press.
Vickery, Amanda. 1993. "Women and the World of Goods: A Lancashire Consumer and Her Possessions—1751–81." In John Brewer and Roy Porter (eds.), *Consumption and the World of Goods,* 127–305. London: Routledge.
Wieder, Alan. 2004. "Testimony as Oral History: Lessons from South Africa." *Educational Researcher* 33 (6): 23–28.

2

Dress, Time, and Space: Expanding the Field through Exhibition Making

GREER CRAWLEY AND DONATELLA BARBIERI

INTRODUCTION

In contemporary exhibitions of historical dress, the perception, interpretation, and representation of time have acquired a new significance. There is recognition that the presentation and interpretation of historical dress involve more than causal explanations and empirical evidence. Material description and empirical investigation are only two of the current museological methodologies. Influenced by postmodernist discourses on historical temporality, memory, and narrative, curators are finding innovative ways to preserve and represent the passage of time. As Susan Stewart has observed in *On Longing,* "time must be seen as concomitant with a loss of understanding, a loss which can be relieved through the reawakening of objects and thereby, a reawakening of narrative" (1993: 142).

This chapter explores notable curatorial attempts to create original temporal narratives and arrangements for historical dress in which historical time becomes human time "to the extent that it is articulated through a narrative mode" (Ricoeur 1984: 52). Rather than fixing and describing a moment in time through dress, these new historical narratives experiment with temporality, spatiality, materiality, and performativity to change the perception of historical dress. Curators are adopting the performative strategies described by Jens Hoffmann and Joan Jonas in *Perform (Art Works)* as "participatory, ephemeral, process-orientated, provisional and conceptual" (2005: 17) to establish a dialogue between the spectator and the dress/object.

The performance in this chapter is that of curated and conserved dress, as museum object, which inevitably refers to a body that is absent and is simultaneously evoked by the curatorial intervention. Philosopher of language John L. Austin (1962) first utilized the word *performative* to describe the difference between words that "do" something rather than "describe" something. The exemplars included in this chapter draw out the "doing" in exhibition through imaginative processes.

THE HISTORICAL IMAGINATION

The presentation of historical dress, as a shared and embodied symbol of past existence, offers its curators interesting dilemmas. Often when historical dress is exhibited, the focus of the displays will be on the quality of the craftsmanship and the spectacle of the social elite that these garments represented. Historical dress is displayed as a way to show reverence and reflect voyeuristic interest and as an object representing a specific time and place within an ordered system. The institutional criteria for the choice of objects to be conserved, interpreted, and exhibited create a cultural, social, and material hierarchy. And in the process of valuing it, the act of conservation embalms the object. In the case of dress this can run counter to the essence of the object itself. In her introduction to *Adorned in Dreams,* Elizabeth Wilson speaks about the eeriness of a museum of costume, where glass cabinets hold silent old gowns that can appear haunted:

> We experience a sense of the uncanny when we gaze at garments that had an intimate relationship with human beings long since gone. . . . They hint at something only half understood, sinister, threatening; the atrophy of the body, and the evanescence of life. (2007: 1)

The "something only half understood" has come as a challenge to contemporary curators of dress. The absent body leaves space for the new interpretation and new understanding not only of historical dress but also of history itself and our relationship to it. Hans Gumbrecht in *Production of Presence* talks about the "historical imagination" and suggests that

> the desire for presence makes us imagine how we would have related, intellectually and with our bodies, to certain objects...if we had encountered them in their historical everyday worlds. Once we feel how this play of our historical imagination can be appealing and contagious, once we lure other persons into the same intellectual process, we have produced the very situation to which we are referring when we say that somebody is capable of conjuring up the past. (2004: 124)

In 1969 Daniel Robbins, director of the Museum of Art of the Rhode Island School of Design, invited Andy Warhol to curate an exhibition of objects from the museum's storerooms. Beginning in the costume collection, the artist made the first in a number of unexpected curatorial moves. He selected the entire reserve collection of shoes along with assorted parasols as costume accessories (Figure 2.1). When asked if he wanted the cabinet in which they were stored as well, he replied, "Oh, yes, just like that." To the question as to whether the museum visitors would be allowed to open and close the doors, Warhol seemed to reply affirmatively, suggesting it as "spectator participation" (Bourdon 1969: 17). The artist also requested that the exhibition catalog contain a

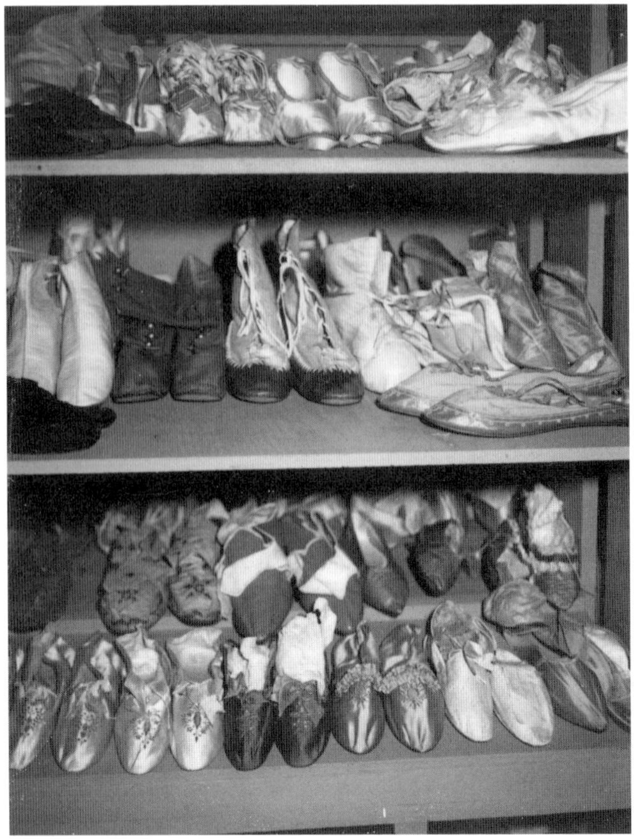

FIGURE 2.1 Andy Warhol, *Untitled* (Three shelves of shoes), 1969. From Raid the Icebox 1 with Andy Warhol, an exhibition selected from the reserve collections of the Museum of Art, Rhode Island School of Design.
Credit: Gift of J. Malcolm and Clarice S. Grear. Photograph by Erik Gould. Courtesy of the Museum of Art, Rhode Island School of Design, Providence.

detailed inventory of all the items with no distinction about relative merit nor regard for provenance. Stephen Ostrow, the chief curator, describes how the catalog itself was conceived as a "neutral entity" with "no historically based organisation." It was simply divided into two categories: single objects and objects in series (Ostrow 1969: 26).

Robbins was initially skeptical about Warhol's instructions and couldn't at first understand the value of Warhol's seemingly willful approach. However, as he was to write in his essay accompanying the exhibition,

> we now understand why: each object is obliged to carry its full set of associations, and a weird poetry results; the combination of pedantry and sentiment that can be read in the entries is the serial image of history. There are personal overtones of almost

> unbelievable poignancy in the now anonymous rubbed kid heels of some fine lady's shoes. (1969: 14)

Robbins also notes how "Warhol's choice will be part of the catalogued record," stating that

> the art that he chose from our reserves will reverberate with all the repressed meaning that the passage of time has left adhering to each piece. . . . Andy Warhol's choice will have become part of their ever expanding meaning. For now, let the contemporary artist decide on the relevancy of the past. (15)

Robbins's enlightened response to Warhol's interventions indicated the director's recognition that Warhol's role was as "an agent of change" (Dorsett 2009: 244).

This extraordinary exhibition, Raid the Icebox 1, established a precedent for museum and curatorial experiments that were to critique museum methodologies and bring more creative approaches to the presentation of museum objects, including dress. In the 1960s, artists were introducing their "expanded field" of radical new artistic practices that were to transform curation and exhibition design. Museums became sites of experimentation through artistic intervention and installation that invited audience participation and engagement in new, accessible ways.

Among those who were influenced by the exhibition was Peter Wollen. In 1993 Wollen included the Warhol museum project in his book *Raiding the Icebox,* in which he discussed the artist's "subversive new sensibility" and the relationship between performance and design. He wrote about the artist's "refusal of hierarchy or consequence or narrative (hierarchy and consequence of events over time)" (1993: 166). Wollen was to co-curate with Fiona Bradley the 1998 exhibition Addressing the Century: 100 Years of Art and Fashion, at the Hayward Gallery. In his introduction to the catalog, Wollen identifies the challenge presented to fashion by artistic practices of installation and performance, and the exhibition was designed by the architect Zaha Hadid to emphasize materiality, visuality, and performativity. Chronology was less important than the transitions, gaps, allusions, and suggestions to be explored and made by the willing and engaged spectator. The scenographic treatment of the space—the layering, juxtaposing, framing, and spotlighting—focused the attention on the material object, its technical innovation, construction, and form. Both analytical and theatrical, the presentation was part stage set, part archaeological landscape of forms "that engulf the visitor and blur the boundaries between spectator and spectacle" (Hadid 2000: 220).

Hadid describes how she "treated the entire building as a three dimensional framework within which the garments and artworks could contain a new site-specific allusiveness." Through "isolating patterns of movement found in the seams of dresses or the weft of fabrics and enlarging them to the level of the galleries" she established the spatial organization for the exhibition. Hadid observed that "the absence of a moving body complementing a garment is alleviated by the dynamism of a gesture that manifests itself as catwalks and stages, settings for the total theatre of art and fashion" (Hadid 2000: 220).

The absence of the body of the wearer offers a discursive opportunity through which to articulate, performatively and spatially, not only the range of ever-changing forms but also the use of the playfulness, questioning, and open-endedness that are at the center of fashion design practice in the way that fashion "plays" with and is haunted by its history.

This was demonstrated more recently in Claire Wilcox's 2012 redesign and curation of the Victoria and Albert Museum fashion gallery. Shoes are once again the focus for disruption and subversion. In the traditional glass cases, the organized presentation is disturbed by a single embodied object—a shoe on its side (Figure 2.2). This tenderly evocative indication of presence enlivens the traditional static displays of dress and museum objects. Clear, informative, and accessible—this single gesture repeated in a number of cases transcends the institutional and introduces an element of the performative that is subtly handled without recourse to the full theatrical repertoire often associated with temporary fashion exhibitions.

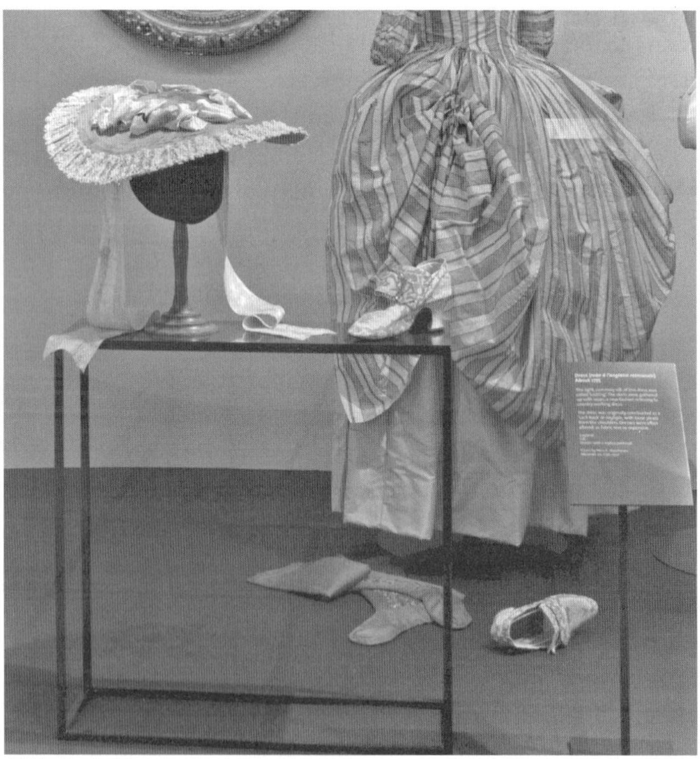

FIGURE 2.2 Display and cropped detail of overturned shoe, 1760–1770, displayed in From Court and Country 1750–1800, V&A Fashion Gallery Permanent Collection.
Credit: © Victoria and Albert Museum, London.

Shoes had also featured in Wilcox's 1991 exhibition Satellites of Fashion at the Crafts Council. For this exhibition of fashion accessories, she wanted to expand the interpretative possibilities of sartorial display. Mirrors strategically positioned at head, waist, and foot height invited the visitor's active and performative engagement with the hats, shoes, and bags, while the objects "acted" out their own performances in animated displays of sound and movement. A suspended silver purse by Emily Jo Gibson, which had a specially commissioned sound composition, was described by Wilcox as an "exploding silver thistle." Shaking slightly in suspension, it seemed to emit the sounds "of glass breaking in the distance."[1] In a review of the exhibition, Christopher Breward described "the sensation of stumbling into a dream scenario peopled by fantastic and expensive commodities," and he saw in the use of performance and the "dramatic set-piece" a "radical museological paradigm for the framing of clothing commodities" (1999: 270–71).

Wilcox's experience as a curator and her studies in literature, ceramics, and painting inform her approach to fashion exhibition and curation. She describes how she reads scenographically, visualizing the narrative, a process that she applies to curatorial

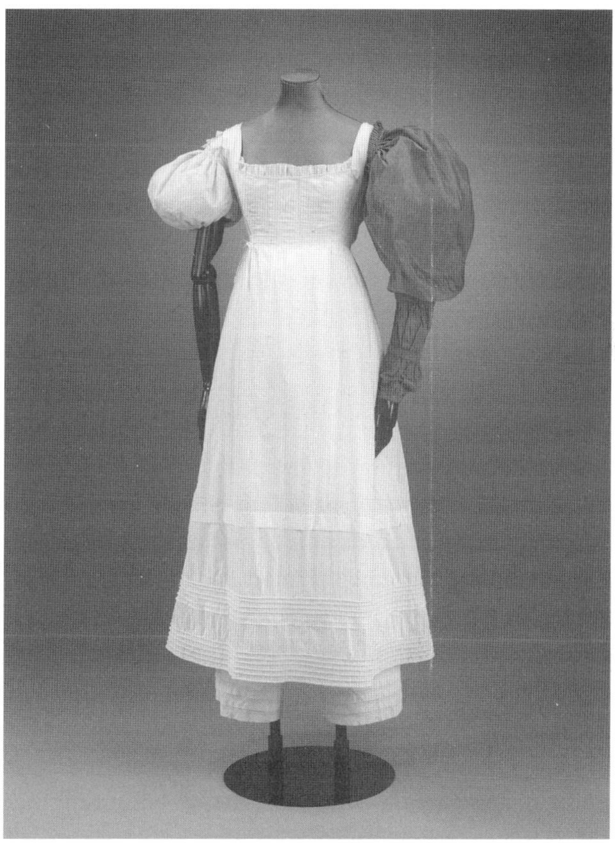

FIGURE 2.3 Sleeve, 1830s, displayed in At Home 1830–1840, V&A Fashion Gallery Permanent Collection.
Credit: © Victoria and Albert Museum, London.

interpretation and presentation. A thorough grounding in object analysis underpins her innovative approaches to display, drawn from theater and art practices. Wilcox is a believer in the power of allusion and the materiality and sensuality of the object. For Wilcox the discovery of a single sleeve of a dress from about 1803 in the Victoria and Albert store is as important as finding an entire dress (Figure 2.3):

> I climbed to the top of the ladder and there in the very top drawer was a single grey silk sleeve, all on its own, with a huge puffed shoulder. I thought I'm going to display it on a figure without the rest of the dress. It's just going to be a stockman with a big grey sleeve on it. And that to me is about history but it's also about time, sort of alluding. I think we slither back and forth in time as curators; we're reading the museological archives or we're reading Virginia Woolf's diaries or we're looking at sleeves in drawers.

Wilcox's scholarly but also playful and personal curation demonstrates her recognition of the unique power of the embodied object that is dress, and the way this enables the viewer to identify with it. It is a curatorial approach that goes beyond the ability to catalog style or historical period or to define provenance. Rather than provide escapism, the new fashion museology now "can move the viewers emotionally and/or challenge or enhance existing experiences and perceptions" like no other object in the museum can (de la Haye 2010: 287).

Museums are today embracing exhibitions of dress with unprecedented ardor, as it has become evident that their appeal is far more universal than that of other objects. Through interdisciplinary inquiry and intervention, the object that is historical dress is being reinvented and rediscovered in a process brought about by the curator as an agent of change.

CRITICAL CONSTELLATIONS

The curator Howard Morphy, writing in *Museum Materialities: Objects, Engagements, Interpretations,* describes how "times of paradigm change are the moments when new tropes replace old and stimulate the direction of discourse." Morphy identifies the shifts in museology as "a turn towards a more phenomenological approach, an emphasis on the body and theories of embodiment and steps towards an anthropology of the senses" (2010: 278). Drawing on the methodologies of cultural history, sociology, anthropology, and ethnography, curators have expanded the interpretive possibilities of their discipline. Jens Hoffmann, the director of the CCA Wattis Institute for Contemporary Art, writing in *The Exhibitionist: Journal of Exhibition Making,* observes that the adoption of a wider interdisciplinary approach in curatorial practice has meant that

> contemporary curating is...almost like anthropology, in the sense that the anthropologist and the curator are both self-reflexive and self-conscious producers of culture.

> They are aware they are not just showing or displaying an object or idea, but that they themselves are operating within a dynamic that actively creates new understandings of what is being shown, seen or represented. (2012: 4)

For these contemporary curators, complex ideas about dress are made evident in the interaction between objects, the compositional narrative of space in which they are placed, and the context of the encounter with the viewer. Their exhibition design methodologies and museological practices present a challenge to the curatorial conventions associated with the interpretation and presentation of historical dress.

Traditionally, the aim of a "museum of costume" with its plinths and vitrines is to project a pristine and unambiguous version of the past. Chronological arrangements in which "the whole universe of style" is "organised, catalogued and contained" (Mackie 1994: 335) make for an easily consumable and unchallenging view of history. However, as the curator Chris Dorsett has pointed out in his essay "Making Meaning beyond Display" (2009), this institutional authority and "calculated order" are being tested by a growing number of critical engagements by artist-curators with museum objects and museum procedures. For example, the fashion exhibition maker Judith Clark challenges the pedestal as a physical and metaphorical space that creates privilege and hierarchies of chosen objects, conserved and interpreted by the institution holding and protecting them. "The exhibitions and collection policies of many museums privilege objects of wonder: rare, valuable (financially and historically) single items that are presented, often literally, on a 'pedestal'" (Clark and de la Haye 2008: 154).

When the Judith Clark Costume Gallery was established in 1997 in Notting Hill, London, it became a center for the dissemination of ideas around new museology and new ways to look at fashion theory. The gallery was to provide a focus for debate and for "creating a new grammar, new patterns of time and reference" (Clark 2002: 147).

For her exhibition Parure de Plumes, held at the gallery in December 1998, Clark exhibited a late 1850s Peacock Dress from the Alsace region of France. Its large, crinolined skirt, covered with a prominent print of scaled-up feathers in the hues of a peacock's tail, made reference to orientalism, art nouveau, Aubrey Beardsley, and Chinese porcelain. By highlighting connections between historical periods, and between geographical places on the same body, Clark intended to reveal how "historical reference in dress has never been about evolution, continuity. . . . In dress, surfaces float free of their histories" (2002: 147).

The following year, Clark explored the transience of objects and their meanings in Be-hind Be-fore Be-yond (October 1999), in which Naomi Filmer's jewelry pieces, made out of ice, marked the passage of time as they melted. The disembodied hands and sections of mannequins that had held the jewelry were left redundant, until replacements were made from refrigerated molds in a repeating circular temporal pattern.

Although historical and chronological narratives can be constructed through the cut, construction, and materiality of dress, more commonly in the twenty-first century the new stories being told in museums and galleries are characterized by temporal fragmentation and drift. The study of historical dress has been expanded by its interaction with fashion, which "disregards the logical progression of linear time, finding a contemporaneity in the past that breaks through to the present" (Nagel 2004: 33). Among those who have had significant influence on the reassessment of historical dress is Vivienne Westwood. Her use and interpretation of historical precedents and references in her process is well documented:

> I take something from the past which has a sort of vitality that has never been exploited—like the crinoline—and get very intense. ... You get so involved with it that in the end you do something original because you overlay your own ideas. (Westwood, quoted in Wilcox 2004: 32)

To Wilcox it seemed that Westwood had a "nostalgia for the future"; that "it was as if she already knew all the historical influences that she incorporated into her collections, that she found them and discovered them and they were new but it was almost as if they were the future, as if time had somehow twisted." It was because of designers such as Westwood that Wilcox believes that she and Clark reunderstood "that fashion was somehow poetic and expressive and could take us back in time as well as into the future." All three recognized the creative and intellectual possibilities in exploring nonlinear ways of looking at history. The panoramic view replaces the single perspective and the temporal becomes spatial.

> We knew that fashion is this most marvellous three dimensional force that's not linear, that's as unsystematic as anything could possibly be, and yet resembles a fashion system. The fashion system could be the commercial imperative but actually the stylistic fashion system is very, very complicated and if you understand, or begin to understand that about contemporary fashion, then you can apply those same principles to historical fashion and start looking at historical fashion in a different way.

The chronological methodologies of the linear continuum are replaced by sampling, bricolage, montage, allusion, association, and juxtaposition. Clark cites among the influences on her curatorial methods Anna Piaggi's "Mitologia" and Aby Warburg's Mnemosyne Atlas, his extraordinary series of screens with arrangements of visual fragments, "an art history without text." In both projects, images are juxtaposed and arranged to create affective associations and resonances across time (Clark 2006). Piaggi and Warburg suggested alternative solutions to chronology, other ideas about spatial, material, and conceptual arrangements. Clark in *Anna Piaggi: Fashion-ology* (2006) noted how in 1949 James Laver, while keeper of prints and drawings at the Victoria and Albert Museum, published *Style in Costume* and advised "we shall proceed not logically but analogically. There will be no attempt to prove anything but only to bring related shapes together in the hope of firing the imagination to a perception of reality behind pattern" (Laver 1949: 7).

Curators like Wilcox and Clark were encouraged by these examples to find new ways of interpreting historical dress. Their research drew them to the experimental projects of artists and curators working outside the field of dress. Clark in her catalog essay describes how the concept for The Art of Fashion: Installing Allusions, at Museum Boijmans Van Beuningen (2009), derived from Harald Szeeman's 1998 A-Historical Sounds, which also took place at the Museum Boijmans Van Beuningen. Szeeman is a pivotal figure in contemporary curatorial interpretation. His arrangements of "a-historical resonances" between objects have created highly influential models of presentation. Clark sees in these arrangements the rehearsals of "connective possibilities that keep us mindful that there is no inevitable logic between any two objects, only temporary groupings." She goes on to say that these could be described as "'movements,' 'collections,' or even, but less fashionably, 'coincidences.' They can be called 'trends' or 'patterns.' For experimental exhibition designer and architect Frederick Kiesler they were 'Galaxies.' For Picasso they became 'constellations'" (2009: 16). These spatial-temporal arrangements have captured the contemporary curatorial imagination and provided an alternative to the linear time line.

> I think of historical dress as like all that detritus that's circulating around us in space, all the fragmented and broken up space capsules and satellites, we're being orbited by a milky way of fragments. We're reconstructing the historical detritus to make a new meaning.[2]

Caroline Evans has described Clark's installation "Locking In and Out" (Figure 2.4) in Spectres: When Fashion Turns Back (2005) as a "critical constellation": "It was not that the past simply illuminated the present, or that the present illuminated the past; rather the two images came together in a 'critical constellation' tracing a previously concealed connection" (2003: 33).

Clark's experimental methods of display, based on a dialogue between dress, space, and ideas that privilege a conceptual approach over an instructive one, had found an important focus in conversations with Evans, a fashion theorist. In the early stages of the planning for Malign Muses: When Fashion Turns Back, the ModeMuseum exhibition that opened in Antwerp in October 2004, Clark was asked to review a final draft of Evans's *Fashion at the Edge: Spectacle, Modernity, and Deathliness.* It was immediately clear to Clark that aspects of this text could provide the textual counterpoint for the visual logic of the installations.[3] The installations themselves became metaphors based on Evans's reading of Walter Benjamin's writings about the relationship between past, present, and future. Benjamin's "Tigersprung" would be a central leitmotif in Malign Muses, which became Spectres: When Fashion Turns Back when the exhibition transferred to the Victoria and Albert Museum in February 2005. Correspondences between

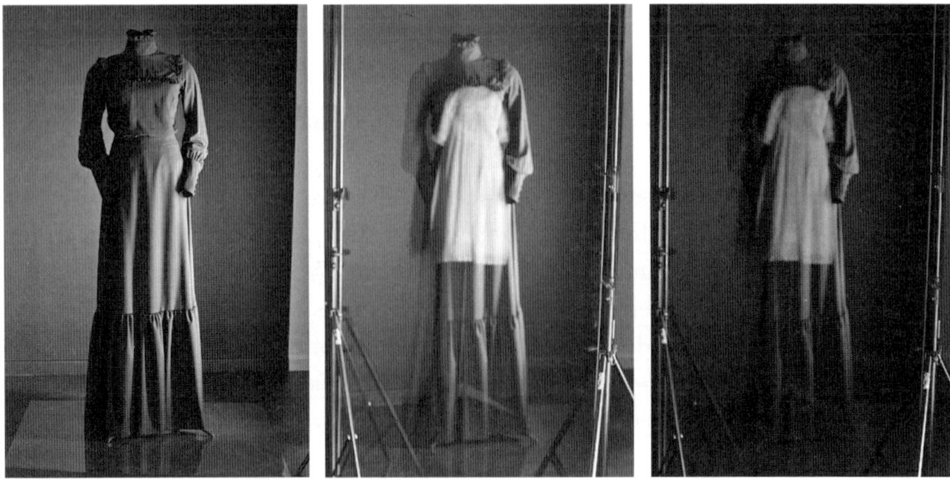

FIGURE 2.4 "Pepper's Ghost" installation in Malign Muses at ModeMuseum, Antwerp, 2004. Veronique Branquinho blouse and skirt, 1999, and baptism robe decorated with torchon lace and bobbin lace, 1900–1950.
Credit: Photograph by Ronald Stoop.

historical periods were also expressed in the visual and spatial allusions of the telescope, the diorama, and the labyrinth, and Evans's quotations were to be found throughout the exhibition providing the theoretical context.

Spectres was composed of a series of separate installations, some with titles suggesting a specific action: "Reappearances: Getting Things Back," "Locking In and Out," "Remixing It: The Past in Pieces," and "Phantasmagoria: The Amazing Lost and Found" (Figure 2.5). These titles draw attention to how connections are made and unmade, how historical references are remembered and forgotten. The idea of a single, fixed perspective on dress was challenged visually and physically. The overlay of historical and contemporary time on the same body was developed using the theatrical device of "Pepper's Ghost." In this installation, a Veronique Branquinho blouse and skirt (spring/summer 1999) glowed intermittently with the ghost of a 1900–1950 baptism robe, in torchon and bobbin lace, through a lighting and reflection trick, devised in the Victorian theater to stage ghosts. Positioned at the end of a long corridor, Clark's "ghost" performed the implied connection between the two objects, one from the present and one from the past, in which the the dress and its historical muse or specter are inextricably linked. This narrative gesture reinforced in the viewer the understanding of the theatrical language deployed in the exhibition.

The associations between historical periods were performed and temporally unfolded in the constructed spaces of the exhibition, and were experienced by the viewer in a "staging" of dress narratives, emerging from conversations between the objects. As in André Malraux's "musee imaginaire," we find "the persisting life of certain forms, emerging ever and again like spectres from the past" (Foster 2003: 31). Historical time was usefully explained through the performed time of the interaction between objects,

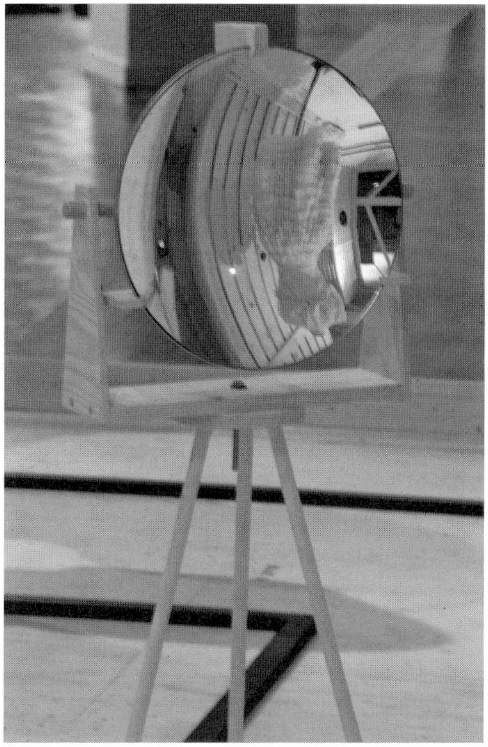

FIGURE 2.5 "Reappearances: Getting Things Back," detail of "Labyrinth" installation, in Malign Muses at ModeMuseum, Antwerp, 2004.
Credit: Photograph by Ronald Stoop.

space, movement, and audience. In "Remixing It: The Past in Pieces," the taking apart of the past and mixing with the new were represented in an installation where segmented bodies and garments from the past and the present appear set as in a sliding block puzzle, suggesting infinite possible rearrangements.

Spectres was representative of a renewed curatorial interest in theatricality, surrealism, cabinets of curiosities (*Wunderkammers*), games, optical devices, and the spectatorial relationship. The spatial, temporal, and optical arrangements of Spectres, like those of the theater and the cabinet of curiosity, were performative and perceptual. Evans describes how "seven views are set up: magnifying, reflecting, selecting, doubling the objects through the peepholes. They remind us of looking games, with each game suggesting different ways a designer might edit the past to create new designs."[4] For Valerie Steele, Malign Muses/Spectres was "paradigm breaking":

> She [Judith Clark] had used all the spatial and visual formulas to make you realise that the way fashion changed over time was so multi-faceted. It shook you out of the normal way of looking at the history which is that things are pre-determined. She freed us up a lot more to think in terms of a theatrical mise-en-scene.[5]

THEATRICALITY AND PERFORMATIVITY: THE MISE-EN-SCÈNE

The theatrical allusion is significant as it reflects what has become the predominant aesthetic and temporal reference for the presentation of historical dress within the museum. The fashion historian Marie Riegels Melchior has described the presentation and perception of fashion in museums in theatrical terms as having a "front-stage" and a "back-stage." The International Council of Museums' guidelines for the handling of dress inform the back-stage activities of conservation and cataloging, while front-stage there is "less focus on the actual piece of clothing, but on creating an atmosphere, feeling or experience" (Melchior 2011).

The historical association between the fashion exhibition and theatricality has been well documented. Particularly notable were the numerous special exhibitions created by Diana Vreeland, the former editor in chief of American *Vogue* (1963–1971), between 1972 and 1989 at the Costume Institute in New York. These controversial fashion exhibitions theatricalized a mixture of historical dress and contemporary assemblage. Steele recognizes the influence of Vreeland in challenging the association of historical dress with its outmoded roots in the Wax Works Museums. According to Steele, Vreeland's innovative concern with creating "fashionable spectacle" has "played a crucial role in conveying the experience of fashion" (2008: 12).

The design teams for fashion exhibitions today can include creative directors, scenographers, theater designers, production designers, and filmmakers. Exhibitions of historical dress and fashion have become dramatic visual narratives. They project the "dramaturgy of style" (Cotter 2012: C23). It is an approach, however, that is not without its critics. There are many historians and theorists who regret what they see as the compromise of authenticity and historical accuracy in the quest for theater. In scholarly and creative debates around historical dress and the creative opportunities it offers, these restagings of historical moments through dress are seen as denying the complexity of the object itself. They also too frequently represent a very narrow interpretation of theatricality, that is, one concerned only with decor and scenic effects.

Contemporary curators of historical dress, however, are expanding their interpretation of the theatrical to create embodied experiences for the museum visitor. Amy de la Haye has observed that dress/costume is representative of "lives lived, performances performed" (quoted in Barbieri 2012), and it is the historian's task to find a way to re-animate those past actors. The immediacy of the "lived experience" has become the temporal objective, with the spectator and the dress/object in visual and physical dialogue across time and space.

Wilcox's Fashion in Motion series, which began in 1999, introduced the performative aspects of the live catwalk show into the museum's presentation and interpretation of dress. Wilcox has described her installations as performance, and the durational element is often explored in her curations. For Radical Fashion (2001) she commissioned *Changelings,* a film about the transience of time, beauty, and fashion. Two models, one about twenty, the other in her seventies, were wearing the same dress and morphed into each other continually, becoming old and then young again. The layering of time became embodied performatively. Another temporal device used by Wilcox in Radical Fashion was the tableau. This dramatic form of presentation emphasizes simultaneous presentation and creates a temporal and spatial narrative through juxtaposition. For the staging of eleven tableaux in Radical Fashion, soundtracks from Paul Schütze, Björk, and David Toop contributed to an immersive spectacle devised to draw the viewer into an active "lived" experience.

The emphasis is less on scenery and props and more on the spatial, temporal, and sensorial relationships between the physical object and the perceiving subject. As with theater, our imaginative engagement with objects is physical, cognitive, and emotional. "To see objects not as background scenery to the drama of human life but as actors within it, bridging the realms of the physical, the social and the mental, has been an important part of the recent turn towards the material" (Dudley 2010: 13). The social anthropologist Sandra Dudley in *Museum Materialities* cites Jules Prown's argument that historical artifacts as materialized events allow past events to "be re-experienced," but she questions that the artifact can be the "event" (12). Instead, Dudley proposes that it is the object-subject engagement that is the event, that

> what matters . . . is the way in which things instigate or trigger a particular set of perceptions and response in the human subject—a repeated set of events perpetually open to change, including once something has become a museum object. (12)

Clark in her essay "Kinetic Beauty: The Theatre of the 1920s" for the *Addressing the Century* exhibition catalog explored the relationship between fashion and theater and the evolution of the stage set from painted backdrop to three-dimensional environment. She described how in futurist dress, clothing was "to become not only an object but an event" (Clark 1998: 79). At the heart of the event is the relationship between the temporal and the material. Sanford Kwinter writes in *Architectures of Time,* his influential study of time and design, that to approach the problem of "the new," one must "redefine the traditional concept of the object and . . . reintroduce and radicalize the theory of time." For Kwinter the object is more than how "it appears." It is saturated and enveloped by physical and historical forces, "constellations of active agencies" (2001: 11). Through the scenographic treatment of the contemporary exhibition space—layering, juxtaposing, and spotlighting—attention is focused on the material object and its constellations of ideas. Along with these scenographic strategies, exhibition design has adopted the temporal leaps and collapsed time spans of theater. Sight lines replace time lines.

CONCLUSION

Working outside a chronological time line allows curators to reveal connections between objects, and also to imagine encounters between the designers of those objects.

For the 2012 exhibition Elsa Schiaparelli and Miuccia Prada's Impossible Conversations, in the Costume Institute of the Metropolitan Museum—organized by Andrew Bolton, curator, with the support of Harold Koda, curator in charge—the director Baz Luhrmann made eight short videos. In the films, an actress playing the part of Schiaparelli is shown seated with Miucca Prada at a dining table. Excerpts from Schiaparelli's autobiography, *Shocking Life,* are edited together with Prada's responses. In this scripted dialogue, the two designers speak to each other across the historical and temporal divide. In Schiaparelli and Prada's impossible and imagined dialogues, one can detect the complexity of dress, its layered ethical, artistic, cultural, and social meanings, in a way that a chronology based on classification of form and style could not contain.

We perceive historical dress within temporal and spatial frameworks that are constructed, and more often than not those frameworks are theatrical. Theater exists in the "now" but references the past. Narrative sequences and scenarios have a temporal elasticity and flexibility; time can be expanded, compressed, or suspended. Historical moments are not singular events that take place along a linear and progressive route. Time is spatial, theatrical, and scenographic.

By applying the performative strategies to the exhibition of historical dress, curators and exhibition makers are broadening further the complex relationship between dress and culture. These performative strategies imply questioning and transgressing, and often setting new norms of practice. Richard Martel, an artist and performance theorist, writes:

> A performance is the updating in front of a potential audience of a variable expressive content; it is at once an attitude to liberalise habits, norms, conditioning, and at the same time a destabilising experience aimed at rewriting the codes of representation, knowledge and conscience. A performance is the staging of materials in a certain context, a destitution of conventional relations and a transformation of stylistic categories. ... The performance usually relates to the context in which it is staged. In some performances the body is totally present, in others the collection of objects tends to be the essential part of the action; at other times, the investigation implies theoretical questioning, while on certain occasions performer and audience interact. (2003: 83, quoted in Mangion 2009: 14)

In the desire to redefine dress and its complex meanings within a framework that encompasses performativity, temporality, spatiality, and materiality, fashion curators find themselves redefined as makers of cultural, artistic, and performative interventions, which nonetheless are rooted in deeply considered curatorial practice. The possibilities that exist in the relationship between history and dress, and its perception and experience in an exhibition context, demonstrate the way in which historical dress sits at the intersection between practices and can only be considered from a multiplicity of perspectives.

NOTES

1. Claire Wilcox, interview with Donatella Barbieri at the Victoria and Albert Museum, January 3, 2012. All quotations from Wilcox are from this source.
2. Ibid.
3. Judith Clark, interview with Donatella Barbieri and Greer Crawley at Judith Clark Studio, November 16, 2011.
4. Quoted from the web page for the exhibition Spectres: When Fashion Turns Back, which ran from February 24 to May 8, 2005, at the Victoria and Albert Museum. http://www.vam.ac.uk/content/articles/s/spectres/ (accessed June 10, 2012).
5. Valerie Steele, interview with Donatella Barbieri at the Fashion Institute of Technology, New York, December 2, 2011.

BIBLIOGRAPHY

Austin, John L. 1962. *How to Do Things with Words.* Oxford: Oxford University Press.

Barbieri, Donatella. 2012. "Encounters in the Archive: Reflections on Costume." *V&A Online Journal,* no. 4 (Summer). http://www.vam.ac.uk/content/journals/research-journal/issue-no.-4-summer-2012/encounters-in-the-archive-reflections-on-costume/ (accessed October 10, 2012).

Bourdon, David. 1969. "Andy's Dish." In *Raid the Icebox 1 with Andy Warhol,* 17–25. Providence: Museum of Art, Rhode Island School of Design.

Breward, Christopher. 1999. "Exhibition Review: *Satellites of Fashion: Hats, Bags, Shoes.* The Craft Council Gallery, London." *Fashion Theory: The Journal of Dress, Body and Culture* 3 (2): 269–72.

Clark, Judith. 1998. "Kinetic Beauty: The Theatre of the 1920s." In Peter Wollen, *Addressing the Century: 100 Years of Art and Fashion,* 78–87. London: Hayward Gallery.

Clark, Judith. 2002. "Statement 1." In Kaat Debo (ed.), *The Fashion Museum Backstage,* 146–51. Ghent, Belgium: Ludion. http://www.judithclarkcostume.com/publications/essays_05.php (accessed September 25, 2012).

Clark, Judith. 2005. *Spectres: When Fashion Turns Back.* London: V&A Publishing.

Clark, Judith. 2006. "Fashion-ology." In *Anna Piaggi: Fashion-ology,* n.p. London: V&A Publishing. http://www.judithclarkcostume.com/exhibitions/victoria_albert_02.php (accessed September 25, 2012).

Clark, Judith. 2009. "Installing Allusions." In Jan Brand and José Teunissen (eds.), *The Art of Fashion: Installing Allusions,* 158–69. Rotterdam: Museum Boijmans Van Beuningen.

Clark, Judith, and Amy de la Haye. 2008. "One Object: Multiple Interpretations." *Fashion Theory: The Journal of Dress, Body and Culture* 12 (2): 137–69.

Cotter, Holland. 2012. "Speaking of Fashion." *New York Times,* May 11.

de la Haye, Amy. 2010. "Introduction: Dress and Fashion in the Context of the Museum." In Joanne B. Eicher (ed.), *Berg Encyclopedia of World Dress and Fashion,* vol. 10, *Global Perspectives,* 285–87. Oxford: Berg.

Dorsett, Chris. 2009. "Making Meaning beyond Display." In Sandra Dudley (ed.), *Museum Materialities: Objects, Engagements, Interpretations,* 241–59. London: Routledge.

Dudley, Sandra. 2010. "Museum Materialities: Objects, Sense and Feeling." In Sandra Dudley (ed.), *Museum Materialities: Objects, Engagements, Interpretations,* 1–17. London: Routledge.

Evans, Caroline. 2003. *Fashion at the Edge: Spectacle, Modernity, and Deathliness.* New Haven, CT: Yale University Press.
Foster, Hal. 2003. *Design and Crime: And Other Diatribes.* London: Verso.
Gumbrecht, Hans U. 2004. *Production of Presence.* Stanford, CA: Stanford University Press.
Hadid, Zaha. 2000. "Internal Terrains." In Alan Read (ed.), *Architecturally Speaking,* 211–32. London: Routledge.
Hoffmann, Jens. 2012. "Overture." *The Exhibitionist* 6: 3–4.
Hoffmann, Jens, and Joan Jonas. 2005. *Perform (Art Works).* London: Thames and Hudson.
Kwinter, Sanford. 2001. *Architectures of Time: Towards a Theory of Event in Modernist Culture.* Cambridge, MA: MIT Press.
Laver, James. 1949. *Style in Costume.* Oxford: Oxford University Press.
Mackie, Erin. 1994. "Fashion in the Museum: An Eighteenth-Century Project." In Deborah Fausch and Paulette Singley (eds.), *Architecture: In Fashion,* 314–42. New York: Princeton Architectural Press.
Mangion, Eric. 2009. "The Fetish-Making Finishing of Performance Art: Interview with Raphaëlle Giangreco." In Eric Mangion and Marie de Brugerolle (eds.), *Not to Play with Dead Things,* 11–30. Zurich: JRP Ringier.
Melchior, Marie Riegels. 2011. "Fashion Museology: Identifying and Contesting Fashion in Museums." Fashion: Exploring Critical Issues, *3rd Global Conference,* Inter-disciplinary.net, Mansfield College, September. http://www.inter-disciplinary.net/wp-content/uploads/2011/08/Oxford_fashion_exploring_critical_issues_PAPER_MarieRiegelsMelchior.pdf (accessed June 18, 2012).
Morphy, Howard. 2010. "Afterword: Museum Materialities: Objects, Engagements, Interpretations." In Sandra Dudley (ed.), *Museum Materialities: Objects, Engagements, Interpretations,* 275–85. London: Routledge.
Nagel, Alexander. 2004. "Fashion and the Now-Time of Renaissance Art." *RES: Anthropology & Aesthetics* 46 (Autumn): 33–52.
Ostrow, Stephen E. 1969. "Catalogue." In *Raid the Icebox 1 with Andy Warhol,* 26–102. Providence: Museum of Art, Rhode Island School of Design.
Ricoeur, Paul. 1984. *Time and Narrative.* Chicago: University of Chicago Press.
Robbins, Daniel. 1969. "Confessions of a Museum Director." In *Raid the Icebox 1 with Andy Warhol,* 8–15. Providence: Museum of Art, Rhode Island School of Design.
Steele, Valerie. 2008. "Museum Quality: The Rise of the Fashion Exhibition." *Fashion Theory: The Journal of Dress, Body and Culture* 12 (1): 7–30.
Stewart, Susan. 1993. *On Longing.* Durham, NC: Duke University Press.
Wilcox, Claire. 2004. *Vivienne Westwood.* London: V&A Publications.
Wilson, Elizabeth. 2007. *Adorned in Dreams: Fashion and Modernity.* London: I. B. Tauris.
Wollen, Peter. 1993. *Raiding the Icebox: Reflections on Twentieth-Century Culture.* London: Verso.

3

New Fashion Times: Fashion and Digital Media[1]

AGNÈS ROCAMORA

INTRODUCTION

On August 21, 2011, popular fashion blogger Sasha Wilkins (LibertyLondonGirl.com) posted a message apologizing for "the unexpected hiatus in posting." I scrolled down the page to see when she had last updated her site, expecting to see a gap of weeks or maybe even months; it turned out she had not posted for three days. Three days only. That she felt obliged to apologize struck me as an illustration of the redefinition of time the field of fashion is currently experiencing; a new time defined by the speeding up of the circulation of material and symbolic goods. It is this process of acceleration, more specifically as articulated on the Internet, that is the object of the present chapter.

In the first section, looking at the work of a range of theorists, I discuss the idea that with the creation in the second half of the twentieth century of new technologies and the proliferation of digital platforms such as the Internet, modernity has entered a new phase, characterized by the intensification of speed and the valuing of immediacy and real time. In the second section I further interrogate the idea of acceleration in light of the field of fashion. Focusing on the fast fashion phenomenon I discuss how it evidences some of the ideas discussed in the first section. In the third and final section I look at the ways new digital media have supported the speeding up of fashion. Throughout, time is understood as a social construct. As Emile Durkheim notes, "That which the category of time expresses is a time common to the group, it is social time. . . . This category is itself a real social institution" ([1912] 2007: 49n6; but see also Elias [1984] 2007). The chapter then discusses some of the ways time has been constructed, appropriated, and represented in the field of fashion to argue that with the rise of new technologies fashion time has speeded up; a new fashion time has emerged defined by acceleration and immediacy.

NEW TIMES: ACCELERATION, IMMEDIACY, PERMANENT PRESENT

Although modernity came into being in the sixteenth century, a central moment in its unfolding is the eighteenth century (Berman 1983; Habermas 1987; Harvey 1990). At the time, and in the context of a nascent industrialism, progress, rationality, and rapid change rose as central values for the development and organization of society (Habermas 1997; Harvey 1990). Time became experienced "as a scarce resource" for the solving of problems (Habermas 1997: 6). Acceleration emerged as a key marker of modernity (Bauman 2000a; Conrad 1998; Rosa 2010; Tomlinson 2007). Thus, Reinhart Koselleck ([1970] 2004: 41), for instance, notes that it is a category clearly in evidence since the 1789 French Revolution. The French upheaval transformed expectations and experiences by heralding the possibility of a future whose coming could be triggered and quickened (41, 59). A new age seemed to have opened up whereby the tempo of events could be accelerated, with change and renewal becoming a tangible reality (41, 59). Thus, "from the eighteenth century on," Koselleck argues, "it was possible to formulate the postulate of acceleration" (238).

For Hartmut Rosa (2010: 28), although accounts of acceleration can be found before the French Revolution—they emerged around 1750, he argues, conveying concerns with an accelerated speed of history—it was with the Industrial Revolution and the introduction of railways that "acceleration" took on a more resonant and visible manifestation (see also Hassan 2003: 228). Time became a central dimension of capitalism, which cemented its value as a commodity and a disciplining tool (Marx [1857/1858] 1971; Thompson 1967), with speed as one of its defining features (Adam 2004: 119). A sense of ephemerality, transience, increasingly pervaded everyday life, making modern existence one marked by constant change. As Karl Marx and Friedrich Engels wrote:

> The bourgeoisie cannot exist without constantly revolutionising the instruments of production, and thereby the relations of production, and with them the whole relations of society. . . . Constant revolutionising of production, uninterrupted disturbance of all social conditions, everlasting uncertainty and agitation distinguish the bourgeois epoch from all earlier ones. All fixed, fast-frozen relations, with their train of ancient and venerable prejudices and opinions, are swept away, all new-formed ones become antiquated before they can ossify. All that is solid melts into air, all that is holy is profaned. ([1848/1888] 2004: 16)

Most apt at capturing and sustaining the central role of time and speed in eighteenth- and nineteenth-century society is the clock, whose diffusion, along with that of watches, became more generalized with the Industrial Revolution's requirement for more synchronized labor (Thompson 1967: 69). Thus Lewis Mumford contends that "the clock, not the steam-engine, is the key-machine of the modern industrial age" (quoted in Lee and Liebenau 2000: 47; see also Thompson 1967). Clocks allowed for the promotion of efficiency and the pursuit of time saving (Eriksen 2001: 53), all in the name of profit. Time and money became "tightly coupled" (53), an idea that Benjamin Franklin's well-known "time is money" conveyed (see Weber [1904–1905] 2001: 14). The clock, as Barbara Adam notes, "changed the meaning of time," which, abstracted from space and rendered seemingly neutral, indeed abstract, became subject to appropriation and calculation (2004: 113, 114). Time could be made an economic asset, speed a factor of profit—an instrument of conquest and power (114, 123–24; see also Virilio 2006).

The Industrial Revolution was also when a "communications revolution" took place with the invention, in 1837, of the electric telegraph, followed by wireless telegraphy at the beginning of the twentieth century (Adam 2004: 120). Speed was its "defining temporal feature," allowing for "instantaneity and simultaneity" to replace "sequence and duration," and for time to be divorced from, and take over for, space: "the global present came into being" (119, 120). Thus, at the end of the nineteenth century, correlative to the changing meaning of time and the acceleration brought about by the French Revolution and the Industrial Revolution was a changing sense of the present. Past and future collapsed into a "thickened" present with simultaneity as its core experiential mode (Kern 2003: 314). At the beginning of the twentieth century the cubists were to vibrantly capture and promote this new sense of time (Kern 2003).

The second half of the twentieth century ushered in a new phase in the history of acceleration. Although many authors agree that, in terms of acceleration, this historical time does not so much signal a rupture with modernity as a new stage in its unfolding, this is a stage so significant, it is argued, that it warrants particular attention. Moreover, although there is no agreement as to when exactly the shift really took place, with some authors arguing that it was in the 1970s, and others in the 1980s, or even later, all concur that the development of new information and communication technologies (ICTs), and in particular computers and the Internet, is a key element in this new stage and in the history of acceleration. This is not to say that one should fall into the trap of technological determinism in the manner of Marshall McLuhan ([1964] 1967) but to acknowledge that while technologies are the product of a particular culture, they also impact on it (Eriksen 2001: 25; Rosa 2010; Tomlinson 2007; Williams [1975] 1990).

Thus, Daniel Bell, for instance, who notes "the quickening change of pace that drives all our lives," identifies computers as core to "the accelerating revolution of our time" ([1973] 1999: 169, 192; see also Kumar 2005: chap. 3). Derrick de Kerckhove also argues that in the 1980s—the decade when personal computers became mass produced (Forrester 1985)—"computers brought in the 'speed culture'" (de Kerckhove 1997: 133). For Jay David Bolter the computer is "the contemporary analog of clocks" in past centuries (quoted in Lee and Liebenau 2000: 48) and, for Yoneji Masuda, writing in the early 1980s about the new emerging "information society," that of the steam engine (1985: 621).

A term often debated, *information society* generally refers to the idea that contemporary society no longer is primarily focused on the production of material goods but instead on the creation and circulation of information, which has drastically increased with the proliferation of new information technologies (Eriksen 2001; Forrester 1985; Webster 2006: 2). Society, it is argued, has moved "from things to signs" (Eriksen 2001: 29), from hardware to software, leading Zygmunt Bauman (2000a, 2000b, 2011) to name the contemporary era a "light," "liquid" modernity made of flows and constant change in contrast to "the era of *hardware,* or *heavy* modernity: the bulk-obsessed modernity" (2000b: 174).

Manuel Castells—who to the notion of "information society" prefers that of "informational society," for, he argues, information has always been central to the functioning of society (2000: 21n31)—agrees that ICTs have reshaped, "at accelerated pace, the material basis of society" (1). Having emerged in the 1970s, a new social structure brought about by the development of new ICTs came to fruition in the late 1990s defined by a "new 'time regime'" (459, drawing on Harold Higgins). Where in modernity time was "linear, irreversible, measurable, predictable" (463), in informational society, time sequences have disappeared. As Bauman also puts it, time

> is no longer cyclical... but not linear either because events and actions succeed each other randomly rather than in a straight line. ...Nowadays we are held together by short-term projects. ...What model of time can be derived from such experience? I suggest a "pointillist" time. Much like canvasses of Sisley, Seurat or Signac, which consist of points only, no broad brushstrokes and no continuities. That is, though, as far as the analogy goes, because in pointillist paintings you have pre-designed and inbuilt meaningful configurations. However, in liquid modern life configurations are not given beforehand. ...Living through the moment, one point in time, you cannot be sure to what configuration you will eventually belong when scrutinized retrospectively. (Bauman, quoted in Deuze 2007: 673)

The regular, repetitive "clock time" of modernity has been taken over by a "timeless time," a time that, born out of new information technologies, cancels out duration (Castells 2000). For, in the informational society, following Castells, capital negates time by relentlessly compressing and breaking it down into units that can be manipulated to promote "at the same time the eternal and... the ephemeral" (2000: 492). Thus, "split-second transactions, flex-time enterprises, variable life working time, the blurring of the life-cycle, the search for eternity through the denial of death, instant wars, and the culture of virtual time, all are fundamental phenomena, characteristic of the network society, which systematically mix tenses in their occurrence" (494). For the informational society is also a "network society" as "it is played out in a global network of interaction between business networks" (77). This "networking logic" has been supported by new information technologies, and in particular the Internet, which Castells singles out as "perhaps the most revolutionary technological medium of the Information Age" (21, 45).

The Internet is the brainchild of the U.S. Department of Defense, which was looking for a way of avoiding the neutralization of American systems of communication in the case of a nuclear attack (Rosa 2010: 250). The aim was to control and slow down the war, not to accelerate it (250). This is at odds, as Rosa points out, with its contemporary use, for the Internet is at the heart of a "new wave" (190) of acceleration that sees, with the speeding up, in the late twentieth century, of information and communication flows, a "radicalisation" (33) of the principles of modernity.

Thus Rosa notes that we are witnessing a new bout of spatiotemporal compression (2010: 190), a concept made famous by David Harvey, for whom the term *compression* captures the idea that "the history of capitalism has been characterized by speed-up in the pace of life, while so overcoming spatial barriers that the world sometimes seems to collapse inwards upon us" (1990: 241). As Bauman also observes, "In the software universe, space may be traversed, literally, in 'no time'; the difference between 'far away' and 'down here' is cancelled. And so space counts little, or does not count at all" (2000b: 177).

Finally, in discussions of the contemporary "new wave" of acceleration, two related notions recur that clearly capture the idea of the intense speeding up of society: "immediacy" and "real time." We have become preoccupied, it is argued, with instantaneity (Agger 2004; Bauman 2000b: 177–78; Harvey 1990: 59) to the extent that real time—the "drive towards instantaneity within and between networks" (Hope 2006: 276)—has become, if not yet a fully accomplished reality, a dominant value society is striving for (Hassan 2003; Hope 2006: 276; Rosa 2010: 97). As Thomas Hylland Eriksen (2001) puts it, in contemporary society the "tyranny of the moment" reigns.

Thus John Tomlinson, for instance, who argues that we live in a "culture of speed," notes that although "mechanical speed" has not disappeared it is on the wane (2007: 89). The late twentieth-century "condition of immediacy" has displaced it (89). It is a condition whereby "the gap between here and there, now and later" is being closed (91). Thus, he notes, immediacy has become the "goal" of contemporary media, immediacy both in the sense that content should reach media users rapidly and in the sense that it should be delivered in a seemingly "live" manner, as if media users were really experiencing the event shown to them (99), as if they were really t/here and now. New technologies and digital networks have been integral to this drive toward "real time" (Hassan 2003: 231–33; Hope 2006; Rosa 2010: 97; Virilio 1991). It is, for instance, a recurring trope of digital fashion platforms, an idea I return to later.

Thus, the principle of "nowness"—tellingly, the name of a fashion website—drives contemporary experiences (Hope 2006: 284). As Adam puts it, "No-where and now-here have become interchangeable" (2004: 146), past and future have collapsed into the present, at once permanent and made of a rapid succession of instants. Time has been detemporalized, turned into a kind of timeless time, as we saw with Castells, an idea

Eriksen also takes up when he writes, "When time is partitioned into sufficiently small pieces, it eventually ceases to exist as duration. All that is ultimately left, is a screaming, packed moment which stands still at a frightful speed" (2001: 150).

FAST FASHION

Charles Baudelaire defined modernity as "the transitory, the fugitive, the contingent" ([1863] 1999: 518). For the French poet, fashion, being inherently ephemeral, is the visual expression and material manifestation of modernity. That fashion is a paradigm of modernity is also captured in the shared etymology—the Latin *modus*—of the French terms *mode* (fashion) and *modernité* and the German *Mode* and *Moderne* (Habermas 1987: 9; Lehmann 2000: xv; Vinken 2005: 43; see also Evans 2007: 8–10).

A key trait of modernity, as discussed earlier, is acceleration, which intensified in the second half of the twentieth century with the coming of new technologies. Such an intensification also took place in the field of fashion with computerized technologies also playing a central role in that process. In that respect too fashion can be seen as paradigmatic of modernity and its changing temporality. The fast fashion phenomenon is exemplary of this.

"Fast fashion," that is, "the retail strategy of adapting merchandise assortments to current and emerging trends as quickly and effectively as possible" (Sull and Turconi 2008: 5), became common parlance at the beginning of the twenty-first century (Hines 2007: 40). However, the ideas behind the concept emerged in 1970s America with the development in the textile and apparel industry of new quick-response (QR) techniques to compete with the rise of low-cost Far Eastern supply countries (40). Fashion companies relying on QR have become known as fast fashion companies. The aim is for manufacturers to be able to quickly replenish the stock of retailers (39). However, once a line has been sold, it is no longer produced (44), making fast fashion goods also ephemeral. The fact that they are built not to last (44) also contributes to this ephemerality.

QR is about optimizing "the flow of information and merchandise between channel members to maximize customer service" (Hines 2007: 39). Central to this are computers (41), as shown by the following description of the designer studio at Zara, a company often singled out as the epitome of fast fashion: "On the immense modern white floor where clothes are sketched, young designers . . . are sitting at large desks next to the sales team. The latter face a computer screen that indicates the instantaneous state of sales in all the shops. The interaction between the designer and the sales personnel is immediate" (Soula 2011: 62).

Also crucial to fast fashion companies is the Internet, which allows them to achieve the goal of "time compression" by developing products faster through the rapid sourcing of suppliers and products without the help of intermediaries (Hines 2007: 40). Thus, while Zara designers work on three collections at the same time—that of the current season, that of the next season, and that of the coming year—the company produces

"30.000 different designs a year," while the cycle of production from the design of goods to their presence in stores takes three weeks only (Soula 2011: 62).

Thus, with high-fashion shows no longer the preserve of an elite but made immediately available on the Internet, an idea I return to later, the styles featured can be easily copied by fast fashion companies to find their way into high-street shops before they reach designer boutiques. The hegemony of high fashion is being confronted by the challenging of its timeliness, with new asynchronic temporalities becoming more predominant. Fashion time does not unfold in a smooth, linear way but is made of various moments that point to its disjointing and acceleration. Witness also the increasingly earlier sales seasons: in London, for instance, the summer 2011 sales started in mid-June, at a time when the summer had barely started. They had been preceded by pre-summer sales, further splitting fashion time from that of actual seasons, as if the turnover and obsolescence of fashion commodities had accelerated so much that the seasons could not catch up with them.

Zara is an archetypal fast fashion company, a post-Fordist one (but see also Kumar 2005 on Benetton). Indeed, fast fashion is a correlate of what many authors have identified as the rise of a new industrial paradigm with the move in the mid-1970s away from Fordism to post-Fordism (see, for instance, Amin 1994; Kumar 2005). Although analyses of this shift encompass a broad range of approaches, key themes recur (Amin 1994; Kumar 2005: chap. 4). Indeed, *Fordism,* coined after Henry Ford, who in the 1920s and 1930s championed new production and management rules in his car factories in the United States, is generally defined as premised on the principles of mass production, which involves long, inflexible production runs, standardized goods, and economies of scale (Amin 1994: 9–10). In contrast, post-Fordism promotes flexibility, small batches, and a rapid response to consumer wants (Agger 2004: 8–9; Amin 1994).

Where Fordism was a regime of "intensive accumulation" (Amin 1994: 9), post-Fordism is a regime of "flexible accumulation" (Harvey 1990). Drawing attention to the idea of acceleration by underscoring the importance of the increasing rate of innovation that typifies post-Fordist companies, Harvey defines "flexible accumulation," his coinage, as

> marked by a direct confrontation with the rigidities of Fordism. It rests on flexibility with respect to labour processes, labour markets, products, and patterns of consumption. It is characterized by the emergence of entirely new sections of production, new ways of providing financial services, new markets, and, above all, greatly intensified rates of commercial, technological, and organizational innovation. (147)

Flexible accumulation has led to a reduction of the turnover time in both production and consumption, to "a much greater attention to quick-changing fashions" (156). As Harvey also puts it, "The relatively stable aesthetic of Fordist modernism has given way to all the ferment, instability, and fleeting qualities of a postmodernist aesthetic that celebrates difference, ephemerality, spectacle, fashion, and the commodification of cultural forms" (156). The use of computers and, more recently, the Internet has supported the putting into practice of post-Fordism and the speeding up of "an already quick capitalism" (Agger 2004: 23).

Fast fashion, then, is a post-Fordist fashion, a fashion of rapid commodity circulation, of quick response to consumer wants, of fast production and fast consumption. However, fashion is made not only of material but also of symbolic goods. In that respect, fast fashion is also fast symbolic fashion, the rapid circulation of fashion images and words, all visual and written information that has supported fashion's participation in the development of the information society. Thus in the late twentieth and early twenty-first centuries, with the proliferation of digital technologies such as the Internet, it can be argued that fashion has entered a new stage, one defined by the proliferation and acceleration of fashion discourse, the speeding up of the signs and symbols of fashion. The rapid flow of commodities has been paralleled by an increasingly rapid flow of immaterial fashion, as I now discuss.

NEW FASHION MEDIA AND THE ACCELERATION OF FASHION TIME

Fashion websites have become key platforms for the circulation of fashion discourse. The following section focuses on these and, more particularly, on fashion blogs. It briefly charts the rise of digital fashion platforms and discusses the ways time is embedded in them. Temporality and the idea of speed, it is shown, are part of the makeup of digital fashion both in terms of the internal organization of digital fashion pages and in terms of their structural linking, that is, the hypertextual and rhizomatic nature of digital texts. In this section, then, I approach time both as a key signifier of fashion discourse as well as an organizing, structural factor.

The first fashion websites appeared in the mid-1990s. In the United Kingdom, for instance, 1995 saw the birth of Vogue.com, with the subsequent years witnessing the launch and proliferation of more websites, including apc.fr (1996), WGSN (1998), Net-a-porter.com (June 2000), SHOWstudio (November 2000), Dazeddigital (November 2006), and Nowness (February 2010) (see also Borelli 2002).

However, a key moment in the history of digital fashion came with the creation in the early twenty-first century of fashion blogs. Among the first was *nogoodforme,* launched in 2003 (see Rocamora 2011). At first the products of nonprofessional and independent individuals, they quickly became appropriated by various fashion institutions as a way of further disseminating their visions and values. They are now central to the field of fashion and have contributed to the speeding up of its discourse, as I argue in the remainder of this section.

Blog posts appear anti-chronologically, with the most recent posts the first to appear on the screen. Their newness is signaled through the display of the date of posting but also, often, through the indication of the time at which a new entry was posted. Indeed, some bloggers update their sites many times a day. On *bryanboy.com,* for instance, the time of posting is clearly indicated above the title of the new post. The digits thereby displayed are evocative of digital clocks.

In his essay on time Norbert Elias reminds us of the symbolic and social dimension of time as captured and constructed in clocks. He asks, "What do clocks really show when we say that they show the time?" ([1984] 2007: 11). Clocks, he argues, communicate meaning. Similarly, the "numerical symbols" (13) shown on blogs and other digital fashion platforms to represent a specific time do not simply indicate hours and seconds. Rather they function as signs: signs of rapidity, of immediacy, of the timeliness and fast pace of fashion blogs, characteristics that are also favored by most other blogs. Indeed, thanks to a web-based technology that allows for the instantaneous editing and updating of blogs (Papacharissi 2007: 24), one of their defining traits resides in their ability to be in the present, to facilitate the rapid, constant communication of information. This is particularly true of the microblogging site Twitter, which is premised on the idea of short, fast, constant news, as indicated in the reference to the time elapsed since a tweet was last sent: "2 minutes ago," "19 minutes ago," and "2 hours ago," for instance.

In 2009 fashion players increasingly started to embrace the Twittersphere with the *Business of Fashion* (hereafter *BOF*) reporting on March 16, 2009, that tweets during the New York Fashion Week were so numerous that "New York Fashion Week actually became the 4th biggest trend in Twitter."[2] For the September 2009 collections they report on a new website, FashionTweek, that aggregated tweets on the New York collections, citing the platform's intention to promote "realtime reaction to the shows, parties and people of Fashion Week NYC."[3] This enthusiasm for the fashion "twitterverse" (*BOF,* September 10, 2009) has gone unabated, with the 2011 collections being punctuated by the constant flow of tweets bloggers and journalists alike posted to publicize their latest encounters, mood, or impressions.

The rapid turnover of information has become a trait, more generally, of online fashion media. Not only have they responded to the popularity of the blogosphere through the launch of their own blogs, but they have also embraced speed and immediacy through the creation of sections that clearly feed into the trend for fast news (see Phillips 2010 on the emphasis on speed in news journalism). Style.com's "the latest" ("The fashion feed: breaking news from across the web"), interviewmagazine.com's "most recent," and Vogue.com's "latest trends" and "breaking news" are but a few examples of fashion media's promotion of fast fashion news. Thus, for instance, in a June 5, 2008, interview with *BOF,* Dolly Jones, editor of the UK site Vogue.com, notes the revamping of the site, launched in 1995:

> We have expanded the news to at least 12 stories per day, along with our daily Vogue.com Loves slot, we've increased the daily beauty updates. ... The entire site has a daily feel,

> with pods around the site updating all the time to show off the latest content—and of course we have the world's first downloadable calendar—that syncs with your own Outlook calendar.[4]

When Bonnier Magazines launched their first digital magazine, *C Mode,* by way of an iPad application in August 2011, rapidity and immediacy were also brought to the fore. The iTunes page states that readers will be able to find out "what is new and what is hot in fashion right now," adding that the magazine, edited by popular fashion blogger Caroline Blomst, "is a fast, fun and up-to-date review of the fashion world" and highlighting "frequency" and "tempo" as core values.[5]

Fashion media's embrace of the rapid passing of time is not new. The ephemeral being at the very core of fashion, the fashion media have always had to reflect, as well as support, this evanescence through the constant updating of their pages, fashion magazines being themselves fashion commodities. In the twentieth century, for instance, and still to this day perhaps, one of the most influential fashion media has been a daily newspaper, *Women's Wear Daily,* founded in 1910 and now also available online. As Rosa (2010: 149) notes, a visible sign of social acceleration in the eighteenth century was the creation of daily newspapers. However, the Internet has instilled a new pace in the media's circulation of news (149). Blogs have disrupted "the temporality of traditional news cycles" through their "real-time virtual feedback loop" (Jason Gallo, quoted in Bruns 2005: 217), which suggests that a daily read is no longer enough (Rosa 2010: 149). Instead, hopping on and off digital sites has become the norm. As Eriksen notes of Internet newspapers and their frequent updates, "This kind of media instils a new rhythm and a new restlessness, and—importantly—new routines in the consumption of news" (2001: 67).

Indeed, studies show that online readers allocate short fragments of time to each text they engage with, favoring a swift movement through web pages. Thus, Jakob Nielson (2011) notes that "the average page visit lasts a little less than a minute. As users rush through Web pages, they have time to read only a quarter of the text on the pages they actually visit." This rapid type of online *passage* has been supported by the introduction of faster, larger broadband networks, which, allowing customers to always be connected, have resulted in frequent short visits to sites and e-mail inboxes (Pavlik 2008: 12). By often being very short, blog posts allow for such swift movements on- and offline and for the rapid flicking through of information.

The writing style of fashion blogs conveys this idea of a quick-paced movement through the blogosphere, that of the bloggers. Indeed, typos, abbreviations, and an informal tone are recurring features of fashion posts (Rocamora 2011). They lend the blogs an air of immediacy, of the now that has become a key professional value (Tomlinson 2007). When asked for some advice on creating a blog, Susie Lau, for instance, of the popular *Stylebubble,* says, "Type at 80 wpm!" and highlights "the beauty of the blogging medium" as "its ability to connect with readers quite quickly. So if writing well researched posts are taking up too much time then perhaps you can pare it back a bit to make it a bit more relaxed."[6] As Tomlinson notes, contemporary media presentation "favours informality, direct conversational modes of address, and a certain assumption of intimacy (sometimes even of ironic complicity) with the audience" (2007: 100). "Pace" is privileged. This results in "the removal of symbolic barriers and conventions (the newsreader's desk) which signal the media as *mediators,* rather than as, say, everyday acquaintances and interlocutors" (100). By favoring a casual, intimate, conversational tone of writing (see Rocamora 2011), bloggers have capitalized on this valuing of immediacy, at the same time as they have reproduced it.

John V. Pavlik observes that "new technologies can transform the nature of storytelling and media content in general" (2008: 4; see also Kern 2003: 115). In the fashion blogosphere, they have paved the way for the frequent production of informal texts whose syntax captures and strengthens fashion and contemporary society's embrace of the ephemeral and of the rapid passing of time.

Transience is also an intrinsic part of blogs' makeup by way of their textuality: a hypertextuality. Indeed, the World Wide Web and fashion websites in particular are hypertexts. These are texts whose limits exceed their immediate content, whose borders are fluid and ever-changing (Landow 1997). They are made of units that, linked to each other, are constantly on the move, shifting and brought together in endless new reconfigurations. Hypertexts are networked texts. Links, also called hyperlinks, are the arborescence through which such networks are formed (Landow 1997). They allow for a rapid movement across an infinite space of words, sounds, and images, a fluidity and rapidity that the idea of surfing through the net aptly captures.

Hypertextuality brings to mind the Deleuzian notion of rhizome, a concept also helpful for reflecting on the structure of the Web, and on the role of fashion blogs in the acceleration of fashion time. A rhizome, following Gilles Deleuze and Félix Guattari, is an a-centered system that is always changing and is made up of units—so-called plateaus—that are linked together in a nonlinear way, in a network formation (1980: 32). "Plateaus can be read in any order and linked to any other plateaus," to which they are joined by "lines" (33). In the blogosphere they are the links that allow Internet users the constant movement from one page to the next, from one site to the next. Indeed, the blogosphere, like the rhizomes Deleuze and Guattari discuss, is a space in a permanent state of becoming, never fixed. Its plateaus are the many pages blogs and the blogosphere are made up of, which, in a perpetual movement of displacement and replacement, open onto a limitless number of sites and signs that allow the reader to be always on the move within a continuously changing textual space.

A rhizome, by virtue of being never fixed, is "a short memory, or an anti-memory" (Deleuze and Guattari 1980: 32), a state that aptly defines fashion with its constant quest for, and production of, the new. In that respect the rhizomatic structure of the blogosphere aptly lends itself to fashion. The latter's logic of renewal of clothes and styles is mirrored in the rapid renewal of posts and the endless replacing of one site by another that links enable. This is a logic of replacement that, as Jay Bolter and Richard Grusin (2000: 43–44) observe, is also that of the Web: each new page takes over another ad infinitum. Thus they argue that "replacement is the essence of hypertext" and the Web "an exercise in replacement" (43), a comment also true of the very content of websites in online fashion. As Geert Lovink puts it, "Technology such as the Internet lives on the principle of permanent change. . . . The 'tyranny of the new' rules" (2008: xi), as it does in the field of digital fashion. Witness, for instance, the "what's new," "just in," and "new arrivals" sections of online fashion shops, in which collections are constantly updated, or the many flash-sale sites that allow buying on very limited timescales, themselves the online manifestation of the trend for ephemeral pop-up stores. Witness also the ubiquitous "now" of commercial digital fashion platforms, which tell readers "what to buy right now" and "view now," invite them to "sign up now" and, of course, to "shop now."[7]

In their constant updating of sites with new posts, fashion blogs feed into this tyranny of the new. The flow of posts replicates the flow of goods, with the posts and goods of today promised to be rapidly overtaken, out-fashioned by newer arrivals that freeze time, and fashion, online into a perpetual present. As Paul Virilio (1991: 14) notes, "Chronological and historical time, time that passes is replaced by a time that exposes itself instantaneously." "It is a pure computer time," which "helps construct a permanent present, an unbounded, timeless intensity" (15; see also Nowotny 1994).

Thus, the short memory of blogs draws attention to the idea of temporality and the role of time in the definition of the blogosphere, and the fashion blogosphere in particular. Contemporary time, Bauman (quoted in Deuze 2007: 673) argues, as mentioned earlier, can be defined as pointillist. Blogs clearly articulate and feed into this conception of time, a time made of fragments, of a succession of brief moments: the moments made of one's encounter with a succession of interlinked web pages and sites; of written texts, images, sounds, and videos; and of the snapshots of life bloggers narrate in their posts. Time as articulated in the blogosphere, a new time of interconnected *points,* time as "a fluid, networked entity" (Fuery 2009: 31), echoes and reproduces the new time of late modernity.

Deleuze and Guattari (1980) encapsulate the rhizome's state of short memory and constant change in the notion of nomadism, which translates into the digital wandering and *flânerie* often constitutive of one's virtual movement through the Web. Within the fashion blogosphere, this flânerie brings to mind another type of flânerie at the heart of fashion: shopping. Where in real life (or IRL, as offline life is also called) consumers move from one shop to the next, wander around, and *browse*—a term that aptly captures the link between shopping and digital deambulation—in the fashion blogosphere they move from one site to the next.

> Instead of Parisian streets, shopping windows, and the faces of the passersby, the virtual flâneur travels through virtual streets, highways, and planes of data; the eroticism of a split-second virtual affair with a passerby of the opposite sex is replaced with the

> excitement of locating and opening a particular file or zooming into the virtual object. Like Baudelaire's flâneur, the virtual flâneur is happiest on the move, clicking from one object to another, traversing room after room, level after level, data volume after data volume. (Manovich 2001: 274–75)

However, where real-life flânerie is leisurely and slow—as Walter Benjamin reminds us, "In 1839 it was considered elegant to take a tortoise out walking. This gives an idea of the tempo of flânerie in the arcades" (2003: 422)—the pace of online flâneurs, their movement from one digital page to the next, takes up the rapidity and instantaneity of flows pertaining to hyperlinks.

Moreover, while flicking through a magazine is akin to flânerie, too, the shopping remains imaginary, a distant project. With blogs it becomes real, thanks to the many links that take readers straight to a digital point of sale, triggering and responding to the desires of "the society of immediate satisfaction" (Laïdi 2000: 115). Zaki Laïdi notes "the logic of never-ending choices to be made on the spot" with which contemporary individuals are confronted. They are "submerged with possibilities. But these possibilities are in open access. They are here. They are no longer a horizon" (115). The Web has intensified this collapsing of the there/later into the here/now, which makes of fashion news in the fashion blogosphere information immediately conducive to the act of buying.

Thus, speed and rapidity of action and interaction are a regular trope of online fashion. Net-a-porter.com, for instance, invites their reader to "shop the entire issue [of the online magazine] with a click of a button!" while stylehive.com tells their readers they can "get updates from your favorite brand, style experts and stylish people from around the world... instantly!" Suddenlee.com, the eloquently named fashion website whose "live support staff... is excited to hear from you and even more excited to help you," states that customers can "enjoy shopping your favourite stores in a matter of minutes." It gives the assurance that "orders placed by 3PM ET Mon–Fri will be delivered tomorrow!"

The recent trend for the live streaming of catwalk shows also illustrates fashion's embrace of speed and immediacy, with fashion websites repeatedly promoting the values of "real-time" "live" fashion. Fashion156.com, for instance, states that they offer "a fresh perspective on fashion in real time with a daily blog" and a "constant stream of information," Ykone.com presents itself as "live fashion," while Paris *Vogue*'s website displays a Twitter section called "Vogue Paris Live."[8] During the September 2011 London shows, London Fashion Week's website announced, "We are live—streaming from the BFC Show Space."[9]

However, not only have live online fashion shows become a staple of digital fashion, but companies such as Burberry have started selling clothes as soon as they hit the catwalk during shows simultaneously streamed online. In September 2011 they led a "Runway to Reality" event in forty-eight stores across the world, during which invitees followed the show live and could preorder certain items with the help of in-store iPads, with the items to be delivered eight weeks later. On Monday, September 19, 2011, they also live-tweeted pictures of their 2012 collection from backstage. Twitter users could see the clothes before they appeared in front of the audience of buyers, journalists, celebrities, and other fashion insiders, putting one more nail in the coffin of the shows' elitism.

CONCLUSION

Acceleration has become a defining trait of contemporary society, with the related notions of immediacy and real-time as two values institutions are striving for, among them fashion companies and the fashion media. With their speeding up of the circulation of both material and symbolic fashion, digital media have supported this process. Fashion discourse as articulated on web pages is more than ever subject to fashion's core principle: evanescence. This speeding up of the words and images of fashion suggests that it might now be as relevant to talk about instant fashion as about fast fashion.

Behind words and images are individuals: those writers, photographers, stylists, and other fashion intermediaries whose role is to feed fashion's symbolic dimension. This chapter has focused on the former by way of a discussion of various digital platforms. However, to fully grasp the acceleration of fashion time, research should also be conducted into actual practices of fashion, and this includes the practices of producing words and images. Light would be shed on the impact of new time constraints on the field of fashion, on the new working conditions related to such redefinitions of time.

Adam notes that "time is lived, experienced, known, theorized, created, regulated, sold and controlled. It is contextual and historical, embodied and objectified, abstracted and constructed, represented and commodified" (2004: 1). Here, then, can one find a programmatic statement for the study of time not as a universally shared given but as a context-dependent product, and this includes the study of time as constructed in the particular field of fashion.

However, not only is time a product, but it is also productive. Therefore, understanding time as articulated in the field of fashion means understanding the many ways through which it is both produced *by* fashion as well as productive *of* fashion, an underexplored approach. Indeed, in studies of fashion it is as if time has been taken for granted, with its workings and formation assumed more than investigated. But because time is so intrinsic to the field of fashion it needs to be interrogated if one is to fully understand fashion. This chapter is a step toward this, but it is also a call for scholars' attention to fashion's temporalities, which in a context of accrued acceleration seems more timely than ever. Only then will the complex relation between fashion and time be fully captured, the better to illuminate the former's temporalities and the latter's characteristic as productive/produced.

NOTES

1. Some passages in the third section of this chapter have appeared in Agnès Rocamora (2012), "Hypertextuality and Remediation in the Fashion Media," *Journalism Practice* 6 (1): 92–106.
2. Vikram Alexei Kansara, "Tweets and Tribes," *Business of Fashion,* March 16, 2009, http://www.businessoffashion.com/2009/03/fashion-20-tweets-and-tribes.html (accessed October 15, 2012).
3. Vikram Alexei Kansara, "Fashion 2.0 | New York Fashion Tweek," *Business of Fashion,* September 10, 2009, http://www.businessoffashion.com/2009/09/fashion-2-0-new-york-fashion-tweek.html (accessed October 15, 2012).
4. Imran Amed, "Q&A | Dolly Jones, Editor-in-Chief of Vogue.co.uk," *Business of Fashion,* June 5, 2008, http://www.businessoffashion.com/2008/06/qa-dolly-jones-editor-in-chief-of-voguecouk.html (accessed September 2, 2012).
5. iTunes Store, https://itunes.apple.com/us/app/c-mode/id448580920?mt=8 (accessed August 16, 2011).
6. Imran Amed, "Q&A: A Conversation with Susie from Style Bubble," *Business of Fashion,* November 12, 2007, http://www.businessoffashion.com/2007/11/qa-a-conversation-with-susie-from-style-bubble.html (accessed September 12, 2011).
7. For example, http://www.matchesfashion.com/ (accessed June 28, 2011), http://www.refinery29.com (accessed July 11, 2011), http://www.asos.com (accessed September 16, 2011), and http://www.theoutnet.com (accessed May 8, 2011).
8. "About Fashion156," Fashion156.com, http://www.fashion156.com (accessed October 10, 2011), http://www.ykone.com/ (accessed September 30, 2011), and http://www.vogue.fr (accessed September 23, 2011).
9. http://www.londonfashionweek.co.uk (accessed September 17, 2011).

BIBLIOGRAPHY

Adam, Barbara. 2004. *Time.* Cambridge, UK: Polity.

Agger, Ben. 2004. *Speeding Up Fast Capitalism.* London: Boulder.

Amin, Ash. 1994. "Post-Fordism: Models, Fantasies and Phantoms of Transition." In Ash Amin (ed.), *Post-Fordism: A Reader,* 1–39. Oxford: Blackwell.

Baudelaire, Charles. [1863] 1999. "Le Peintre de la Vie Moderne." In *Baudelaire: Ecrits sur L'Art,* 503–52. Paris: Poche.

Bauman, Zygmunt. 2000a. *Liquid Modernity.* Cambridge, UK: Polity.

Bauman, Zygmunt. 2000b. "Time and Space Reunited." *Time and Society* 9 (2–3): 171–85.

Bauman, Zygmunt. 2011. *Culture in a Liquid Modern World.* Cambridge, UK: Polity.

Bell, Daniel. [1973] 1999. *The Coming of Post-industrial Society.* New York: Basic Books.

Benjamin, Walter. 2003. *The Arcades Project.* London: Belknap Press of Harvard University Press.

Berman, Marshall. 1983. *All That Is Solid Melts into Air.* London: Verso.

Bolter, Jay David, and Richard Grusin. 2000. *Remediation.* Cambridge, MA: MIT Press.

Borelli, Laird. 2002. *Net Mode.* London: Thames and Hudson.

Bruns, Axel. 2005. *Gatewatching.* New York: Peter Lang.

Castells, Manuel. 2000. *The Rise of the Network Society.* Oxford: Blackwell.

Conrad, Peter. 1998. *Modern Times, Modern Places.* London: Thames and Hudson.

de Kerckhove, Derrick. 1997. *The Skin of Culture.* London: Kogan Page.

Deleuze, Gilles, and Félix Guattari. 1980. *Mille Plateaux.* Paris: Minuit.

Deuze, M. 2007. "Journalism in Liquid Modern Times: An Interview with Zygmunt Bauman." *Journalism Studies* 8 (4): 671–79.

Durkheim, Emile. [1912] 2007. *Les Formes Elémentaires de la Vie Religieuse.* Paris: CNRS.

Elias, Norbert. [1984] 2007. *An Essay on Time.* Dublin: University College Dublin Press.

Eriksen, Thomas Hylland. 2001. *Tyranny of the Moment.* London: Pluto.

Evans, Caroline. 2007. *Fashion at the Edge.* London: Yale University Press.

Forrester, Tom (ed.). 1985. *The Information Technology Revolution.* Oxford: Blackwell.

Fuery, Kelli. 2009. *New Media.* New York: Palgrave.

Habermas, Jürgen. 1987. *The Philosophical Discourse of Modernity.* Cambridge, UK: Polity.

Harvey, David. 1990. *The Condition of Postmodernity.* Oxford: Blackwell.

Hassan, Robert. 2003. "Network Time and the New Knowledge Epoch." *Time and Society* 12 (2–3): 225–41.

Hines, Tony. 2007. "Supply Chain Strategies, Structures and Relationships." In Tony Hines and Margaret Bruce (eds.), *Fashion Marketing,* 27–53. Oxford: Butterworth-Heinemann.

Hope, Wayne. 2006. "Global Capitalism and the Critique of Real Time." *Time and Society* 15 (2–3): 275–302.

Kern, Stephen. 2003. *The Culture of Time and Space: 1880–1918.* London: Harvard University Press.

Koselleck, Reinhart. [1970] 2004. *Futures Past.* New York: Columbia University Press.

Kumar, Krishan. 2005. *From Post-industrial to Post-modern Society.* Oxford: Blackwell.

Laïdi, Zaki. 2000. *Le Sacre du Présent.* Paris: Flammarion.

Landow, George P. 1997. *Hypertext 2.0.* Baltimore: Johns Hopkins University Press.

Lee, Heejin, and Jonathan Liebenau. 2000. "Time and the Internet at the Turn of the Millenium." *Time and Society* 9 (1): 43–56.

Lehmann, Ulrich. 2000. *Tigersprung.* London: MIT Press.

Lovink, Geert. 2008. *Zero Comments.* London: Routledge.

Manovich, Lev. 2001. *The Language of New Media.* Cambridge, MA: MIT Press.

Marx, Karl. [1857/1858] 1971. *Grundrisse.* London: Macmillan.

Marx, Karl, and Friedrich Engels. [1848/1888] 2004. *Manifesto of the Communist Party.* Proofed and corrected against 1888 English Edition by Andy Blunden. Citizens of the American Constitution. http://citizensoftheamericanconstitution.net/Tyranny%20Files/Additional%20Resouces/Additional%20Resouces/Communist%20Manifesto.pdf (accessed September 10, 2011).

Masuda, Yoncji. 1985. "Parameters of the Post-industrial Society." In Tom Forrester (ed.), *The Information Technology Revolution,* 620–34. Oxford: Blackwell.

McLuhan, Marshall. [1964] 1967. *Understanding Media.* London: Sphere.

Nielson, Jakob. 2011. "How Long Do Users Stay on Web Pages?" Nielsen Norman Group, September 12. http://www.useit.com/alertbox/page-abandonment-time.html (accessed October 4, 2011).

Nowotny, Helga. 1994. *Time: The Modern and Postmodern Experience.* Cambridge, UK: Polity.

Papacharissi, Zizi. 2007. "Audience as Media Producers: Content Analysis of 260 Blogs." In Mark Tremayne (ed.), *Blogging, Citizenship, and the Future of the Media,* 21–38. New York: Routledge.

Pavlik, John V. 2008. *Media in the Digital Age.* New York: Columbia University Press.

Phillips, Angela. 2010. "Old Sources: New Bottles." In N. Fenton (ed.), *New Media, Old News: Journalism and Democracy in the Digital Age,* 87–101. London: Sage.

Rocamora, Agnès. 2011. "Blogs Personnels de mode: Identité et Sociabilité dans la Culture des Apparences." *Sociologie et Sociétés* 43 (1): 19–44.

Rosa, Hartmut. 2010. *Accélération: Une Critique Sociale du Temps.* Paris: Découverte.

Soula, Claude. 2011. "Quand Zara Révolutionne le Textile." *Le Nouvel Observateur,* July 28, 62–63.

Sull, Donald, and Stefano Turconi. 2008. "Fast Fashion Lessons." *Business Strategy Review,* Summer, 11–15.

Thompson, Edward Palmer. 1967. "Time, Work-Discipline, and Industrial Capitalism." *Past and Present* 38 (1): 56–97.

Tomlinson, John. 2007. *The Culture of Speed.* London: Sage.

Vinken, Barbara. 2005. *Fashion Zeitgeist: Trends and Cycles in the Fashion System.* Oxford: Berg.

Virilio, Paul. 1991. *Lost Dimension.* New York: Semiotext(e).

Virilio, Paul. 2006. *Speed and Politics.* Los Angeles: Semiotext(e).

Weber, Max. [1904–1905] 2001. *The Protestant Ethic and the Spirit of Capitalism.* London: Routledge.

Webster, Frank. 2006. *Theories of the Information Society.* Oxon: Routledge.

Williams, Raymond. [1975] 1990. *Television.* London: Routledge.

4

Fashion, the Body, and Age

JULIA TWIGG

INTRODUCTION

Clothes lie at the interface between the body and its social presentation, one of the ways whereby bodies are made social, given identity and meaning. Dress thus needs to be understood, in Joanne Entwistle's (2000) words, as "situated body practice," in which getting up and dressed is a process of preparing the body for the social world, both an intimate experience of the body and a public presentation of it. When we get dressed we do so within the bounds of a culture and its particular norms. These norms include ones in relation to age.

Within popular culture, and the related medicalized accounts that have come to dominate perception, age is primarily seen as a product of physiology, something rooted in the processes of bodily decline, evidenced in outward signs such as wrinkles, graying hair, and changes in figure and stance. But aging also needs to be understood as a social and cultural construct. As analysts of the political economy school have shown (Arber and Ginn 1991; Estes 1979; Estes and Binney 1989; Phillipson 1998; Phillipson and Walker 1986; Townsend 1986), many of the key features of later years are determined as much by social as physiological processes. Critical cultural gerontologists like Margaret Gullette (1997, 1999) and Kathleen Woodward (1999, 2006) have extended the critique to show how individuals are aged by culture, exploring the network of meanings and practices within which later life is experienced and understood.

In this chapter I explore the role that dress plays—and has played historically—in the constitution of age. In particular, I look at the idea that the relationship between age and dress is changing and that traditional assumptions have been eroded with the result that dress is no longer age ordered in the way it once was. Have the rise of consumption culture and the democratization of fashion meant that older people are no longer expected to dress in distinctive ways? What role might the body play in this?

What Counts as Old?

The point at which people become "old" varies historically and across cultures, as it does by gender and social class also (Calasanti and Slevin 2006). In current Western society, the entry to old age is conventionally marked by retirement: this is how it is defined in official statistics. But as we shall see, in recent years the boundaries have become more fluid with the destabilization of the normative life course and the wider reconstitution of age. As a result chronological age has increasingly given way to versions rooted in lifestyle. Aging also needs to be understood as specific to distinctive cultural spheres, so that what counts as old or older varies according to the cultural context. In relation to high fashion, aging sets in early, certainly by the late twenties. Fashion is, in general, a youth-oriented cultural field, and these judgments reverberate through it at all levels. For the purposes of this chapter, however, I will largely be addressing late middle age and older, broadly conceived as fifty plus.

Gender

In this chapter I mostly look at the question of age and dress in relation to women. This reflects both the scope of the literature and the wider cultural perception of the field. Fashion and dress have long been culturally constituted as feminized areas, their discourses predominantly embodied in the lives of women. Thus women, in the past and today, are more engaged with fashion: spending more money on clothes and more time shopping, paying more attention to reading about the topic. Preoccupation with dress in men has traditionally been viewed negatively (at least since the period of the great masculine renunciation; Flugel 1930), though this is changing with the current spread of interest in fashion among younger men. It remains the case, however, that older men as a group are largely disengaged from the sphere of fashion. However, they too wear clothes, buy garments in the market, and are subject to many of the cultural pressures that bear on women in relation to age. They have, however, received little attention in the literature, which when it does address age—and that is rare—concentrates almost exclusively on women.

THE NEGLECT OF AGE AS A SOCIAL CATEGORY

There is a long-established link in dress studies between clothing and social identity, with extensive work exploring the intersections of dress with gender, ethnicity, social class, and sexuality (Davis 1992; Holliday 2001; Khan 1993; Rolley 1993; Tarlo 2010), as well as with distinctive, often transgressive subcultural styles (Polhemus 1994; Wilson 1985). Clothes are indeed, as Christopher Breward (2000) notes, one of the ways in which social difference is made concrete and visible. Such perspectives have, however, rarely been extended to age. Though age is one of the master identities and a source of significant social and cultural differentiation, it has been neglected within sociology and cultural studies. It is often omitted from debates on intersectionality (Anthias 2001). It remains taken for granted in the same way that gender was until the 1980s: treated as something so obvious, so naturalized in biology, that its social significance is neglected. But how we are perceived, who we socialize with, how we are judged and ordered socially, what deserts are deemed appropriate for us, are all crucially determined by our age or our location within an age categorization. It is indeed a key social division (Calasanti and Slevin 2006; Laws 1995; Laz 1998, 2003). We should not be surprised, therefore, to find it expressed in and through dress.

The neglect of age within fashion studies has been particularly marked. This is partly the result of a general omission within the related field of cultural studies, but it also reflects the specific values of the fashion world. Fashion is strongly—perhaps inherently—youth oriented. It is beautiful, young bodies that designers aspire to dress and that are featured throughout the fashion system (Fine and Leopold 1993). This presents an idealized world in which age does not feature, or where it represents a dereliction, a corruption of the vision, a falling off and failure, something to be excluded and ignored. Aging here takes on the features of Julia Kristeva's (1982) abjection, something to be feared, repelled, cast into darkness. From the perspective of mainstream fashion, age is simply not attractive or sexy. Fashion is indeed closely linked to the erotic, so much so that for some theorists the constant play of eroticism is the engine force of fashion and the key to its meaning and deep appeal. Older people, particularly women, are regarded to be beyond the erotic, and indeed, particularly in the eyes of the young, beyond sex itself.

A more sympathetic approach exists within social anthropology, which has a long tradition of taking clothing and dress seriously (Crane and Bovone 2006; Hansen 2004). This has received further impetus from the material turn in anthropology and sociology, in which clothing and dress are part of the creation of symbolic values and their attribution to material culture. Daniel Miller and others have explored the ways in which material objects, like the physical surroundings of the home, become significant in meaning making, representing aspects of distributed personhood (Guy, Green, and Banim 2001; Miller 1987, 1998; Weber and Mitchell 2004; S. Woodward 2007). Clothes are part of this: indeed, for Miller, getting dressed is an almost Hegelian process of self-actualization. Among these meanings are ones relating to age.

AGE ORDERING

The clearest way we can observe the links between age, dress, and identity is through the long-established pattern of age ordering. By this I mean the systematic patterning of cultural expression according to an ordered and hierarchically arranged concept of age. It is clearest to see in relation to children, where at least since the late eighteenth century, and often before, children have worn distinctive age-related forms of dress. The degree to which childhood is marked out in this way has varied historically (Marshall 2008). It is associated in particular with the romantic movement and the new cult of childhood that emerged in the nineteenth century with its emphasis on children as social beings in their own right, expressed through distinctive dress. Daniel Cook (2004) traces this development into the early twentieth century with the emergence of retailing specifically aimed at children, particularly based in department stores. More recently, the trend has been for children's clothes to be less, rather than more, distinctive, with the spread to young girls in particular of adult female styles, as part of a more general extension of consumption culture to this group.

In relation to old age, there has been a similar pattern of structured expectations, expressing norms about what is appropriate—or, more significantly, inappropriate—dress for people as they age. Such patterning is observable historically in manuscripts, portraits, woodcuts, and book illustrations, and it is vividly present in classic pyramidal images of the ages of man or woman, in which dress is used to convey social and bodily change across the life course (Thane 2005). Though always subject to historical specificity, certain features recur in relation to dress and age: more covered-up styles, higher necklines, tighter-drawn linen, and longer skirts, or for men the adoption of the long robe. Colors tend to be darker and more sober, styles less showy. There is a widespread sense—persisting today—that old age is a time for pulling back from overt display. The pressure to tone down, to retreat from being visible, was reported even in Samantha Holland's (2004) study of women who had adopted radical, transgressive styles of dress. Such strictures focus in particular on sexuality. Old women wearing ultrafashionable or sexually explicit dress have long been the mainstay of misogynistic imagery that draws on the Vanitas tradition (Tseëlon 1995). In more muted form it is found in the cultural trope of mutton dressed as lamb (Fairhurst 1998). Lastly, the traditional dress of age is often presented as shabby and worn, as well as dull and dark, reflecting the structural association of age with poverty.

These features of age-associated clothing point to the ways in which dress makes manifest deeper ideological structures. As Malcolm Barnard (1996) argues, clothes are ideological, part of the process whereby social groups establish, sustain, and reproduce positions of power, relations of domination and subordination. They contribute to how inequity is made to seem natural, proper, and legitimate. This perception has largely been developed in relation to gender and class, but it applies also to age. Many of the features noted above—the drabness, the self-effacement, the retreat from social claims to fashionability and display—reflect the wider social marginalization of the old. Many older women report becoming invisible (Gibson 2000; Greer 1991; K. Woodward 2006). Such forms of dress thus underwrite the structural exclusion and poverty imposed on many older people, naturalizing at a bodily level processes that are essentially social.

More recently, however, there has been a growing sense that norms are changing; that age-related rules of dress have gone, or are at least fading fast. A number of elements underlie this. The first relates to changes in the clothing system itself, with the decline, over the long historical period, of status-related forms of dress, so that, for example, marital status in women or professional standing in men are no longer overtly marked in dress as they once were—though of course they are still reflected in subtler ways. The requirement to express age in dress has thus weakened in line with general developments in the dress code.

Significant changes have also occurred in relation to the social position of older people. Demographic change in the twentieth century has reweighted the population toward older groups: between 1901 and 2003 the proportion of the UK population aged fifty and over increased from 15 to 30 percent, and it is projected to rise to 41 percent in 2031 (Tomassini 2005). Increased longevity, rising living standards, and new fluidities in social roles have supported the emergence of the Third Age as a new cultural space (Gilleard and Higgs 2000; Phillipson 1998). A period of post-retirement, free from the constraints of work and, to some degree, family responsibility, it represents a time of leisure, pleasure, and self-development. Peter Öberg and Lars Tornstam (1999, 2001) suggest that later life is best conceptualized as an extended plateau of middle years that ceases only with the irruption of ill health and disability. They argue that modern cultures are marked by a declining salience of age ordering at all stages of life, with adulthood increasingly forming an undifferentiated period between childhood and frail old age. In this reconfiguration of later years, consumption plays a significant role. Many middle-aged and older people have high disposable incomes (though many do not), and this has supported the use of consumption as a means of agency and identity formation in later years, as in younger stages. Within an increasingly individuated culture, consumption also performs an integrative function, acting to integrate people within a common culture of lifestyle. For better-off older people it thus offers a concrete means of integration with the mainstream, helping to undermine the marginalization traditionally associated with age. Clothing can be part of this.

Lastly, in parallel with these developments in relation to older people have been changes in the fashion industry itself, which has undergone major restructuring with the development in the late twentieth and early twenty-first century of fully globalized supply, resulting in massive growth in productive capacity (Aspers 2010; Jones 2006). This has stimulated the active creation of new markets through the extension of the fashion cycle to groups previously excluded from the mainstream, notably children and older people.

"MOVING YOUNGER": THE NEW OLD

Across the field of fashion and age there is a pervasive language of "moving younger." There is a sense that older people today are "different" from earlier cohorts. Those currently in their fifties and sixties—sometimes loosely termed the baby boomers—are often presented as a pioneer generation (Gilleard and Higgs 2002, 2007; Phillipson 2007), the cohort that grew up with youth culture in the 1960s and matured with the consumption boom of the 1980s and 1990s. Accustomed to consumption, they see no reason to abandon its pleasures—including those of wearing attractive, fashionable dress. Furthermore, most older women in this cohort have worked, or are working, and this has given them access to income and opportunities to shop. As a result they represent a generation, it is suggested, who are in some sense "younger" than previous ones—a feature captured in the popular media phrase of "sixty as the new fifty," or even forty—and they have no interest in adopting "frumpy" age-related styles.

Retailers certainly share this view. As the design manager for George at Asda, a UK value supermarket, noted in an Economic and Social Research Council study of clothing and age:

> When I first started working 30 years ago, there was a point in time when people, the majority of people, would switch into that way of dressing, into classic dressing, because they felt that was appropriate to their age. But that is gone. ... This is a massive change, I mean, it's a huge change in my lifetime. (Twigg 2013: 130)

The marketing director of Edinburgh Woollen Mill, a UK retailer focused on the older market, similarly commented in the study:

> I don't think people who are in their 50s see themselves as being 50. They actually see themselves as being a lot younger. ... Our customer was telling us, you know, we might be 55, we might be 65, but we actually don't wanna look like grannies, you know. We don't feel like grannies in our head. We're looking for something younger, slightly more fashionable. (Twigg 2012a: 1047)

These changes have largely been presented in positive terms, reflecting new social confidence among older people. The freedom to wear stylish mainstream dress is seen as a form of empowerment, of resistance to the traditional culture of marginalization and invisibility. The media in particular have been fascinated by imagery of middle-aged and older women "shopping till they drop," or refusing to give up their Manolos. These themes are particularly strongly present in magazines or newspapers aimed at—and crucially written by—women in their forties, fifties, and sixties. This defiant consumption-driven vision dominates the popular media account.

These developments are, however, also open to more negative interpretation. Like many cultural phenomena, the spread of fashionability to older women is Janus faced. As the culture extends new opportunities, it also imposes new demands, new requirements—that they be fashionable. Dress can be part of a wider process of governmentality in relation to women's bodies in which they are increasingly subject to disciplinary demands regarding appearance. We are familiar with these pressures in terms of younger women, with widespread regimes of slimming, exercise, and cosmetic surgery through which they are required to discipline and control their bodies (Bordo 1993; Gimlin 2002; Shilling 2005; Wolf 1990). Increasingly these demands are spreading to older women too (Furman 1997; Hurd Clarke 2011). The requirement to be fashionable, to avoid age-stigmatized clothing, can thus be seen as part of the wider set of Foucauldian techniques of the self, through which the bodies of older people are disciplined, ordered, and made subject to cultural norms, in which successful aging is increasingly interpreted as aging without the appearance of doing so (Katz 1996; K. Woodward 2006). These new versions of "successful" or "positive aging," however, implicitly act to silence other versions, other ways of being old—of "not bothering," of "giving up," of using the invisibility imposed on older women, as Germaine Greer (1991) suggests, as a screen behind which to develop a new life, one freed from the demands of appearance and of the disciplinary practices of normative femininity.

"MOVING YOUNGER": CONSUMPTION AS ASPIRATIONAL

There are, however, two other ways in which we can understand the pervasive language of "moving younger." The first relates to the aspirational nature of consumption. Clothes are part of consumption culture, aspirational goods promoted in terms of a dream of an idealized self. This is the central dynamic that fuels the constant pursuit of goods, and it is of particular significance in the case of clothing, where retailers are selling into a saturated market. Part of that dream is of a younger self. As a result retailers persistently present their goods as aimed at a younger market than is in fact the case, and they certainly try to avoid association with an older one. This produces a dynamic whereby everyone in the field is "moving younger": using young models to display their clothes, selecting promotional settings that emphasize youthful zest, weeding their ranges to lift the offer visually. A similar dynamic operates in the field of fashion magazines, where the target readership is systematically described as younger than the actual age profile revealed in the marketing data (Twigg 2010, 2012b, 2013). This allows the magazine to perform its classic role of reflecting back to readers a visual world that is an idealized version of the one they inhabit, allowing them to identify at a fantasy level with a self that is younger—just as it is slimmer, smarter, and richer—than the reality (Gough-Yates 2003; Hermes 1995; Winship 1987).

In addressing the gray market, retailers face an essential tension: how to build a brand around a negative identity. As the editor of UK *Vogue,* Alexandra Shulman, commented in the Economic and Social Research Council study:

> I think at some level nobody wants to be older. Nobody wants to be fat and nobody wants to be old. You don't want to be poor either. There's lots of things that nobody wants to be, and actually older is just, in general, one of them. So to sort of create a kind of niche whereby if you buy it you're saying, "I am older," you can kind of see why people don't necessarily want to do that. (Twigg 2013: 126)

Nonetheless, she added, "I'm not convinced that there isn't a way round dealing with it, that we don't quite seem to have got."

Retailing analysts concur with this, and there is a widespread sense that the older market is badly served. Through the late 1990s and early 2000s older women were repeatedly identified as "frustrated shoppers," unable to find attractive clothes aimed at them (Mintel 2000). Marketeers are certainly very conscious of the potential of the gray market (Gunter 1998; Key Note 2006; Lavery 1999; Mintel 2006; Moschis 1996; Sawchuk 1995; Verdict 2008). They are aware of the spending power of this group, or at least sections of it. Nick Long (1998) describes the over forty-fives in the United Kingdom as having nearly 80 percent of all financial wealth and being responsible for about 30 percent of consumer spending. Harry Moody and Sanjay Sood (2010) in their account of age branding describe the over fifty-fives in the United States as having twice the discretionary income of younger groups (18–49). Market research reports in the United Kingdom (Key Note 2006) point to the relative affluence of those in their fifties and sixties. But retailers find it difficult to address this market effectively. Part of the problem is that "older people," as David Metz and Michael Underwood (2005) and others note, are as diverse in their circumstances, values, and lives as younger groups. Though attempts have been made to develop market segmentation based around lifestyle rather than chronological age, these have not proved successful (Easey 2002; Gunter 1998; Hines and Quinn 2007; Lavery 1999; Mintel 2000; Moschis 1996; Otieno, Harrow, and Lea-Greenwood 2005). Attempts to reconstitute the older population in terms of lifestyle are also open to the criticism that they act to hide significant differences rooted in class, income, race, and sexuality. Stephen Katz and Barbara Marshall (2003) note how the discourses of marketing with their emphasis on silver surfers and zoomers ("boomers who zoom") allow structural differences in the population to disappear into market niches.

Retailers thus face a problem in signaling their relevance to this group, which remains in a vague, undifferentiated state that the companies are reluctant to define. Some used coded terms such as "classic" to indicate the market. Occasionally a brand will use humor, such as Not Your Daughter's Jeans, to suggest a cut aimed at the older figure. What they all avoid, however, is direct reference to age.

The aspiration of "moving younger" needs to be set in the context of a pervasive culture of ageism, in which looking "ten years younger" (the title of a popular makeover show in the United Kingdom) has become a central cultural ideal. This supports a vast international industry of antiaging, promoted through pills, diets, exercise regimes, cosmetics, pharmaceuticals, and aesthetic surgery (Gilleard and Higgs 2000; Hurd Clarke 2011). Clothing and dress can be part of this, and one of the persistent themes of magazine makeovers is how to achieve this younger look. The process of wearing "younger" clothes to look younger, however, has its limits. Though youthful and fashionable dress can create a more youthful style, particularly where it reflects body styles that are more casual and relaxed in a "modern" way, extremely youthful styles act only to point up the aging body that wears them. Styles that are frilly, girly, pretty, or overtly sexy are all marked by this quality of emphasizing age rather than diluting it. They each point to a particular version of embodied femininity that centers on youthful sexuality. As Toni Calasanti and Kathleen Slevin (2006) have argued, the dominant cultural concept of femininity is itself youthful. Youth here becomes part of the unmarked category, the dominant neutral that is the assumed state, the standard against which other versions of femininity are judged as lacking.

"MOVING YOUNGER": AGE AS STYLE DIFFUSION

There is, however, a third, and different, way in which we can understand the language of "moving younger," and this is in terms of the processes of fashion themselves, and in particular the dynamics of style diffusion. From classic sociological accounts, starting with the works of Thorstein Veblen ([1899] 1953) and Georg Simmel ([1904] 1971), we are familiar with fashion as a tool of class competition, part of a dynamic of competitive emulation and display in which styles are taken up and abandoned by elites as they are transferred down the social hierarchy. Elites display their distinction through repeatedly marking themselves off from lower orders (Bourdieu 1984). More recently, the dominance of class in the dynamic of fashion has been questioned, with the rise of a plurally based fashion system, in which alternative sources such as street fashions, music styles, and youth cults are increasingly influential (Davis 1992; Entwistle 2000; Polhemus 1994). As part of this shift, Diane Crane argues, youth has replaced class as the engine of fashion. With the wider democratization of fashion, she argues, class is no longer the key driver. Although the analysis centers on youth, her insight is also significant for age:

> Instead of the upper class seeking to differentiate itself from other social classes, the young seek to differentiate themselves from the middle aged and the elderly. As trends diffuse to older age groups, younger age groups adopt new styles. (2000: 198)

By this interpretation, age ordering has not gone. It is still significant; it is just that it has taken on a new form. Rather than simply denoting social position as in the past, it is now caught up in the dynamic of fashion itself. What we are observing, therefore, is not that the dress of older people is moving younger but that styles are diffusing older, as they pass from the center of fashionability in the youth market to the periphery in the older one. It is this that underlies the sense that ultrafashionable styles look "odd," "unsuitable," "ridiculous," or "sad" on older people. The sharpness of their fashionability has to be blunted before they can be adopted by older wearers. Thus in the 1980s leggings initially emerged on the fashion scene promoted by Vivienne Westwood, carrying a sense of shock and sexual frisson, then moved into the youthful mainstream, and from there on to middle-aged housewives on peripheral housing estates, thus making the diffusional journey in terms of both age and class (until, of course, they were revived again in the youthful market in the mid-2000s). There is a parallel here with James Laver's (1937: 40) celebrated account of the fashion cycle, in which styles are indecent ten years before their time, daring one year before, chic in their time, dowdy three years later, hideous twenty years after, amusing thirty years after, romantic a hundred years later, and beautiful in a hundred and fifty years; however, since the 1930s, the cycle has speeded up. Part of the diffusion to the status of dowdiness and out-of-dateness relates to age. Anthony Freitas and colleagues (1997), for example, in their study of college-aged young people's views found that they associated styles for older people with being out-of-date and were keen to mark themselves off from them.

Sometimes the process of style diffusion rests on a cohort effect, with the meaning of styles altering with the aging of the cohort that wears them. For example, in the 1950s tweed sports jackets in the United Kingdom were worn by young men—undergraduates or young teachers—and were associated with a youthful, easygoing approach. Although in photographs today they appear conservative, that was not their meaning in the 1950s and 1960s. By the 1980s such jackets—classically in gray herringbone—become standard wear for conservative, middle-aged male academics, representing sober, sensible garb that stopped short of the formality of a suit. By the early twenty-first century, the tweed jacket and tie has gone from the world of work and is to be found in older people's clubs and retirement homes, worn by men in their seventies and eighties. A parallel pattern occurs in relation to pleated skirts for women. Young and fresh in the 1950s and 1960s, they have become increasingly age coded, until in the early 2000s they are emblems of age; retailers like Jaeger in the United Kingdom refuse to stock them because they "age the range" (though in the ever restless nature of a fashion, they are enjoying a revival at the younger end; Twigg 2013).

AGING AND THE BODY: ADJUSTING THE CUT

So far we have—rightly—treated clothing and age as cultural phenomena. But we need to recognize the ways in which the dress styles in relation to age also reflect the ways in which the body alters. The female body, as it ages, changes: waists thicken, busts lower, stomachs expand, shoulders move forward (Goldsberry, Shim, and Reich 1996). Part of the skill of a designer is accommodating these changes so that the garment fits, but in ways that do not detract from its fashionability and that—ideally—subtly alter the presentation of the body, assisting the wearer to appear nearer the fashionable norm—in the case of older women, nearer the body of a slim young woman. Designers sometimes add details that adjust or "help" with such presentation; for example, shoulder pads in a blouse or jersey can restore the body nearer the youthful norm, allowing the garment to hang better. Clothes have always performed this function, enabling individual bodies with their idiosyncrasies to be presented publicly in a form nearer the current norm, and these reflect systematic ideals about the body. The history of English tailoring for men, as it developed from the end of the eighteenth century in the context of elite, wool-based clothing, is a testimony to these processes whereby an idealized masculine figure is produced through the judicious use of tailoring, cut, and padding.

Adjusting the cut to make it fit better can, however, have the effect of "aging" the garment, writing into its very structure information about the sort of body that is meant to inhabit it. This is most clearly visible in ranges aimed at distinctly older women, where the cut is markedly different, with lower bust seams and undefined waists. Certain features such as elasticized waists come to be associated with age, and retailers aiming at a less age-identified look try to avoid these, substituting, for example, drawstrings. Retailers can also adjust the cut in the degree to which it is close to the body, with ranges aimed at those in their fifties and sixties more closely shaped than those aimed at people in their seventies and eighties. Retailers sometimes also try to finesse the issue by featuring styles that are looser and softer and that draw on Japanese influences. Some of the most successful and "modern"-looking ranges for the older market deploy this approach (Twigg 2012a).

Adjusting the cut is also often about preventing the exposure of the body in ways that are deemed "unattractive" and that may violate norms about the visibility of older bodies, in particular where this is linked to expressed sexuality. Avoiding such exposure can present difficulties for designers, for example, when fashion dictates sleeveless dresses, so that adding sleeves detracts from fashionability, aging the garment and, by implication, the wearer. Here, of course, although the features of the body they are designing to are rooted in physiological aging, the meanings accorded to them are not. There is no inherent reason why low necks, or loose arms, should not be displayed, except as part of a desire to hide something that is deemed culturally shameful. A range of work has explored the ways in which older, particularly female, bodies are rarely on view within modern visual culture. Such images, particularly if they involve nakedness, can be strongly transgressive, as Emmanuelle Tulle-Winton (2000) showed in her analysis of the photo essay *Pretty Ribbons,* in which a model in her eighties was depicted in conscious glamour shots photographed in hard, clear light. Dress can thus be part of a set of processes whereby the bodies of older women are disciplined, made subject to cultural assumptions about what may or may not be on view that are internalized by the women themselves and by those designing for them. Particularly sensitive are aspects of the body that express sexuality. Here women's bodies, as we have noted, are judged against a cultural norm that equates sexuality with youthfulness and presents older bodies as inadequate, flawed, or failed and best kept covered up.

A third way in which cut is adjusted for the aging body concerns sizing. As people age, they tend to put on weight. One of the marked features of ranges aimed at older customers is that they have a "generous" cut, so much so indeed that one of the ways one can recognize such ranges is through sizing. Though all UK manufacturers use standard schemes such as 10, 12, and 14, how they operationalize these varies: a size 12 in a youth shop is very different from one in a shop oriented to the over fifties. This is partly in order to flatter and reassure older customers, but it also reflects changes in the shape of the body. Manufacturers tend to treat sizing data as commercially confidential, reflecting their detailed knowledge of their market (Apeagyei 2010). More systematic data have, however, recently become available through the Size UK study that scanned 11,000 members of the UK population.[1] This established a distinctive "mature" figure type that is available for manufacturers to use as a basis for sizing.

As a result of these changes in the body, slimming is often pursued as an antiaging technique. Extreme slimness means having a body more like that of a young woman, at least of a young fashion model, with the ultraslim androgynous figure favored by the industry. In particular, it means not having the problematic aspects of the female body once it has aged, when the bust has enlarged and lowered, the hips spread, and flesh in general lost its tone. Having little or no flesh thus enables ultraslim older women to fit into fashionable dress in a way that is denied to most women as they age. Paradoxically, therefore, remaining "youthful" rests on avoiding a very feminine figure earlier in life.

CONCLUSION

As we have seen, dress is closely implicated in the expression of identity, one of the means whereby this is made concrete and visible. Though dress studies have explored these links in relation to classic dimensions such as gender, class, and sexuality, it has neglected age, despite its cultural significance. As we have noted, age ordering is a long-established feature of Western dress. More recently, however, claims have been made for its demise. There is certainly evidence to support a sense that its rigor has lessened. This has occurred in conjunction with wider changes in the social location of older people, indeed with a general dissolution of the boundaries that once defined old age as a distinctive period. Cultural forms such as consumption have played a part in this—certainly for the better-off. But as we noted, there are other ways in which we can understand the persistent sense that older people are "moving younger" in their dress choices. One of these relates to the aspirational nature of consumption and of the related cultural fields of the media and advertising, which project dreams in which people's lives are reflected back to them in improved and aspirational forms. In a culture saturated with fear of aging, this means showing them as younger. "Moving younger" can also be understood in terms of changes in the fashion system itself, with the shift in the dynamic of fashion diffusion away from class toward age. Age ordering has taken on a new form. Rather than simply denoting social position as in the past, it is now caught up in the dynamic of fashion itself. It is not that the dress of older people is moving younger but that styles are diffusing older.

As we have noted, most of the academic work addressing fashion has omitted age from its view, and most of the work on age has similarly ignored these areas of consumption, performance, and identity. Recently, welcome developments have attempted to bridge this gap in analysis. Debates around appearance, the commodification of antiaging, and the tensions of age denial and age resistance have emerged as part of the wider cultural turn in gerontology. In a parallel way, dress studies, particularly under the influence of anthropological and sociological approaches, have begun to extend their remit to the population as a whole and to the everyday nature of clothing as situated body practice (Entwistle 2000). Further work linking clothing and age would allow these developments to come to fuller fruition.

NOTE

1. "SizeUK—Results from the UK National Sizing Survey 2012," University of the Arts London, http://www.fashion.arts.ac.uk/research/projects-collaborations/archive/size-uk/ (accessed May 7, 2013).

BIBLIOGRAPHY

Anthias, Floya. 2001. "The Concept of Social Division and Theorising Social Stratification: Looking at Ethnicity and Class." *Sociology* 35 (4): 835–54.

Apeagyei, Phoebe R. 2010. "Application of 3D Body Scanning Technology to Human Measurement for Clothing Fit." *DCTA: International Journal of Digital Content Technology and Its Applications* 4 (7): 58–68.

Arber, Sara, and Jay Ginn. 1991. *Gender and Later Life: A Sociological Analysis of Resources and Constraints.* London: Sage.

Aspers, Patrik. 2010. *Orderly Fashion: A Sociology of Markets.* Princeton, NJ: Princeton University Press.

Barnard, Malcolm. 1996. *Fashion as Communication.* London: Routledge.

Bordo, Susan. 1993. *Unbearable Weight: Feminism, Western Culture and the Body.* Berkeley: University of California Press.

Bourdieu, Pierre. 1984. *Distinction: A Social Critique of the Judgement of Taste.* London: Routledge & Kegan Paul.

Breward, Christopher. 2000. "Cultures, Identities, Histories: Fashioning a Cultural Approach to Dress." In Nicola White and Ian Griffiths (eds.), *The Fashion Business: Theory, Practice, Image,* 23–36. Oxford: Berg.

Calasanti, Toni M., and Kathleen F. Slevin. 2006. "Introduction." In Toni M. Calasanti and Kathleen F. Slevin (eds.), *Age Matters: Realigning Feminist Thinking,* 1–17. New York: Routledge.

Cook, Daniel T. 2004. *The Commodification of Childhood: The Children's Clothing Industry and the Rise of the Child Consumer.* Durham, NC: Duke University Press.

Crane, Diana. 2000. *Fashion and Its Social Agendas: Class, Gender, and Identity in Clothing.* Chicago: University of Chicago Press.

Crane, Diana, and Laura Bovone. 2006. "Approaches to Material Culture: The Sociology of Fashion and Clothing." *Poetics* 34: 319–33.

Davis, Fred. 1992. *Fashion, Culture and Identity.* Chicago: University of Chicago Press.

Easey, Mike (ed.). 2002. *Fashion Marketing.* Oxford: Blackwell.

Entwistle, Joanne. 2000. *The Fashioned Body: Fashion, Dress and Modern Social Theory.* Cambridge, UK: Polity.

Estes, Carroll L. 1979. *The Aging Enterprise.* San Francisco: Jossey-Bass.

Estes, Carroll L., and Elizabeth A. Binney. 1989. "The Biomedicalization of Aging." *The Gerontologist* 29 (5): 587–96.

Fairhurst, Eileen. 1998. "'Growing Old Gracefully' as Opposed to 'Mutton Dressed as Lamb': The Social Construction of Recognising Older Women." In Sarah Nettleton and Jonathan Watson (eds.), *The Body in Everyday Life,* 258–75. London: Routledge.

Fine, Ben, and Ellen Leopold. 1993. *The World of Consumption.* London: Routledge.

Flugel, John C. 1930. *The Psychology of Clothes.* London: Hogarth.

Freitas, Anthony, Susan Kaiser, Carol Hall, Jung-Won Kim, and Tania Hammidi. 1997. "Appearance Management as Border Construction: Least Favourite Clothing, Group Distancing, and Identity… Not." *Sociological Inquiry* 67 (3): 323–35.

Furman, Frieda K. 1997. *Facing the Mirror: Older Women and Beauty Shop Culture.* New York: Routledge.

Gibson, Pamela Church. 2000. "'No One Expects Me Anywhere': Invisible Women, Ageing and the Fashion Industry." In Stella Bruzzi and Pamela Church Gibson (eds.), *Fashion Cultures: Theories, Explorations and Analysis,* 79–90. London: Routledge.

Gilleard, C. J., and Paul Higgs. 2000. *Culture of Aging: Self, Citizen and the Body.* London: Prentice Hall.

Gilleard, C. J., and Paul Higgs. 2002. "The Third Age: Class, Cohort or Generation?" *Ageing & Society* 22: 369–82.

Gilleard, C. J., and Paul Higgs. 2007. "The Third Age and the Baby Boomers: Two Approaches to the Social Structuring of Later Life." *International Journal of Ageing and Later Life* 2 (2): 13–30.

Gimlin, Debra L. 2002. *Body Work: Beauty and Self-Image in American Culture.* Berkeley: University of California Press.

Goldsberry, Ellen, Soyeon Shim, and Naomi Reich. 1996. "Women 55 Years and Older: Part I Current Body Measurements as Contrasted to the PS 42–70 Data." *Clothing and Textiles Research Journal* 14 (2): 108–20.

Gough-Yates, Anna. 2003. *Understanding Women's Magazines: Publishing, Markets and Readership.* London: Routledge.

Greer, Germaine. 1991. *The Change: Women, Ageing and the Menopause.* London: Hamish Hamilton.

Gullette, Margaret M. 1997. *Declining to Decline: Cultural Combat and the Politics of Midlife.* Charlottesville: University of Virginia Press.

Gullette, Margaret M. 1999. "The Other End of the Fashion Cycle: Practising Loss, Learning Decline." In Kathleen Woodward (ed.), *Figuring Age: Women, Bodies, Generations,* 34–58. Bloomington: Indiana University Press.

Gunter, Barrie. 1998. *Understanding the Older Consumer: The Grey Market.* London: Routledge.

Guy, Ali, Eileen Green, and Maura Banim (eds.). 2001. *Through the Wardrobe: Women's Relationships with Their Clothes.* Oxford: Berg.

Hansen, Karen Tranberg. 2004. "The World in Dress: Anthropological Perspectives on Clothing, Fashion and Culture." *Annual Review of Anthropology* 33: 369–92.

Hermes, Jake. 1995. *Reading Women's Magazines: An Analysis of Everyday Media Use.* Cambridge, UK: Polity.

Hines, Tony, and Lee Quinn. 2007. "Segmenting Fashion Consumers: Reconstructing the Challenge of Consumer Complexity." In Tony Hines and Margaret Bruce (eds.), *Fashion Marketing: Contemporary Issues,* 73–88. Oxford: Butterworth-Heinemann.

Holland, Samantha. 2004. *Alternative Femininities: Body, Age and Identity.* Oxford: Berg.

Holliday, Ruth. 2001. "Fashioning the Queer Self." In Joanne Entwistle and Elizabeth Wilson (eds.), *Body Dressing,* 215–32. Oxford: Berg.

Hurd Clarke, Laura. 2011. *Facing Age: Women Growing Older in Anti-aging Culture.* Toronto: Rowman and Littlefield.

Jones, Richard M. 2006. *The Apparel Industry.* Oxford: Blackwell.

Katz, Stephen. 1996. *Disciplining Old Age: The Formation of Gerontological Knowledge.* Charlottesville: University Press of Virginia.

Katz, Stephen, and Barbara Marshall. 2003. "New Sex for Old: Lifestyle, Consumerism and the Ethics of Aging Well." *Journal of Aging Studies* 17 (1): 3–16.

Key Note. 2006. *Market Assessment: Grey Consumer.* London: Key Note.

Khan, Naseem. 1993. "Asian Women's Dress: From Burqah to Blogs." In Juliet Ash and Elizabeth Wilson (eds.), *Chic Thrills,* 61–74. Berkeley: University of California Press.

Kristeva, Julia. 1982. *Powers of Horror: An Essay on Abjection.* New York: Columbia University Press.

Laver, James. 1937. *Taste and Fashion.* London: Harrap.

Lavery, Kevin (ed.). 1999. *The Definitive Guide to Mature Advertising and Marketing.* Shipley, UK: Millennium.

Laws, Glenda. 1995. "Understanding Ageism: Lessons from Feminism and Postmodernism." *The Gerontologist* 35 (1): 112–18.

Laz, Cheryl. 1998. "Act Your Age." *Sociological Forum* 13 (1): 85–113.

Laz, Cheryl. 2003. "Age Embodied." *Journal of Aging Studies* 17: 503–19.

Long, Nick. 1998. "Broken Down by Age and Sex—Exploring the Ways We Approach the Elderly Consumer." *Journal of Market Research Society* 40 (2): 73–92.

Marshall, Noreen. 2008. *Dictionary of Children's Clothes: 1700 to Present.* London: V&A Publishing.

Metz, David, and Michael Underwood. 2005. *Older, Richer, Fitter: Identifying the Customer Needs of Britain's Ageing Population.* London: Age Concern.

Miller, Daniel. 1987. *Material Culture and Mass Consumption.* Oxford: Blackwell.

Miller, Daniel. 1998. *A Theory of Shopping.* Cambridge, UK: Polity.

Mintel. 2000. *The UK Clothing Market.* London: Mintel.

Mintel. 2006. *Fashion for the Over 45s—UK.* London: Mintel

Moody, Harry R., and Sanjay Sood. 2010. "Age Branding." In Amy Drolet, Norbert Schwarz, and Carolyn Yoon (eds.), *The Aging Consumer: Perspectives from Psychology and Economics,* 229–45. New York: Routledge.

Moschis, George P. 1996. *Gerontographics: Life Stage Segmentation for Marketing Strategy Development.* Westport, CT: Quorum Books.

Öberg, Peter, and Lars Tornstam. 1999. "Body Images among Men and Women of Different Ages." *Ageing & Society* 19: 629–44.

Öberg, Peter, and Lars Tornstam. 2001. "Youthfulness and Fitness—Identity Ideals for All Ages?" *Journal of Aging and Identity* 6 (1): 15–29.

Otieno, Rose, Chris Harrow, and Gaynor Lea-Greenwood. 2005. "The Unhappy Shopper: A Retail Experience Exploring Fashion, Fit and Affordability." *International Journal of Retail and Distribution Management* 33 (4): 298–309.

Phillipson, Chris. 1998. *Reconstructing Old Age: New Agendas in Social Theory and Practice.* London: Sage.

Phillipson, Chris. 2007. "Understanding the Baby Boomer Generation: Comparative Perspectives." *International Journal of Aging and Later Life* 2 (2): 7–11.

Phillipson, Chris, and Alan Walker (eds.). 1986. *Ageing and Social Policy: A Critical Assessment.* Aldershot, UK: Gower.

Polhemus, Ted. 1994. *Streetstyle: From Sidewalk to Catwalk.* London: Thames and Hudson.

Rolley, Katrina. 1993. "Love, Desire and the Pursuit of the Whole: Dress and the Lesbian Couple." In Juliet Ash and Elizabeth Wilson (eds.), *Chic Thrills,* 30–39. Berkeley: University of California Press.

Sawchuk, Kim A. 1995. "From Gloom to Boom: Age, Identity and Target Marketing." In Mike Featherstone and Andrew Wernick (eds.), *Images of Aging: Cultural Representations of Later Life,* 173–87. London: Routledge.

Shilling, Chris. 2005. *The Body in Culture, Technology and Society.* London: Sage.

Simmel, Georg. [1904] 1971. "Fashion." In *On Individuality and Social Forms: Selected Writings,* trans. D. C. Levine, 294–323. Chicago: University of Chicago Press.

Tarlo, Emma. 2010. *Visibly Muslim: Fashion, Politics and Faith.* Oxford: Berg.

Thane, Pat (ed.). 2005. *The Long History of Old Age.* London: Thames and Hudson.

Tomassini, Cecilia. 2005. *Focus on Older People: Demographic Profile.* London: Office of National Statistics.

Townsend, Peter. 1986. "Ageism and Social Policy." In Chris Phillipson and Alan Walker (eds.), *Ageing and Social Policy: A Critical Assessment,* 15–44. Aldershot, UK: Gower.

Tseëlon, Efrat. 1995. *The Masque of Femininity.* London: Sage.

Tulle-Winton, Emmanuelle. 2000. "Old Bodies." In Philip Hancock, Bill Hughes, Elizabeth Jagger, Kevin Paterson, Rachel Russell, Emmanuelle Tulle-Winton, and Melissa Tyler (eds.), *The Body, Culture and Society,* 64–83. Buckingham, UK: Open University Press.

Twigg, Julia. 2010. "How Does *Vogue* Negotiate Age? Fashion, the Body and the Older Woman." *Fashion Theory: The Journal of Dress, Body and Culture* 14 (4): 471–90.

Twigg, Julia. 2012a. "Adjusting the Cut: Fashion, the Body and Age on the UK High Street." *Ageing & Society* 32 (6): 1030–54.

Twigg, Julia. 2012b. "Fashion and Age: The Role of Women's Magazines in the Constitution of Aged Identities." In Virpi Ylänne (ed.), *Representing Ageing: Images and Identities,* 132–46. Basingstoke, UK: Palgrave Macmillan.

Twigg, Julia. 2013. *Fashion and Age: Dress, the Body and Later Life.* London: Bloomsbury.

Veblen, Thorstein. [1899] 1953. *The Theory of the Leisure Class: An Economic Study of Institutions.* New York: Mentor.

Verdict. 2008. *Clothing and Footwear 2008: Verdict Forecast.* London: Verdict.

Weber, Sandra, and Claudia Mitchell (eds.). 2004. *Not Just Any Dress: Narratives of Memory, Body and Identity.* New York: Peter Lang.

Wilson, Elizabeth. 1985. *Adorned in Dreams: Fashion and Modernity.* London: Virago.
Winship, Janice. 1987. *Inside Women's Magazines.* London: Pandora.
Wolf, Naomi. 1990. *The Beauty Myth.* London: Vintage.
Woodward, Kathleen M. (ed.). 1999. *Figuring Age: Women, Bodies, Generations.* Bloomington: Indiana University Press.
Woodward, Kathleen M. 2006. "Performing Age, Performing Gender." *NWSA Journal* 18 (1): 162–89.
Woodward, Sophie. 2007. *Why Women Wear What They Wear.* Oxford: Berg.

SECTION II

Fashion, Identity, and Difference

Introduction

JOANNE ENTWISTLE

So much has been written about fashion and identity that it has become something of a cliché to say that fashion articulates identity. Indeed, this theme has probably the longest history within fashion studies as a topic of intellectual investigation, and it may seem that there is little one can add to this. And yet it remains an enduring aspect both in daily dress practices and in academic considerations of them, such that no fashion handbook can be complete without some reflection on this core issue. What one finds when considering the more recent scholarship in this area is that the subject is vastly more complex and nuanced than anything that has preceded it.

From the earliest days of sociological writings on the topic via Georg Simmel and John C. Flugel to the flurry of literature on fashion coming out of the emerging fashion studies of the 1980s and 1990s to the present day, we have had continual reminders of the significance of fashion for marking out identities of various kinds. Indeed, the formation of modern subjectivity seems bound up with various forms of dress and self-presentation, as some histories and contemporary studies of the self have shown (Davis 1994; Entwistle 2000a, 2000b; Entwistle and Wilson 2001; Finkelstein 1991; Hall and Jefferson 1976; Hebdige 1979; Laver 1968; Paulicelli and Clark 2009; Sennett 1977). Hence, we have had accounts of the rise of dandies, bohemians, dress reformers, subcultures, lesbians, gay men, career women, and a whole cast of characters whose dress was in some way significant in their forms of identity and self-expression. Moreover, identities are themselves are *performed through* the forms of dress adopted.

The essays in this section take as their focus three key dimensions of identity and dress—class, gender, and sexuality. This is by no means the sum of work in this area—there might have been many more papers examining race, ethnicity, age, occupation, and so on (the list could go on). However, while space would not allow us to examine all of these, the three we have chosen do have particular resonance, both as elements of analysis that refer back to a much larger literature from within fashion studies and also as topics of great currency in academic debates on fashion today.

Much of the existing fashion literature takes as its focus class and gender. The former has often been implicit in many accounts of fashion—especially histories of fashion that have described aristocrats and dandies, ladies and their maids—while the latter has often been very explicitly analyzed. How is it that class, so crucial a dimension of fashion and dress, has been more implicit than overtly examined? This is the focus of Katherine Appleford's paper. Her argument highlights the critical significance of class to the many evaluations, judgments, opinions, and practices of fashion and dress, especially in the United Kingdom, where class remains a national preoccupation. Yet while labels like "chav" are used to label and ridicule particularly lower-class styles of dress, and while studies of subculture have attended to some of the class dimensions inherent in the style of particular subcultural groups, there has been surprisingly little academic attention paid to the importance of class in accounts of fashion and dress. This is all the more remarkable when one considers the strong association between class, forms of taste, and consumption practices. It is apparent that distinctions and demarcations in class positions and practices are prevalent in everyday dress practices in the United Kingdom, as evidenced in the mainstream media. Meanwhile, academics writing on class itself have tended to skirt around the issue of dress, while literature on dress has tended to focus on other dimensions of identity that are, perhaps, more "spectacular," or at least more prominent, such as gender, race, and ethnicity. Appleford's work, therefore, highlights the importance of attending to class, first by revisiting early and classic studies that have examined fashion and class through the idea of "emulation." Although a much-discredited argument, this idea has been particularly influential and remains one of the most clearly articulated attempts to understand the way in which fashion might demarcate class identities. More recent thinking has, of course, shown that contemporary consumer culture has opened up fashionable expression beyond any elite group and thus provides a much more complex backdrop against which class identities are played out. This does not mean, as Appleford clearly argues, that fashion's association with class has disappeared or been eradicated. Instead, the lines of demarcation are much more subtle, and a new theoretical and methodological framework needs to be properly articulated. Her own work thus shows the relevance of Pierre Bourdieu's analysis to understand the ways status and distinction are articulated through dress practices that form part of class habitus. This is evident particularly in the evaluations and discourses on identity in the popular media in the United Kingdom, where dress often works to define working-class identities—"chav" being the obvious one—which are articulated as against an assumed middle-class standard of dress taken as self-evidently the norm. No longer are the upper and middle classes concerned with elaborate fashions of the day, but their implicit good taste has become the unspoken norm against which the elaborate, fashion-driven, and "vulgar" tastes of the working classes are evaluated.

If class has been an oft-neglected component of identity within the literature on fashion and dress, this is in dramatic contrast to gender, which is perhaps the most examined aspect of all within fashion literature. This concern with gender in fashion studies may have a lot to do with the fact that fashion has, by association, always been gendered; seen as something "feminine." Indeed, much of the literature on fashion history has seen fashion and dress playing a critical part in the historical emergence of a gender regime that sharply differentiates male and female through styles of masculine and feminine dress. Significant in accounts of the emergence of this gender order has been work from historians of eighteenth-century fashion, who, as Jennifer M. Jones in this section puts it, "realized not only that clothing was deeply gendered but that fashion culture itself was deeply tied to important historical questions about gender, consumer culture, power, and the modern self." Hence, gender has played a critical part in the fashion studies literature, although often neglected in other historical accounts until the 1980s.

In her paper, Jones examines in detail the way this eighteenth-century history has been constituted through a careful analysis of the shifts in fashion and other histories of the period. As she notes, the dominant paradigm for analysis has been Flugel's "great masculine renunciation," which tells a story of the disassociation of men from fashion and the subsequent association of femininity with it. This model of increasing gender differentiation has been relayed by numerous scholars, as Jones summarizes, because it makes sense of transformations in dress over the eighteenth and nineteenth centuries, providing causal explanations in relation to political and social change and dovetailing with an emerging concern in the 1970s and 1980s with the idea of "separate spheres." As Jones notes, growing criticism of Flugel's model helped develop a more nuanced account of gender and fashion. In addition, histories of eighteenth-century consumption produced in the 1980s and 1990s, emerging out of Daniel Roche's influential work, began to attend to the material culture of fashion through the use of inventories. Alongside this, and as part of a growing recognition across a range of disciplines, a concern with materiality and with production has emerged of late; as Jones notes, historians need to attend to the "cut and construction of the clothing." For example, histories of female seamstresses and their battle for recognition within the guilds in the seventeenth century underscore the need to examine production and distribution as well as consumption if we are to fully understand the production of identities within the fashion industry.

If gender has long been theorized in terms of fashion, sexual identities have not been attended to until relatively recently, although particular styles of dress have long enjoyed associations with lesbian identity. Indeed, as Vicki Karaminas in this section argues, butch and femme styles have long been practiced, dating back to at least the early twentieth century and possibly earlier. In addition, a long-standing association of lesbians with "poor fashion sense" on the one hand and "mannish" style on the other persists. These associations are traced in Karaminas's chapter, and her analysis also takes us on a colorful and stylish journey through the boulevards of Paris, to the cafés and bars of Berlin and the cabaret venues of Greenwich and Harlem in New York, in search of the lesbian dandy and bohemian. The styles of lesbian dress Karaminas describes in the early and mid-twentieth century took on a new complexion when feminism of the "second wave" emerged to challenge fashion altogether. As she notes, among many lesbians as well as feminists, fashion was to be rejected, and, so too were gendered forms of dress, in favor of androgynous dress. Such a clear articulation of political affiliations with the "sisterhood" through a rejection of fashion per se was commonly felt beyond lesbian communities, with women, lesbian or not, who refused this antifashion stance subject to criticism.

Toward the end of the twentieth century, such a stance was not sustainable or indeed required. As postmodernism and poststructuralism took hold in the academy, and as mainstream practices began to shift, ideas of authenticity and stable political categories and identities were increasingly challenged. A new playfulness with gender and sexuality began to emerge over the 1980s and 1990s and, along with it, a new acceptance of lesbian, gay, and queer style in the mainstream. As this playfulness made its way through popular music and media, through the likes of Madonna, for example, the very terms of debate about, and the very style of fashion dress, and identity itself, were opened up. Whereas once gender and sexuality had been considered fixed categories of identity, a more fluid, hybrid, and less rigid sense of style emerged that "mixed it up." Alongside this, recognition of gender as drag further challenged our notions of stable sexual identities.

So while heterosexual men might wear skirts in the form of "metrosexual" man, as the media would have him labeled and embodied by the likes of soccer player David Beckham, "lipstick lesbians" could finally be seen enjoying fashion and style in popular television and film. Karamanis's chapter provides a careful analysis of the ways in which lesbian sartorial style has been played out against the changing social scene from the early twentieth century through to today. Ironically, the downside of such absorption into the mainstream of "lesbian chic" may be a blurring of the codes that signaled lesbian identity in the first place.

Fashion may be closely associated with particular, discrete identities and identity formation, but today's literature demonstrates a concern with more nuanced accounts of the ways in which identities are fashioned through dress. Not only have the historical stories of class, gender, and sexual identities (along with many other dimensions of identity) still to be told, but theorists and students of fashion have also to contend with a vastly expanded field of research within fashion studies that has moved beyond simple models like "emulation" or the "great masculine renunciation" to understand and analyze complex flows of meaning and more highly differentiated practices. As such, we have moved far beyond simple theories and associations between fashion, dress, and identity and find ourselves on much more interesting theoretical terrain.

BIBLIOGRAPHY

Davis, Fred. 1994. *Fashion, Culture and Identity.* Chicago: University of Chicago Press.

Entwistle, Joanne. 2000a. *The Fashioned Body: Fashion, Dress and Modern Social Theory.* Cambridge, UK: Polity.

Entwistle, Joanne. 2000b. "Fashioning the Career Woman: Power Dressing as a Strategy of Consumption." In Mary R. Andrews and Mary Margaret Talbot (eds.), *All the World and Her Husband: Women, Consumption and Power,* 224–38. London: Continuum International.

Entwistle, Joanne, and Elizabeth Wilson (eds.). 2001. *Body Dressing.* Oxford: Berg.

Finkelstein, Joanne. 1991. *The Fashioned Self.* Cambridge, UK: Polity.

Hall, Stuart, and Tony Jefferson (eds.). 1976. *Resistance through Rituals: Youth Subcultures in Post-war Britain.* London: Hutchinson.

Hebdige, Dick. 1979. *Subculture: The Meaning of Style.* London: Methuen.

Laver, James. 1968. *Dandies.* London: Weidenfeld and Nicolson.

Paulicelli, Eugenia, and Hazel Clark. 2009. "Introduction." In Eugenia Paulicelli and Hazel Clark (eds.), *The Fabric of Cultures: Fashion, Identity, Globalization*, 1–12. Oxford: Taylor and Francis.

Sennett, Richard. 1977. *The Fall of Public Man.* New York: Alfred A. Knopf.

5

Fashion and Class Evaluations

KATHERINE APPLEFORD

In 1977 Ivan Reid's study of social class differences in the United Kingdom found that over half of the women interviewed rated dress and behavior as the clearest indication of class position. Over thirty years on it seems not much has changed. Britain is still obsessed with class (Arnold 2001; Jones 2011; McRobbie 2004; Solomon and Rabolt [2004] 2009), and fashion's use as a means of classifying and communicating "social worth and status" appears to have continued (Barnard [1996] 2002: 61; Vinken 2005). British newspapers continually identify a relationship between fashion and social class in terms of retail outlets and fashion trends (e.g., Gold 2011; Mills 2009), and celebrities and their fashions are frequently evaluated in terms of class background (I. Tyler and Bennett 2010; White 2011), while reality fashion programs often have class at their core (McRobbie 2004; Palmer 2004).

Indeed, it seems that within the United Kingdom at least, "fashions remain … class fashions" (Vinken 2005: 15), enabling the British public "to distinguish the superordinate from the subordinate" (McCracken 1985: 46): the posh from the "chav," the "classy" from the "tarty" (Fox 2004). Yet while authors often note that "clothes are one of the main ways … in which class is recognised" (Lurie [1981] 1992: 117), within contemporary sociology few actually explore just how fashion communicates social class. In fact, with the exception of Dick Hebdige's ([1979] 2006) and Stuart Hall and Tony Jefferson's ([1976] 2000) discussions of working-class subcultures, Beverley Skeggs's (1997) work on working-class respectability, and Merl Storr's (2003) research into Anne Summers lingerie, it seems that the association between class and fashion has been largely overlooked. Certainly, contemporary theories that deal specifically with the everyday associations between fashion and class are limited.

Consequently, the aim of this chapter is to highlight the pivotal role that class has traditionally played in understanding British fashion consumption and, more important, to demonstrate its continuing significance for an understanding of mainstream fashion practices and discourses in Britain today. The chapter is divided into three parts. The first part begins by exploring traditional theories of fashion and class, which rely heavily on notions of emulation. Though largely outdated, these theories still provide a useful starting point for this discussion as they offer ideas on how the current fashions may be used as a means of classification and distinction. Moreover, their critiques provide some explanation as to why sociologists have tended to neglect the relationship between fashion and class in favor of gender, race, and subculture. The second part of the chapter looks more closely at the relationship between fashion and identity. It explores the traditional argument, laid out by Georg Simmel ([1901] 2004), that fashion signifies union with one group and thus differentiation from others, and argues that, within Britain at least, fashion is still a key way in which class identity is evaluated and discussed. The third, and final, section of the chapter explores how sociology might renew theories of fashion and class for today's society. It suggests how more modern class theories, such as Pierre Bourdieu's *Distinction* ([1984] 2005), could be used to further examine the role that fashion plays in terms of classification and differentiation, and similarly to assess the role that class plays in informing fashion tastes and practices.

PART I: TRADITIONAL IDEAS ON FASHION AND CLASS

Historically class has played a central role in theories of fashion, with several authors suggesting that the fashion cycle is fueled by the need for class differentiation. Indeed, Simmel ([1901] 2004), Herbert Spencer ([1902] 2004), Ferdinand Tönnies ([1909] 2004), and Thorstein Veblen ([1899] 1994) all suggest that "fashion is a product of class distinction," arguing that fashion is used to "signify union" (Simmel [1901] 2004: 29) and at the same time differentiate social classes during periods of social change, or where there is the potential for social mobility (Polhemus and Procter 1978; Simmel [1901] 2004; Wilson [1985] 2007). Often referred to as "trickle-down" theories, their essays suggest that fashion is the innovation or pursuit of the upper class and is subject to emulation by the middle class in a bid for social status. "Models of the few are imitated by the many" (Tönnies [1909] 2004: 335), motivated by a desire to belong to that group, or class, and in an attempt to advance up the social hierarchy. But as the nature of fashion "demands that it should be exercised at one time only by a portion of the given group," universal adoption means styles of dress lose their exclusivity and fashionable status, and consequently the fashion soon dies out (Simmel [1901] 2004: 295). At the same time, the imitation and mass appropriation of fashionable dress compromises fashion's role as a means of class identification and therefore causes the "higher set [to] throw aside a fashion the moment a lower set adopts it" (306), replacing it with new fashions in an attempt to reestablish class boundaries. And so the cycle continues, with fashion changes and appropriation both being driven by social class.

Although a popular explanation of fashion adoption at the beginning of the twentieth century, these trickle-down theories have faced substantial criticism from more contemporary authors. Colin Campbell ([1987] 2005), Diana Crane (2000), and Fred Davis (1994), for example, maintain that with contemporary fashion, and fashion media, so much more widely available, trickle-down theories are just too simplistic an explanation of the fashion cycle and place too much emphasis on the communication of class identity. The "diffusion of fashion today is highly complex," Crane (2000: 16) argues, and while the "top down model was characteristic of Western societies until the 1960s" (Crane 1999a: 15), it is naive and overdeterministic to suggest, first, that fashion is exclusively the innovation of the upper class or even fashion designers; second, that fashion change is driven by a need for class distinction; and, third, that fashion adoption is driven solely by emulation.

Fashion today, she suggests, is "consumer fashion" rather than "class fashion." It incorporates "tastes and concerns of all social groups" and all social classes (Crane 2000: 135) and emanates from a "multiplicity" of sources. "The product of a chain of activities which are industrial, economic and cultural, as well as aesthetic" (Entwistle [2000] 2004: 220), fashion is diverse, heterogeneous, and unpredictable (Braham [1997] 2003), and its adoption is motivated by a range of factors including social identity and personal taste (Crane 1999a; Davis 1985, 1994). Today's fashion industry is composed of a complex system of fashion designers, fabric and clothing manufacturers, and retailers (Braham [1997] 2003; Breward 2003; Entwistle [2000] 2004). There are fashion capitals all over the globe, including Paris, London, New York, Milan, and Tokyo, and fashion designers with teams of assistants from different countries and different continents are producing new designs at any given moment (Crane 1999a: 15). The increasingly global nature of fashion means that there can be a number of fashionable trends at any one time. And, in fact, there is often "little consensus about the direction in which fashion is moving" (Crane 2000: 161) as biannual fashion collections, used to generate publicity for luxury clothing firms, generate a host of possibilities for fashion trends, which fashion editors, forecasters, and buyers then have to select from for the industrial fashion market.

Rather than there being one design disseminated down the social hierarchy, as the trickle-down model suggests, fashion innovation and fashion production are increasingly differentiated. Today the luxury fashion market caters for the wealthy aristocracy through to the avant-garde, while at the same time generating ideas for mainstream consumer trends. In a bid to satisfy celebrities, professionals, executives, and the very rich, designers produce an array of products that are on the one hand highly conformist and on the other "so highly coded that they are not easily understood by the general public" (Crane 2000: 162). This diversity means that luxury fashion no longer simply represents the styles worn by the upper classes, and while "an elite may influence the direction of taste" (Entwistle [2000] 2004: 222), rarely is it expected that these fashions will be adopted by the mass public.

Instead, "some designers develop cult followings among very specific segments of the upper and upper middle class" (Crane 1999a: 20) or within certain working-class subcultures (de la Haye and Dingwall 1996), such as the chavs' adoption of the Burberry tartan (Martin 2009). For others, aspects of their work may develop subtle tendencies within more mainstream industrial fashion production and high street clothing manufacture. In fact, Braham ([1997] 2003) argues that couture fashion houses are still significant influences among ready-to-wear collections; for those fashion houses owned by multimillion-dollar corporations it is even more important that their designs are "popular and simple enough to be easily translated into mass produced high-street designs" (Entwistle [2000] 2004: 224).

Moreover, although some fashion trends or tendencies may emerge from luxury fashion at the top of the status hierarchy, contemporary fashion innovators can equally be found at the lower end of the social scale. Indeed, the "bubble-up" model suggests that widely accepted fashions can be generated out of lower socioeconomic groups, in particular youth and music subcultures (Blumer [1969] 1981; Davis 1994; Halnon 2002; Polhemus 1994). The process starts with a "genuine streetstyle innovation" (Polhemus 1994: 10) either started by middle-class strata such as homosexual and artistic groups (Crane 1999a: 15) or more typically created by adolescents or young adults within a subculture. Through media coverage such as music videos and magazine articles these fashion innovations are picked up by others in different cities and countries around the world. As their popularity flourishes, they are adopted by increasing sections of the population, and eventually they work their way into the collections of top fashion designers. As a result, "styles which start life on the street corner have a way of ending up on the backs of top models on the world's most prestigious fashion catwalks" (Polhemus 1994: 8), and items that were once subcultural emblems, such as the Bronx leather jacket, become mainstream fashionable alternatives for all (11–12).

Moreover, as Crane (1999a) argues, the emergence of "electronic fashion worlds" means that this type of fashion cycle is becoming more and more common, particularly within the urban music scene. She suggests that popular music corporations, in elevating new bands, also promote and develop new styles of clothing, primarily among adolescents and young people. Aided by the advancement of cable television, they are able to rapidly transmit "street-generated clothing trends" to a wide range of social audiences within localities and across the globe, which consequently leads to more widespread adoption (20). The development of the Internet has intensified this still further, not only enabling individuals to become even more involved in subcultures (Hodkinson 2005: 565), but also operating as a "facilitating network" that allows the global spread of information and ideas, such as fashion trends, at a much greater pace. Indeed, Ruth Marciniak and Margaret Bruce argue that "fashion e-tailing" is becoming more and more popular, and despite "continued speculation over the ability to sell clothes online, the volume of sales of clothing and footwear sold via the Internet has grown steadily" ([2001] 2007: 259). Alongside traditional media formats, then, fashion trends are spreading by "word of mouse" (303) in Internet chat rooms, notice boards, blogs, and online stores as well as through music, clubs, offices, and advertising.

The overall consequence is that today's fashion is much more pluralized and polycentric than the trickle-down model would suggest (Braham [1997] 2003; Davis 1994). Fashion innovation does not simply exist within upper classes, or even couture fashion houses, and it is no longer centrally located, or controlled, and then diffused out to the periphery, or down the social hierarchy (Polhemus and Procter 1978: 16). Rather, fashion leaders sit within all strata of society (Sproles 1985), and there are "multiple fashion systems in which fashion moves up, down and along from a variety of starting positions and in several directions" (Braham [1997] 2003: 145). Fashion is the innovation of designers, subcultures, students, pop icons, ethnic minorities, and haute couture. It is global, local, and electronic, and, consequently, the way in which it is marketed is increasingly diverse and the pace at which it changes has accelerated dramatically.

The substantial development of the fashion industry means that today it is mediated by a great variety of organizations and departments including fashion designers, editors, marketing groups, buyers, and advertisers (Blumer [1969] 1981; Braham [1997] 2003: 134; Entwistle and Rocamora 2006). Fashion "selection" is not simply a reflection of upper-class tastes but a "collective selection" that "represents an effort to choose from among competing styles of models those which match developing tastes" (Blumer [1969] 1981: 52). "Consumers can select from a wide range of current and classic designs and still be entirely 'in fashion' regardless of the particular selection she makes" (King [1963] 1981). What is important is that a style corresponds to the "incipient taste of the fashion consuming public" (Blumer [1969] 1981: 52). Rather than answering a need for class differentiation or prestige, fashion is arguably adopted because it is considered fashionable (Blumer [1969] 1981: 52), and its appropriation is a matter of "personal choice" (Polhemus and Procter 1978: 16). Although a style might be heralded by the elite as the up-and-coming new trend, this does not necessarily mean it will be widely appropriated.

As Crane argues, for clothing companies "to be successful, fashion clothes have to be synchronized with media culture as expressed in television, film and popular music" (1999a: 18). Fashion editors, buyers, and marketers choose styles that will be in keeping with popular media culture as well as developing tastes (18), while at the same time the producers and retailers rely on television media, fashion magazines, and increasingly the Internet to democratize these fashion trends. Programs such as *Sex in the City,* for example, have been fundamental in publicizing particular brands and designs, such as Jimmy Choo and Manolo Blahnik, while simultaneously influencing the production of new fashion designs (König [2004] 2007: 301). Moreover, the growth in fashion magazines such as *Grazia, Look,* and *Glamour* over the past decade, as well as of television programs such as *What Not to Wear, How to Look Good Naked,* and *Ten Years Younger,* has significantly increased knowledge of fashionable styles and awareness of catwalk designs among women across all social classes. This has arguably led to a dramatic rise in consumer demand, as women seek to constantly update their wardrobes with the latest designer trend or fashionable style, often imitating celebrities' looks (Finkelstein 1996; Gibson 2010). Indeed, websites such as ASOS (As Seen On Screen) are marketed precisely on this type of demand.

The increased democratization of fashion trends, combined with the emergence of new "fast fashion" retailers such as Primark and the entry of supermarkets such as Asda, Sainsbury's, and Tesco into the fashion market, means there is far greater competition between traders, and with the rise of mass production, the British fashion cycle has accelerated rapidly. Though it has always been true that the "essence of fashion" lies in its endless need to change and update (Bell [1947] 1976; Simmel [1901] 2004), "nowadays a new fashion may well have difficulty in surviving for a season, let alone for several seasons" (Braham [1997] 2003: 131). According to Liz Barnes and Gaynor Lea-Greenwood, the "'fast fashion' concept has become a mainstay of the UK fashion industry" (2006: 259), and within Britain the fashion cycle has been dramatically reduced as retailers attempt to produce and distribute new fashion products as quickly as possible. This has led to fashion production being outsourced to countries such as Turkey, where "trend fabric" is more readily available and production costs are lower, ultimately "resulting in as many as 20 'seasons' per year" (261). As a result "the lag time for vertical flow of fashion adoption at the consumer level is almost non-existent" (King [1963] 1981: 33), which is yet another reason why trickle-down models can no longer apply.

PART II: FASHION AND (CLASS) IDENTITY

While contemporary authors argue that fashion adoption is driven by "collective selection," media influence, and consumer tastes, they also suggest that fashion is highly concerned with the production of different social identities (Crane 1999a, 2000; King [1963] 1981) and one's sense of self (Crane 1999a: 18; Davis 1994; Woodward 2007). In writing about women and their wardrobes, for instance, Sophie Woodward (2007) argues that clothing enables women to construct social identities and enact certain personality traits. Women use fashion to extend their sense of self and, depending on the social context, "bring out" particular aspects of their character. Fashion production may be increasingly diverse, and fashion adoption may be driven by popularity, or personal taste, but ultimately the clothes people wear still provide "one of the most ready means through which individuals make expressive visual statements about their identities" (A. Bennett 2005: 103), and part of that social identity is a class identity.

But whereas traditional trickle-down theories focus solely on class identity and ignore other aspects such as age, gender, ethnicity, sexuality, and political affiliations, to name but a few, contemporary sociology appears to have gone in the opposite direction. In fact, recent work has been reluctant to acknowledge the important relationship fashion still maintains with social class and has preferred instead to concentrate on the relationships between fashion and subcultures, fashion and gender (Woodward 2007), dress and ethnicity (Eicher 1995), or more recently fashion and religion (Tarlo 2010). Yet within these discussions are the basic arguments for the continued association between fashion and class, as they demonstrate quite clearly that fashion is still used as a means of constructing a social character and classifying individuals. Indeed, the literature on subcultures shows quite plainly that fashion is still an important means of "union" and "isolation," just as Simmel ([1901] 2004: 291) suggested, signifying "union with those in the same class" and at the same time excluding those from "all other groups."

Stuart Hall and Tony Jefferson ([1976] 2000), Dick Hebdige ([1979] 2006), and Ted Polhemus (1994), for instance, all agree that fashion is often a crucial aspect in the construction of subcultural identities, used to create a spectacle and mark them out from the mainstream. Whether it be the distinctive "tribal" hair and makeup of punks; the black velvet, lace, and tightly laced corsets of goths (Polhemus 1994); or the bootlace ties and velvet-collared drape jackets of the Teddy Boys (Hebdige [1979] 2006: 96), clothing and possessions are used to identify individuals as belonging to a group or class and at the same time to distinguish them from all others both inside and outside of the community (Entwistle [2000] 2004: 137).

Moreover, within their discussions, these authors also acknowledge an association between fashion and class, arguing that mods and rockers, skinheads and Teddy Boys are all considered to be working-class groups (Hall and Jefferson [1976] 2000; Hebdige [1979] 2006; Polhemus 1994; Polhemus and Procter 1978). As a result, their work suggests not only that these fashion choices work to communicate subcultural identity but also that fashion is concerned with class identity, too. In fact, Hall and Jefferson suggest that "in modern societies the most fundamental groups are the social classes" ([1976] 2000: 12), while Hebdige suggests that fashion communicates class not only within subcultures but in the context of mainstream conventional society too:

> The conventional outfits worn by the average man and woman in the street are chosen with the constraints of finance, "taste," preference, etc. and these choices are undoubtedly significant. Each ensemble has its place in an internal system of differences—the conventional modes of sartorial discourse—which fit a corresponding set of socially prescribed roles and options. These choices contain a whole range of messages which are transmitted through the finely graded distinction of a number of interlocking sets—class and status, self-image and attractiveness, etc. ([1979] 2006: 101)

That is not to say that fashion is not concerned with personality, individual choice, or even other forms of social identity. Even Simmel acknowledges that "while fashion postulates a certain amount of general acceptance, it nevertheless is not without significance in the character of the individual, for it emphasises his personality" ([1901] 2004: 297). But at the same time, despite the diversity in contemporary British fashion and the increased availability of fashion trends, fashion choices still operate as an important means of evaluation in terms of wealth and class (Fischer-Mirkin 1995; Storr 2003). And as Bernard Barber and Lyle S. Lobel argue,

> At least on first glance we all apply the following equation: consumption equals wealth or income, wealth or income equals occupational position, occupational position equals social class, and therefore consumption equals social class position. ([1952] 1993: 130)

This association between fashion and class, and this form of class evaluation, is clearly evident in British press and popular culture, with celebrities such as Jade Goody, Kerry Katona, and Katie Price often being branded as working class or "chavy" on the basis of their dress (Skeggs and Wood 2012a, 2012b; I. Tyler and Bennett 2010). At the same time, programs such as *The Only Way Is Essex; Made in Chelsea; Snog, Marry, Avoid;* and *My Big Fat Gypsy Wedding* work to reinforce the "haves and chavs" divide (Duncan 2011). As Dale Southerton (2002), Merl Storr (2003), and Imogen Tyler (2008) suggest, it seems that fashion is used to create distinction between "us" and "them," not only within the media but within everyday life; in fact, the very emergence of the "chav" phenomenon demonstrates the clear class evaluations that are made on the basis of dress.

According to Antoinette Renouf, *chav* was originally a Romany term for a young child, which first emerged in English texts in the 1990s. In 2004, however, the term was revised and used by the press to refer to a "British person of low education, having insufficient means to live away from home, though sufficient to indulge in the purchase and wearing of hitherto socially prestigious clothing, such as *Burberry* Caps" (Renouf 2007: 75). Indeed, today "chavs" are identified by their "excessive participation in forms of... consumption" and in particular by their dress (Hayward and Yar 2006: 14). Their "branded or designer casual wear and sportswear" and excessive makeup and jewelry, including "chunky gold rings and chains" (2006: 14) and "hoop earrings" (I. Tyler 2008: 26), operate as class markers, allowing them to "not only recognise themselves" but "crucially" to be "recognised by others" (Haywood and Yar 2006: 14). In the same way that punks are distinguishable by their quiffs and leather jackets, and mods by their absurd neatness (Hebdige [1979] 2006), chavs too are chiefly differentiated from other groups and mainstream society on the basis of their dress.

Moreover, as I argue elsewhere (see Appleford 2011) chavs are often cited by middle-class women as a point of distinction, in order to establish themselves as respectable and simultaneously create distance from any working-class connotations of sexuality and/or deviance. This relationship between fashion, class, and respectability is highlighted in the work of Stephanie Lawler (2005a), Skeggs (1997), and Storr (2003). Arguing that notions of femininity are created and performed within a classed context, they suggest that there are clear class distinctions in the way in which femininity is understood and performed by women. Moreover, whereas middle-class performances of femininity are regarded as the "real thing, the (quint)essence of femininity" (C. Tyler 1991: 57), and thus considered normal, appropriate, and respectable, working-class practices tend to be classified as something "other" and are often considered to be morally inferior as a result (Sayer 2002; Sennett and Cobb 1972; C. Tyler 1991).

Though Lawler (2005a), Skeggs (1997), and Storr (2003) do not look specifically at everyday fashion consumption or tastes, their discussions nevertheless suggest that there are important class differences in women's fashion practices and attitudes, as femininity is, in part, "performed" through fashion (Evans and Thornton 1989: 13; MacDonald [1995] 2004). Again, then, their work demonstrates that although fashion may be concerned with self-identity, gender, race, sexuality, or subculture, it is at the same time concerned with class identity. Indeed, as with other areas of social life (Crenshaw 1991), it seems that these different categories intersect in terms of individuals' fashion choices, but all too often sociologists have overlooked the class aspect of social identity. How then can sociology move on and redress the balance? And what exactly do sociologists need to explore?

PART III: RENEWING THEORIES OF FASHION AND CLASS

Although class has tended to be viewed as outdated, particularly during the 1980s and 1990s (Smith 2000), over the last decade the concept has had something of a renaissance, and within sociology it has become a much more popular topic for social research (see, for example, Casey 2008; Lawler and Byrne 2005; Savage 2000; Savage, Bagnall, and Longhurst 2001; Taylor 2008; Tomlinson 2003). Indeed, for Rosemary Crompton (1998, 2008), Fiona Devine and Mike Savage and colleagues (Devine 1997; Devine and Savage 2005; Savage 2000; Savage, Bagnall, and Longhurst 2001), Stephanie Lawler (2005b), and Beverley Skeggs (2004, 2005), class remains "central to the sociological enterprise" (Crompton 2008: 1). But, they argue, the way in which we understand class has changed. Rather than evaluating class solely on the basis of occupation, they suggest that sociology adopts a more Bourdieuian approach to class that acknowledges cultural practices and tastes (Bourdieu [1984] 2005).

In the 1970s changes in Western employment structures, including increased feminization of the workforce and a growing service sector industry, made occupational class distinctions much less clear (Pakulski and Waters 1996). Traditional class models were brought into question (Crompton 1993, 2008; Devine 1997; Savage 2000), and sociologists argued that society was increasingly individualized and stratified on the basis of lifestyle (e.g., Bauman 1982; Beck 1992; Giddens 1991; Pahl 1989; Pakulski and Waters 1996). Attention turned to other forms of stratification such as gender, race, and subculture (Smith 2000). The importance of class as a means of explaining attitudes and practices waned (Walkerdine, Lucey, and Melody 2001), and some authors argued that class had been brought "to a point of decomposition" (Pakulski and Waters 1996: 24) and western Europe had moved "beyond a class society" (Beck and Beck-Gernsheim 2002: 30).

However, while Crompton (1993, 1998) and others accept that traditional class models, which differentiate groups solely on the basis of occupation, are somewhat limited, they argue that class distinctions through cultural practices and tastes persist and have in many ways become more definite (Bottero 2004). "Class is a word with a number of meanings," including "prestige, status, culture or lifestyle" (Crompton 2008: 15), and it is in this sense that class is still relevant (Savage 2000; Savage, Bagnall, and Longhurst 2001; Skeggs 1997, 2004). Instead of taking a Marxist view of class that centers on production, as Jan Pakulski and Malcolm Waters (1996) do, Crompton and others claim that contemporary understandings of class must acknowledge that class is not only concerned with our economic position, or what Bourdieu terms the "conditions of existence," but also consumption habits and practices, or "dispositions" (Bourdieu [1984] 2005: 53).

It is in Bourdieu's *Distinction* ([1984] 2005) that he "develops a systematic theory of symbolic power and its relations to economic and political power" (Brubaker 1985: 747). By linking stratification by status to stratification by class, through the notion of lifestyle, he demonstrates how class-based inequalities are apparent in "everyday consumption practices" (749). Instead of defining class simply on the basis of production, Bourdieu takes a much broader view, arguing that one's position in the social space is dependent on "capital," which can take "*three* fundamental guises" (1986: 243). The first is economic capital, which is the traditional basis for class distinctions and refers to income and wealth, or ownership of property. The second is "cultural capital," which can be either embodied in perspectives, movements, and mannerisms; objectified in the form of cultural goods, such as books and musical instruments; or institutionalized in the form of educational qualifications. Third, there is social capital. This refers to the social networks and acquaintances that bring some form of "credential," either economic or cultural.

Together, these various forms of capital provide the basis for "conditions of existence," defined as our distance "from necessity" and "practical urgencies" (Bourdieu [1984] 2005: 53). Expressed through lifestyles, Bourdieu argues that "conditions of existence" give rise to diverse practices and "dispositions," such as the "concern for conformity" or a desire for functionalism and practicality (331). The "aesthetic disposition," for instance, reflects an ability to fulfill basic necessities and practicalities and consequently concentrates on the "mode of representation" and "style," demonstrated through a "practice of activities which are an end in themselves, such as scholastic exercise or the contemplation of works of art" (54).

Not only do "conditions of existence" result in differing lifestyles, however; they also produce different "habitus" (Bourdieu [1984] 2005, 1990). This is a structure that "generates" internalized practices and perceptions, which operate as "distinctive signs" or "classifiable" acts, and simultaneously allows individuals "to differentiate and appreciate these practices and products (tastes)" ([1984] 2005: 170). "Taste classifies, and it classifies the classifier" (6). Indeed, anything, from our ways of eating, drinking, talking, or walking to even the most "automatic gestures," such as "blowing our nose," are, according to Bourdieu, a product of our class habitus and as such operate as a means of classification (466).

Moreover, as well as structuring individual practices, Bourdieu argues that the habitus also operates as a "structuring structure" ([1984] 2005: 170), locating individuals in a social hierarchy, as the appropriation of cultural goods and knowledge demonstrates their "taste of freedom," while distance from necessity brings with it "legitimated superiority" (56). As a result, their cultural practices and tastes, indeed their lifestyle, become what Max Weber terms "stylisation of life" ([1948] 1970: 191): a sign of honor and status, associated with the most socially and economically privileged, while "dispositions" become a means of distinction. Consequently, "social class comes much closer to that of status group than does the conception of purely economic class" (Giddens [1973] 1980: 48) and is therefore identified on the basis of differences in leisure activities, food, and clothing.

Since suggesting that class can be identified through our cultural practices, attitudes, and dispositions, several authors have demonstrated how class informs, and is made apparent, through musical tastes and newspaper readership (T. Bennett et al. 2010), preferences in food (Tomlinson 1994), gambling habits (Casey 2008), and even gardening activities (Taylor 2008).The emergence of the "chav" phenomenon further demonstrates the links between consumption and class, with emphasis placed on consumer goods and cultural preferences in relation to cars, mobile phones, pets, television programs, and fashion (Jones 2011; Lawler 2005b; Nayak 2006; I. Tyler 2008; I. Tyler and Bennett 2010).

But, as already noted, the role that class plays in informing fashion choices, and the way in which fashion is used to make class evaluations today, has been largely ignored. Even within Bourdieu's *Distinction* ([1984] 2005), the discussion of fashion specifically is limited to just a few sections, and instead greater credence is given to cultural distinctions in terms of food, art, and music. And yet at the same time authors continue to claim that fashion is a key way in which class is evaluated (e.g., Barnard [1996] 2002; Forsythe, Drake, and Hogan 1985; Fox 2004; Mount 2004) and further suggest that there are marked class differences in consumer practices (Miller et al. 1998; Solomon and Rabolt [2004] 2009).

Even if we just follow Bourdieu's argument that taste is a marker of class ([1984] 2005: 12), it seems reasonable to suggest that people's fashion choices, their knowledge of fashion, and their consumption practices will operate as a means of class distinction, no matter how democratized or pluralized fashion is. Arguably determined by our "conditions of existence" and social origins, fashion dispositions are informed by class location. Although individuals may have a greater awareness of fashion through magazines, television, or the Internet, and may be influenced by any number of fashion leaders, there will still be class differences in terms of their fashion adoption, preferences, and tastes. For instance, Angela Partington claims that even when social classes adopt the same styles of dress, they are still able to "articulate class identities" by using "deliberately different appropriation," thus creating a different version of a given fashion and providing it with a new meaning (1992: 146). Further, as Daniel Miller and colleagues (1998) and Michael Solomon and Nancy Rabolt ([2004] 2009) both suggest, there are general differences in the buying criteria of the middle and working classes.

Though Bourdieu ([1984] 2005) does not write extensively about fashion, his work does suggest that the practices and consumption of the working and middle classes are significantly different and that these general distinctions are made evident through their clothing choices. For example, he argues that while the middle class has a "habitus of order" that places emphasis on formality, restraint, and propriety, members of the working class have much greater concern for "practical urgencies" and thus "seek 'value for money,' and choose what will last" (201). These differences have crucial implications for the clothes they wear. In fact, he suggests that the working class has a functional approach to clothing and buys items on the basis of practicality, whereas the middle class, anxious over the judgments made by others, looks for "fashionable and original garments" (247).

Although the idea that contemporary working-class individuals buy only practical and functional clothing or that the middle classes look particularly for "fashionable" items is, as I have discussed elsewhere (Appleford 2011), vastly outdated, the notion that there are clear class differences in practices and dispositions is still salient. The increase in mass production, the outsourcing of fashion manufacturing, and the development of "fast" and "disposable" clothing have made fashion more democratized and affordable. "Well made apparel is available for everyone" (Solomon and Rabolt [2004] 2009: 263), and the working class is much more able, therefore, to engage with, and consume, fashionable goods and clothing (Partington 1992; I. Tyler 2008). Indeed, as I have previously shown (Appleford 2011), today's British working-class women have a keen desire to follow fashion. No longer restricted by a "taste of necessity," they are eager to buy fashionable trends at low cost and quickly dispose of them. But this does not mean that class distinctions do not remain. For while working classes seem keen to buy fashion cheaply, it seems that middle-class purchases are by contrast motivated much more by a desire for practicality and longevity, with their buying criteria focusing much more heavily on notions of quality, cut, and "classic" styles. Indeed, fashion may be more democratized, but it seems that class distinctions in terms of fabric, color, and cut strongly persist, with middle-class women preferring more neutral colors and natural fabrics, as opposed to their working-class counterparts, who look for trend-led and conspicuous items.

It is not only in relation to buying criteria that there are important class distinctions, however. Bourdieu's work also suggests that perceptions of social audiences differ between class groups and that this has implications for fashion adoption, too. Arguing that the middle classes are highly aware of the judgments made by others, he suggests that they have an immense desire to be "seen in a good light." This leads to a "disposition towards the bluff," which causes them to imitate or "usurp" the social identity of higher social classes in order to give a "self representation normally associated with those in a higher position" ([1984] 2005: 253). In many respects his assertion is similar to those made by emulation theorists, as he argues that the middle classes imitate the "symbolic goods" of those with "distinction," thereby "forcing the possessor of distinctive properties…to engage in an endless pursuit of new properties through which to assert their rarity" (251–52). As such, his argument is subject to the same criticisms leveled at Simmel ([1901] 2004) and Veblen ([1899] 1994). But at the same time it highlights how different perceptions or dispositions lead to differences in practice, and further suggests that there are significant distinctions in the ways in which the middle and working classes view audiences and themselves.

Since Bourdieu's work is based on 1960s France, the extent to which his specific ideas are still accurate in terms of contemporary British practice is questionable. For one, Britain has a peculiar obsession with class (Ringen 1996), and therefore his explanation of fashion and class, based on French society, will not necessarily accurately represent the relationship in today's United Kingdom (Archer 1993). In addition, the nature of fashion and consumption has changed considerably in recent years (Crane 1999a, 1999b, 2000; Lipovetsky 1994; Slater 1997), and increased affluence across all social classes has also enabled the working class to engage much more in fashionable consumption (Partington 1992). So it is unlikely that working-class consumption is driven only by a "taste of necessity" or, indeed, that fashion consumption is only determined by class identity (Davis 1994; Rocamora 2002; Slater 1997).

But although Bourdieu's specific explanations may be less convincing today, the general premise that there are different criteria for fashion purchases, different fashion tastes, and different perceptions of social space between the classes is arguably still salient, as demonstrated by the popular British press. In 2010, for example, a number of news articles reported Tesco's ban on shoppers entering the store in their nightwear, because it was considered "offensive" and "embarrassing" to others in the store (Hornby 2010). While it had been regular attire for some of their working-class customers, who did not perceive the space as public, when "popping in" to buy a small number of items (Hornby 2010), it was considered inappropriate by Tesco because, within the context of the middle class, it was deemed to be a space that necessitated a more "public" form of dress.

Although these distinctions have been noted by the media, within sociology the relationship between fashion, class, and space has not been fully explored. Malcolm Barnard ([1996] 2002: 115) and Angela McRobbie (1994), for example, both discuss the common conception that working-class and middle-class individuals dress differently for different social spaces and social audiences, but they do not fully explain just *how* fashion, class, and space are linked. Similarly, Efrat Tseëlon (1992, 1995) argues that there is an important relationship between fashion, space, and femininity. But, again, she neglects the role that class plays in terms of the perceptions of space and audiences.

There is a definite gap in the literature, which sociology needs to explore. Fashion has become an area of much greater interest to sociology in recent years. The journal *Fashion Theory* and a variety of other publications, including *The Fashioned Body* (Entwistle [2000] 2004), *Fashioning the City* (Rocamora 2009), *Why Women Wear What They Wear* (Woodward 2007), and *Clothes* (Harvey 2008), demonstrate its growing popularity as a topic for inquiry. In fact, in the last twenty years or so, "the study of fashion... has been transformed" (Entwistle and Wilson [2001] 2005: 1), and the important role it plays in regard to consumption and identity has been much more widely acknowledged. But the equally important role that class plays in relation to fashion consumption and identity needs to be recognized and fully examined.

CONCLUSION

As a form of visual culture, fashion plays an important role in terms of distinguishing and distancing individuals and groups within mainstream, ordinary society. "Always in evidence" (Veblen [1899] 1994: 102), fashion offers an immediate means of recognition and differentiation, and although distinctions may be less overt than they have been in the past, they are still no less important. Moreover, with class theorists arguing that cultural practices and tastes play an increasingly important role in determining class location and classifying individuals, it seems even more crucial that the relationship between fashion and class is properly acknowledged. Class is about distinctions in cultural knowledge, attitude, and practices. It "is not based on recognising oneself as belonging to a given position, but as differentiating oneself from others in a field" (Devine and Savage 2005: 14), and fashion, as the literature on subcultures shows, offers one of the most instantly accessibly ways of creating and constructing those dividing lines of "us" and "them" (Southerton 2002).

BIBLIOGRAPHY

Appleford, Katherine. 2011. "Classifying Fashion and Fashioning Class." PhD diss., London College of Fashion, University of the Arts London.

Archer, Margaret. 1993. "Bourdieu's Theory of Cultural Reproduction: French or Universal?" *French Cultural Studies* 4 (12): 225–40.

Arnold, Rebecca. 2001. *Fashion, Desire and Anxiety: Image and Morality in the 20th Century.* New York: I. B. Tauris.

Barber, Bernard, and Lyle S. Lobel. [1952] 1993. "Fashion in Women's Clothes and the American Social System." In Bernard Barber, *Constructing the Social System*, 127–43. New Brunswick, NJ: Transaction.

Barnard, Malcolm. [1996] 2002. *Fashion as Communication.* London: Routledge.

Barnes, Liz, and Gaynor Lea-Greenwood. 2006. "Fast Fashioning the Supply Chain: Shaping the Research Agenda." *Journal of Fashion Marketing and Management* 10 (3): 259–71.

Bauman, Zygmunt. 1982. *Memories of Class: The Pre-history and After-life of Class.* London: Routledge & Kegan Paul.

Beck, Ulrich. 1992. *Risk Society: Towards a New Modernity.* London: Sage.

Beck, Ulrich, and Elizabeth Beck-Gernsheim. 2002. *Individualization: Institutionalized Individualism and Its Social and Political Consequences.* London: Sage.

Bell, Quentin. [1947] 1976. *On Human Finery.* London: Hogarth.

Bennett, Andy. 2005. *Culture and Everyday Life.* London: Sage.

Bennett, Tony, Mike Savage, Elizabeth Bortolaia Silva, Alan Warde, Modesto Gayo-Cal, and David Wright. 2010. *Culture, Class, Distinction.* London: Routledge.

Blumer, Herbert. [1969] 1981. "Fashion: From Class Differentiation to Collective Selection." In George B. Sproles (ed.), *Perspectives of Fashion,* 49–57. Minneapolis: Burgess.

Bottero, Wendy. 2004. "Class Identities and the Identity of Class." *Sociology* 38 (5): 985–1003.

Bourdieu, Pierre. [1984] 2005. *Distinction: A Social Critique of the Judgement of Taste.* London: Routledge & Kegan Paul.

Bourdieu, Pierre. 1986. "The Forms of Capital." In John G. Richardson (ed.), *Handbook of Theory and Research for the Sociology of Education,* 241–58. London: Greenwood.

Bourdieu, Pierre. 1990. *The Logic of Practice.* Cambridge, UK: Polity.

Braham, Peter. [1997] 2003. "Fashion: Unpacking a Cultural Production." In Paul Du Gay (ed.), *Production of Culture, Cultures of Production,* 119–76. London: Sage.

Breward, Christopher. 2003. *Fashion.* Oxford: Berg.

Brubaker, Rogers. 1985. "Rethinking Classical Theory: The Sociological Vision of Pierre Bourdieu." *Theory and Society* 14 (6): 745–75.

Campbell, Colin. [1987] 2005. *The Romantic Ethic and the Spirit of Modern Consumerism.* Oxford: Blackwell.

Casey, Emma. 2008. *Women, Pleasure and the Gambling Experience.* Aldershot, UK: Ashgate.

Crane, Diana. 1999a. "Diffusion Models and Fashion: A Reassessment." *Annals of the American Academy of Political and Social Science* 566 (1): 13–24.

Crane, Diana. 1999b. "Gender and Hegemony in Fashion Magazines: Women's Interpretations of Fashion Photographs." *Sociological Quarterly* 40 (4): 531–63.

Crane, Diana. 2000. *Fashion and Its Social Agenda: Class, Gender, and Identity in Clothing.* Chicago: University of Chicago Press.

Crenshaw, Kimberle. 1991. "Mapping the Margins: Intersectionality, Identity Politics and Violence against Women of Colour." *Stanford Law Review* 43 (6): 1241–99.

Crompton, Rosemary. 1993. *Class and Stratification: An Introduction to Current Debates.* Cambridge, UK: Polity.

Crompton, Rosemary. 1998. *Class and Stratification: An Introduction to Current Debates.* 2nd ed. Cambridge, UK: Polity.

Crompton, Rosemary. 2008. *Class and Stratification.* 3rd ed. Cambridge, UK: Polity.

Davis, Fred. 1985. "Clothing and Fashion as Communication." In Michael R. Solomon (ed.), *The Psychology of Fashion,* 15–77. Lexington, MA: Lexington Books.

Davis, Fred. 1994. *Fashion, Culture and Identity.* Chicago: University of Chicago Press.

de la Haye, Amy, and Cathie Dingwall. 1996. *Surfers, Soulies, Skinheads and Skaters: Subcultural Style from the Forties to the Nineties.* New York: Overlook.

Devine, Fiona. 1997. "Towards a Classless Society." In H. Jones (ed.), *Towards a Classless Society,* 201–24. London: Routledge.

Devine, Fiona, and Mike Savage. 2005. "The Cultural Turn, Sociology and Class Analysis." In Fiona Devine, Mike Savage, John Scott, and Rosemary Crompton (eds.), *Rethinking Class: Culture, Identities and Lifestyles,* 1–23. Basingstoke, UK: Palgrave.

Duncan, Amy. 2011. "Made in Chelsea Gang Confuse *The Only Way Is Essex* Stars on Twitter." *The Metro* (London), May 18.

Eicher, Joanne B. 1995. *Dress and Ethnicity: Change across Space and Time.* Oxford: Berg.

Entwistle, Joanne. [2000] 2004. *The Fashioned Body.* Cambridge, UK: Polity.

Entwistle, Joanne, and Agnès Rocamora. 2006. "Field of Fashion Materialised: A Study of London Fashion Week." *Sociology* 40 (4): 735–51.

Entwistle, Joanne, and Elizabeth Wilson. [2001] 2005. "Introduction." In Joanne Entwistle and Elizabeth Wilson (eds.), *Body Dressing,* 1–12. Oxford: Berg.

Evans, Caroline, and Minna Thornton. 1989. *Women in Fashion: A New Look.* London: Quartet.

Finkelstein, Joanne. 1996. *After a Fashion.* Carlton South, Australia: Melbourne University Press.

Fischer-Mirkin, Toby. 1995. *Dress Code: Understanding the Hidden Meaning of Women's Clothes.* New York: Clarkson Potter.

Forsythe, Sandra M., Mary Frances Drake, and Jane H. Hogan. 1985. "Influences of Clothing Attributes on the Perception of Personal Characteristics." In Michael R. Solomon (ed.), *The Psychology of Fashion,* 267–78. Lexington, MA: Lexington Books.

Fox, Kate. 2004. *Watching the English: The Rules of English Behaviour.* London: Vintage.

Gibson, Pamela Church. 2010. "Actors and Actresses' Impact on Fashion." In Valerie Steele (ed.), *Berg Companion to Fashion,* 4–5. Oxford: Berg.

Giddens, Anthony. [1973] 1980. *The Class Structure of the Advanced Societies.* London: Hutchinson.

Giddens, Anthony. 1991. *Modernity and Self Identity: Self and Society in the Late Modern Age.* Stanford, CA: Stanford University Press.

Gold, Tanya. 2011. "Is Anyone Safe from World War Twee?" *The Telegraph* (London), June 24.

Hall, Stuart, and Tony Jefferson. [1976] 2000. *Resistance through Rituals: Youth Subcultures in Post-war Britain.* London: Routledge.

Halnon, Karen Bettez. 2002. "Poor Chic: The Rational Consumption of Poverty." *Current Sociology* 50 (4): 501–16.

Harvey, John Robert. 2008. *Clothes.* Stocksfield, UK: Acumen.

Hayward, Keith, and Majid Yar. 2006. "The 'Chav' Phenomenon: Consumption, Media and the Construction of a New Underclass." *Crime Media Culture* 2 (1): 9–28.

Hebdige, Dick. [1979] 2006. *Subculture: The Meaning of Style.* London: Routledge.

Hodkinson, Paul. 2005. "Communicating Goth." In Ken Gelder (ed.), *The Subcultures Reader,* 564–74. Oxford: Routledge.

Hornby, Gill. 2010. "Tescos and Nightwear: A Wake-Up Call for Jim-Jam Masses." *The Telegraph* (London), January 29.

Jones, Owen. 2011. *Chavs: The Demonization of the Working Class.* London: Verso.

King, Charles W. [1963] 1981. "A Rebuttal to the Trickle-Down Theory." In George B. Sproles (ed.), *Perspectives of Fashion,* 31–39. Minneapolis: Burgess.

König, Anna. [2004] 2007. "Sex and the City: A Fashion Editor's Dream." In Linda Welters and Abby Lillethun (eds.), *The Fashion Reader,* 130–43. Oxford: Berg.

Lawler, Stephanie. 2005a. "Disgusted Subjects: The Making of Middle Class Identities." *The Editorial Board of the Sociological Review* 2005: 429–46.

Lawler, Stephanie. 2005b. "Introduction: Class Culture and Identity." *Sociology* 39 (1): 797–806.

Lawler, Stephanie, and David Byrne (eds.). 2005. "Class, Culture and Identity." Special issue, *Sociology* 39 (5).

Lipovetsky, Gilles. 1994. *The Empire of Fashion: Dressing Modern Democracy.* Princeton, NJ: Princeton University Press.

Lurie, Alison. [1981] 1992. *The Language of Clothes.* London: Bloomsbury.

MacDonald, Myra. [1995] 2004. *Representing Women: Myths of Femininity in Popular Media.* London: Edward Arnold.

Marciniak, Ruth, and Margaret Bruce. [2001] 2007. "Fashion E-tailing." In Tony Hines and Margaret Bruce (eds.), *Fashion Marketing: Contemporary Issues,* 259–77. Oxford: Elsevier.

Martin, Greg. 2009. "Subculture, Style, Chavs and Consumer Capitalism: Towards a Critical Cultural Criminology of Youth." *Crime Media Culture* 5 (2): 123–45.

McCracken, Grant D. 1985. "The Trickle Down Theory Rehabilitated." In Michael R. Solomon (ed.), *The Psychology of Fashion,* 39–54. Lexington, MA: Lexington Books.

McRobbie, Angela. 1994. *Postmodernism and Popular Culture.* London: Routledge.

McRobbie, Angela. 2004. "What Not to Wear and Post-feminist Symbolic Violence." *The Sociological Review* 52 (s2): 97–109.

Miller, Daniel, Peter Jackson, Nigel Thrift, Beverley Holbrook, and Michael Rowlands. 1998. *Shopping, Place and Identity.* London: Routledge.

Mills, Simon. 2009. "How the Posh Hoodie Came of Age." *The Guardian,* January 7. http://www.guardian.co.uk/lifeandstyle/2009/jan/07/hoodies-fashion-retailers (accessed January 12, 2009).

Mount, Ferdinand. 2004. *Mind the Gap: The New Class Divide in Britain.* London: Shortbooks.

Nayak, Anoop. 2006. "Displaced Masculinities: Chavs, Youth and Class in the Post-industrial City." *Sociology* 40 (5): 813–31.

Pahl, Raymond Edward. 1989. "Is the Emperor Naked?" *International Journal of Urban and Regional Research* 13 (4): 711–20.

Pakulski, Jan, and Malcolm Waters. 1996. *The Death of Class.* London: Sage.

Palmer, Graham. 2004. "The New You: Class Transformations in Lifestyle Television." In Susan Holmes and Deborah Jermyn (eds.), *Understanding Reality Television,* 173–90. London: Routledge.

Partington, Angela. 1992. "Popular Fashion and Working Class Affluence." In Juliet Ash and Elizabeth Wilson (eds.), *Chic Thrills: A Fashion Reader,* 145–61. London: HarperCollins.

Polhemus, Ted. 1994. *Street-Style: From Sidewalk to Catwalk.* London: Thames and Hudson.

Polhemus, Ted, and Lynn Procter. 1978. *Fashion and Anti-fashion: Anthropology of Clothing and Adornment.* London: Thames and Hudson.

Reid, Ivan. 1977. *Social Class Differences in Britain.* London: Open Books.

Renouf, Antoinette. 2007. "Tracing Lexical Productivity and Creativity in the British Media: 'The Chav and the Chav-Nots.'" In J. Munat (ed.), *Lexical Creativity, Text and Context,* 61–89. Amsterdam: John Benjamins.

Ringen, Stein. 1996. "The Truth about Class Inequalities." *Czech Sociology Review* 42 (3): 475–92.

Rocamora, Agnès. 2002. "Fields of Fashion: Critical Insights into Bourdieu's Sociology of Culture." *Journal of Consumer Culture* 2 (3): 341–62.

Rocamora, Agnès. 2009. *Fashioning the City: Paris, Fashion and the Media.* London: I. B. Tauris.

Savage, Mike. 2000. *Class Analysis and Social Transformations.* Buckingham, UK: Open University Press.

Savage, Mike, Gaynor Bagnall, and Brian Longhurst. 2001. "Ordinary, Ambivalent and Defensive." *Sociology* 35 (4): 875–92.

Sayer, Andrew. 2002. "'What Are You Worth?' Why Class Is an Embarrassing Subject." *Sociology Research Online* 7 (3). http://www.socresonline.org.uk/7/3/sayer.html (accessed May 16, 2006).

Sennett, Richard, and Jonathan Cobb. 1972. *Hidden Injuries of Class.* New York: Knopf.

Simmel, Georg. [1901] 2004. "Fashion." In Daniel Leonhard Purdy (ed.), *The Rise of Fashion: A Reader,* 294–323. Minneapolis: University of Minnesota Press.
Skeggs, Beverley. 1997. *Formations of Class and Gender: Becoming Respectable.* London: Sage.
Skeggs, Beverley. 2004. *Class, Self and Culture.* London: Routledge.
Skeggs, Beverley. 2005. "The Making of Class and Gender through Visualizing Moral Subject Formation." *Sociology* 39 (5): 965–82.
Skeggs, Beverley, and Helen Wood. 2012a. *Reacting to Reality TV: Performance, Audience and Value.* Oxford: Routledge.
Skeggs, Beverley, and Helen Wood. 2012b. *Reality Television and Class.* London: British Film Institute.
Slater, Don. 1997. *Consumer Culture and Modernity.* Oxford: Blackwell.
Smith, Neil. 2000. "What Happened to Class?" *Environment and Planning A* 32: 1011–32.
Solomon, Michael, and Nancy J. Rabolt. [2004] 2009. *Consumer Behaviour in Fashion.* Upper Saddle River, NJ: Pearson/Prentice Hall.
Southerton, Dale. 2002. "Boundaries of 'Us' and 'Them.'" *Sociology* 36 (1): 171–90.
Spencer, Herbert. [1902] 2004. "Fashion." From *The Principles of Sociology.* In Daniel Leonhard Purdy (ed.), *The Rise of Fashion: A Reader,* 328–32. Minneapolis: University of Minnesota Press.
Sproles, George B. 1985. "Behavioural Science Theories of Fashion." In Michael R. Solomon (ed.), *The Psychology of Fashion,* 15–28. Lexington, MA: Lexington Books.
Storr, Merl. 2003. *Latex and Lingerie.* Oxford: Berg.
Tarlo, Emma. 2010. *Visibly Muslim: Fashion, Politics and Faith.* Oxford: Berg.
Taylor, Lisa. 2008. *A Taste of Gardening: Classed and Gendered Practices.* Hampshire, UK: Ashgate.
Tomlinson, Mark. 1994. "Do Distinct Class Preferences for Foods Exist? *British Food Journal* 96 (7): 11–17.
Tomlinson, M. 2003. "Lifestyles and Social Class." *European Sociological Review* 19: 97–111.
Tönnies, Ferdinand. [1909] 2004. "Customs: An Essay on Social Codes." In Daniel Leonhard Purdy (ed.), *The Rise of Fashion: A Reader,* 333–40. Minneapolis: University of Minnesota Press.
Tseëlon, Efrat. 1992. "Self Presentation through Appearance: A Manipulative vs. Dramaturgical Approach." *Symbolic Interaction* 15 (4): 501–13.
Tseëlon, Efrat. 1995. *The Masque of Femininity: The Presentation of Woman in Everyday Life.* London: Sage.
Tyler, Carole-Anne. 1991. "Boys Will Be Girls: The Politics of Gay Drag." In Diane Fuss (ed.), *Multiculturalism: A Critical Reader,* 32–70. Oxford: Blackwell.
Tyler, Imogen. 2008. "'Chav Mum, Chav Scum': Class Disgust in Contemporary Britain." *Feminist Media Studies* 8 (1): 17–34.
Tyler, Imogen, and Bruce Bennett. 2010. "Celebrity Chav: Fame, Femininity and Social Class." *European Journal of Cultural Studies* 13 (3): 375–93.
Veblen, Thorstein. [1899] 1994. *Theory of the Leisure Class.* London: Dove.
Vinken, Barbara. 2005. *Fashion Zeitgeist: Trends and Cycles in the Fashion System.* Oxford: Berg.
Walkerdine, Valerie, Helen Lucey, and June Melody. 2001. *Growing Up Girl: Psychosocial Explorations of Gender and Class.* London: Palgrave.

Weber, Max. [1948] 1970. "Class, Status, Party." In Hans Heinrich Gerth and Charles Wright Mills (eds.), *From Max Weber: Essays in Sociology*, 190–95. Boston: Routledge.

White, Michael. 2011. "The Class War: Why Everyone Feels Insecure." *The Guardian*, May 30. http://www.guardian.co.uk/politics/2011/may/30/michael-white-political-briefing-class-war (accessed January 20, 2012).

Wilson, Elizabeth. [1985] 2007. *Adorned in Dreams: Fashion and Modernity*. London: I. B. Tauris.

Woodward, Sophie. 2007. *Why Women Wear What They Wear*. Oxford: Berg.

6

Gender and Eighteenth-Century Fashion

JENNIFER M. JONES

Eighteenth-century French fashion calls to mind images of the voluminous silk sack dresses sported by aristocratic women in Jean-Antoine Watteau's *fête galante,* Madame de Pompadour's *robe à la française* flowing over impossibly wide hoops to fill François Boucher's canvases, and the sky-high confections of Marie Antoinette's *marchande de modes,* Rose Bertin, who teased and tightly wound hair over a scaffolding of wool and gauze, laced it with ribbons and jewels, and finished the coiffure with a powdering of the finest white flour. Eighteenth-century French fashions permitted elite French women literally to embody the style of Louis XV and cloak themselves in the aesthetic of rococo.

Yet, until the 1980s and 1990s, eighteenth-century French fashion was a topic that few historians felt compelled to engage seriously as an academic subject. When French fashion entered the narrative of French history, it was as a story of aristocratic refinement descending into frivolity and decadence heading inevitably toward the guillotine. Fashion was a story that historians happily neglected, leaving the world of hoopskirts and hairstyles to art historians, fashion and textile historians, museum directors, collectors, and connoisseurs.

All that began to change, however, in the 1980s, when social historians, women's historians, and historians inspired by the new "cultural turn"[1] in history discovered that shopgirls and seamstresses made fitting subjects for historical inquiry; that mantuas, corsets, and wigs had stories to tell; and that Pompadour's silks and Marie Antoinette's poufs were linked to major transformations in consumption. Historians became interested in the history of eighteenth-century fashion when they realized not only that clothing was gendered but that fashion culture itself was deeply tied to important historical questions about gender, consumer culture, power, and the modern self.

This essay explores the recent history of historians' engagement with the history of clothing and fashion, particularly focusing on scholarship that examines eighteenth-century French women's relationship to clothing, as well as the broader "gendering" of fashion as a feminine realm by the eve of the French Revolution. I seek to introduce students to the leading questions, paradigms, and debates with which historians have wrestled as they rethink the role of clothing and patterns of consumer behavior as important artifacts of human culture that demand attention in historical narratives. I begin with an exploration of historians' use of John C. Flugel's model of the "great masculine renunciation" (1930), then move to an exploration of how social historians in the 1970s and 1980s transformed the historians' understanding of the potential of small fragments from history—like clothing inventories—to recast existing narratives about gender roles and modernity. Next, I explore the rich scholarship on women's work in the clothing trades and the explosion of new research on the history of early modern female consumer culture. Finally, I consider new directions in the history of eighteenth-century fashion: new approaches for understanding the connections between fashion, sexuality, and performance; situating the history of fashion within both local and global narratives; and integrating the history of fashion and clothing into political history.

HISTORIANS AND THE GREAT MASCULINE RENUNCIATION

In the nineteenth century, the history of clothing constituted a fundamental part of the tradition of narrating the *la petite histoire* of private life and local histories; details about clothing were woven into historical accounts by female historians, amateur historians, and even professional scholars writing for a broad popular readership. In the hands of Edmond and Jules de Goncourt, the fashions of Madame de Pompadour and Marie Antoinette served as fitting symbols of the power of women's patronage of the arts and an evocative reminder of the sweet splendors of the rococo (Goncourt and Goncourt 1862). As the study of history became professionalized in the nineteenth and early twentieth centuries, historians relegated both the history of clothing and the world of courtesans and queens to the back of the closet.[2] Like many other aspects of "private life," nineteenth- and early twentieth-century historians viewed clothing and fashion as little more than historical ephemera, at best a gauzy reflection of social values, but not a constitutive part of the main narratives of society, culture, politics, and, most important, the nation. Yet, by the mid-twentieth century, as many historians of eighteenth-century Europe embraced the methods and paradigms of social history and the *Annales* school, they turned their focus away from political narratives and intellectual history to explore the deep structures of the economy, environment, social life, and *mentalité*. In the 1960s and 1970s, the history of clothing came back into focus as a valuable area of historical inquiry. Still, the history of clothing and fashion did not gain wide acceptance from historians as a significant part of the historical narrative until the 1990s and 2000s.

The reentry of the history of fashion into the mainstream historical narrative resulted from three major developments that energized and transformed the historical profession between the 1970s and 1990s: the emergence of women's history, new approaches to the history of consumer culture, and new and more theoretically engaged histories of gender and sexuality.

For much of the twentieth century, the starting place for historians who sought to chart the transformation of men's and women's relationship to fashion was a broad examination of shifts in clothing styles, fabrics, and silhouettes across the centuries. When viewed from the perspective of a mid-nineteenth-century culture in which bourgeois men's sober three-piece suits departed dramatically from the aesthetic of women's hoopskirts, elaborate silks, and fanciful trim, eighteenth-century men's and women's fashions looked by contrast strikingly similar: both aristocratic men and women in the eighteenth century embraced an aesthetic of powdered wigs, dainty heels, embroidered silks, and lace ruffles. Noting the growing dimorphism of men's and women's clothing styles between 1750 and 1850, many historians of fashion embraced the view of psychologist John C. Flugel, who contended in *The Psychology of Clothes* that the period after the French Revolution had witnessed a "great masculine renunciation" of fashion (1930).

The core ideas of Flugel's "great masculine renunciation"—that by the nineteenth century bourgeois men were relatively uninterested in fashion, that men's fashions changed relatively little compared to women's styles, and that men had a sober, steady, and practical relationship to their clothing in contrast to their wives' and sisters' mania for each passing fashion trend—remain to this day a dominant paradigm among gender historians and fashion historians. Indeed, much of the most exciting work on eighteenth- and nineteenth-century fashion in recent decades uncritically adopted Flugel's model, accepting male disinterest in fashion as a foundational truth. Writing men out of the story of fashion's evolution in the nineteenth century threw the spotlight instead on the female consumer. Dozens of important books and articles in the past thirty years, including Elizabeth Wilson's *Adorned in Dreams: Fashion and Modernity* (1985), Erika Rappaport's *Shopping for Pleasure: Women in the Making of London's West End* (2000), and Susan Hiner's *Accessories to Modernity: Fashion and the Feminine in Nineteenth-Century France* (2010), focus on women's fashions and the emergence of the modern female consumer. Victoria de Grazia's edited collection, *The Sex of Things: Gender and Consumption in Historical Perspective* (1996), offers a snapshot of the state of the field of the history of fashion and consumption in the mid-1990s, as nearly every article in the collection reveals the enduring influence of Flugel's model of the "great masculine renunciation."

Many of the scholars included in de Grazia's collection had begun their research on fashion and consumer culture in the 1980s, at a moment when older models that explained the history of fashion through Thorstein Veblen's theory of conspicuous consumption (1899) or Norbert Elias's "trickle-down" model of popular emulation of elite courtly styles (1983) felt increasingly one-dimensional, especially as historians moved away from theoretical models that emphasized class as the primary category of analysis and motor of history. Sociologist Pierre Bourdieu's *Distinction: A Social Critique of the Judgment of Taste* (1984) provided a conceptually rich analysis of the role of fashion and material goods in the maintenance of status hierarchies but offered little insight into the gendering of consumption. Other theories, such as James Laver's "shifting erogenous zones" (1937: 200), inspired some fashion historians but offered little to engage broader historical narratives and were generally kept at arm's length by historians suspicious of psychological theory. Even Roland Barthes's seminal work, *The Fashion System* (1983; first published in French in 1967) had limited influence on historians because Barthes focused almost exclusively on the discourse in fashion magazines rather than the transformation in real clothing or actual consumption patterns. For historians, the enduring usefulness of Flugel's model rested on three factors: (1) its broad chronological framework for making sense of transformations in the history of fashion; (2) its loose model of causation, which left room for historians to debate the roles of politics, class, and culture in social change; and (3) the ways in which Flugel's paradigm dovetailed with the growing interest among women's historians in the 1970s and 1980s in exploring the roots of the nineteenth-century "separate spheres" ideology.

Although many historians continue to refer to the "great masculine renunciation" as though it were an incontrovertible fact, important scholarly work in the past two decades has questioned many of the details of Flugel's model and significantly enriched and qualified his argument. David Kuchta's *The Three-Piece Suit and Modern Masculinity: England, 1550–1850* (2002) questions Flugel's chronology and causal model and pushes the beginnings of men's modern relationship to clothing back to the seventeenth century, situating it within English debates over republicanism and civic virtue. Art historian Ann Hollander argued in *Sex and Suits: The Evolution of Modern Dress* (1994) that men's fashions, and not women's, were inherently modern, achieving a streamlined male aesthetic that was ultimately copied by women. Hollander contends that "male dress was always essentially more advanced than female throughout fashion history, and tended to lead the way, to set the standard, to make the esthetic propositions to which female fashion responded" (6). Other historians, myself included, have reframed Flugel's question: instead of asking why men "renounced" fashion, they have asked instead why women so avidly embraced the new ideology of the femininity of fashion in the eighteenth century (J. Jones 2004).

More recently, historians have fundamentally called into question the outlines of Flugel's model. Historians of both eighteenth- and nineteenth-century men's fashion have sought to correct Flugel by arguing for men's persistent participation in fashion culture (Shannon 2006). In a particularly subtle and important intervention, Michael Kwass (2006) explores eighteenth-century French men's relationship to wigs. Kwass disrupts the standard narrative in which late eighteenth-century bourgeois men abandoned the courtly and aristocratic practice of wearing wigs on their path to sartorial modernity. Far from eschewing wigs, Kwass argues, men of all social ranks embraced them. Commenting on the ubiquity of the male wig, eighteenth-century social critic Louis-Sebestian

Mercier noted in 1782 that male shopkeepers, clerks, and even male kitchen servants now sported wigs. Men's wigs were big business, Kwass observes, and a fitting example of men's active participation in the burgeoning eighteenth-century consumer economy. Accessories such as wigs and cosmetics were a particularly dynamic sector of this emerging economy. Kwass argues that men did not buy wigs primarily to emulate the aristocracy. He notes that wigmakers marketed their wigs as a convenient, useful, and healthy alternative to natural hair that allowed men a degree of self-expression. Kwass concludes, "The success of the wig reminds us that eighteenth century fashion consumption was not always gendered feminine. Indeed, the moralist critique that wigs symbolized the increasing effeminacy of men and should therefore be rejected does not seem to have had much purchase on the minds of male consumers before the very end of the century" (2006: 659).

HISTORIANS EMBRACE THE HISTORY OF FASHION

Although in the 1970s and early 1980s women's historians, cultural historians, and social historians had begun to appreciate the possibilities of integrating the history of clothing and material culture into their narratives, the history of fashion would not have entered the mainstream narrative of eighteenth-century French politics and the Enlightenment without the inspiration of French historian Daniel Roche's seminal research on the history of clothing and consumption. More than any other historian, Roche brought the history of fashion into the mainstream of eighteenth-century French history. Roche's research on the material culture of the popular classes of Paris culminated in *The People of Paris: An Essay in Popular Culture in the 18th Century* ([1981] 1987), which piqued historians' interest in the history of French clothing and material culture and laid the foundation for much of the scholarship on the history of eighteenth-century French material culture over the past thirty years. *The People of Paris* revealed to historians the possibilities of the notarial archive for bringing to life the world of ordinary Parisians.[3] As notaries recorded postmortem inventories of the deceased's belongings, they revealed intimate details about Parisians' living conditions—the size of their apartments, the number of books on their shelves, and, most important for fashion historians, the numbers and items of clothing in their closets and cabinets. Roche found that in the period from 1700 to 1715 the wardrobes of lower-class women consisted of five main garments: the skirt, petticoat, mantua/mantel, apron, and bodice/corset. Undergarments were uncommon, and accessories were limited to simple head coverings and cotton or muslin stockings. Shoes, scarves, and gloves were all rare. Silk and cotton fabrics were rare and stiff, and somber wool and coarse linen or hemp dominated women's wardrobes. Men of the lower classes wore four main garments: shirts, jackets, breeches, and jerkins. Men owned few accessories (collars, cuffs, and cravats), and shoes were found in only 37 percent of inventories after a person's decease. Men's apparel, like their wives' and sisters', was dark and somber. In the final quarter of the eighteenth century, however, Roche finds that popular dress changed dramatically, ushering in nothing less than a "sartorial revolution." The popular classes began to wear more colorful clothing, lighter fabrics, and dozens of new accessories as they embraced a fashion culture based on novelty and new forms of display and social distinction. From a careful archival reconstruction of wardrobes, Roche constructed a conceptually powerful model of how material goods expressed and contributed to cultural change. Reading Roche's work, many historians began to realize that clothing could be a "maker" as well as a "marker" of change.[4]

Roche's argument for an eighteenth-century "vestimentary revolution" culminated in his magisterial study, *La Culture des apparences* (1989). Translated into English as *The Culture of Clothing: Dress and Fashion in the Ancien Régime* (1994), this book remains the most important and comprehensive treatment to date of the history of eighteenth-century clothing. Roche explores the history of clothing and fashion in eighteenth-century France holistically, surveying the full social and economic spectrum, charting changing clothing styles, the creation of new items of clothing, new practices of hygiene, transformations in soldiers' uniforms, the birth of the fashion press, and the discourse on fashion and clothing in Enlightenment tracts and novels. Roche's work complemented the work of early modern British historians such as Neil McKendrick, John Brewer, and J. H. Plumb (1982), who transformed historians' understanding of early modern economy and society in the 1980s by arguing that the eighteenth century witnessed a profound consumer revolution that preceded industrialization. Roche also offered historians a new narrative and chronology of how the consumer revolution of the eighteenth century transformed men's and women's identities and social relationships. In the quarter century before the French Revolution, Roche argues, France had already undergone the birth of a modern consumer culture of fashion, in which an older connection between social status and dress was supplanted by a new, more fluid culture in which people began to create and express their identity through fashion. "The great political Revolution did not so much transform practices," Roche argues, "as accelerate certain changes" (1994: 148).

Roche's research not only provided hard data to document the complex relationship of different classes to the new culture of fashion but also allowed historians to study the differential relationship of men and women to fashion. "Sexual bimorphism," Roche argued, "was emphasized by the pioneering and bold behavior of women, as compared with the more conservative behavior, and even resistance to innovation, of men" (1994: 148). To be sure, Roche's research suggested that men participated actively in the consumer revolution, but his careful distinction between male and female wardrobes underscored a striking shift in the eighteenth century that cut across all social classes: whereas in the late seventeenth century the value of men's wardrobes surpassed that of their wives, daughters, and sisters, by the end of the eighteenth century that pattern had been reversed. In a dramatic transformation, by the late eighteenth century women across a range of classes not only spent more money on clothing than the men of their social class but also owned considerably more items and types of clothing. Thus, Roche's archival research provided solid data that women's and gender historians (Crowston 2001; J. Jones 2004; Martin 2009) interpreted and analyzed in an outpouring of new gender histories of eighteenth-century French fashion in the 1990s and 2000s.

For Roche, interpreting the meaning of fashion entailed more than analyzing eighteenth-century language, ideas, and discourse. It also required understanding the technical details of clothing production. To this end, Roche encouraged historians of fashion to explore the entire "vestimentary system," which included the making and selling of clothing. His analysis enabled two distinct historiographic traditions—social histories of women's work and histories of fashion and consumption—to join together to explore the feminization of fashion and clothing in eighteenth-century France.

THE CLOTHING AND FASHION TRADES

At the same time that Roche was calling for a more holistic study of the entire "vestimentary system," other practitioners of the new social history were turning their attention to the history of women's work in the early-modern world and their roles in the transition to industrialization and mass production. Nowhere were the fruits of this research more apparent than in the pathbreaking books and articles published on the clothing trades. The feminist movement of the 1960s and 1970s sparked a new interest in the history of women's work in the textile arts and clothing trades. Feminist art historian Rozsika Parker's exploration of the gendering of embroidery in her classic *The Subversive Stitch: Embroidery and the Making of the Feminine* (1984) offered a provocative exploration of the history of women's often ambivalent relationship to needlework. Parker argues that the gradual relegation of women's embroidery to the status of craft, as opposed to the fine arts, worked to marginalize women's work and women's creative expression. In France, feminist anthropologist Yvonne Verdier's *Façons de dire, façons de faire: la laveuse, la couturièrem la cuisinière* (1979) explored the workaday world and mentality of female dressmakers in twentieth-century rural Burgundy. Although Verdier listened in on the lives of contemporary seamstresses, her now classic study offered feminist historians a model for reconstructing the voices of female workers in the past. The pioneering work of social historians such as Olwen Hufton (1975) and Louise Tilly and Joan Scott (1978) helped historians understand the ways in which women's work, often in the weaving and textile trades, took place in the family economy, and they chronicled the impact of proto- and early industrialization on female workers. Case studies by historians Gay Gullickson (1986) and Tessie P. Liu (1994) on rural spinners and weavers helped historians understand the ways in which rural textile production was transformed by industrialization. Historians have been particularly interested in exploring women's relationship to the guilds that organized production in many early-modern cities in France. Daryl Hafter's (2007) and Cynthia Truant's (1995) studies of women in the textile and clothing trades are particularly valuable for historians who seek to understand the powers and limitations of women working within guilds. In 1996 Judith

Coffin offered a powerful new narrative of the transformation of women's work experience in the garment trades, beginning with the mid-eighteenth-century guild and culminating with the widespread adoption of the sewing machine by the beginning of the twentieth century.

Although the careful studies of the textile trades and women's guilds are essential for historians' understanding of women's roles in the production of clothing and fashion, few historians have command of the knowledge of both the economic and political organization of production and the material process of cutting and sewing clothing. That is to say, historians have been very good at tallying items of clothing in probate inventories and explaining the legal privileges that structured women's work within the clothing trades, but they have been less successful in understanding the actual technical processes of crafting clothing. Even less have historians succeeded in linking together the transformation in clothing production, clothing styles, and broad cultural attitudes toward fashion and gender roles. As a result, a gap divides the history of clothing and the history of fashion, and the material history of clothing appears to have little importance in the story of eighteenth-century fashion. The history of clothing has been subsumed, perhaps too completely, by larger narratives about transformations in women's work, the birth of consumer culture, and the birth of the modern self. And in that process, historians have too often neglected the clothing itself.

To make clothing tell stories, historians need to understand the cut and construction of the clothing. To that end, historians need to learn to make better use of the internal histories of clothing provided by textile historians and clothing historians. In France, Nicole Pellegrin's work offers a detailed understanding of the technique of clothing production. Pellegrin's *Les Vêtements de la Liberté: Abécédaire des pratiques vestimentaires françaises de 1780–1800* (1989) provides an essential dictionary of fashion with references and technical details for the late eighteenth century. Costume historians Aileen Ribeiro (1984, 1988) and Madeleine Delpierre (1997) also provide useful introductions to eighteenth-century dress that offer insights into the technical details of cut, pattern, and textiles. Visits to major costume collections (the Musée de la Mode et du Textile and the Musée Galliera in Paris, the Costume Institute at the Metropolitan Museum of Art in New York City, the Los Angeles County Museum, the art museums at Colonial Williamsburg, and the Victoria and Albert Museum in London, to name just a few of the leading collections) to study the construction of eighteenth-century clothing are invaluable to an understanding of clothing construction. In lieu of actual visits to museums, show catalogs and newly available online research sources also offer excellent ways to begin to master the technical details of clothing and fashion. Eighteenth-century fashion engravings are particularly rich primary sources. Raymond Gaudriault's *Répertoire de la gravure de mode française des origines à 1815* (1983) provides a comprehensive catalog of all French fashion engravings with information about their location in French libraries and archives. Modern reconstructions of eighteenth-century patterns such as Linda Baumgarten's *Costume Close-Up: Clothing Construction and Pattern, 1750–1790* (1999) are also valuable resources for historians.

Clare Haru Crowston's social history of the seamstresses' guild in seventeenth and eighteenth-century France, *Fabricating Women: The Seamstresses of Old Regime France, 1675–1791* (2001), offers an innovative model for fashion historians as she grounds her analysis of fashion in the technical details of clothing construction and deeply integrates the histories of women's work, clothing, and fashion consumption. *Fabricating Women* provides a rich social history of the most important female guild in Old Regime France and narrates the protracted legal battle of female seamstresses against male tailors and male clothing workers who claimed that they, and not women, had the exclusive privilege to make many items of clothing for women. Parisian seamstresses were incorporated as a guild in 1675 but continued to battle male workers for their turf in the fashion trades. Key to the seamstresses' rhetorical arguments for their trade was their contention that women had a right to be dressed by women. Yet, at the time of their guild's incorporation in 1675, the king maintained and protected the male tailors' monopoly on making whalebone dress bodices (*corps de robes*) and dress skirts (*bas de robes*). The dress bodice, reinforced with whalebone, provided the elegant and distinctive look of aristocratic female attire: it kept the spine erect, flattened the stomach, and pushed up the breasts. The dress bodice cost a small fortune, thanks to the laborious technique of embedding whalebone in the bodice. Forbidding seamstresses to make this key and lucrative item of women's wardrobes dealt a huge blow to the fledgling seamstresses' guild.

Crowston's research suggests that female seamstresses met this challenge with a mixture of resiliency and creativity that ultimately helped spark an entirely new aesthetic and social trend in fashion, the playful and informal mantua (in French, *le manteau*) that would dominate fashion by the eighteenth century. The mantua was based on the casual one-piece, kimono-like dressing gowns that had originally been worn informally inside the house as a form of *déshabillé,* or undress. Seamstresses were allowed to make these informal dressing gowns. And within a decade of the seamstresses' guild's incorporation, elite women in France and throughout Europe adopted the new style of the mantua as their preferred form of dress for public outings, shopping, and social visits. The advantages of the mantua over the traditional skirt and boned bodice combination was readily apparent to female consumers, who sought comfort, affordability, and elegance: lightweight silks replaced heavy boned bodices; women could now buy more dresses and vary their wardrobes more frequently; and with the corset no longer built into each dress's bodice, women could now buy a single pair of boned stays that could be worn with any dress. In addition, Crowston argues that the mantua began the process of breaking down the distinction between elite and common clothing as women of all social groups began to adopt the mantua. Indeed, not only did the mantua spread throughout France, but by the late seventeenth century it had spread to England and throughout Europe (2001: 36–41).

Crowston's understanding of the cut and construction of the clothes, as well as the legal and social context in which clothing was produced in the seamstresses' guild, allows her insights into the connections between the histories of production and consumption that are often obscure to, or neglected by, historians. Connecting the dots between new patterns of production and new patterns of consumption, Crowston attributes a shared agency to both female seamstresses and their clients in revolutionizing fashion:

> In the 1679s, as the mantua appeared on the streets of the capital, the Parisian seamstresses emerged from long years of illicit labor with the status of an independent guild. Needleworkers who had formerly engaged in clandestine work could now openly seek female clients. They took up the mantua eagerly, as a garment they were authorized to produce and one which was not to difficult to create. Producing thousands of these gowns in workshops across Paris, the seamstresses propagated a novel form of dressing for women, using it to establish a niche in the high-end of the garment trades and to spread the new taste to other social groups. Like Coco Chanel in her day, seamstresses prospered by rendering casual, comfortable garments into a new style for elite women and their social inferiors. (2001: 40)

Crowston persuasively argues that the seamstresses of Old Regime France helped revolutionize fashion by helping to spark the vogue for the mantua, a new, less expensive dress style that was well suited to a clientele that desired novelty in clothing. But she also argues that seamstresses played a crucial role in the feminization of fashion: by the eighteenth century their participation in a shared female world of producers and consumers helped to render fashion as feminine. As they defended their privilege as women to sew, seamstresses helped fabricate a new vision of womanhood itself.

FROM CLOTHING TO CONSUMER CULTURE

Women's historians' insistence on placing the story of female workers front and center in their narratives of the gendering of clothing and fashion has opened up important avenues for research; in many ways Crowston's *Fabricating Women* stands at the pinnacle of that tradition of the social history of clothing production. Yet the last twenty years have also seen great strides in understanding the role that consumers and consumer culture played in the feminization of fashion in eighteenth-century France and the Western world. Indeed, studying the intersection between the history of clothing and the history of consumer culture has sparked a series of lively scholarly debates over questions of chronology, human agency, and the interpretation of cultural artifacts, debates that continue to define academic study of eighteenth-century fashion.

A first generation of historians researching consumer behavior and consumer culture were largely interested in questions of chronology, and they focused on the relationship of the emergence of modern consumer behavior to grand narratives like "industrialization" or "the rise of capitalism." Many historians assumed that modern consumption, with its attendant behaviors and psychology, was produced by the Industrial Revolution. For example, Michael Miller's *The Bon Marché: Bourgeois Culture and the Department Store, 1869–1920* (1981) and Rosalind Williams's *Dream Worlds: Mass Consumption in Late Nineteenth-Century France* (1982) encouraged historians to place the birth of modern consumer culture squarely in the mid- to late nineteenth century with the rise of the department store and new retailing techniques. Yet by the early 1980s British historians Neil McKendrick, John Brewer, and J. H. Plumb (1982) were already challenging that model by arguing that the mania for colorful calicos and cheap cottons in the eighteenth century inspired the Industrial Revolution. Other scholars, such as Chandra Mukerji in her influential *From Graven Images: Patterns of Modern Materialism* (1983), questioned the entire concept of a "consumer revolution" by arguing that many of the features we associate with modern consumerism—materialist desires to indulge in comforts and frivolities—were well-established behaviors in the West as early as the fifteenth and sixteenth centuries.

For historians who want to tease out what is new and distinctive about the relationship of consumers to fashion in the eighteenth century, these debates over chronology are still relevant. But among scholars today the urgency of the "when" question has been replaced by a more complex set of "how" questions about consumption. When the Marxist paradigm, which posited economic production as the generating motor of history, slowly loosened its grip on the historical profession in the 1980s, historians began to conceptualize consumption as an active force in history that could be interpreted broadly to include a vast range of behaviors from the reading of fashion magazines to travel and tourism. Both the "linguistic turn" and the "cultural turn" in the historical profession in the 1980s also suggested new ways of analyzing female consumers. For many historians, anthropologist Grant McCracken's *Culture and Consumption: New Approaches to the Symbolic Character of Consumer Goods* (1988) provided an inspiring guide to the emerging field of the cultural study of consumption. In particular, he introduced students to the anthropological literature on interpreting the expressive power of goods, including clothing (McCracken 1988: 57).

The promise of the new scholarship on the gender of consumption was fulfilled by a series of important works on consumption in eighteenth-century England that were published in the 1990s, including Elizabeth Kowaleski-Wallace's *Consuming Subjects: Women, Shopping and Business in the Eighteenth Century* (1997) and Erin Mackie's *Market à la Mode: Fashion, Commodity, and Gender in* The Tatler *and* The Spectator (1997). Reed Benhamou's (1997) research on fashion coverage in *Le Mercure Galant*, an official organ of the royal court published from 1672 to 1791, traces the growing awareness of fashion by the early eighteenth century as a "female failing." And in an article titled "Repackaging Rousseau: Femininity and Fashion in Old Regime France" (J. Jones 1994), I argue that the French fashion press in the 1780s played an active role in reshaping Rousseau's gender ideology in order to persuade women that shopping, spending, and adornment were compatible with proper femininity.

Because so many of the key studies of the gendering of consumption focus on the English example, it is important for historians of eighteenth-century France to find ways to incorporate British scholars' research while remaining attentive to the particular context of French fashions. French commercial culture in the eighteenth century seemed to lag behind British consumerism; for example, the first French magazine to focus exclusively on fashion, Jean Antoine Brun's *Cabinet des modes,* did not begin publication until 1785. French peasants are often depicted as "resistant to consumption" (Fairchilds 1993: 228). Leading historian of French consumer culture Colin Jones (1991) argues that France did not embrace fashion and commercial culture later than Britain but embraced modern consumer culture differently. In France, before 1789, complex legal and social codes regulated a society based on privileges rather than rights. Where other historians have seen a stagnant preindustrial economy rooted in privilege and consumption based on rank in the social order, Jones sees the stirrings of a market mentality and consumer choice growing up among the cracks in the economy of Old Regime France. Historian Cissie Fairchilds made an important intervention in debates about French consumption by coining the word *populuxe* to refer to the distinctive style of much of eighteenth-century consumption among the popular classes. According to Fairchilds, cheap knockoffs of aristocratic goods were the salient feature of French consumer culture. As she observes, "English tourists to Paris were astonished at the propensity of the Parisian lower class to spend on fashionable luxuries" (1993: 228).

Rose Bertin, Marie Antoinette's marchande de modes, provides another useful illustration of the distinctive path of French consumer culture as it grew up within an aristocratic culture of privilege. The marchande de modes was a new type of fashion retailer in the late eighteenth century; unlike the seamstresses with their hard-won guild status, marchandes de modes largely worked outside the guild structure, creatively carving out a realm of legal employment by decorating dresses, trimming hats, and arranging hair, all tasks that did not require a legal privilege. Yet Bertin's entire advertising campaign depended on the system of aristocratic privilege that pervaded Old Regime France. She became famous because of her haughty demeanor, her ornate shop filled with royal portraits under the sign "Au grand mogul," and her patronage by Marie Antoinette, which earned her the title "First minister of Fashion" (J. Jones 2004: 168–69).

NEW DIRECTIONS IN THE STUDY OF EIGHTEENTH-CENTURY FRENCH FASHION

For the past thirty years, historians have actively researched and debated the ways in which and the reasons why clothing production, clothing consumption, and clothing itself were gendered as masculine or feminine in the course of the eighteenth century. New avenues for research that have the potential to challenge existing narratives of eighteenth-century history and historians' interpretation of material objects point in several directions. Deeply inspired by Judith Butler's groundbreaking work on gender and performativity in *Gender Trouble: Feminism and the Subversion of Identity* (1990), historians are beginning to place more emphasis on interpreting the history of clothing and fashion through the lens of gender performativity. An outstanding example of this approach is historian Gary Kates's (1995) engaging study of the cross-dressing Chevalier d'Eon, a French diplomat and spy who spent the first half of his life dressed as a man and the second half as a woman. Caroline Weber's *Queen of Fashion: What Marie Antoinette Wore to the Revolution* (2006) offers the most finely tuned portrait to date of the ways in which an individual eighteenth-century woman performed and shaped her identity through fashion. Weber argues that Marie Antoinette used clothing to perform a tortuous and ultimately ill-fated dance at court as she asserted her power and navigated between factions through her use of new hairstyles and hoopskirts.

Weber's focus on fashion, performance, and politics at Versailles signals that the history of fashion has in a sense "come of age." No longer exclusively interested in narratives from social and economic history, historians of fashion now directly interrogate the relationship of clothing to politics and political culture. The engagement of historians of fashion with political history has enormous potential for posing new questions, drawing attention to the performative nature of politics and the ways in which the creation of citizens in the late eighteenth century took place through the experience of a gendered material culture as well as through the written and spoken word. A spate of recent studies on eighteenth-century politics explore fashion as a key site of political culture, debate, and identity formation. Kate Haulman's *The Politics of Fashion in Eighteenth-Century America* (2011), an example of this new direction in the American context, joins a growing body of work on dress and the political culture of the French Revolution (Cage 2009; Fairchilds 2000; Heuer 2002; Hunt 1998; Wrigley 2002).

The explosion of research on the history of eighteenth-century fashion in the past thirty years, and historians' creation of nuanced interpretations of the ways in which clothing and fashion are connected to broad transformations in gender roles, the economy, politics, and the creation of the modern self, positions the history of fashion at the heart of eighteenth-century historiography in the early twenty-first century. But there remains much work for fashion historians to do. Fashion historians need to do even more to move beyond the context of national history to global history, posing new questions about the experience of global trade, the stimulation of desires for exotic goods, and the creation of new norms for clothing the Western body. Historians of clothing and fashion also need to continue to deepen their engagement with historians in other fields and to broaden their engagement with scholars in other disciplines, to create new ways to study material culture, and to find new ways to make noncanonical sources—like wigs and fashion magazines—speak volumes.[5]

NOTES

1. For background on the so-called cultural turn in the historical profession, see Victoria E. Bonnel and Lynn Hunt's *Beyond the Cultural Turn: New Directions in the Story of Society and Culture* (1999).
2. On the professionalization of history in the nineteenth and twentieth centuries, see Bonnie G. Smith (2000).
3. For an excellent example of the use of the probate inventory to explore English material culture in the eighteenth century, see works by Amanda Vickery (1998, 2009).

4. Mary Louise Roberts (1993) makes an important and influential distinction between fashion as "maker" and "marker" in one of the pioneering attempts to wed the history of fashion to larger narratives regarding gender, politics, and cultural change.
5. On the importance of historians' learning to interpret material culture, see Leora Auslander's essay "Beyond Words" (2005).

BIBLIOGRAPHY

Auslander, Leora. 2005. "Beyond Words." *American Historical Review* 110 (4): 1015–45.

Barthes, Roland. 1983. *The Fashion System.* New York: Hill and Wang.

Baumgarten, Linda. 1999. *Costume Close-Up: Clothing Construction and Pattern, 1750–1790.* Williamsburg, VA: Colonial Williamsburg Foundation with Quite Specific Media Group.

Benhamou, Reed. 1997. "Fashion in the *Mercure:* From Human Foible to Female Failing." *Eighteenth-Century Studies* 31 (1): 27–43.

Bonnel, Victoria E., and Lynn Hunt (eds.). 1999. *Beyond the Cultural Turn: New Directions in the Story of Society and Culture.* Berkeley: University of California Press.

Bourdieu, Pierre. 1984. *Distinction: A Social Critique of the Judgment of Taste.* Cambridge, MA: Harvard University Press.

Butler, Judith. 1990. *Gender Trouble: Feminism and the Subversion of Identity.* New York: Routledge.

Cage, Claire. 2009. "The Sartorial Self: Neoclassical Fashion and Gender Identity in France, 1797–1804." *Eighteenth-Century Studies* 42 (2): 193–215.

Coffin, Judith G. 1996. *The Politics of Women's Work: The Paris Garment Grades, 1750–1915.* Princeton, NJ: Princeton University Press.

Crowston, Clare Haru. 2001. *Fabricating Women: The Seamstresses of Old Regime France, 1675–1791.* Durham, NC: Duke University Press.

de Grazia, Victoria (ed.). 1996. *The Sex of Things: Gender and Consumption in Historical Perspective.* With Ellen Furlough. Berkeley: University of California Press.

Delpierre, Madeleine. 1997. *Dress in France in the Eighteenth Century.* New Haven, CT: Yale University Press.

Elias, Norbert. 1983. *The Court Society.* Oxford: Blackwell.

Fairchilds, Cissie. 1993. "The Production and Marketing of Populuxe Goods in Eighteenth-Century Paris." In John Brewer and Roy Porter (eds.), *Consumption and the World of Goods,* 228–48. London: Routledge.

Fairchilds, Cissie. 2000. "Fashion and Freedom in the French Revolution." *Continuity and Change* 15 (3): 419–33.

Flugel, John C. 1930. *The Psychology of Clothes.* London: Hogarth.

Gaudriault, Raymond. 1983. *Répertoire de la gravure de mode française des origines à 1815.* Paris: Les editions de l'amateur.

Goncourt, Edmond de, and Jules de Goncourt. 1862. *La femme au dix-huitième siècle.* Paris: Firmin Didot frères.

Gullickson, Gay. 1986. *Spinners and Weavers in the Auffay: Rural Industry and the Sexual Division of Labor in a French Village, 1750–1850.* Cambridge: Cambridge University Press.

Hafter, Daryl. 2007. *Women at Work in Preindustrial France.* University Park, PA: Penn State University Press.

Haulman, Kate. 2011. *The Politics of Fashion in Eighteenth-Century America.* Chapel Hill: University of North Carolina Press.
Heuer, Jennifer. 2002. "Hats on for the Nation! Women, Servants, Soldiers and the 'Sign of the French.'" *French History* 16 (1): 28–52.
Hiner, Susan. 2010. *Accessories to Modernity: Fashion and the Feminine in Nineteenth-Century France.* Philadelphia: University of Pennsylvania Press.
Hollander, Anne. 1994. *Sex and Suits: The Evolution of Modern Dress.* New York: Alfred Knopf.
Hufton, Olwen. 1975. "Women and the Family Economy in 18th-Century France." *French Historical Studies* 9 (1): 1–22.
Hunt, Lynn. 1998. "Freedom of Dress in the French Revolution." In Sara E. Melzer and Kathryn Norberg (eds.), *From the Royal to the Republican Body,* 224–49. Berkeley: University of California Press.
Jones, Colin. 1991. "Bourgeois Revolution Revivified: 1789 and Social Change." In Colin Lucas (ed.), *Rewriting the French Revolution,* 71–100. Oxford: Oxford University Press.
Jones, Jennifer M. 1994. "Repackaging Rousseau: Femininity and Fashion in Old Regime France." *French Historical Studies* 18: 939–61.
Jones, Jennifer M. 2004. *Sexing La Mode: Gender, Fashion and Commercial Culture in Old Regime France.* Oxford: Berg.
Kates, Gary. 1995. *Monsier d'Eon Is a Woman: A Tale of Political Intrigue and Sexual Masquerade.* New York: Basic Books.
Kowaleski-Wallace, Elizabeth. 1997. *Consuming Subjects: Women, Shopping and Business in the Eighteenth Century.* New York: Columbia University Press.
Kuchta, David. 2002. *The Three-Piece Suit and Modern Masculinity: England, 1550–1850.* Berkeley: University of California Press.
Kwass, Michael. 2006. "Big Hair: A Wig History of Consumption in Eighteenth-Century France." *American Historical Review* 111 (3): 631–59.
Laver, James. 1937. *Taste and Fashion: From the French Revolution to the Present Day.* London: Harrap.
Liu, Tessie P. 1994. *The Weaver's Knot: The Contradictions of Class Struggle and Family Solidarity in Western France, 1750–1914.* Ithaca, NY: Cornell University Press.
Mackie, Erin. 1997. *Market à la Mode: Fashion, Commodity, and Gender in* The Tatler *and* The Spectator. Baltimore: Johns Hopkins University Press.
Martin, Morag. 2009. *Selling Beauty: Cosmetics, Commerce and French Society, 1750–1830.* Baltimore: Johns Hopkins University Press.
McCracken, Grant. 1988. *Culture and Consumption: New Approaches to the Symbolic Character of Consumer Goods.* Bloomington: Indiana University Press.
McKendrick, Neil, John Brewer, and J. H. Plumb. 1982. *The Birth of a Consumer Society: The Commercialization of 18th-Century England.* Bloomington: Indiana University Press.
Miller, Michael. 1981. *The Bon Marché: Bourgeois Culture and the Department Store, 1869–1920.* Princeton, NJ: Princeton University Press.
Mukerji, Chandra. 1983. *From Graven Images: Patterns of Modern Materialism.* New York: Columbia University Press.
Parker, Rozsika. 1984. *The Subversive Stitch: Embroidery and the Making of the Feminine.* London: Women's Press.

Pellegrin, Nicole. 1989. *Les Vêtements de la Liberté: Abécédaire des pratiques vestimentaires françaises de 1780–1800.* Aix-en-Provence, France: Alinea.

Rappaport, Erika D. 2000. *Shopping for Pleasure: Women in the Making of London's West End.* Princeton, NJ: Princeton University Press.

Ribeiro, Aileen. 1984. *Dress in Eighteenth-Century Europe, 1715–1789.* New Haven, CT: Yale University Press.

Ribeiro, Aileen. 1988. *Fashion in the French Revolution.* New York: Holmes and Meier.

Roberts, Mary Louise. 1993. "Samson and Delilah Revisited: The Politics of Women's Fashions in 1920s France." *American Historical Review* 98 (3): 657–84.

Roche, Daniel. [1981] 1987. *The People of Paris: An Essay in Popular Culture in the 18th Century.* Berkeley: University of California Press.

Roche, Daniel. 1994. *The Culture of Clothing: Dress and Fashion in the Ancien Régime.* Cambridge: Cambridge University Press.

Shannon, Brent Alan. 2006. *The Cut of His Coat: Men, Dress, and Consumer Culture in Britain, 1860–1914.* Athens: Ohio University Press.

Smith, Bonnie G. 2000. *The Gender of History: Men, Women, and Historical Practice.* Cambridge, MA: Harvard University Press.

Tilly, Louise, and Joan Scott. 1978. *Women, Work, and Family.* New York: Holt, Rinehart and Winston.

Truant, Cynthia. 1995. "Parisian Guildswomen and the (Sexual) Politics of Privilege." In Dena Goodman and Elisabeth Goldsmith (eds.), *Going Public: Women and Publishing in Early Modern France,* 46–61. Ithaca, NY: Cornell University Press.

Veblen, Thorstein. 1899. *The Theory of the Leisure Class: An Economic Study of Institutions.* New York: Macmillan.

Verdier, Yvonne. 1979. *Façons de dire, façons de faire: la laveuse, la couturièrem la cuisinière.* Paris: Gallimard.

Vickery, Amanda. 1998. *The Gentleman's Daughter.* New Haven, CT: Yale University Press.

Vickery, Amanda. 2009. *Behind Closed Doors: At Home in Georgian England.* New Haven, CT: Yale University Press.

Weber, Caroline. 2006. *Queen of Fashion: What Marie Antoinette Wore to the Revolution.* New York: Henry Holt.

Williams, Rosalind. 1982. *Dream Worlds: Mass Consumption in Late Nineteenth-Century France.* Berkeley: University of California Press.

Wilson, Elizabeth. 1985. *Adorned in Dreams: Fashion and Modernity.* London: Virago.

Wrigley, Richard. 2002. *The Politics of Appearances: Representations of Dress in Revolutionary France.* Oxford: Berg.

7

Lesbian Style

VICKI KARAMINAS

A stereotype exists of lesbians having poor fashion sense, which is rooted in cultural prejudices about the "mannish woman" as unnatural and ugly. Although lesbian style is not exclusively about masculine attire, the idea that lesbians tend to dress like men has persisted through representations in popular culture. There has never been one type of lesbian style, whether local or international, underground or visible, femme or butch. Lesbian style reflects a mix of cultural forms and multiethnic styles.

The historical and social formation of lesbian subjectivities and their association with a sartorial style has been, since the early twentieth century, framed around butch versus femme identities. It is difficult to determine how long lesbians have practiced butch and femme roles. Prior to the middle of the twentieth century in Western culture, gay, lesbian, and queer societies were mostly underground or secret. Butch and femme roles and the importance of elements of styling—mannerism and clothing—date back at least to the beginning of the twentieth century, although the exact origins of the butch and femme identities are unknown. Before the twentieth century, women passed as men by dressing and acting like men for either sexual or economic reasons or simply for adventure. It comes as no surprise, then, that after years of feminist scholarship and political interventions, from the Stonewall Riots of 1969 to the feminist movements of the 1970s and the establishment of queer theory and postfeminism in the 1990s, lesbian style has now become more fluid as gender and sexual binaries have become increasingly blurred.

In "The Femme Question," Joan Nestle writes that both butches and femmes have a history of ingenuity in the creation of a personal style and that it is "easy to confuse innovative or resisting style with a mere replica of the prevailing custom" (1987b: 141). As Nestle notes, both butches and femmes created very distinct styles that, although they seem to replicate heterosexual gender roles and styles, were in fact "rewriting" them in order to signify their desires and sexualities. A butch woman who dressed in men's clothing was still a woman, but the creation of a particular style was used to "signal to other women what she was capable of doing—taking erotic responsibility" (141). A femme woman, although dressed in clothing that signaled conventional femininity in order to "attract men," was in fact subverting this convention and attracting women. However, the emergence in the 1990s of a new, sexy, and glamorous style, coined "lipstick lesbianism" by the media, reflected deeper questions about identity, gender, and politics. This article traces lesbian sartorial style of the twentieth century by drawing on popular culture and established lesbian scholarship to uncover the impact that dress and appearance have in constructing lesbian identities.

MANNISH LESBIANS AND SALON DANDIES

In the late nineteenth and early twentieth centuries, there was greater visibility and cultural presence of lesbian identities in major urban cities such as London and Paris. However, those who had the freedom to dress this way were primarily middle-class women who were economically independent and privileged because they had received a family inheritance and did not depend on marriage as a means of daily survival. These women enjoyed the privileges and economic power that nobility and class offered and were drawn into literary and artistic circles.

Such women included the Duchesse de Clermont-Tonnere (Elizabeth de Gramont), the artist Gluck (Hannah Gluckstein), Una Vincenzo, and Radclyffe Hall, who were the epitome of the lesbian style of the period. The cigarette, the monocle, the cropped short haircut, the tuxedo, and the fedora hat were the most recognizable accessories and sartorial displays of the "mannish" lesbian culture of London and Paris.

The representation of the mannish lesbian portrayed in Radclyffe Hall's novel *The Well of Loneliness* (1928), writes Esther Newton, "was and remains an important symbol of rebellion against male hegemony, and... of one significant pattern in lesbian sexuality and gender identification" (1990: 281). The protagonist of the novel, Stephen Gordon, is a woman who from birth finds herself "different," somehow masculine in appearance and personality while female in body. In her essay "Forbidden Love," Elizabeth Wilson writes of Stephen as embodying a masculinity that is infused with a sense of danger and power, one that is attributed to a "doomed" personality. "The lesbian," she writes, "resembles the archetypal Romantic movement hero, the doomed rebel, often an artist, often sexually ambiguous" (1984: 214). Like her protagonist Stephen, Hall's appearance reflected the model of the "sexual invert" offered by sexologists. The *Birmingham Post* described her in April 1927 as

> [a] well-known figure at all the interesting parties and public occasions and [she] is easily recognizable by her distinctive appearance, tall, slim, and very well groomed. Miss Hall affects a mannish mode of dress, and has what many people consider the

best shingle in London. Her hair is of gold, and cropped as closely as a man's, a natural ripple in it being the only break in its sleek perfection. (quoted in Jennings 2007: 119)

"The high-fashion clothing of women like Radclyffe Hall [Figure 7.1], the Marquise de Belbeauf (Collette's lover), Romaine Brooks, and Una Vincenzo was in part an extension of the costume of the male dandy," writes Marjorie Garber (1992: 153). Upper-class women dressed in tuxedos and cravats in public and often wore a monocle and smoked a cigarette or a cigar. Women belonging to the lower classes wore mannish clothes only in the evening, concealed under a coat while on their way to a lesbian venue. Lesbian styles of the 1920s, writes Garber, "men's formal dress, top hats and tails—popularized onstage by entertainers like Marlene Dietrich and Judy Garland, became high fashion statements, menswear for women re-sexualised as straight (as well as gay) style" (158).

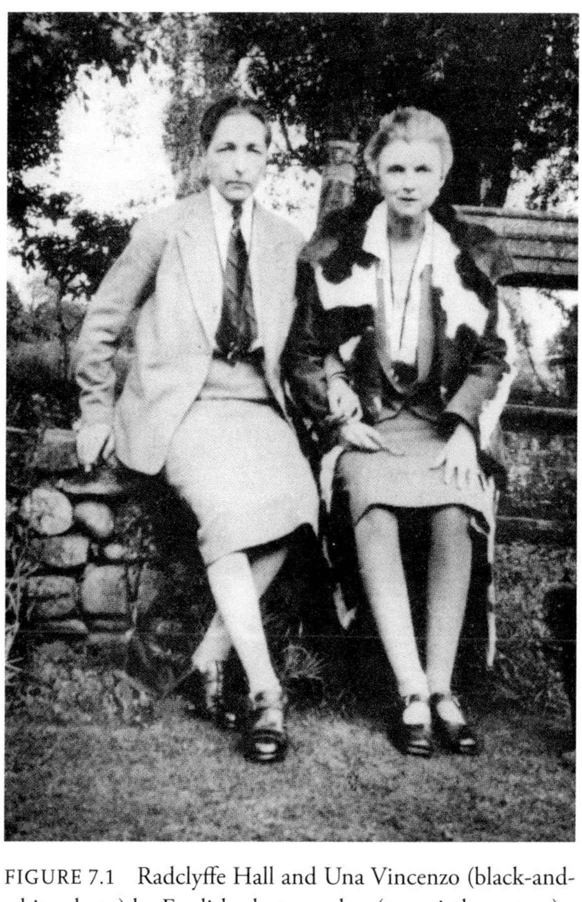

FIGURE 7.1 Radclyffe Hall and Una Vincenzo (black-and-white photo) by English photographer (twentieth century). *Credit*: Private collection/the Bridgeman Art Library.

Although scholars contextualize lesbian style at the time as masculine, or mannish, Laura Doan argues that masculine dress in the 1920s was not necessarily an indication of the wearer's sexuality and challenges the image of the tuxedoed, crop-haired, cigarette-smoking woman as a lesbian. In her article "Passing Fashions: Reading Female Masculinities in the 1920s," Doan discusses the fashion trend toward a "masculine style," particularly in Britain and Paris. She makes implicit the assertion that caution should be taken when pinning down the cultural significance of monocles, short hair (the Eton crop), and cigarettes to any one effect. Cross-dressing women of all sexual persuasions, she argues, were merely being fashion conscious, and such stylistic accessories were also symbols of the freedom and decadence that women embraced after World War I, when women wore trousers for the first time.

This type of boyish or masculine look came to be known by a variety of names, including hard-boiled flapper, boyette, boy-girl or modern girl, and can be traced by fashion historians to about 1918. "The phenomenon of masculine fashion for women with its concomitant openness and fluidity," writes Doan,

> allowed some women, primarily the middle and upper classes, to exploit the ambiguity that tolerated, even encouraged, the crossing over of fixed labels and assigned categories, such as a female boy, women of fashion in the masculine mode, lesbian boy, mannish lesbian and female cross-dresser. (1998: 670)

According to Doan, lesbians seem to follow the fashion and stylistic trends of the time and did not single out any particular accessory or garment as a sign of sexual identity. "Radclyffe Hall," writes Doan, "rarely wore trousers in public, and women such as Vita Sackville-West would normally only wear them [trousers] in the privacy of their own home. Only Gluck continued to wear trousers publically" (1998: 677–79). The doubling of meaning associated with masculine dress at the time, as modern chic and lesbianism, enabled women such as Una Vincenzo and Radclyffe Hall to simultaneously appear as lesbians and as women of fashion. However, by 1928, the masculine mode of style was gradually on the wane and was being replaced by a more feminine look.

Although Doan cautions the reader that "masculine style" should not be taken as synonymous with lesbian subjectivity, a new cultural and social presence of self-fashioning lesbians was emerging in the early twentieth century. Women with same-sex desires began forming vibrant lesbian communities in major urban metropolises such as Paris, Berlin, Harlem, and Greenwich Village in New York.

The lesbian, writes Elizabeth Wilson, "is an inhabitant of great cities, first glimpsed by Baudelaire in Paris" (1984: 213). From the late nineteenth century until the 1940s, Paris was a center of sexual freedom and same-sex sexual cultures. Lesbian American and European expatriates and French lesbian writers and artists created a bohemian social, sexual, and creative milieu. They were drawn to the city because it offered an escape from English and American conservative values. Paris's cultural milieu accepted homosexual practices to some degree, provided that they were restricted to the elite and aristocratic salons or to secluded working-class bars.

In his writings, the photographer Gyula Halasz Brassai describes the city of Paris as the "Sodom and Gamorrah" where the lesbian bar The Monocle, on the Boulevard Edgar-Quinet, was "the capital of Gamorrah," one of "the first temples of Sapphic love" (1976: 68). "From the owner, known as Lulu de Montparnasse, to the barmaid," he writes,

> from the waitress to the hat-check girl, all the women were dressed as men, and so totally masculine in appearance that at first glance one thought that they were men. A tornado of virility had gusted through the place and blown away all the finery, all the tricks of feminine coquestry, changing women into boys, gangsters and policemen. Gone the trinkets, ruffles! Pleasant colors, frills!... they wore the most sombre uniforms; black tuxedos... and of course their hair—women's crowning glory—abundant, waved, sweet smelling, cured—had also been sacrificed on Sappho's alter. The customers of Le Monocle wore their hair in the style of a Roman emperor or Joan of Arc. (69)

The wealthy American playwright, poet, and novelist Natalie Clifford Barney established a salon from the 1890s to the 1960s that attracted a coterie of lesbian writers and artists such as Collette, Romaine Brooks, Renèe Vivien, Gertrude Stein, Alice B. Toklas, and Radclyffe Hall. Flamboyant and self-confident, Barney was openly lesbian, declaring, "Albinos are not reproached for having pink eyes and whitish hair, why should they [society] hold it against me for being a lesbian? It's a question of nature: my queerness isn't a vice, isn't deliberate and harms no one" (quoted in Rupp 2006: 241). Gertrude Stein's salon at 27 rue de Fleurus, frequented by artists George Braque, Henri Matisse, and Pablo Picasso and poet Max Jacobs, also flourished at that time, cultivating a circle of significant relationships with well-known members of the avant-garde artistic and literary world. Barney's and Stein's salon society supported subversive sexuality and cultural practices and was considered by the dominant French aristocracy as bohemian. While their status as expatriate artists and writers allowed these women to participate in subversive behavior and dress, French dominant society still considered homosexuality as "deviant" and needing to be hidden.

Berlin was also home to a vibrant lesbian community in the 1920s until the Nazi rise to power in the late 1930s. It boasted a number of lesbian bars, balls, circles, and groups as well as prominent lesbian publications such as *Die Freundin* ("The Girlfriend") between 1924 and 1933, and *Garçonne* specifically for male transvestites and lesbians. According to Leila J. Rupp, both periodicals featured "photographs and illustrations of a variety of lesbians: some crossdressed, some in butch-femme couples, some entirely feminine" (2006: 244). Clubs varied from large establishments so popular that they were tourist attractions to small neighborhood cafés where only local women went to find other women (Figure 7.2).

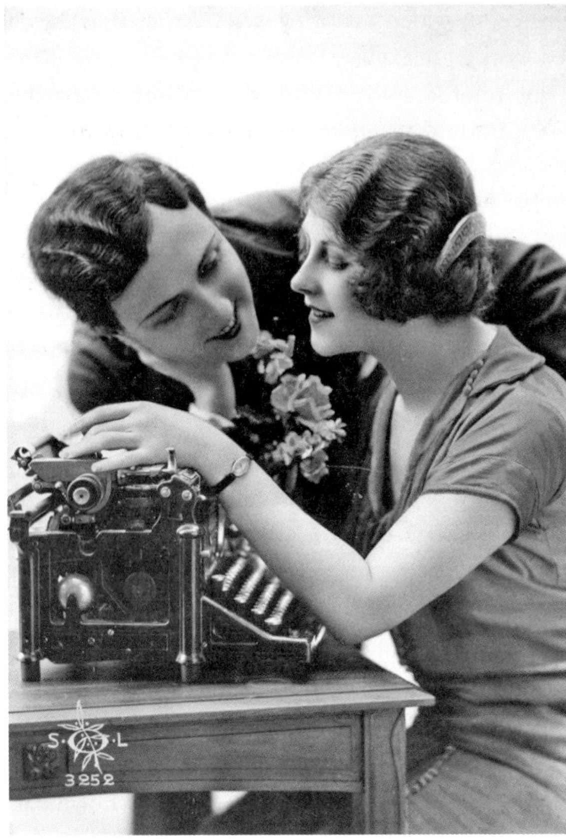

FIGURE 7.2 *At the Office* (color photo), ca. 1930, by French School (twentieth century).
Credit: Private collection/Archives Charmet/the Bridgeman Art Library.

By the 1920s neighborhoods such as Greenwich Village and Harlem in New York had established reputations as hubs of lesbian activities. Like Paris and Berlin, these two districts were bohemian enclaves that attracted subversive crowds. During what is called the "Harlem Renaissance" period, from about 1920 to 1935, African American lesbians were meeting each other, socializing in cabarets and rent parties, and creating a language that spoke of lesbian love and erotica among women. The most popular lesbian (and gay) venue was the Clam House, a long, narrow room on 133rd Street's Jungle Alley. Popular lesbian celebrities such as Libby Holman and her lover Louisa Carpenter du Pont Jenny, who often dressed in matching bowler hats, were regulars among the crowd. The Clam House presented live stage acts, drag queen performers, and the mannish impresario Gladys Bentley, who dressed in a tuxedo and top hat and sang popular songs of the day. Other lesbian or mixed gay bars included Yeahman and The Garden of Joy and Ubangi, which featured a female impersonator who went by the name of Gloria Swanson (E. Garber 1990: 23–25). Like Paris and Berlin, Harlem's lesbian venues reflected a zone where sartorial display and extravagance were a key indicator of the diversity of sexual identities and the politics of subcultural style.

BAR CULTURE OF THE 1940S AND 1950S

Femme and butch styles were particularly prominent in the working-class lesbian bar culture of the 1940s, 1950s, and early 1960s where butch-femme relationships were the norm. In the 1940s in the United States, most butch women had to wear conventionally feminine dress in order to maintain their jobs, wearing their heavily starched shirts, large cuff links, ties, and oxford shoes only on weekends to go to bars or parties.

The 1950s saw the rise of a new generation of butches who refused to live double lives and wore butch attire full-time, or as close to full-time as possible. Their wardrobes consisted of casual wear for weekends such as sports jackets, chino pants, and Western shirts. Penny loafers were also popular and were worn with argyle socks as well as cowboy boots. From the late 1950s, sweaters, cardigans, and V-necks became trendy among butches. Tuxedo shirts and ties were popular for evening wear as well as low-cut men's dress boots. Their visibility usually limited the butches to a few jobs, such as factory work and taxi driving, which had no dress codes for women. Because of their increased visibility, combined with the antigay rhetoric of the McCarthy era, violent attacks on lesbians increased, while at the same time the strong and defiant bar culture became more willing to respond with force. Although femmes also fought back, it became primarily the role of butches to defend against attacks and hold the bars as lesbian space. While in the 1940s the prevailing butch image was severe but gentle, it became increasingly tough and aggressive as violent confrontation became an aspect of life. In "Butch-Femme Relationships: Sexual Courage in the 1950s," one of the first groundbreaking essays in defense of butch-femme roles, Nestle (1987a) argues that such role-playing made lesbian communities visible and paved the way for sexual liberation in the 1960s and 1970s (Kennedy and Davis 1993: 124).

The most publicly visible sign of lesbianism in the 1950s was the appearance of the butch or "stud" lesbian, with her stylized short hair, men's tailored suit or blue jeans, and boots, loafers, or sneakers (Kennedy and Davis 1993: 157). She held doors for her femme women, paid the bill when on a date, and lit the femme's cigarettes. Femmes appeared glamorous and wore makeup, tight dresses and skirts (rarely pants), pantyhose, and high-heeled shoes. The importance of dressing up continued throughout the 1950s; however, the style changed as they reflected dress styles and trends in mainstream culture. These changes also reflected developments in the lesbian community. "White tough bar lesbians, Black tough lesbians, and the primarily white upwardly mobile lesbians projected different images" (158).

In their study of a pre-1960s working-class lesbian community in Buffalo, New York, Kennedy and Davis noted that white American tough bar butches cultivated working-class masculine looks and modeled themselves on popular musicians of the emerging rock and roll scene, such as Elvis Presley, Ritchie Valens, and Buddy Holly, whose slicked-back hair, pouted lips, and smoldering eyes all became models of style for aspiration. Young butches greased their hair in the popular DA, or "duck's ass," and wore black leather jackets, white T-shirts, and blue jeans, a look that was popularized by James Dean and Marlon Brando. "It was a style that was at once tough and erotically enticing; simultaneously careless and intense" (1993: 159).

African American butches adopted more formal wear than white studs did, especially for evening attire. They wore starched white shirts with formal collars and dark dress pants. They preferred men's Florsheim dress shoes, which they wore with dark nylon socks. Their hair was processed, combed back on the sides and cut square at the top. Mannerisms for both black and white butches continued to form an important part of lesbian style; "Mannerism... The way they was [sic] dressed... they [sic] way they talk [sic], the way they acted... was a tough, rough and ready style" (Kennedy and Davis 1993: 164).

Lesbian bars in the 1940s and 1950s were very important meeting places for lesbians and went hand in hand with the development of lesbian sexuality and paved the way to liberation. Lesbian bars such as Rainard's on King Street in Sydney and Tommy's Place in San Francisco were essential meeting places in the construction of a lesbian community and acted as "safe" spaces from an often hostile and homophobic world. In Philadelphia, Barone's and Rusty's were popular among butch and femme lesbians.

FEMINIST ANTISTYLE

If there was such a thing as lesbian style in the 1960s and early 1970s, it was essentially "antistyle," a refusal to submit to mainstream culture's standards of feminine beauty, behavior, and fashion and a rejection of the strict butch-femme role-playing of earlier decades (reclaimed among lesbians in the 1980s). To the politically oriented lesbian-feminists, butch-femme roles seemed to mimic the repressive male/female binary of patriarchal society, which suppressed and objectified women. Scholars such as Lillian Faderman (1991) critique butch-femme roles as replicas of heterosexuality instead of being unique and potentially subversive. She does not negate the way that butch-femme roles have shaped lesbians' lives but attempts to understand how these roles shaped lesbians' identity.

Rather than endorsing butch-femme dress codes, the lesbian-feminist community promoted an androgynous style of dress characterized as comfortable and loose fitting, such as flannel shirts, loose jackets, and baggy pants. Hair was worn cut short, and tennis shoes, Birkenstocks, or fry boots were also considered part of this lesbian "clone" style, which was strictly policed by lesbian feminists. As Karen Everett notes in her film documentary, *Framing Lesbian Fashion* (1992), this perceived androgynous style became known as a "uniform" and was a way for lesbians to identify one another in solidarity. To most lesbian feminists, this style spoke about self-identity and belonging to the "sisterhood" and the women's liberation movement. "In a world where feminist energies were channelled into the creation of battered women's shelters," writes Arlene Stein, "anti-pornography campaigns, or women's festivals, primping or fussing over your hair was strictly taboo" (1997: 478). According to Barbara Creed, lesbians who rejected the feminist model of androgyny were given a difficult time: "some of us who refused the lesbian uniform were labelled 'heterosexual lesbians,'" she writes, "an interesting concept that constructs a lesbian as an impossibility" (1999: 123).

Mainstream fashion also drew inspiration from the subversive image of the androgyne with slicked-back hair and a mannish suit photographed by Helmut Newton. The photographic image, which draws on the erotic representation of Marlene Dietrich, is shot in the dimly lit street and contains suggestions of desire and power. Designed in 1966 by Yves Saint Laurent, le Smoking, which drew inspiration from popular culture and the women's movement, was the first of its kind to earn attention in the fashion world. Le Smoking was designed as part of Saint Laurent's Pop Art collection, in the shape of a black jacket and trousers in *grain de poudre* with four button-down pockets, over a white organdy blouse. The suit was adored by a chic collective of style icons, including Catherine Deneuve, Betty Catroux, Francoise Hardy, Liza Minelli, LouLou de la Falaise, Lauren Bacall, and Bianca Jagger.

Many feminist lesbians of the 1960s and 1970s also associated gendered fashion with a return to the strictly coded butch-femme culture of the 1930s, 1940s, and 1950s, of "forbidden love in smoky bars" (Stein 1997: 478). The politically correct feminist style of androgynous clothing, which first applied to identifiable butches and later to all women, was interpreted by mainstream dominant culture as meaning either that women wanted to be men, and aspired to "maleness" in their appearance, or that *all* feminists were man-hating, bra-burning, hairy lesbians and sexual outlaws of a kind. Even this cultural definition was and continues to be extremely useful because, as Elizabeth Wilson explains in her article "Forbidden Love" (1984), it places women in a position to destabilize, by their very existence, the categories of male and female and to challenge the social construction of gender roles.

CROSS-DRESSING AND ANDROGYNOUS STYLE

Many scholars have noted that butch-femme pairing, perceived in the 1960s by feminist lesbians as oppressive and mimicking masculine and feminine roles, became prominent again in the 1980s. Young lesbians began to reconceptualize role-playing and the stylistic cues that accompany gender identities and envisioned these roles as challenging dominant culture. The resurgence of the butch-femme binary, writes Alice Solomon, "was marked primarily by a playful reassertion of sexual freedom through gender switching, cross-dressing, and gendered role playing" (1993: 264).

Madonna, the quintessential female fashion and gay icon of the 1980s, reinforced gender ambiguity in her performances by traversing the space between the sexual mainstream and the sexual fringes of culture. Her 1990 video for her song "Vogue" celebrated queer subcultural style and was a tribute to the underground dance form known as voguing, which first found popularity in the gay bars and discos of New York City. Consciously referencing gay and lesbian discourses and lifestyle in her work, Madonna signified (and continued to do so well into the 1990s) an affirmation of lesbian (and gay) culture as well as contributing to the politics of queer identity and sex.

As a fashion icon, Madonna constantly reinvented herself with codes and signifiers of lesbian style and identity. Her performances onstage and in video clips were explicitly homoerotic, borrowing from cues and styles from Hollywood icons such as Marlene Dietrich and Greta Garbo. "Where else, apart from a Madonna video," writes Sonya Andermaher, "can millions of women see two women kissing on prime-time television?" (1994: 32). Madonna was both butch and femme with a stylized edge, constantly reinventing and embracing a look that asserted sexual and physical autonomy. When Madonna first rose to prominence in the 1980s, she was clothed in leather and accessorized with bows, lace, fishnet stockings, and religious effigies draped around her neck—a stylized "virginal rebel" with platinum locks and a fashion sense that was a slew of edgy plus girly. This "Material Girl" image later morphed into a dominatrix when Jean Paul Gaultier designed her corseted cone bra for her Blond Ambition tour (1990). The pink corset over a stylized version of a man's suit made reference to both the breasts and the phallus. Madonna went from virgin to dominatrix to überwoman through the 1980s and into the 1990s literally overnight. According to Andermaher, this überfemininity "could be intimidating as well as seductive, reinforcing the fluidity of gender identities, and taking control of their identities" (1994: 109). This subversive feminine, even macho, performance can be best described as *gender fuck,* a term that was coined and circulated in the 1980s when subversive and transgressive music celebrities like Adam Ant, Boy George, and Marilyn (Peter Robinson) and pop bands Duran Duran and Spandau Ballet gained global popularity with their flirtation with the dissolution of sartorial codes. Along with the emergence of MTV (music television, launched in 1981), the entertainment industry recognized the value of fashion and style as forms of visual codification in gaining audience popularity. "At both ends of the fashion spectrum," writes Andermaher, "couture and subcultural style, there is a space for experimentation, for transgression and revolt" (109).

Madonna's popularity as a lesbian icon was endorsed by her obsession with drag and camp. Drag is the personification of the instability of gender par excellence, where masculine and feminine signs reveal both dress and gender as performance and masquerade. As Judith Butler argues in the same vein, "There is no original or primary gender that drag imitates, but gender is a kind of imitation for which there is no original" (1991: 21). Within the context of lesbian culture, Madonna's deployment of drag (and camp) as a disguise, as simulation and artifice, acts as a mode of engagement with her audience, while simultaneously positioning her as inside and outside of culture, simultaneously straddling sexual borders.

Drag and androgyny, with its obsession with details, grooming, gestures, accessories, and cosmetics, also highlights the contradictory qualities of fashion. Androgyny had been fashionable many times in history, but it was not until the 1990s that lesbian and bisexual women embraced androgynous style as a political force in queer culture. Until then, cross-dressing had been a recurrent theme in lesbian culture; however, it was closely aligned to sexual disorder or perversion and was bound to marginal underground identities (Entwistle 2000: 176). Even though the history of cross-dressing is bound to gay and lesbian identity, in terms of "drag" and "voguing," Marjorie Garber argues in her analysis of cross-dressing as a site of cultural anxiety (1992) that studies fail to take into account the foundational role that it has played in queer identity and queer style.

In 1984 Annie Lennox, the vocalist for the pop duo Eurythmics (with Dave Stewart), appeared at the Grammy Awards ceremony as the reincarnation of Elvis Presley. Wearing a black suit, white leather belt, silk black shirt, and a gold knit lamé tie, along with Presleyesque coiffure and facial hair, Lennox was impersonating the "King of Rock 'n' Roll" himself as she stepped onto the stage to perform her musical hit "Sweet Dreams (Are Made of This)." As a rock icon, Elvis is instantly recognizable by his own performance, which involves a gyrating pelvis and elaborately sequined and embroidered costumes. In what can best be described as a diva/camp moment, Lennox, via her gender-bending performance, became an instant gay icon. Lennox's androgynous style, which drew parallels between her and male performers Boy George and David Bowie, was characterized by her endless transformations, constantly reinventing herself with various masculine and feminine personas: as a high-class blond call girl; as Earl, a working-class Elvis lookalike with a confident charm; as a sexually repressed housewife; as a camp angel in a French rococo drama; and as a sadomasochistic dominatrix—characters that have now become quintessential drag king personas.

While Lennox dressed as a man, she also performed as a woman dressed as a man dressed as a woman. She played with traditional markers of femininity (dresses, aprons, and lace) and juxtaposed these markers with a raunchy confident sexuality (black leather studded catsuit). The sexual ambiguity prevalent in the Lennox's performance style is, as Graber (1992) points out, a type of subversive behavior that was prevalent and popular, especially with cross-dressing girls in the 1980s. Emerging from the social consciousness-raising movements of the 1960s and 1970s, feminism, civil rights, and the rising influence of gay lifestyle politics, "gender bending" possessed enormous influence in popular culture and paved the road for greater diversity in representations of sexuality. "By the middle of the decade [1980s]," writes Richard Middleton, "particularly male style for girls was ubiquitous fashion" (1995: 476).

Performers such as Madonna and Annie Lennox with their fashionable androgynous style became poster girls for a generation of lesbian women who were looking toward popular culture for style icons and positive role models. References to lesbianism were rife in popular culture, from singer-songwriter Melissa Etheridge, who began performing in lesbian bars in Los Angeles in the 1980s (a gay rights activist who came out publicly in 1993); to Tracy Chapman; to Madonna, who shared a passionate kiss with her backup vocalist; to tennis player Martina Navratilova, who admitted to being a lesbian. Until the 1980s, fashion was one of the most important signifiers of lesbian sexuality and consisted of clear definitions of identities such as femme and butch. Many women in the 1970s and 1980s played an active part in the second-wave feminist movement and wanted to reject dominant models of femininity. "Feminist lesbians, visibly fought fashion as a constraining and feminizing force of capitalism and heteropatriarchy," write Entwistle and Wilson, "although fashion has always had a place within femme lesbian and bisexual cultures" (2001: 6).

By the early 1990s, lesbian style ascendancy was so entrenched in glamour that the French declared lesbians as officially chic, and terms such as *lipstick lesbian, neo femme,* and *stone* and *diesel* butch began gaining currency as identity categories. Lesbian sexuality began to break free from the restrictive binary of femme-butch and to play and explore the boundaries of representations (via dress, accessories, and stylistic codes) in mainstream and underground culture. After her visit to the lesbian sauna Dykes Delight in London, Isabell Wolff wrote in a June 1993 edition of the *Evening Standard,* "Forget the old dungarees image, the latest lesbians are bright, chic and glamorous. . . . Everywhere you look, the joys of dykedom are being vigorously and joyfully extolled" (quoted in Sender 2003: 359).

Lesbian style and desirability were embodied by such style icons as butch country singer k.d. lang, who appeared in 1992 on an American late-night talk show hosted by Arsenio Hall wearing a long, lacy gown (and barefoot) to sing the song "Miss Chatelaine." Lang, who was known at this point in her career as an "out" lesbian, shocked Hall and television audiences alike, who expected her to appear and perform in butch attire. Lang's "femme-ness" was a conscious political strategy of self-representation that she deployed to debunk cultural stereotypes about lesbians and the way they look, behave, and dress. In 1990 a young lang appeared in the Gap's ongoing advertisement campaign Individuals of Style, photographed by Herb Ritts. Wearing Gap stone-washed denim jeans and jacket and cowboy boots and looking dreamily out into the distance, lang's image spoke to a generation of lesbians about popular fashion and style. To stone butches, she was a fashion icon to mimic and admire; to femmes, she was a heartthrob pinup girl to fantasize about and swoon over. Lang relied on fashionable garments and accessories to visually represent and articulate a queer identity, often appearing on stage cross-dressed in masculine attire, while her performative style was inscribed with lesbian meaning. Arlene Stein (1993: 107) wrote of lang as "probably the butchest woman entertainer since Gladys Bentley," and *Vanity Fair* journalist Leslie Bennetts (1993: 50) described her in the following way:

> This was a woman who was clearly born to perform. Not that you'd necessarily know she's a woman at first sight. Tall and broad shouldered, wearing a black cutaway coat flecked with gold, black pants, her favourite steel-toed black rubber shit-kicker work boots, she looks more like a cowboy.

Lang's 1993 appearance with supermodel Cindy Crawford on the cover of the August issue of *Vanity Fair* magazine, also photographed by Herb Ritts, is another example of lang "camping on her butchness" (Rodger 2004: 26). Dressed in a three-piece pin-striped suit, tie, and brogues, lang sits on a traditional barber's chair while being shaved by supermodel (and straight woman) Cindy Crawford, who is dressed in a maillot. The *Vanity Fair* cover spread was a result of a growing trend in popular culture: lesbianism had now become fashionable. The media frenzy over "lesbian chic," note Entwistle and Wilson (2001: 1–12), "possibly fuelled by panic over the erosion of visible differentiation between straight and queer women, has inspired some (middle-class) women to reclaim fashion, and to muscle in on some of the 'boyz fun' organised around the plethora of new clubs and bars."

DESIGNER DYKES AND LESBIAN CHIC

> We've arrived. The postmodern lesbian: not only butch and not totally lipstick chic but definitely demographically desirable—and Showtime's banking on it, big time. It's called *The L-Word.* That's right, folks, L for lesbian—say it out loud, say it proud.
>
> —Kate Nielson (2004: 9)

In the 1990s, Calvin Klein was looking for an androgynous model to represent his new scent CK One and enlisted Japanese American supermodel Jenny Shimizu. A former mechanic, Shimizu went on to model for designers Versace, Anna Sui, Prada, Jean Paul Gaultier, and Yohji Yamamoto and was featured in beauty campaigns for Clinique and Shiseido. CK One was tagged "the fragrance for a man or a woman. A fragrance for everyone," and the black-and-white media campaign featured young, hip, androgynous models casually conversing in small groups and laughing coyly at the camera. The script reads, "The sexy one, the nasty one, the wild one, the male one, the female one, CK One, a fragrance for everyone." The advertisement ends with Shimizu dressed in faded blue Calvin Klein jeans, a white masculine singlet, and a black leather wristband, with a large tattoo of a woman astride a giant phallic wrench on her bicep. Shimizu's appeal lay in her assertive and confident androgynous femininity, which became representative of butch style in the lesbian club culture of the 1990s but was also indicative of a lesbian chic that was being circulated in the mainstream media.

In the May 1993 issue of *New York,* Jeanie Kasindorf's article on "lesbian chic" describes a lesbian bar called Henrietta Hudson in New York City:

> Outside the front stands the bouncer, a short young woman with a shaved head and a broad, square body. She is covered in loose black cotton pants, and looks like an out-of-shape kung fu instructor.... [Inside] sits a young woman straight from a Brooks Brothers catalogue—wearing a conservative plaid jacket and matching knee high pleated skirt, a white blouse with a peter pan collar, and a strand of pearls. She chats with her lover while they sip white wine and rub each other's backs. Across from

> them, at the bar, sits a group of young women in jeans and black leather, all with cropped hair.... The Brooks Brothers woman and her lover leave, and are replaced by two twenty-six-year-old women with the same scrubbed, girl-next-door good looks. (quoted in Ciasullo 2001: 593)

The bouncer is coded with butch and masculine signifiers; her "shaved head and broad, square body" are marked as undesirable, shapeless, and menacing: "an out of shape kung fu instructor," rather than being feminine, curved, warm, and inviting like the lesbians inside the bar. A binary of outside/inside is firmly established of what is acceptable and desirable in lesbian looks and beauty. The description of the lesbians inside the bar as "Brooks Brothers" women equates lesbian looks with consumption and ideal fashionable icons on the pages of a shopping catalog. As Sherrie Inness states, "By emphasizing that lesbians are beautiful, well dressed, and born to shop...writers build up an image of lesbians as being 'just like us,' in other words, 'homosexual=heterosexual'" (Inness 2004, quoted in Ciasullo 2001: 593).

Lesbian and queer lifestyle media did not remain immune to the hype that surrounded this new "mediated" identity. Rena Lewis writes that "for lesbian magazines, which often inherited a feminist perspective, the inclusion of fashion was a conspicuous departure from previous feminist publications, whose opposition to the fashion industry is legendary" (1997: 93). Magazines such as *Diva, Girlfriend, OUT/LOOK,* and *Curve* (formally *Deneuve*) had an ambivalent attitude toward fashion imagery and spending and emphasized images of women participating in everyday activities. They portrayed women playing sports, gardening, hanging around the park, tinkering under the hoods of their cars, playing pool, or relaxing by the pool or at the beach. The models pose casually, immersed in their activities, with an air of indifference to the camera. By and large, "the images appearing in magazines targeted to lesbian readers," writes Linda Dittmar, "are indifferent to the corporate chic of mainstream magazines" (1998: 335). It must also be noted that in these images the majority of the women engaged in an aspirational lifestyle, whether skiing in the Alps or vacationing in Asia, tend to be white and middle class. Whether straight or queer, when acknowledged, the Other is exoticized: "*Vogue* and its counterparts continue to give us the tigress, slave, tribal woman and the other myths of the primitive," writes Dittmar, "while *Curve* and its companions give us the ghetto kid, queen of the blues, and the bull dagger menace" (335). Even lesbian photography posits whiteness as the norm.

This is not to say that the queer press regulates lesbian style or that lesbians do not participate in mainstream fashion magazines' construction of a lesbian subjectivity (albeit a femme one) via viewing positions. Writers (Lewis 1997; Lewis and Rolley 1996) have commented on how lesbian viewers of fashion magazines respond to images of women as narcissistic and objectifying. While editorials of women are intended to invoke buying power and promote consumption, for the lesbian viewer the photographs may also evoke desire for the image and desire to be the image. If the lesbian gaze is based on recognition and identification, then the pleasure of looking is simultaneously experienced as the pleasure of being looked at by another woman. This analysis can also be applied to the pleasures of looking at films that depict lesbian characters and story lines, such as *When Night Is Falling* (1996), an unabashed lipstick lesbian feast, with women who look like goddesses rolling around in crushed velvet, and the neo-noir crime thriller *Bound* (1996), directed by the Wachowski brothers, about a woman (Jennifer Tilly) who longs to escape her relationship with her Mafia boyfriend (Joe Pantoliano). When she meets the alluring ex-prison inmate (Gina Gershon) hired to renovate the next-door apartment, the two women begin an affair and hatch a scheme to steal $2 million of Mafia money. Such films are intended for a mainstream audience, but they star lesbian characters and are coded with lesbian plots.

When Showtime's *The L Word* debuted in 2004, many lesbian viewers complained that the characters were all too "femmey" and that the fashion was too unrealistic. Viewers argued that rather than being inclusive of all women, regardless of class and ethnicity, the cast of lesbians were depicted as glamorous, middle-class professional women with the occasional token Asian, African American, and Latino American lesbian cast for political correctness. Cynthia Summers, costume designer for the series, stated that the show's creator and executive producer Ilene Chaiken wanted *The L Word* to be a show that spoke about fashion.

The series is based on the lives and loves of a group of lesbian friends who are glamorously affluent and ambitious, some talented and others creative lesbians, living in Los Angeles. The cast, which consists of lesbian, bisexual, and straight characters, depicts a sexually flexible style characterized as either "L.A. tomboy" or "lesbian chic." The narrative of lesbian fashion and style in the series marks an important aspect of understanding lesbian visibility (or invisibility) as a form of subcultural identity. "The unease born out of the overwhelming femininity of the lesbians in *The L Word,*" writes Aviva Dove-Viebahn, "originates from the extraordinary emphasis placed within the lesbian community on a style that runs counter to mainstream notions of women's fashion" (2007: 73).

In 2010, following in the same vein as *The L Word,* the British Broadcasting Commission (BBC) screened the first season of *Lip Service,* a lesbian drama/romance series set in Scotland that follows the lives of a group of friends in their early twenties searching for love. In March 2011 the Australian production company Freehand launched an eight-part reality Web series, *Generation L: The Road to Mardi Gras,* that documents the lives of a "new generation" of lesbian women.

The discourse of lesbian chic, a constructed phenomenon of the 1990s media representation and a fashion advertising and marketing trend, placed lesbian identity in the mainstream cultural landscape and produced a particular lesbian representation while erasing others (Figure 7.3). Some critics (Ciasullo 2001; Cottingham 1996; Dittmar 1998) argue that the emergence of the lipstick lesbian, or the femme, has normalized, heterosexualized, or even "straightened out" lesbian sexuality in order to make it more palatable to a straight audience.

What is of importance in any critique of lesbian chic is that it raises (or does not raise) issues concerning the construction of beauty, glamour, gender, sexuality, and style.

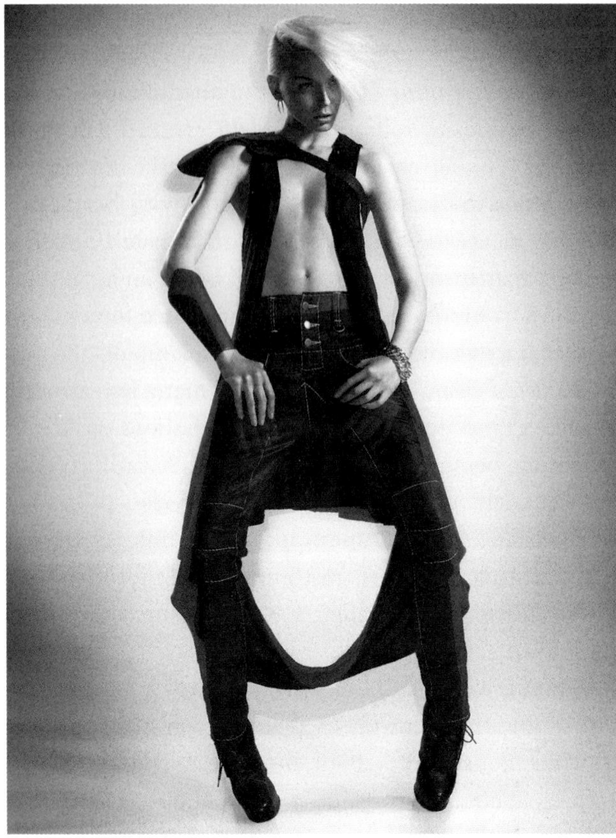

FIGURE 7.3 Lesbian style. Jeans, Opus 9 by Justine Taylor, Gary Bergini extended wool jacket, Demon Leather shoulder piece and cuff, AF Vandervorst boots.
Credit: Photographer Michele Aboud, stylist Bex Sheers, makeup by Angie Barton, hair by Alan White. Model: Anna@CHIC Management.

The "masculinized" power wielded by this new, attractive, and assertive women demanded that she be incorporated into heteronormativity because she was not amenable to it. Imbued with a dynamism that melded traditional femininity with assertiveness, writes Dittmar, this woman evoked lesbian codes of quasi-cross-dressing and female bonding but remained open to heterosexual readings of "power dressing and cosmopolitan sophistication." "Rendered both queer and safe," Dittmar points out, "this new chic at once allowed heterosexuals the *frisson* of bisexual and lesbian desire, and opened up for lesbians—notably middle class and upwardly mobile white lesbians—a hospitable new space for self definition" (1998: 320).

Several critics have argued that the construction of a lesbian chic by marketers is due in part to the rise in income, social mobility, and class standing among lesbian women since the 1980s. A *New York Times Magazine* (1982) article reported that the peak advertisers were attracting the lesbian market. The high-end magazines *Vogue, Newsweek,*

Cosmopolitan, and *Esquire* also echoed such findings, and the *Wall Street Journal* confirmed this in 1994 with the article "More Marketers Aiming Ads at Lesbians." In her article "The Straight Goods: Lesbian Chic and Identity Capital on a Not-So-Queer Planet" (1998), Dittmar writes that this new lesbian look called "chic" is a category defined by class, not sexuality, whose main purpose is to encode power and to give women a place at the crossroads of femininity and authority. "Like so many other cultural products which sustain our economy and safeguard dominant ideology," writes Dittmar, "the sartorial design and photography that constitutes the 'lesbian chic' phenomenon absorbs lesbians into heterosexuality even as they invite straight women to tour lesbian terrains" (323). High-end designer brands such as Ralph Lauren, Gucci, Emanuel Ungaro, Calvin Klein, and Prada, to name a few, took the opportunity to market their designs to appeal to a lesbian sartorial taste. This media-hyped style has codes and subtexts that corresponded to lesbian subculture, while simultaneously reaching out to a dominant heterosexual market (Figure 7.4).

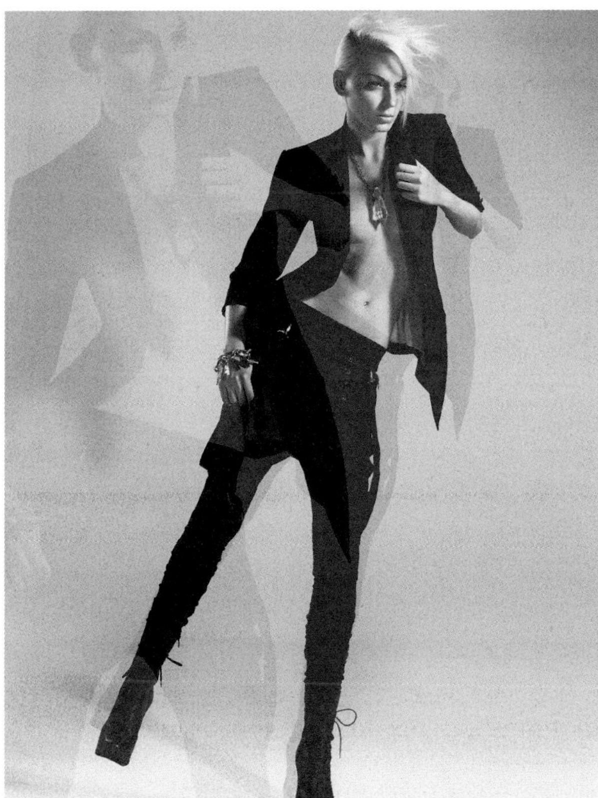

FIGURE 7.4 Lesbian style. Pants, Opus 9 by Justine Taylor, Alexander McQueen jacket, AF Vandervorst boots, Chanel bracelet, Raphael Mhashikar crystal pendant.
Credit: Photographer Michele Aboud, stylist Bex Sheers, makeup by Angie Barton, hair by Alan White. Model: Anna@ CHIC Management.

CONCLUSION

In the field of fashion studies, little attention (if any) has been paid to the dynamics and symbolism of lesbian dress in constructing identities and subcultural style. From the salon dandies of the 1920s, to the strictly encoded femme/butch dress codes of the 1950s, and through to the "lipstick lesbians" of the 1990s, lesbian fashion continues to parody and subvert the associated oppositions between masculinity and femininity. Lesbian style is influenced by mainstream fashion and the trends that appear in fashion magazines, on the film screen, in advertisements, and on the catwalks. In the twenty-first century, politics have become more diversified, and the divide between butch and femme identities has now become blurred and watered down.

What makes the study of fashion and style so important to lesbian identity is the role of clothing in constructing material identity and its shaping of personal and social space. Patrizia Calefato is eloquent on this idea, writing that

> fashion has turned the body into a discourse, a sign, a *thing*. A body permeated by discourse, of which clothes and objects are an intrinsic part, is a body exposed to transformations, to grotesque openings toward the world; a body that will feel and taste all that the world feels and tastes, if it simply lets itself open up. (1997: 72)

The study of style with respect to lesbians allows for these "tastes." For lesbianism is something far more lived, experienced, enjoyed, and suffered than theorized. In the last twenty years, studies have highlighted the intersections between gender, class, race, and sexuality and their impact on the body and style. The politics of appearance is about the process of becoming, a statement that is politically and aesthetically charged. Calefato describes how a look functions as an image and an expression of one's outlook on the world. She argues that a look articulates "a way of being in the world and creating a social universe" and that the "worldliness" of a clothed body conveys rational values, by virtue of a sort of category of Otherness (71). In other words, style is about identity; it is a way of being in the world. Style is a strategy of resistance, of "talking back" and drawing attention to oneself. It is a state of refusal and revolt.

NOTE

This chapter is a revised version of the chapter "Lesbian Style: From Mannish Women to Lipstick Dykes," in Adam Geczy and Vicki Karaminas, *Queer Style* (London: Bloomsbury, 2013).

BIBLIOGRAPHY

Andermaher, Sonya. 1994. "A Queer Love Affair? Madonna and Gay and Lesbian Culture." In Diane Hamer and Belinda Budge (eds.), *The Good, the Bad, and the Gorgeous: Popular Culture's Romance with Lesbianism,* 28–40. London: HarperCollins.

Bennetts, Leslie. 1993. "k.d. lang Cuts It Close." *Vanity Fair,* August, 46–93.

Brassai, Gyula Halasz. 1976. *The Secret Paris of the Thirties.* Trans. Richard Miller. London: Thames and Hudson.

Butler, Judith. 1991. "Imitation and Gender Subordination." In Diana Fuss (ed.), *Inside/Out: Lesbian Theories, Gay Theories,* 345–87. London: Routledge.

Calefato, Patrizia. 1997. "Fashion and Worldliness: Language and the Imagery of the Clothed Body." *Fashion Theory: The Journal of Dress, Body and Culture* 1 (1): 69–90.

Ciasullo, Anne M. 2001. "Making Her (In)visible: Cultural Representations of Lesbianism and the Lesbian Body in the 1990s." *Feminist Studies* 27 (3): 577–608.

Cottingham, Laura. 1996. *Lesbians Are So Chic... That We're Not Really Lesbians at All.* London: Cassell.

Creed, Barbara. 1999. "Lesbian Bodies: Tribades, Tomboys and Tarts." In Janet Price and Margrit Shildrick (eds.), *Feminist Theory and the Body: A Reader,* 111–24. Edinburgh: Edinburgh University Press.

Dittmar, Linda. 1998. "The Straight Goods: Lesbian Chic and Identity Capital on a Not-So-Queer Planet." In Deborah Bright (ed.), *The Passionate Camera: Photography and Bodies of Desire,* 319–39. London: Routledge.

Doan, Laura. 1998. "Passing Fashions: Reading Female Masculinities in the 1920s." *Feminist Studies* 24 (3): 663–700.

Dove-Viebahn, Aviva. 2007. "Fashionably Femme: Lesbian Visibility. Style and Politics in *The L Word.*" In Thomas Peele (ed.), *Queer Popular Culture: Literature, Media, Film and Television,* 71–83. New York: Palgrave Macmillan.

Entwistle, Joanne. 2000. *The Fashioned Body: Fashion, Dress and Modern Social Theory.* Cambridge, UK: Polity.

Entwistle, Joanne, and Elizabeth Wilson. 2001. "Introduction: Body Dressing." In Joanne Entwistle and Elizabeth Wilson (eds.), *Body Dressing,* 1–12. Oxford: Berg.

Everett, Karen (dir.). 1992. *Framing Lesbian Fashion: A Documentary.* Davis, CA: Wolfe Video.

Faderman, Lillian. 1991. *Odd Girls and Twilight Lovers: A History of Lesbian Life in Twentieth Century America.* New York: Penguin.

Garber, Eric. 1990. "A Spectacle in Color: The Lesbian and Gay Subculture of Jazz Age Harlem." In Martin Duberman, Martha Vicinus, and George Chauncery Jr. (eds.), *Hidden from History: Reclaiming the Gay and Lesbian Past,* 318–32. New York: Meridien.

Garber, Marjorie. 1992. *Vested Interests: Cross-Dressing and Cultural Anxiety.* London: Penguin.

Inness, Sherrie. 2004. *Action Chicks: New Images of Tough Women in Popular Culture.* London: Palgrave.

Jennings, Rebecca. 2007. *Tomboys and Bachelor Girls: A Lesbian History of Post-war Britain, 1945–71.* Manchester: Manchester University Press.

Kasindorf, Jeanie. 1993. "Lesbian Chic." *New York Magazine,* May 10, 30–37.

Kennedy, Elizabeth Lapovsky, and Madeline D. Davis. 1993. *Boots of Leather, Slippers of Gold: The History of a Lesbian Community.* New York: Routledge.

Lewis, Reina. 1997. "Looking Good: The Lesbian Gaze and Fashion Imagery." *Feminist Review* 55: 92–109.

Lewis, Reina, and Katrina Rolley. 1996. "Ad(dressing) the Dyke: Lesbian Looks and Lesbian Looking." In Peter Horne and Reina Lewis (eds.), *Outlooks: Lesbian and Gay Sexualities and Visual Cultures,* 178–90. London: Routledge.

Middleton, Richard. 1995. "Authorship, Gender and the Construction of Meaning in the Eurythmics Hit Recording." *Cultural Studies* 9 (3): 465–85.

Nestle, Joan. 1987a. "Butch-Femme Relationships: Sexual Courage in the 1950s." In *A Restricted Country.* Ithaca, NY: Firebrand.

Nestle, Joan. 1987b. "The Femme Question." In Joan Nestle (ed.), *The Persistent Desire: A Femme-Butch Reader,* 138–46. Boston: Alyson.

Newton, Esther. 1990. "The Mythic Mannish Lesbian: Radclyffe Hall and the New Woman." In Martin Duberman, Martha Vicinus, and George Chauncery Jr. (eds.), *Hidden from History: Reclaiming the Gay and Lesbian Past,* 281–93. New York: Meridien.

Nielson, Kate. 2004. "Lesbian Chic. Part Deux." *The Advocate,* February 17, 9.

Rodger, Gillian. 2004. "Drag, Camp and Gender Subversion in the Music and Videos of Annie Lennox." *Popular Music* 23 (1): 17–29.

Rupp, Leila J. 2006. "Loving Women in the Modern World." In Robert Aldrich, *Gay Life and Culture: A World History,* 223–47. London: Thames and Hudson.

Sender, Katherine. 2003. "Sex Sells: Sex, Taste and Class in Comercial Gay and Lesbian Media." *GLQ: A Journal of Lesbian and Gay Studies* 9 (3): 331–65.

Solomon, Alisa. 1993. "It's Never Too Late to Switch: Crossing toward Power." In Lesley Ferris (ed.), *Crossing the Stage: Controversies on Cross-Dressing,* 144–53. London: Routledge.

Stein, Arlene. 1993. "Androgyny Goes Pop: But Is It Lesbian Music?" In Arlene Stein (ed.), *Sisters, Sexperts, Queers: Beyond the Lesbian Nation,* 96–109. London: Penguin.

Stein, Arlene. 1997. *Sex and Sensibility: Stories of a Lesbian Generation.* Davis: University of California Press.

Wilson, Elizabeth. 1984. "Forbidden Love." *Feminist Studies* 10 (2): 213–26.

SECTION III

Spaces of Fashion

Introduction

AGNÈS ROCAMORA

Scholars have shown that different cultures have different spatial organizations and that space is a historical and social product. It is not a homogeneous pre-given container ready to be filled with things and bodies; rather, it is the product of social relations and practices, an assemblage of places, things, individuals, institutions, and points of view (see Certeau 1988; Foucault [1967] 1984; Kern 2003; Lefebvre 1991; Massey 2005; Thrift 1996).

The social relations and practices that constitute space are themselves embedded in, and shaped by, specific fields, as Pierre Bourdieu has shown of the field of art, the academic field, and the field of fashion (Bourdieu 1975, 1996a, 1996b; for discussions of the field of fashion, see also Entwistle and Rocamora 2006; Rocamora 2002). Thus, understanding space as a social product also means understanding space as produced by particular fields, spaces rather than space, with the field of fashion then active in the making of this plurality. The present section focuses on some of the spaces of fashion.

Moreover, fashion is the outcome, and the producer, of specific systems of representation, production, and consumption, articulated in particular spaces and places, whether they be, for example, textual spaces such as magazines or films or urban spaces such as the high street or the shopping mall, Paris or New York. There are, then, many "species of spaces" (Crang and Thrift 2000: 3, after Perec [1974] 2000): three-dimensional as well as two-dimensional, geographical and material as well as representational and imagined. Thus, looking at the spatial formation of fashion means not only looking at its particular geography, as authors who have discussed fashion cities and related urban spaces have done (see, for instance, Arnold 2008; Breward 2004; Breward and Gilbert 2006; O'Neill 2007; Rappaport 2000; Rocamora 2009; Rocamora and O'Neill 2008; Steele 1998), but also looking at the many "species of spaces" that it is made of, generates, or appropriates. Indeed, the spaces of fashion are numerous, and although various authors have attended to some of them, most notably John Potvin's 2009 edited collection *The Places and Spaces of Fashion, 1800–2007* (but see also, for instance, Quinn 2003), there are still many to be interrogated. The present section is a step in that direction.

Thus, in "Border Crossings: Fashion and Film/Fashion in Film," Paul Jobling draws on Henri Lefebvre's (1991) conceptualization of space as perceived, conceived, and lived—that is, in Lefebvre's terms, respectively, spatial practice, representations of space, and representational spaces—to explore the dialogue between fashion and film. Through his appropriation of Lefebvre's conceptual framework, Jobling interrogates the relation between the two-dimensional space of the screen and the three-dimensional spaces of the cinema theater, the workplace, and the retail environment. This allows him to engage not only with the role of clothing in the "metaphysical space" of the film but also with issues of audience reception, consumption patterns, and dynamics of work and retail. The relation between fashion and film, he shows, is articulated across a range of spaces that cross over on- and off-screen. In doing so, he draws attention to the gendered and ethnic hierarchies that structure the design studio and the manufacturing of costume, to the porosity of borders between "the space of fashion-in-film" and "the space of material culture and the retail environment," and to costume in film as the locus for the playing out of various identities and the confluence of internal and external bodily experiences.

By showing how fashion crosses borders between two- and three-dimensional spaces Jobling shows that the spaces of fashion are not clear-cut but overlap and feed into each other. There is a symbiosis between the perceived, the conceived, and the experienced; that is, space is not a rigid or fixed formation. But neither is fashion, for it moves and changes across spaces: across the two-dimensional space of the cinema screen and the three-dimensional space of the design studio and retail environment, as Jobling shows. Whereas Jobling focuses on the spaces of cinema and the retail environment, in her chapter Regina Lee Blaszczyk looks at the "hidden spaces of fashion production" in an approach evocative of the work of Erving Goffman (1990). Indeed, in his study of the presentation of the self in everyday life, the American scholar makes a distinction between front and back regions. Front regions are spaces where only "end products... something that has been finished, polished, and packaged" are presented to an audience, while back regions are where the "dirty work," "the long, tedious hours of lonely labour" involved in the making of products, takes place (1990: 52–53). Goffman developed these terms in relation to the study of the presentation of the self in everyday life, but the concepts are useful for making sense of fashion as a spatialized formation, that is, as a field split into front and back regions (Breward 2006; Rocamora 2009). The front regions of fashion, for instance, include the windows of a department store, a brand's advertising campaign, or, indeed, a film where the creations of a designer are worn, as Jobling reminds us with respect to Edith Head, for instance. The back regions of fashion include, for instance, a department store's alterations department, the sweatshops in which a product is manufactured, and the many other hidden spaces where fashion is assembled, negotiated, and kept out of the consumer's sight.

However, fashion studies, Blaszczyk argues, has tended to neglect the behind-the-scenes business activities involved in the making of fashion. In her chapter she shows that business history is useful for attending to this neglect. In the mid-1990s a cultural turn took place in business history that paved the way for a series of studies of fashion, including hers. Thus, in contrast with the term *fashion system,* which, she observes, privileges "the cultural production of meaning," she coins the notion "fashion-industrial complex," informed by the new business history, to insist on the importance of researching behind-the-scenes fashion activities. The term attends to the many individual and institutional players involved in "the design, manufacture, wholesaling, distribution, promotion, and retailing of fashion." Among them are the many invisible fashion intermediaries in charge of the decisions that will determine what products are on offer on the shop floor. In her chapter, Blaszczyk discusses both the nineteenth-century and post–World War II American fashion-industrial complexes by focusing on two types of invisible intermediaries, "practical men," who were involved in the design of fabrics, and fiber makers. She draws attention to the web of flows, practices, and intermediaries involved in the making of fashion, dense yet hidden from sight.

Blaszczyk reminds us that fashion is not just about spectacular and highly visible practices of display and consumption; it is also about the less visible because less glamorous practices of production. Understanding fashion means understanding its front but also its back regions, bringing the hidden spaces of fashion to the fore of academic knowledge—a task she convincingly undertakes.

With José Teunissen's "Fashion: More Than Cloth and Form," we return to the front regions of fashion to look at some of the changes that have informed the display of fashion. Indeed, the second half of the twentieth century, the author notes, witnessed the emergence of new spaces for the conceptualizing and experiencing of fashion. In the 1960s designers started engaging with fashion on a more conceptual plane, giving commodities an accrued immaterial and abstract dimension. As a result, new platforms for the display of fashion appeared, among them galleries and museums—spaces normally reserved for the legitimated arts of painting or sculpture. Designers have also revisited the traditional spaces of fashion such as the catwalk and the store to convey their vision. Such changes have led to the redefinition of "the 'performance' of fashion": from the catwalk to the shop floor, "the label itself has (been) turned into a spectacle."

By bringing together realms that are commonly seen as antinomic—art and commerce, high and low culture—Teunissen argues that designers have turned the catwalk and the shop floor into hybrid spaces, as is the case, for instance, with Rei Kawakubo's "poetics of space." The Japanese designer has reconfigured the traditional setting of the fashion show to allow for a greater proximity between clothes and the audience. She has also turned her boutiques into gallery-like spaces for the display of her highly conceptual creations. As Prada's New York store also illustrates, fashion shops have become points of confluence between the realms of architecture, design, and art. What matters is the range of experiences—visual, haptic, and even olfactory—that shopping in specific locations engenders, rather than the particular aesthetic of the products on display.

Teunissen's discussion underscores the idea that space is always open to appropriation and redefinition. Once the preserve of the traditional arts, galleries and museums are now open to fashion, which turns them into less formal and elite spaces. This appropriation also helps fashion to recreate itself as a legitimate art, which shows the importance of space in the definition of fields of culture such as that of fashion. As Lefebvre (1991) notes, space is a productive product; that is, it is both a product of fashion and productive of fashion, an idea Patrik Aspers's "Markets as Fashion Spaces" also supports. Indeed, Aspers focuses on the idea of the market to show that "spatiality is both constituted by fashion and helps to constitute fashion." To discuss the importance of markets in the coordination of fashion, he problematizes their spatial dimension by making a distinction between physical and virtual markets. The former include the marketplace such as the traditional spaces of the market square but also specific locations such as London's Carnaby Street and other shopping clusters; the latter include the virtual space of the Internet, the new form of the contemporary fashion market space. The fashion market is made up of both. Markets allow for the enabling and controlling of free choice that is central to the logic of fashion. They are also premised on a series of social interactions and practices productive of fashion: the observation of others, the relation between buyers and sellers, the enacting of choice, competition. Fashion is not the product of either one or the other but the outcome of all in their unfolding in the fashion market.

By insisting on the relational dimension of the particular space of the market, Aspers reminds us that, as Doreen Massey also observes, space must be understood relationally. For it is made of "multiple trajectories, a simultaneity of stories-so-far" (Massey 2005: 24). These are the stories and trajectories of the designers who show their clothes in the front regions of the cinema screen, the store window, the museum, or the Internet but also those of the fabric designers, fiber makers, fashion buyers, and other invisible fashion intermediaries without whom fashion cannot happen. The following chapters show that the spaces of fashion are numerous and networked, formed by and formative of fashion; that to fully understand fashion's logic these spaces must be interrogated. This is a task left wanting in much of the literature on fashion. However, this section attends to setting the ground for further studies of the many spaces of fashion.

BIBLIOGRAPHY

Arnold, Rebecca. 2008. *The American Look.* London: I. B. Tauris.

Bourdieu, Pierre. 1975. "Le Couturier et sa Griffe. Contribution à une Théorie de la Magie." With Y. Delsaut. *Actes de la Recherche en Sciences Sociales* 1: 7–36.

Bourdieu, Pierre. 1996a. *Homo Academicus.* Cambridge, UK: Polity.

Bourdieu, Pierre. 1996b. *The Rules of Art.* Cambridge, UK: Polity.
Breward, Christopher. 2004. *Fashioning London.* Oxford: Berg.
Breward, Christopher. 2006. "Fashion's Front and Back: 'Rag Trade' Cultures and Cultures of Consumption in Post-war London c. 1945–1970." *London Journal* 31 (1): 15–40.
Breward, Christopher, and David Gilbert (eds.). 2006. *Fashion's World Cities.* Oxford: Berg.
Certeau, Michel de. 1988. *The Practice of Everyday Life.* Berkeley: University of California Press.
Crang, Mike, and Nigel Thrift. 2000. "Introduction." In Mike Crang and Nigel Thrift (eds.), *Thinking Space,* 1–28. London: Routledge.
Entwistle, Joanne, and Agnès Rocamora. 2006. "The Field of Fashion Materialised: A Study of London Fashion Week." *Sociology* 40 (4): 735–51.
Foucault, Michel. [1967] 1984. "Des Espaces Autres." *Architecture, Mouvement, Continuité* 5 (October): 46–49.
Goffman, Erving. 1990. *The Presentation of the Self in Everyday Life.* London: Penguin.
Kern, Stephen. 2003. *The Culture of Time and Space: 1880–1918.* London: Harvard University Press.
Lefebvre, Henri. 1991. *The Production of Space.* Oxford: Blackwell.
Massey, Doreen. 2005. *For Space.* London: Sage.
O'Neill, Alistair. 2007. *London—After a Fashion.* London: Reaktion.
Perec, Georges. [1974] 2000. *Espèces d'Espaces.* Paris: Galilée.
Potvin, John. 2009. *The Places and Spaces of Fashion, 1800–2007.* London: Routledge.
Quinn, Bradley. 2003. *The Fashion of Architecture.* Oxford: Berg.
Rappaport, Erika D. 2000. *Shopping for Pleasure: Women in the Making of London's West End.* Princeton, NJ: Princeton University Press.
Rocamora, Agnès. 2002. "Fields of Fashion: Critical Insights into Bourdieu's Sociology of Culture." *Journal of Consumer Culture* 2 (3): 341–62.
Rocamora, Agnès. 2009. *Fashioning the City: Paris, Fashion and the Media.* London: I. B. Tauris.
Rocamora, Agnès, and A. O'Neill. 2008. "Fashioning the Street: Images of the Street in the Fashion Media." In E. Shinkle (ed.), *Fashion as Photograph: Viewing and Reviewing Images of Fashion,* 185–99. London: I. B. Tauris.
Steele, Valerie. 1998. *Paris Fashion: A Cultural History.* Oxford: Berg.
Thrift, Nigel. 1996. *Spatial Formations.* London: Sage.

8

Border Crossings: Fashion in Film/Fashion and Film

PAUL JOBLING

PROLOGUE: SURVEYING THE FIELD

For a long time the relationship between fashion and film was overlooked or underdeveloped in fashion and film studies alike. Even though Oscars for costume design were introduced in 1948 and BAFTA (British Academy of Film and Television Arts) Awards in 1964, many cinema critics, historians, and theorists have marginalized the role of costume in their writing (Higson 1993; Mulvey [1976] 1989). It is as if dress is somehow a distraction from dealing with the film's text and context. Certain directors, including Alfred Hitchcock, have likewise argued that an emphasis on apparel simply encourages a superficial or fetishistic relationship between spectators and star images, and on this level clothing acts as a kind of decoy or mask to the "true" character beneath (Chierichetti 2003: 125–26). Indeed, the fashion industry itself has been the subject of satire in several films. Recent examples include Robert Altman's *Ready to Wear* (1994) and David Frankel's *The Devil Wears Prada* (2007), but blazing the trail was fashion photographer William Klein's *Qui Etes Vous, Polly Magoo?* (1966). Starring his favorite female model, Dorothy McGowan, the film was a *succès d'estime,* garnering a cult following on account of its op art–inspired geometric designs and its antifashion message. Klein excoriates the fashion system as vacuous and artificial; for instance, the models who are sent down the catwalk wearing aluminum costumes to rapturous applause by the audience (featuring cameos of fashion photographers Richard Avedon and Jeanloup Sieff, and a spoof on *Vogue*'s editor Diana Vreeland), and whose skin is left grazed and bleeding by the sharp edges of their metal outfits, symbolize the stupidity of those involved in promoting the latest period style at any cost.

Nor did film fare much better in the history of fashion and dress, usually because it was assumed most Hollywood historical dramas took great liberties with period costume and proffered, therefore, an inaccurate perspective on how clothes both appeared and were worn that was directly opposed to documentary evidence such as Pathé and Gaumont fashion shorts of the early twentieth century, and amateur and ethnographic film (Leese [1976] 1991: 9; Taylor 2002: 186–88). Thus powdered hair came to be shorthand for the eighteenth century and the "Juliet Cap" for the Renaissance, even though the latter did not exist in the sixteenth century and was invented by actor Theda Bara in 1916 to wear in J. Gordon Edwards's silent film *Romeo and Juliet* (Wilson 1985: 170). To be sure, many interwar designers in Hollywood regarded taking liberties with historical dress as the raison d'être for their work. Travis Banton and Adrian were two of the designers who most blatantly traduced period style, simultaneously observing authenticity in historical dress and departing from it. Several of the low-cut dresses with hooped skirts and frills that Banton designed for Marlene Dietrich in *The Scarlet Empress* (Josef von Sternberg, 1934), a film about Catherine of Russia's rise to power in the 1760s, do pay a passing resemblance to those worn by ladies at the Russian court during the rococo period of the mid-eighteenth century. But he also exceeded historical detail considerably by including gowns trimmed with ostrich feather collars and nightgowns made of chiffon with frosted fur trim. Likewise, Adrian's costumes for Norma Shearer in *Marie Antoinette* (W. S. van Dyke, 1938), reputedly based on Madame Vigée-LeBrun's portraits, were accurate in regard to their intricate embroidery but eschewed the drop-waist chemise popularized by the French queen between 1774 and 1793 in favor of an extravagant pannier silhouette (Gaines and Herzog 2005: 19, 24).[1]

It is with some justification, therefore, that Anne Hollander contends, "A whole fake history of costume, almost entirely composed of stage conventions, has come to exist" (1978: 342–43). Yet in their heyday between the 1930s and 1960s, the big studios usually spent huge amounts on research to get the period details of dress right, and in this regard Banton's stylistic flourishes contrasted negatively with Paul Czinner's more realistic use of costume in Alexander Korda's 1934 biopic, *Catherine the Great* (Cook 1996: 75). It was not until the 1970s, however, that creative license in period costume for film came to be a solecism and designers aimed for authenticity. Hence, the Oscar-winning designs by Ulla-Britt Søderlund and Milena Canonero for *Barry Lyndon* (Stanley Kubrick, 1975) and by James Acheson for *Dangerous Liaisons* (Stephen Frears, 1988) were exact copies of eighteenth-century clothes.[2]

The issue of authenticity and hybridity is also the leitmotif of two exhibitions and their accompanying catalogs: Hollywood and History, curated by Edward Maeder at the Los Angeles County Museum of Art in 1987 (see Maeder 1988), and Film und Mode—Mode in Film, conceived by Regine and Peter W. Engelmeier for the Deutsches Filmmuseum, Frankfurt, in 1990. While the latter was modeled thematically on Elizabeth Leese's pioneering *Costume Design in the Movies* ([1976] 1991), the former propounded a fresh understanding of the eclecticism of historical dress in contemporary cinema, which was subject to the interests and constraints of designers, directors, studio budgets, and prevailing tastes.[3] Engelmeier and Maeder were among the first to cross borders between film and fashion studies, but several scholars in Britain and North America soon followed suit, opening up clothing in all genres of film—not just costume drama—as a fecund space for the analysis of the relationship of fashion and dress to gender, class, and race identities. Their task, nonetheless, was hampered by the fact that the archival paper trail concerning motion picture costume design is diffuse or nonexistent, as Deborah Landis discovered when she was researching *Dressed: A Century of Hollywood Costume Design* (2007: xvi).

Jane M. Gaines of Columbia University, in particular, has done much to illuminate and revise how we regard fashion in film/fashion and film, and her trenchant work on the costume designer Adrian constitutes an important methodological strand of my paper. While Gaines has been strategic in setting the bar for writing and research on the nexus of fashion to film, this is not to suggest that she was single-handedly responsible for doing so. Some of her work, for instance, is the result of a long-standing collaboration with Charlotte Herzog, such as *Fabrications: Costume and the Female Body* (1990), an edited anthology of essays mostly about the role and representation of women in classic Hollywood cinema that embraces debates on the relationship of costume to narrative, the costume designer, body discipline, commerce and film, and visual pleasure. Similarly, she has been the lodestar for several other authors. Thus Stella Bruzzi's *Undressing Cinema: Clothing and Identity in the Movies* (1997) deals with issues of gender, sexuality, and race in British, American, and European cinema, mostly after 1980, while in *Fashioning the Nation: Costume and Identity in British Cinema* (1996) Pam Cook explores the relationship of past to present, masquerade, and nationality and gender in Gainsborough costume drama of the 1940s and the designs of Elizabeth Haffenden. More recently, Marketa Uhlirova has curated the Fashion in Film Festival, whose focus in 2006, *Between Stigma and Enigma*, ranged across issues such as posing, fetishism and eroticism, while in 2008 its theme examined fashion and crime in cinema with *If Looks Could Kill*.

Although each of these writers argues her own agenda, there is a cluster of overarching points that unites them in the way they approach costume in cinema. In *The Production of Space* ([1974] 1991), Henri Lefebvre postulates a compelling dialectic on spatialization and socialization that involves everyday practices and perceptions (*le perçu*), representations (*le conçu*), and the relationship of embodied space and time (*le vécu*). His ideas have been highly influential to urban theory and psychogeography, but I want to apply them here as a productive framework for coordinating the authors cited in this essay and negotiating the relationship between fashion and film in terms of production and reproduction in several ways. Accordingly, on one level I want to deal with the dialectic of le perçu, le conçu, and le vécu in film as a two-dimensional or metaphysical space, interrogating how dress plays a crucial part in mise-en-scène and narrative on the extradiegetic level as described by Gérard Genette (1980: 228–31), that is to say, how the actors and the costumes they wear function as storytellers in and of the film text. On another level, I want to examine how Lefebvre's dialectic is manifested in crossing the border from the two-dimensional space/time of the film to the three-dimensional social and temporal spaces of the cinema theater (or, as André Breton put it in the *First Surrealist Manifesto* [1924], the darkened room as an arena for dreams). This entails modes of spectatorship and audience involvement with extradiegetic clothing, and the developmental workplace and the retail environment, considering the creation of film costume as a matter of women's writing and the way it spills over into consumption patterns.

FILM COSTUME: A CREATIVE SPACE FOR WOMEN

The majority of authors who have concentrated on the role of fashion in film and its relationship to consumerism are female, and the way they opened up an analytical space to assess it coincided, to a greater or lesser degree, with the idea of *l'écriture féminine,* or women's writing, which had emerged in France by the mid-1970s. Thus psychoanalytical feminists like Julia Kristeva and Luce Irigaray challenged the patriarchal ideology of phallogocentrism, which invests power of speech in the male subject, and posed instead significant questions about sexual difference and empowerment in terms of women's polyvocality:

> Is it . . . that having started with the idea of difference, feminism will be able to break free of its belief in Woman, Her power, Her writing, so as to channel this demand for difference into each and every element of the female whole, and, finally, to bring out the singularity of each woman, and beyond this, her multiplicities, her plural languages, beyond the horizon, beyond sight, beyond faith itself? (Kristeva 1986: 208)

Although she does not cite these authors in *Fabrications,* nevertheless Gaines attests to the impact of women's writing on film studies, claiming in a similar vein, "What was produced was a much more risky and recalcitrant idea of women's potent pleasure, produced in the plural to suggest that it didn't stop with the body but that it spread to transform other 'indulgences' into powers" (Gaines 1990b: 5). This theoretical position also underpins her interrogation of Adrian's costume design for *Queen Christina* and *Madam Satan,* to which I return later.

Henceforth, then, the issue at stake for women—and men as well—was to cross over from the flat horizon of gender as biologically and socially determined to the more modulated and challenging terrain of labile sex and gender identities by considering, who does the speaking and from which position?

On this level, women's work is not peripheral but central to making meaning in film and, indeed, in the guise of the costume designer and dressmaker, is crucial to the production of film itself. In the early days of Hollywood, costumes were organized by the female cast. Sometimes, this involved commissioning specific outfits—Lillian Gish, for example, had her mother design and make up the garments she wore in *Birth of a Nation* (D. W. Griffith, 1915). Mostly, however, it involved stars relying on their own wardrobes or hiring historical dress from theatrical outfitters or costume agencies (Nielsen 1990: 161). By the early 1920s Hollywood began to hire wardrobe mistresses and specialist personnel on short-term contracts, and by the mid-1920s the studio behemoths—MGM, Paramount, and 20th Century Fox—had their own costume departments, staffed full-time and employing costume designers, milliners, tailors, and seamstresses (Landis 2007: 30, 2012). Several of the key designers of the period were, of course, men: between 1924 and 1927 Paramount's costume department was headed by Howard Greer, who had previously worked for Lucille (alias Lady Duff Gordon) in New York, and between 1927 and 1938 by Travis Banton, who was responsible for much of Marlene Dietrich's on- and off-screen wardrobe (Engelmeier 1990: 19). Meanwhile, Gilbert Adrian (Adolphe Greenberg), who had studied costume and scene design in Paris at the Parson School of Applied Arts and Design, was MGM's leading costumer between 1928 and 1942. And yet it was Edith Head, a protégée of Greer, who became one of the most prolific and versatile designers in Hollywood's male-dominated film industry, with the longest career of any costumer to date.

Head started off as a sketch artist in 1924, eventually supervising costume at Paramount between 1938 and 1967 and afterward at Universal until her death in 1981. She witnessed, therefore, the change from monochrome to color stock and the challenges of designing for each: orthochromatic black and white, for example, made reds and yellows look unnaturally dark, and blues and greens much lighter (Chierichetti 2003: 17). Involved with 781 films (Head and Calistro [1983] 2008: 247–90) and winning a total of eight Oscars between 1949 and 1973, she produced designs for major female stars such as Dorothy Lamour (*The Jungle Princess,* William Thiele, 1936), Marlene Dietrich (*A Foreign Affair,* Billy Wilder, 1948), Grace Kelly (*Rear Window,* Alfred Hitchcock, 1954), and Ginger Rogers (*Lady in the Dark,* Mitchell Leisen, 1944).[4] This activity and inventiveness is well accounted for in three biographical texts about her, by Head and Calistro ([1983] 2008), Chierichetti (2003), and Jorgensen (2010). Largely, however, these are works of encomium, narrating the tale of the "ugly duckling" that made good, witness Chierichetti's (2003: 6) description of her: "She was short and dark, and bow-legged, and behind her thick glasses her right eye was slightly crossed."

Head asseverates that much of her success was due to the fact that the costumer, in contrast to the couturier, was a collaborative employee of the film studio and usually had to work much more closely with the script and director, characterizing the look of the film's apparel in its entirety: "I do not design the costumes all by myself, I work in close cooperation with all concerned. I do not design *for* people, but *with* people" (Engelmeier 1990: 21). Just how much she cooperated "with people," however, is a matter of debate. Certainly, Head was *prima inter pares* when it came to understanding costume as embodied and the ways it could discipline and disguise a star's physical shortcomings. Speaking about the challenge of designing sarongs for an overweight Lamour in *The Jungle Princess,* for example, Head observed, "She had a terrible figure, and we were supposed to make her look so sexy" (Chierichetti 2003: 50). But by any measure, her own status as a costume designer stood in marked contrast to the subordinate working conditions of Gile Steele and Charles LeMaire, codesigners on *The Heiress* (William Wyler, 1949) and *All about Eve* (Joseph L. Mankiewicz, 1950) respectively, for which Head won the Oscar for best costume, as well as seamstresses and costumers like Agnes Henry and Georgina Grant, all of whom were laboring tirelessly behind the scenes.

This is the theme of Elizabeth Nielsen's 1990 essay, which provides a broader perspective for Head's creativity and dispels the myth of the autonomous star designer. She relates how the motion picture industry replicated the division of labor in the household, restricting women to certain areas of low-paid work such as sewing, handling costumes, and gluing films together, with cramped conditions and round-the-clock shifts the norm (1990: 160, 167). Yet she illuminates how the manufacture of garments involved transnational expertise as well, relying as it did on ethnic minorities and immigrant workers: German Jewish tailors, Mexican beaders, Armenian crochet workers, Japanese and Chinese embroiderers, and lace makers from Ireland, Portugal, and Spain (167–68). Absent, however, were black women, who, with the notable exception of tendered-out employment in nonunion specialty shops, were not admitted directly to the Hollywood costume departments until race labor reform in the 1970s. Furthermore, as Nielsen points out, such manufacture was more accurately a form of custom creating, carried out by a team of highly skilled artisans: "people with job titles such as cutter, fitter, figure maker, table lady, draper, finisher, tailor, beader, milliner, and shoemaker, who can transform raw sketches and bolts of every conceivable kind of material into finished garments" (161).

Looking at film costume design in these terms enables us to appreciate both the diversity of expertise behind its production and the different hierarchies of studio space and craftspeople operative in Hollywood. It means, therefore, we have to acknowledge the rivalry that existed between women like Head at Paramount and Helen Rose at MGM,[5] and between them and male costume designers like Adrian. By extension, as press and public interest in the screen style of individual actors burgeoned, it invites us to consider how film costume design was reproduced in everyday dress and the concomitant crossover between watching fashion in the cinema and consuming it in the retail tie-up.

FROM SCREEN SPACE TO SHOP SPACE: THE FILM AND FASHION TIE-UP

Since the mid-1920s there has been a long line of Hollywood stars who have become role models for the public, and whose looks and clothes have afforded various levels of identification to picture-goers and fans (Cook and Hines 2005; Herzog and Gaines 1991; Landis 2007; Moseley 2002; Wilson 1985). Indeed, so persistent has been the interdependence between costume and film in the creation of fashionable identities, and so rapid the pace of stylistic change, that fashion designer Bella Freud contends, "Fashion has become so fashionable that it has reached a pinnacle. It has to reinvent itself again so it's looking to film as its new medium" (quoted in Dyson 1999: 90).[6] The commodity tie-up, therefore, proffers a self-reflexive experience of and encounter with cinema and clothing that, as Freud intimates, involves a reciprocal border crossing between le perçu and le conçu, enabling fashion to reproduce itself in the image of film and vice versa. This dialectic between production and reproduction and the way it extends the space of fashion-in-film to the space of material culture and the retail environment via the shopwindow, the shopping mall, the fashion show, the magazine fashion feature, and advertising is amplified by Charles Eckert (1978), Jeanne Allen (1980), Robert Gustafson (1982), Mary Ann Doane (1989), and Jane Gaines and Charlotte Herzog (Gaines 1989; Gaines and Herzog 1990; Herzog and Gaines 1991).

As Hollywood designers were producing costumes at least one year before any film was released, their creations (apart from period costume) were often mobilized by the fashion industry to forecast style trends (Eckert 1978: 8; Herzog and Gaines 1991: 81). Gustafson (1982) probes how successful Edith Head was in meeting such a style challenge by considering press reports and publicity relating to her designs. He examines the body of work she produced between 1934 and 1954, and his research reveals that there were only two instances when her costumes were sufficiently prescient to strike a chord with the public. In 1936 the sarong she had designed for Dorothy Lamour in *The Jungle Princess* set off a fashion craze for tropical materials and motifs for several years, and ads and articles about the sarong appeared in American magazines like *Good Housekeeping, Colliers, Ladies' Home Journal,* and *Vogue* until as late as July 1954 (Gustafson 1982: 10). And a tight, buttonless jacket closed by a cluster of pearls, designed for Lamour in *Moon over Burma* (Louis King, 1940), proved equally popular since its decorative element enabled women to compensate for the rationing of material, controlled between 1942 and 1945 by the U.S. government's war order L85 (12). It is instructive, however, that Gustafson concludes both designs were "very different from the prevailing fashions," and we should also not regard Head as solely responsible for popularizing them (14).

The collaborative business between the film and retail industries Gustafson alludes to is underscored by Eckert in his pioneering—though speculative—article, "The Carole Lombard in Macy's Window," where he argues, "If one walked into New York's largest department stores towards the end of 1929 one could find abundant evidence of the penetration of Hollywood fashions, as well as a virulent form of moviemania" (1978: 8). To this end, he cites how Bernard Waldman's Modern Merchandising Bureau played a pivotal mediating role between the film studios and stores, so that by 1937 there were 400 of its official Cinema Fashion franchises nationwide, with the largest at Macy's, New York (8). In his telling, Macy's most popular film tie-up was one of Adrian's designs for Joan Crawford in *Letty Lynton* (Clarence Brown, 1932). This white starched chiffon gown with ruffles and puff sleeves reputedly sold over half a million copies in the United States and, according to one fashion buyer, was even plagiarized in Paris by "all the cheap little shops which have sprung up like weeds in the Champs-Elysees [sic]" (quoted in Eckert 1978: 6).

While certain authors have amplified Eckert's hypothesis about consumer tie-ups (Cook 1996: 46–47; Doane 1989: 26), Herzog and Gaines dispute it. They share common ground with him in addressing the impact that tie-ups had on the ready-to-wear industries and in giving the "fashion-conscious" woman democratic access to star styles in the interwar period. But they contest any straightforward transition from film costume to mass consumption, asserting there is little hard evidence to corroborate such large sales of the *Letty Lynton* dress or the exponential proliferation of Waldman's Cinema Fashion shops across the United States in the 1930s and proposing that both "are wishful accounts of the tie-up phenomenon" (Herzog and Gaines 1991: 88). This is not to argue that tie-ups and their attendant publicity either had limited public impact or should not be counted as "valid historical discourse" (88). Rather, the way that certain Hollywood fashions became the subject of considerable media hype in fan and fashion magazines alerts us to the fact that the commodity aesthetic of the film and fashion tie-up generates different types of consumerism and more borderline forms of shopping, whereby it is not always easy to distinguish "the commodity host from the commodity parasite" (Gaines 1989: 38). In this sense, then, the separate spaces of the cinema and shopwindow could also function symbiotically and allow the consumer to fulfill what Walter Benjamin called a "utopian wish-image" instead of the purchase of the commodity itself (Gaines 1990b: 12)—something that applied as much to the *Sex and the City* (Michael Patrick King, 2008) tie-up in the recession-hit 2000s as it did to *Letty Lynton* in the Depression era.[7] Thus the shopwindow replicates and reciprocates the spectacle of the cinema screen, affording the public the opportunity to perform the projective fantasy of ownership in which, to coin Allen's apt phrase, possession was "awarded only to the eye" (1980: 482).

One of the most interesting accounts of the crossover between visual access (le conçu) and actual possession (le vécu), and the way that the cinema and window shopping could offer the same spatial experience of "browsing without obligation to buy," is Gaines's appraisal of the promotion of gowns based on Adrian's historical dress for Greta Garbo in *Queen Christina* (Rouben Mamoulian, 1933) in Macy's Cinema Shop (Gaines 1989: 35). Historical clothing such as this posed a specific marketing problem when it passed from its extradiegetic context on the screen to the retail space, and as Gaines reminds us, the woman's fashion trade of the period often found Hollywood costumes too extravagant, intricate, or outlandish to copy wholesale, referring to them as "spinach" (53). Thus the sober seventeenth-century-styled garments that Adrian designed for *Queen Christina* would seem to be matter out of place in the 1930s United States and somewhat idiosyncratic for contemporary commodification. Yet it is probable Macy's merchandised them during the Depression to strike a realistic chord with cash-strapped consumers by promoting a sensible rather than a glamorous Hollywood dress style. Accordingly, they copied the puritanical use of black material and white starched collars and cuffs, but the full-skirted, long gowns were slimmed down to a 1930s silhouette, and the hemlines rose to midcalf to appeal to modern taste.[8] But, analyzing the role of a cross-dressing monarch, Gaines's essay is more remarkable still in interrogating the complex issue of the different forms of spectatorship it engendered for mainstream and subcultural audiences; as Doane (1989: 32) puts it, therefore, "One must ask at this point, 'Whose gaze is ultimately addressed?' and 'Who profits?'"

LOOKING AT COSTUME IN FILM AND LOOKING INTO COSTUME FILM

First published in 1976, Laura Mulvey's ideas about the cinematic gaze have shaped much subsequent writing on the sexual dynamics of looking at—and looking in—film. In this economy of spectatorial pleasure, men are foregrounded as active and women as passive. Accordingly, the female star is put on display on two levels: as an erotic object for the male characters in the film space as well as for the male spectators in the cinema space (Mulvey [1976] 1989: 19). Taking a Freudian position on Hitchcock and Sternberg, she insists, therefore, that looking at the female star's body becomes an act of control for men because it enables them to deflect their castration anxiety onto women. On the one hand, this means that men assert control through voyeurism, whereby women must be punished for evoking such anxiety (as in film noir). On the other, it means they sublimate their castration anxiety by objectifying the female body as a reassuring fetish, concentrating on its physical beauty or certain items of clothing—a process Mulvey calls fetishistic scopophilia.

Stella Bruzzi reappraises this psychosexual tack in analyzing *Picnic at Hanging Rock* (Peter Weir, 1976) and *The Piano* (Jane Campion, 1999). Here, she argues, looking at clothing evinces a "genderised territory that centres on the erotic" (Bruzzi 1997: 36), but one in which female display becomes a matter of appeasing the desires and anxieties of women as well as men. In the case of *Picnic at Hanging Rock,* then, she maintains that the scenes of the schoolgirls donning white dresses and lacing corsets represent the "idealisation of femininity through clothes and female sexuality," to wit, "the film's masculinisation of the voyeuristic and fetishistic impulses" (43, 44). By contrast, in *The Piano* she argues that Ada's independent sexuality and the way she allows Baines to touch her skin through the hole in her woolen stocking connote both Victorian women's ability to use restrictive clothing as the locus of sexual fulfillment and "a complex feminist displacement of the conventionalised objectification of the woman's form via scopophilia and fetishism" (58). Pam Cook likewise qualifies visual pleasure in *Fashioning the Nation,* where she foregrounds what Mulvey overlooks or "looks through"—clothing, and the way film costume in general affords the spectator, whether male or female, an extradiegetic space for trying on and discarding different identities (1996: 50). Both authors, therefore, extend our understanding of how clothing in film crosses the border from guise to disguise, from le perçu to le conçu. But as I have already suggested, it is Gaines (1989, 2000) who opens up film as a space for an entirely different way of looking at and into fashion and dress, and she achieves this in her magisterial explorations of *Queen Christina* (Rouben Mamoulian, 1933) and *Madam Satan* (Cecil B. DeMille, 1930), both costumed by Adrian.

Adrian's opulent approach to film costume was the antithesis to Head's, embodying the idea of costume as "pure spectacle" (Gaines 1989: 40); witness the sumptuous and sensuous garments he designed for Joan Crawford, such as the *Letty Lynton* dress and the sequined chiffon gown she wore in the finale of *Dancing Lady* (Robert Leonard, 1933), and Greta Garbo's outfits in *Camille* (George Cukor, 1936). In her essay on *Queen Christina,* Gaines appraises this "pure spectacle" through the lens of queer looking and the ways in which Adrian's androgynous costumes for Queen Christina, who had been raised as a prince and inherited the Swedish throne in 1633 with the official title of king, "sowed the seeds of an oppositional aesthetic" (1989: 40). Based on a close reading of the relationship of costume to narrative and Garbo's performative body hexis as a monarch who wore masculine dress and refused to marry, Gaines illustrates how the gender ambiguities of character and costume contest the normative dynamics of spectatorship: "in romantic cuts, she is heterosexual; in drag... she articulates male homosexuality" (43). Thus the film crisscrosses the threshold between straight and gay desire, enacting in Gaines's lapidary phrase "a homosexual/heterosexual flip flop" for actors and audiences alike (40). This imbrication of identities and of le perçu and le conçu is evident in two related sequences involving dress and undress. In the first, wearing breeches, doublet, and riding boots, Christina is (mis)taken for a man by an innkeeper and the Spanish envoy, Don Antonio Pimentel, who is en route to Stockholm. Forced to share a bed owing to a shortage of rooms, s/he eventually reveals her anonymous female identity to Pimentel in disrobing, and they become lovers. In the second, ladies-in-waiting assist her in putting on a jewel-encrusted velvet gown to meet him at court, to his pleased astonishment this time as queen of Sweden.

By contrast, in the second essay Gaines analyzes the material threshold between costume and human flesh and the ways in which this embodies female pleasure and power in phenomenological terms. She focuses on *Madam Satan,* in which Angela Brooks (Kay Johnson) sets out to win back her adulterous husband by posing as the eponymous seductress at a masquerade ball. In particular, she unravels how Adrian's revealing design for Angela's party dress, effectively a flesh-colored body stocking supporting a deconstructed black bodice and a skirt split at the knee, was a matter both of circumventing the Hays Code dictum on how much skin could be exposed in film and of not just seeing her body but seeing through it as well. Mobilizing Maurice Merleau-Ponty's intricate ideas on the sensible and sentient (or objective and phenomenological) body and the reciprocal inscription of the visible in the tangible it elicits, alongside Vivienne Sobchak's on how film both embodies experience and is itself embodied experience, Gaines elaborates a dense argument concerning the cooperation of seeing and touching—indeed, the way film attempts to appeal to the sense of touch that it is technically not able to represent.

That is to say, cloth, and in particular cloth worn on the human body, has an instrumental part to play in the coalescence of touch and sight, such that the person who wears it, and sees and feels himself/herself wearing it, is simultaneously seen and felt wearing it by others. Moreover, Angela's diaphanous dress orchestrates the dialectic not only of looking and touching but also of doing so from the inside out and the outside in. Wearing an eye mask and see-through outfit she literally becomes a liminal body: a subject in control from the inside, who from under cover of her double skin (her own and that of the dress) watches herself being admired, as well as an object that is touched from the outside—physically by the garment and metaphysically by the eyes of the film's actors and spectators, who can look at and into her body through the dress. Certainly, this is a complex and convoluted argument, and one that could easily capsize under the weight of its theoretical framework.[9] But not only does Gaines manage to make a compelling intervention into viewing fashion from the threshold of le perçu and le conçu, as with her analysis of *Queen Christina,* but from that of le vécu as well. What is more, she draws our attention to the final point that I want to discuss: namely, the border crossing clothing enacts between the extradiegetic narrative of the film itself and the spatiotemporal dynamic of the costume plot.

CLOTHING AND NARRATIVE

As Adrian's costumes for *Queen Christina* and *Madam Satan* demonstrate, clothing can reinforce a film's plot, theme, or mood and act as a metaphor for a certain character type. This was especially important in silent movies, where costume could be mobilized to say something about someone as a replacement for speech itself. But the idea of using dress as a speech act to delineate character was also transported into the sound era of classical realist cinema. Thus Edith Head argued that clothing in the talkies should carry enough information about character that, if the sound were turned down, the audience would still get the point (Gaines 1990a: 188).

This extradiegetic interdependence of costume, narrative, and character is also central to arguments by Cook and Bruzzi. Hence, Cook amplifies how Elizabeth Haffenden's costume designs for Gainsborough period drama in the 1940s never aimed to reconstruct the past accurately, arguing instead they were "historical travesties... more concerned with presenting history as masquerade" (1996: 75, 77). On this basis, she examines how the exotic costume narrative of Arthur Crabtree's *Madonna of the Seven Moons* (1944), set in late 1930s Italy, and *Caravan* (1946), set in nineteenth-century England and Spain, reinforced a sense of either conforming to or transgressing both gender and national identities in the context of World War II. Bruzzi's (1997) project is more eclectic and ambitious in its remit, examining costume in Hollywood, British, and European films such as *Shaft* (Gordon Parks, 1971), *American Gigolo* (Paul Schrader, 1982), *The Crying Game* (Neil Jordan, 1992), and *Kika* (Pedro Almodóvar, 1993). Nonetheless, she ranges across similar territory concerning the nexus of clothing to gender, sexuality, and race, arguing in the case of movies such as *Scarface* (Howard Hawks, 1932) that the mutual and fetishistic admiration between gangsters for each other's clothes and appearance is a signifier of "obvious homoerotic undertones" (Bruzzi 1997: 75).

But she also introduces another important aspect concerning the relationship of costume to narrative, that is, the role of iconic clothes, which she contends function as visual exclamation marks (Bruzzi 1997: 17). On this level, costume occupies a spectacular filmic space of its own and thereby distracts the viewer from the main narrative, as in *Kika,* where Jean Paul Gaultier's outlandish designs are deliberatively obtrusive, not merely reflecting the meaning of the film's narrative but imposing their own identity on it. This is what Gaines calls the costume idiolect, and she associates it mostly with melodrama—or "women's pictures"—between the 1920s and 1950s. As she argues, directors and designers adhered to a general code such that actresses "should be dressed down for the high emotional scenes and dressed up for the less significant moments" (1990a: 205). Thus in mundane scenes like answering the telephone or writing a letter, the female lead usually wore visually stunning clothes. In such instances, it is the garments' cut, texture, and color that become important to the spectator, suspending or transgressing the extradiegetic narrative, if only temporarily:

> The costume plot organises an idiolect with its own motifs, variations, surprises, anticipations and resolutions which unfold in a temporality which does not correspond with narrative developments, whose climaxes occur in alternation with key dramatic scenes, in the undramatic moments. (205)

A brief scene in *Far from Heaven* (Todd Haynes, 2003), costumed by Sandy Powell, illustrates the point. Kathy Whitaker (Julianne Moore), the archetypal American housewife of the late 1950s, and her husband Frank (Dennis Quaid) are on holiday in Miami for Christmas. At the New Year's ball she wears a green taffeta and chiffon décolleté gown, and he calls both her and it ravishing just before they dance and kiss. But the idyllic costume plot goes against the grain of the main drama as it unfolds: Frank is gay and has also just exchanged furtive glances with a young man, with whom he subsequently falls in love, abandoning Kathy and his family for him.[10]

Hence, iconic clothes contest director George Cukor's idea that if costume "knocked your eye out" it was not good, for a particular scene or the entire film (Gaines 1990a: 195). But the costume idiolect itself has intradiegetic status, dependent on and entwined in the main dramatic drive while also taking an alternative angle on it (Genette 1980: 228). Thus there are moments when clothing both occupies the extradiegetic space-time of the narrative and punctuates it intradiegetically as spectacle. This is evident in the party scene in *Madam Satan* but equally applies to the extended fashion shoot in *Funny Face* (Stanley Donen, 1957), which showcases Hubert de Givenchy's eight stunning outfits for Jo (Audrey Hepburn) and coterminously complements the narrative thrust. At this stage in the film, Jo, a gamine bookseller in Greenwich Village who has been discovered by photographer Dick Avery (Fred Astaire) and taken by him and magazine editor Maggie Prescott (Kay Thompson) to model outfits in Paris, fledges into a confident young woman, while also beginning to fall in love with Dick. In an earlier catwalk scene, wearing a sack-back-style dress by Givenchy, she remarks, "It doesn't feel like me," after the fashion designer Paul Duval calls her a "bird of paradise"; in contrast, in the fashion shoot she increasingly realizes and asserts her independence, subverting the normative dynamic of the active photographer and passive fashion model. Spontaneously marching down the steps of the Louvre in a stunning red New Look evening gown, therefore, she raises her arms and pashmina to mimic the pose of the *Victory of Samothrace* behind her and enjoins Dick three times to "take the picture!"

EPILOGUE

Alexander Walker (1999: 13) regards *Funny Face* as "an amorous photo session of the utmost elegance," and yet the film is not just a visual feast or merely a love story. For its narrative transacts fashion with fashion photography and thus highlights a significant intertextual relationship that writing on cinema costume has overlooked to date: Megan Williams (2000), for instance, addresses this nexus only tangentially in her essay about Michelangelo Antonioni's *Blowup* (1966). Furthermore, *Funny Face* subverts the simplistic idea that clothing and the transformation of personae it enables are trivial. It is, after all, through fashion that Jo is both lost and found, and performatively in or out of control of who she wants to be. Thus, in common with the arguments by Gaines, Bruzzi, and Cook analyzed here, the role of fashion in *Funny Face* reminds us that dress exists on the threshold of identities and does not function straightforwardly as the external sign of some internal essence. Such liminality is as much the concern of the characters portrayed within the film space as it is for those outside it—actors, whose screen style spills into their personal life, and spectators, who "buy into" and imitate the look of the stars they admire. Hepburn herself, for instance, wore Givenchy in public, and as Rachel Moseley (2002) demonstrates, her dress sense has been influential for many young women since the 1950s. Consequently, the spatial and temporal correspondences of fashion and film in terms of both production and consumption are a matter of permeability and transitivity that involve border crossings, on- *and* off-screen, between le perçu, le conçu, and le vécu in relation to designers, actors, and directors; stars and spectators; studios and retailers; and the extradiegetic film and intradiegetic costume plots.

NOTES

1. Sofia Coppola's *Marie Antoinette* (2006), although booed at the Cannes Film Festival, was more accurate in this sense, winning an Academy Award for Milena Canonero's costumes in the process.

2. Most Oscars for costume design have been awarded to films with historical subjects. The first Oscar for costume design, in 1949, was awarded to Edith Head for the nineteenth-century melodrama *The Heiress,* while in 2011 it went to Colleen Atwood for *Alice in Wonderland.*
3. Predating both exhibitions was Diana Vreeland's Romantic and Glamorous Hollywood at the Costume Institute of the Metropolitan Museum, New York. As Taylor (2002: 178) states, its original catalog was, however, a "modest, unillustrated listing."
4. She was awarded Oscars for the following: *The Heiress* (William Wyler, 1949), *Samson and Delilah* (Cecil B. DeMille, 1949), *All about Eve* (Joseph L. Mankiewicz, 1950), *A Place in the Sun* (George Stevens, 1951), *Roman Holiday* (William Wyler, 1953), *Sabrina* (Billy Wilder, 1954), *The Facts of Life* (Edward Stevenson, 1960), and *The Sting* (George Roy Hill, 1973).
5. Rose won two Oscars—for *The Bad and the Beautiful* (Vincente Minnelli, 1951) and *I'll Cry Tomorrow* (Daniel Mann, 1955)—in comparison to Head's eight.
6. Freud was commenting on the revival of the college-girl look that had been designed by Alice Manougian Martin for Ali McGraw in *Love Story* (Arthur Hiller, 1971).
7. *Sex in the City* costumer Patricia Field styled an autumn 2008 collection for Marks & Spencer.
8. In turn, the pinstripes and wide trousers of 1930s men's clothing were popularized in the 1970s after Edith Head's authentic designs for *The Sting* and Theoni V. Aldredge and Ralph Lauren's for *The Great Gatsby* (Jack Clayton, 1974).
9. Gaines compounds this approach in her essay "Wanting to Wear Seeing: Gilbert Adrian at MGM" (2011).
10. *Far from Heaven* is a loving homage to Douglas Sirk's *Magnificent Obsession* (1954) and *All That Heaven Allows* (1955). Bruzzi analyzes the role of costume in these films in "'It Will Be a Magnificent Obsession': Femininity, Desire and the New Look in 1950s Melodrama" (2011).

BIBLIOGRAPHY

Allen, Jeanne. 1980. "The Film Viewer as Consumer." *Quarterly Review of Film and Video* 5 (4): 473–90.

Breton, André. 1924. "First Surrealist Manifesto." In Charles Harrison and Paul Wood (eds.), *Art in Theory 1900–1990: An Anthology of Changing Ideas*, 432–39. Oxford: Blackwell.

Bruzzi, Stella. 1997. *Undressing Cinema: Clothing and Identity in the Movies.* London: Routledge.

Bruzzi, Stella. 2011. "'It Will Be a Magnificent Obsession': Femininity, Desire and the New Look in 1950s Melodrama." In Adrienne Munich (ed.), *Fashion in Film,* 160–80. Bloomington: Indiana University Press.

Chierichetti, David. 2003. *Edith Head.* New York: Perennial.

Cook, Pam. 1996. *Fashioning the Nation: Costume and Identity in British Cinema.* London: British Film Institute.

Cook, Pam, and Claire Hines. 2005. "'Sean Connery Is James Bond': Re-fashioning British Masculinity in the 1960s." In Rachel Moseley (ed.), *Fashioning Film Stars,* 147–59. London: British Film Institute.

Doane, Mary Ann. 1989. "The Economy of Desire: The Commodity Form in/of the Cinema." *Quarterly Review of Film and Video* 11: 23–33.

Dyson, Jenny. 1999. "Fashion Goes to Hollywood." *Elle* (UK), September, 90.

Eckert, Charles. 1978. "The Carole Lombard in Macy's Window." *Quarterly Review of Film Studies* 3 (1): 1–21.

Engelmeier, Regine. 1990. *Fashion in Film.* Munich: Prestel.

Gaines, Jane. 1989. "The Queen Christina Tie-Ups: Convergence of Show Window and Screen." *Quarterly Review of Film and Video* 11: 35–60.

Gaines, Jane. 1990a. "Costume and Narrative: How Dress Tells the Woman's Story." In Jane Gaines and Charlotte Herzog (eds.), *Fabrications: Costume and the Female Body,* 180–211. London: Routledge.

Gaines, Jane. 1990b. "Introduction: Fabricating the Female Body." In Jane Gaines and Charlotte Herzog (eds.), *Fabrications: Costume and the Female Body,* 1–27. London: Routledge.

Gaines, Jane. 2000. "On Wearing the Film: *Madam Satan* (1930)." In Stella Bruzzi and Pamela Church Gibson (eds.), *Fashion Cultures: Theories, Exploration and Analysis,* 159–77. London: Routledge.

Gaines, Jane. 2011. "Wanting to Wear Seeing: Gilbert Adrian at MGM." In Adrienne Munich (ed.), *Fashion in Film,* 139–59. Bloomington: Indiana University Press.

Gaines, Jane, and Charlotte Herzog (eds.). 1990. *Fabrications: Costume and the Female Body.* London: Routledge.

Gaines, Jane, and Charlotte Herzog. 2005. "Norma Shearer as Marie Antoinette: Which Body Too Much?" In Rachel Moseley (ed.), *Fashioning Film Stars,* 11–26. London: British Film Institute.

Genette, Gérard. 1980. *Narrative Discourse: An Essay in Method.* Ithaca, NY: Cornell University Press.

Gustafson, Robert. 1982. "The Power of the Screen: The Influence of Edith Head's Film Designs on the Retail Fashion Market." *The Velvet Light Trap* 19: 8–15.

Head, Edith, and Paddy Calistro. [1983] 2008. *Edith Head's Hollywood.* Santa Monica, CA: Angel City Press.

Herzog, Charlotte, and Jane Gaines. 1991. "'Puffed Sleeves before Tea-Time': Joan Crawford, Adrian and Women Audiences." In Christine Gledhill (ed.), *Stardom: Industry of Desire,* 74–91. London: Routledge.

Higson, Andrew. 1993. "Re-presenting the National Past: Nostalgia and Pastiche in Heritage Film." In Lester Friedman (ed.), *British Cinema and Thatcherism: Fires Were Started,* 109–29. London: UCL Press.

Hollander, Anne. 1978. *Seeing through Clothes.* New York: Viking.

Jorgensen, Jay. 2010. *Edith Head: The Fifty-Year Career of Hollywood's Greatest Costume Designer.* Philadelphia: Running Press.

Kristeva, Julia. 1986. "Women's Time" [1981]. In Toril Moi (ed.), *The Kristeva Reader,* 187–213. London and New York: Routledge.

Landis, Deborah N. 2007. *Dressed: A Century of Hollywood Costume Design.* New York: Collins.

Landis, Deborah N. 2012. *Filmcraft: Costume Design.* East Sussex, UK: Ilex.

Leese, Elizabeth. [1976] 1991. *Costume Design in the Movies.* New York: Dover.

Lefebvre, Henri. [1974] 1991. *The Production of Space.* Oxford: Blackwell.

Maeder, Edward. 1988. *Hollywood and History: Costume Design in Film.* London: Thames and Hudson.

Moseley, Rachel. 2002. *Growing Up with Audrey Hepburn.* Manchester: Manchester University Press.
Mulvey, Laura. [1976] 1989. "Visual Pleasure and Narrative Cinema." In *Visual and Other Pleasures,* 14–28. Basingstoke, UK: Macmillan.
Nielsen, Elizabeth. 1990. "Handmaidens of the Glamour Culture: Costumers in the Hollywood Studio System." In Jane Gaines and Charlotte Herzog (eds.), *Fabrications: Costume and the Female Body,* 160–79. London: Routledge.
Taylor, Lou. 2002. *The Study of Dress History.* Manchester: Manchester University Press.
Uhlirova, Marketa. 2008. *If Looks Could Kill.* London: Koenig Books.
Walker, Alexander. 1999. *Hot Tickets* (London), November 19–25, p. 13.
Williams, Megan. 2000. "A Surface of Forgetting: The Object of History in Michelangelo Antonioni's *Blowup.*" *Quarterly Review of Film and Video* 17 (3): 245–59.
Wilson, Elizabeth. 1985. *Adorned in Dreams: Fashion and Modernity.* London: Routledge.

FILMOGRAPHY

Alice in Wonderland (Tim Burton, 2011)
All about Eve (Joseph L. Mankiewicz, 1950)
American Gigolo (Paul Schrader, 1982)
The Bad and the Beautiful (Vincente Minnelli, 1951)
Barry Lyndon (Stanley Kubrick, 1975)
Birth of a Nation (D. W. Griffith, 1915)
Blowup (Michelangelo Antonioni, 1966)
Camille (George Cukor, 1936)
Caravan (Arthur Crabtree, 1946)
Catherine the Great (Alexander Korda, 1934)
The Crying Game (Neil Jordan, 1992)
Dancing Lady (Robert Leonard, 1933)
Dangerous Liaisons (Stephen Frears, 1988)
The Devil Wears Prada (David Frankel, 2007)
The Facts of Life (Edward Stevenson, 1960)
Far from Heaven (Todd Haynes, 2003)
A Foreign Affair (Billy Wilder, 1948)
Funny Face (Stanley Donen, 1957)
The Great Gatsby (Jack Clayton, 1974)
The Heiress (William Wyler, 1949)
I'll Cry Tomorrow (Daniel Mann, 1955)
The Jungle Princess (William Thiele, 1936)
Kika (Pedro Almódovar, 1993)
Lady in the Dark (Mitchell Leisen, 1944)
Letty Lynton (Clarence Brown, 1932)
Love Story (Arthur Hiller, 1971)
Madam Satan (Cecil B. DeMille, 1930)
Madonna of the Seven Moons (Arthur Crabtree, 1944)
Marie Antoinette (W. S. van Dyke, 1938)

Marie Antoinette (Sofia Coppola, 2006)
Moon over Burma (Louis King, 1940)
The Piano (Jane Campion, 1999)
Picnic at Hanging Rock (Peter Weir, 1976)
A Place in the Sun (George Stevens, 1951)
Queen Christina (Rouben Mamoulian, 1933)
Qui Etes Vous, Polly Magoo? (William Klein, 1966)
Ready to Wear (Robert Altman, 1994)
Rear Window (Alfred Hitchcock, 1954)
Roman Holiday (William Wyler, 1953)
Romeo and Juliet (J. Gordon Edwards, 1916)
Sabrina (Billy Wilder, 1954)
Samson and Delilah (Cecil B. DeMille, 1949)
Scarface (Howard Hawks, 1932)
The Scarlet Empress (Josef von Sternberg, 1934)
Sex and the City (Michael Patrick King, 2008)
Shaft (Gordon Parks, 1971)
The Sting (George Roy Hill, 1973)

9

The Hidden Spaces of Fashion Production

REGINA LEE BLASZCZYK

The vibrant field of fashion history is heavily invested in cultural narratives about clothing, culture, and consumption. Journals such as *Fashion Theory*, exhibition venues such as the Victoria and Albert Museum, and research hubs such as the Centre for Fashion Studies at Stockholm University support this important approach to exhibitions, public programs, and publications. However, there are many approaches to fashion and fashion production. Recent scholarship rooted in business history offers a complementary viewpoint based on economic and cultural themes such as entrepreneurship, corporate strategy, design and innovation, and marketing practice.

The objects of fashion, whether calico prints from the Lowell mills of the 1850s or the easy-care mod ensembles of the 1960s, are the result of technical innovations, backroom negotiations, hit-or-miss marketing, and consumer whimsy. Consumers purchase fashionable clothing for personal "identity kits" that also include houses, cars, music, and electronics (Blaszczyk 2009). Fashion is promoted and displayed in public, but before the product is even worn by the consumer, it has traveled through textile factories, design ateliers, wholesale markets, and photo shoots. Discussions of these businesses and business practices, which are hidden from public view, are often missing from the fashion studies literature (Blaszczyk 2008b). This essay presents several examples of behind-the-scenes business activities to demonstrate why a deeper historical understanding of processes such as design and marketing is crucial to the advancement of the discipline of fashion studies.

BUSINESS PRACTICES AND HIDDEN SPACES

Business history has not always been open to the study of the fashion and style industries. From the 1960s through the early 1990s, the field was dominated by

Alfred D. Chandler Jr., a prolific historian at the Harvard Business School whose Pulitzer Prize–winning book, *The Visible Hand,* sought to explain how big business came to dominate the United States and the world (John 1997). Chandler and his followers focused on major firms, such as General Motors and other Fortune 500 companies that were the engines of the economy. Firms in the creative sectors, such as clothing manufacturers and department stores, were not studied on account of their small size and perceived irrelevance to economic growth.

This focus began to change in the mid-1990s with the "cultural turn" in business history. Historians who pioneered this approach were inspired by the emerging field of cultural history and an older tradition of narrative economic history exemplified by the work of Thomas Cochran, who analyzed the cultural dimensions of business and entrepreneurship in the United States in the nineteenth century (Lipartito 1995). One example of the new business history that is especially relevant to fashion studies is Pamela Walker Laird's *Advertising Progress: American Business and the Rise of Consumer Marketing* (1998). This study of nineteenth-century advertising shows how a judicious review of trade and industry journals, credit reports, and business ephemera can shed light on the design process in the creative industries. By focusing on American advertising before the rise of Madison Avenue in the 1920s, Laird examines how a close working relationship between printers and customers, combined with the spread of the new chromolithographic technology, gave birth to a distinctive style in Victorian advertising. Trade cards, posters, and placards all celebrated the idea of "progress," using brilliant colors and symbolic motifs like the billowing smokestack to celebrate the culture of abundance. While collectors' books point to the genius of the artists at Currier & Ives, Laird shows that printed pictures were the result of a give-and-take exchange between the printer and the client. That give-and-take took place behind closed doors and is not visible to scholars examining the pictures alone.

My own scholarship on the business of design, fashion, and consumer society has identified the "fashion intermediary" as the agent who worked behind the scenes to link designers, manufacturers, retailers, and consumers (Blaszczyk 2000). Before market research techniques were perfected and codified in the 1920s, the companies that made and sold consumer goods needed some way to understand public taste. Long before anyone coined the term *segmented market,* the world of potential customers was divided according to income, taste, geography, race, gender, ethnicity, subculture, social class, and other factors. In 1850 or 1900, there were no door-to-door surveys, mail-in questionnaires, or geodemographic data-mining programs to give manufacturers and distributors hard data about what consumers wanted. Instead, producers relied on the experience and intuition of fashion intermediaries to give them the heads-up on popular taste (Blaszczyk 2000, 2009).

As a springboard for understanding the internal workings of fashion production, I offer the concept of the "fashion-industrial complex" as an alternative to the "fashion system." Scholars of material culture, such as the anthropologist Grant McCracken (1988), have used Roland Barthes's (1983) concept of the fashion system as an analytical tool for understanding the cultural production of meaning. This theory is built around a self-perpetuating cultural loop, which infers the complicity of creators and the helplessness of consumers. Fashion is seen as a cultural phenomenon dependent on the media's manipulation of texts and images in public spaces.

By contrast, the fashion-industrial complex is a concept rooted in the new business history and is dependent on the judicious review of the primary sources and the analysis of the structure and operations of the industry. This framework focuses on behind-the-scenes activities within the production-consumption continuum to develop a deeper understanding of historical realities (Blaszczyk 2008b). It considers the full spectrum of individuals, firms, and organizations that are involved in the design, manufacture, wholesaling, distribution, promotion, and retailing of fashion. Fashion production is contingent on relationships among intermediaries throughout the supply chain, from the chemical companies that make synthetic fibers to the retailers who stock and promote global brands. These fashion intermediaries make crucial decisions about fabrics, textures, colors, and silhouettes that affect the look of goods that consumers purchase to display their identities.

Business historians define *fashion* inclusively, using the term to describe the goods that are used to protect and adorn the body and to display social position and cultural status (Blaszczyk 2008b; Polese and Blaszczyk 2012). Fashion in this sense is not limited to the historical output of French couture houses or the international luxury brands by Moët Hennessy-Louis Vuitton that dominate today's high-end global market. Fashion includes moderately priced clothing sold by retailers like Macy's in the United States, Marks & Spencer in the United Kingdom, Monoprix in France, and C&A in Germany. It includes bespoke and off-the-rack suits for men, plus and petite sizes for women, and fast fashion by Zara and H&M. It includes licensed brands, house brands, and merchandise like woolen overcoats, leather shoes and handbags, Victorian ladies' hats, spandex bras and girdles, denim jeans, and rayon dresses.

Innovation within the fashion-industrial complex has always been remarkably vibrant, and as Laird's work on advertising shows, new designs or images are not the product of a genius designer working alone but the end result of a creative process that involves a complex network of actors. Innovation networks have intrigued cultural geographers like Norma Rantisi, who has studied the relationships among space, economics, and creativity in the New York garment industry. In mapping the locations of garment houses or "cutters," Rantisi (2002, 2004) showed that garment makers were part of a complex web of industries and subindustries, each with its own highly developed approach to design, production, and distribution. The garment trade benefited from the free flow of ideas and information. Nancy Green's (1997) comparative labor history of garment manufacturing in Paris and New York makes similar points.

THE WORLD WE HAVE LOST: WHEN FABRICS WERE FASHION

The nineteenth-century way of producing fashion presents an interpretative challenge to fashion studies. The Victorian fashion-industrial complex didn't look anything like our global fashion-business network, with its electronically connected world of designers, manufacturers, retailers, and the digital media operating 24–7. Historically, the development of stylish clothing has involved layer upon layer of visibly invisible actors, such as patternmakers, sketch artists, entrepreneurs, colorists, cutters, wholesalers, retail buyers, window-display artists, newspaper editors, and trade associations. The American example is a case in point.

For starters, the major media outlets were the local newspapers, which published several editions each day, all in black and white. Consumers learned where to shop for fashion from these papers, from advertisements painted on the sides of buildings, from handbills circulated on the streets, and from the popular pastime of window-shopping. The commercial streets of every good-sized city or town were lined with stores, and shopkeepers filled their windows with merchandise as a form of advertisement and enticement (Blaszczyk 2009).

In the nineteenth century, the ready-made clothing industry was in its infancy, but it was by no means unsophisticated. The menswear trade was the first to industrialize, with slop shops in the major ports offering cheap clothes to sailors, artisans, and frontiersmen by the eighteenth century. With urban growth, businesses in such sectors as banking, insurance, importing, and shipping needed armies of clerks to handle the paperwork, and young men rushed to these new office jobs. Ambitious clerks who wanted to climb the corporate ladder, or at least fit in behind the desk, adopted the new professional uniform: a dark three-piece sack suit and a bright white shirt with a detachable white collar and cuffs. This style evolved out of the plain dark suit worn by London dandies during the Regency period (Blaszczyk 2009; Kidwell and Christman 1974; *Perfect Fit* 2005).

As the sack suit gained popularity, the menswear industry developed techniques for streamlining production, cutting costs, and reducing prices. In major garment hubs such as New York, Philadelphia, Baltimore, Chicago, and New Orleans, the tailoring trade was dominated by Jewish immigrants who had been trained in European cities such as Berlin, Vienna, and London (Zakim 2003). Early assembly lines and the division of labor did not necessarily translate into a standardized look. Male consumers had the freedom of choice and could work with their tailors to create a personal style based on the selection of fabrics, colors, patterns, buttons, trim, and cut. This was true for New York bankers who frequented the upscale Brooks Brothers store and for the little bookkeeper who relied on the corner tailor. Thus, men's fashion was created in the hidden space of the tailor's store, through intimate interactions between the manufacturer and the customer (Blaszczyk 2009; *Perfect Fit* 2005). We see the vestiges of this system today in made-to-measure menswear stores or Internet sites that rely on distant factories to assemble the shirt or suit from a warehouse of materials.

While the production of male business attire was streamlined, female fashions continued to depend on a high degree of stylistic variety. Ever since the time of Louis XIV, France had been the trendsetter in women's luxury goods. Paris was a major design and production center long before Charles Frederick Worth introduced the idea of the genius male dressmaker, or couturier, who presented female clients with models, or prototypes, from which to choose (Steele 1988). American consumers learned about the latest Paris styles from the daily newspapers, from fashion plates in magazines like *Godey's Lady's Book* and *Graham's Magazine,* from mail-order catalogs, and from dry-goods emporiums, millinery shops, and, from the mid-1870s on, the early department stores. They also sized up the local fashion elite, watching the wives of physicians, politicians, and factory owners promenade in the park and down Main Street after church on Sunday (Blaszczyk 2009). Only the wealthiest Americans could afford Paris fashion; the semiannual transatlantic voyages and the custom-made wardrobe cost a small fortune (Amnéus 2003).

Dresses were difficult to make because of the form-fitting styles, which were tight at the bodice and had a large bell shape from the waist to the floor. The average female consumer had a wardrobe that consisted of a few simple homemade garments, a handful of store-bought ready-made items such as a shawl or a cloak, and one or two good dresses cut to her measurements by a local dressmaker. Everyone from the mill girl to the stay-at-home mom aspired to own one good dress, and the rich had more (Blaszczyk 2009). Regardless of their place in the social hierarchy, women knew that "fashion" was synonymous with the fabrics, ribbons, and other "dry goods" that were purchased and sewn up into a garment (Blaszczyk 2012).

This fashion-industrial complex, characterized by close contact among makers and customers, seems alien to us, given the contemporary global world of fast fashion and throwaway fashion. How do we start to understand innovation in this foreign land of hand-colored fashion plates and stores that sold ribbons? We have already touched on the intimate relationship between the man and his tailor, which was similar to that of a woman and her dressmaker. But to understand the nineteenth-century fashion-industrial complex, we need to take a step back from the sewing and look at the production and distribution of textiles.

PRACTICAL MEN, STYLE SERVICES

How did the monster fabric mills in a New England textile city like Lawrence, Massachusetts, determine what colors and patterns were fashionable in Paris and interpret these in ways that would appeal to American tailors, dressmakers, and consumers? To explore this question, we must look at design practice. In the nineteenth century, the United States had no superstar fashion designers, but it did have a vibrant creative economy that depended on layer upon layer of fashion intermediaries. No one spoke about fashion intermediaries, but the term *practical man* was on the tip of everyone's tongue.

Some of these practical men worked in between producers and consumers, and we can learn a good deal about fashion production by going behind the scenes to see how they designed fabrics (Blaszczyk 2000, 2012).

In industry on both sides of the Atlantic, the practical man—an apprentice-trained craftsman who designed everything from furniture to fabrics—was schooled to know the market. It took many years for a practical man to master his trade, gaining some knowledge from secondary schools dedicated to the applied arts and some know-how from on-the-job training. Some practical men worked in highly technical positions such as that of the works chemist, but others had oversight of design and development. The practical man with an entrepreneurial bent could hook up with a *capitalist*—a partner whose financial assets and managerial abilities complemented his craft skills—to form a small workshop. Most of these ventures failed, but a few grew into substantial factories (Blaszczyk 2000, 2012; Locke 1984).

Every good-sized factory that produced style goods had someone in charge of monitoring tastes and watching the competition. Often the salesmen played an active role, since they traveled around the country and observed local and regional tastes. In terms of the design process, this was often a collaborative effort among the factory owner, the salesmen, and the practical man who did the sketches, made the models, or oversaw the creative aspects of manufacturing. The factory designer read the fashion magazines and was known to pester the stylish typists in the front office about the latest trends. Like the salesman, he was an avid people watcher, and when on business in a nearby metropolis like Boston or New York, he might visit the dry-goods emporiums to study the merchandise and size up the shoppers. An astute designer could learn a lot in the stores, noting how the customers handled the merchandise and when they asked the clerk to show them a different color, pattern, or texture (Blaszczyk 2000, 2012).

But by the time a bolt of fabric landed in a dry-goods store, the design was already old news. If a mill were to compete in the cutthroat fashion world, the textile designer had to know trends before they hit the shelves. The trade journals and consumer magazines had very few color illustrations, and journalistic style reports often consisted of florid descriptions. The skilled reader could pick up on the cultural cues and get the general idea. But the fashion reports often focused on what European elites—queens, princesses, and duchesses—were wearing and on how the bourgeoisie emulated them. The journalists said little about the millions of yards of ordinary fabrics generated by the mills in Manchester, Lyon, or Łódź. How did the textile designer for the American mass market secure advance information about the newest calico prints or silk colors that had been created with the average consumer or dressmaker in mind? (Blaszczyk 2012; Fagan Affleck 1987; Sykas 2005).

Textile designers had to keep up with fashion trends as they created new weaves, patterns, and shades for target markets. They needed good reference materials to do their work. Designing fabrics for the mass market depended less on artistic originality and more on the ability to synthesize trends and repackage colors that were already popular.

The textile and fashion industries developed sophisticated methods for sending, receiving, and storing trend reports, so that designers could have timely, reliable information at their fingertips. In Europe and North America, textile mills kept extensive libraries of engravings, illustrated books, and giant scrapbooks filled with swatches (Fagan Affleck 1987; Sykas 2005). These swatch books held samples of the factory's designs, cuttings of competitors' fabrics, and secret alphanumeric codes that could be deciphered by those in the know. Scrapbooks filled with thousands of swatches systematically collected over the years were invaluable to designers, who used them to study trends and reinterpret them for the mill's customers (Blaszczyk 2012).

Paris was the major design center for textiles in the early nineteenth century, and practical men from Europe and North America looked there for inspiration. Fabric design was part of the Parisian fashion-industrial complex of dressmakers, textile mills, dyers, and countless firms in ancillary businesses—the shoemakers, milliners, corset makers, stocking knitters, jewelers, parasol shops, beaders, ribbon makers, feather dyers, and more. Foreign businessmen visited Paris to understand industry trends or hired resident agents to survey the scene and collect samples on their behalf (Blaszczyk 2012).

By the 1830s in Paris, style services emerged, charging fees to gather textile swatches from European fashion centers and ship them to customers abroad, often in the United Kingdom or the United States. Around this time, François and Victor Jean-Claude opened their Paris design studio, and within a few years, they ran a swatch service that mailed cuttings of the current styles to foreign manufacturers. By the late 1800s, J. Claude Frères et Cie was the leading fabric subscription bureau in Paris, offering twenty-nine different services classified by textile and end use. Subscriptions were costly, but it was far less expensive for a textile mill to buy swatches than to support a resident agent in Paris who then had to travel to style centers like Berlin and Vienna. In textile mills, the design department typically glued the swatches into the scrapbooks, forming a record of new fashions to be copied, modified, or combined into new designs. Using this system, a calico design printed in Europe could be copied in the United States within three weeks (Blaszczyk 2012).

ANOTHER SPACE HIDDEN FROM SIGHT: HOW FIBERS SHAPED FASHION

Another example of creative interaction hidden from public view comes from the United States and Europe after World War II and involves fiber makers, fashion designers, and apparel manufacturers. Synergies among the U.S. chemical industry and French and Italian couturiers led to the widespread adoption of synthetic fibers and advanced a fashionable new aesthetic based on informality, practicality, and comfort. The main players were E. I. du Pont de Nemours and Company, the world's largest fiber manufacturer; La Chambre Syndicale de la Couture Parisienne, the Paris trade association for haute couture; the major couturiers in Paris and Florence; and the garment manufacturers in New York. By going behind closed doors to scrutinize the interactions among these groups, we can understand the importance of chemical companies as the invisible powerhouses in fashion production.

In the postwar era, New York's garment cutters, located in the industrial district around Seventh Avenue, sewed most of the clothes worn by ordinary Americans, but Paris continued to set trends and shape taste (*Perfect Fit* 2005). Synthetic fibers counted among the new "miracle materials" of the postwar world. Although American consumers appreciated many new high-tech products like plastics, they were largely unfamiliar with the performance and aesthetics of the "miracle fibers" created by the DuPont Company. Eager to get in touch with these consumers, DuPont's Textile Fibers Department invested heavily in market research and public relations (Blaszczyk 2006, 2008a). As one executive summarized, DuPont adapted to postwar prosperity by transforming the "relatively simple 'art' of selling fabric" into the "complicated 'science' of marketing" (Blaszczyk 2006: 495).

By the early 1950s, DuPont had an impressive merchandising operation. In the company's home base of Wilmington, Delaware, the firm's product developers created fabric prototypes, which they shared with textile mills that were anxious to learn about the new synthetic fibers. In New York, DuPont's extensive sales office in the Empire State Building, at the edge of the Seventh Avenue fashion district, promoted synthetic fibers to textile mills and garment cutters. A 1952 market research report, "The Dress Industry," encouraged DuPont marketers to push the envelope by engaging the "Parisian couturiers in helping to develop and use new fabrics." DuPont "could materially benefit from such an action," which could set the "fabric style" in high-end clothing (Hobbs 1952). The fashion-fiber connection was not new. In the 1920s, DuPont's rayon operation employed a fabric expert to collect textile samples in Europe and share them with the customers. In the 1930s, DuPont and other rayon manufacturers aggressively promoted man-made fibers through product-placement programs with the Hollywood studios and through New York fashion shows (Blaszczyk 2006: 507).

These strategies and tactics were updated for the postwar context, when DuPont hitched its star onto Paris fashion. For decades, style-conscious Americans had turned to Paris for inspiration in women's fashions. In the 1880s, high-end department stores like John Wanamaker in Philadelphia had started importing couture, selling the originals to wealthy customers—often altering them to fit—and creating spin-offs to market in a range of sizes at lower prices. Rodman Wanamaker, the son of the founder, oversaw an extensive importing operation from the store's luxurious buying office in Paris (Blaszczyk 2011).

Luxury retailers like John Wanamaker were haute couture's most important customers. Every year, buyers from the major department stores flocked to the semiannual shows of the Paris dressmakers who worked under the auspices of the Chambre Syndicale. The couture houses set up elaborate salons to welcome the buyers (Golbin 2006). Admission to the couture houses was allowed only to those who possessed a "buyer's card" issued by the syndicate. American buyers ogled the elegant live mannequins who paraded the new dresses and afterward met with the *vendeuse,* or saleswoman, to buy models, or garment prototypes, for shipment back to the United States. By the 1910s, stores like John Wanamaker celebrated the arrival of the new Paris originals, mounting large-scale fashion shows that made good copy for local style journalists (Blaszczyk 2011). They collaborated with garment manufacturers to make line-by-line copies and adaptations. Through this system, luxury department stores like John Wanamaker in Philadelphia and Marshall Field's in Chicago catered to two groups of fashion-conscious shoppers: wealthy consumers who purchased the French originals in their couture salons and emulative shoppers who sought "cachet" at lower prices on the store's ready-to-wear racks. The association with Paris, the legendary European style hub, established the department store as the city's style leader (Palmer 2001).

After World War II, the allure of Paris fashion diminished briefly for Americans until a new generation of designers invigorated haute couture. Most prominent was Christian Dior, whose 1947 collection popularized a romantic silhouette, dubbed the "New Look" by *Harper's Bazaar* editor Carmel Snow. American retailers again sent their buyers to Paris. In New York, Ohrbach's department store flew couture originals to the United States, engaging top Seventh Avenue manufacturers to produce line-for-line copies that went on sale within a few weeks. With the synthetics boom, fiber manufacturers entered the picture (Blaszczyk 2007).

Beginning in the early 1950s, DuPont established a relationship with the Chambre Syndicale so that haute couturiers would collaborate with DuPont merchandisers to integrate synthetic fibers into the Paris collections. Each year, the Paris couture houses introduced designs featuring French textiles made from DuPont synthetics. In turn, DuPont purchased couture samples, hired well-respected photographers to snap pictures in Paris, and generated an endless flow of publicity. These pieces showed the public that haute couture was attuned to high-tech textile technology and, in turn, that American synthetics met the exacting standards of the world's most discriminating dress designers. Haute couture benefited from the association with American big business, while French designs added a glamorous glow to synthetic fibers and an immeasurable amount of prestige to the DuPont brand (Blaszczyk 2006, 2007).

Between 1952 and 1954, DuPont launched this couture venture through collaborations with Christian Dior and Hubert de Givenchy, who visited corporate headquarters in Wilmington to meet DuPont managers, study the new synthetics, and tour the laboratories. By recruiting Dior and Givenchy, DuPont linked itself with two important faces of haute couture: the conservative look favored by leading society ladies and the chic style aimed at younger consumers (Blaszczyk 2006).

DuPont's new fibers made headway in high fashion in February 1954 when Givenchy included Orlon acrylic in his collection. DuPont's head publicist visited the Paris openings and described Givenchy's use of French fabric blends of Orlon acrylic and silk. Intrigued by Orlon's remarkable performance capabilities, the young couturier introduced a series of casual outfits, including a "revolutionary" variation of the shirtwaist dress that fit loosely around the body, and showcased the fabric's suppleness, good draping characteristics, and washability. The dresses came in pastel shades of turquoise, yellow, and rose, colors made possible by Orlon's improved dyeing capabilities. More remarkably, the pleats on several garments were guaranteed to hold even after they had been washed. Givenchy's designs epitomized high-tech chic. His popularity in the United States, especially his appeal among younger women, led DuPont to hope that U.S. dress manufacturers would reproduce these models. A month later, when more established couturiers put on their shows, the older Dior and the grand dame Coco Chanel, in her first Paris show in sixteen years, introduced collections that featured French fabrics made from DuPont nylon (Blaszczyk 2006).

In June 1954, the Chambre Syndicale gave synthetics further blessing by sponsoring, in conjunction with the First International Congress of Man-Made Fibers in Paris, a fashion show reiterating the symposium's "Textiles of Tomorrow" theme. The French couturiers agreed that synthetics had definitely "made it," providing stylists with "greater scope for inspiration" (Blaszczyk 2007: 208).

By the late 1950s, DuPont had perfected a formula for using haute couture to publicize and sell synthetic fibers. The Textile Fibers Department continued to work with members of the Chambre Syndicale to integrate synthetics into the Paris collections. The bargain struck between high fashion and the test tube benefited both parties. Once Givenchy and Dior had demonstrated how synthetics could serve haute couture, the list of French designers using DuPont fibers expanded. Shimmering fibers like Mylar polyester films added a distinctive luster to evening wear, while few fabrics could reproduce the delicate, yet durable, net of nylon tulle. Couturiers could hardly resist the opportunities for elegance and distinctiveness offered by the new synthetics. By 1958 Pierre Balmain, Coco Chanel, Pierre Cardin, Jean Dessès, Jacques Heim, Lanvin-Castillo, Guy Laroche, and Yves Saint Laurent all used fabrics made from DuPont fibers, including rayon, acetate, nylon, acrylic, and polyester (Blaszczyk 2007: 209).

These developments took place behind closed doors, but they reached newspapers and magazines through the efforts of DuPont's Public Relations Department. The New York office assembled an impressive couture collection that could be seen by textile designers, Seventh Avenue cutters, and out-of-town buyers. The couture collection was a tool for product development, sales, and public relations, a fitting complement to DuPont fashion shows with themes such as "Orlon in Paris." DuPont also lent its couture models to fashion shows sponsored by the Fashion Group, the leading professional organization for women in apparel and related businesses, with chapters in New York and other cities around the country. These efforts clinched DuPont's reputation in the fashion business (Blaszczyk 2007: 210).

By the late 1950s, Seventh Avenue cutters were reproducing French designs using DuPont fibers at mass-market prices. In 1959 DuPont circulated a series of press releases and fashion stills showing how this was done. At the Paris winter shows, couturier Jacques Heim had introduced a short gown in white DuPont nylon tulle sprinkled with black DuPont nylon velvet dots. DuPont imported a model, and Seventh Avenue got to work. Within a few months, the New York cutter Martini was making line-for-line copies in American fabrics woven from DuPont nylon, to be sold by better retailers for $110. The story continued with Cristóbal Balenciaga and the House of Ricci, whose DuPont-owned originals were copied by the garment manufacturers Habley Barber Company, Abe Schrader, and Suzy Perette in nylon, rayon, and polyester-cotton. In March and April, DuPont's public relations staff traveled around the United States, soliciting orders for these couture knockoffs on behalf of garment makers. DuPont sales staff showed one Ricci tunic suit, copied by Abe Schrader at 530 Seventh Avenue, to buyers at Saks Fifth Avenue in Los Angeles, Julius Garfinkle in Washington, D.C., and more than a dozen other department stores throughout the country (Blaszczyk 2007: 210–11).

Through these activities, DuPont helped to usher in a transformation in the American fashion business. In the high-style game, the fiber maker assumed some of the functions that had once been the exclusive purview of major retailers, serving as fashion intermediary between French couturiers and American apparel manufacturers. DuPont was not alone in this transition. The entry of big businesses into the textile and garment trade recast the industry. These heavily capitalized giants had enormous market power, which they used to promote synthetic fibers. The Celanese Corporation of America, a major cellulose-fiber manufacturer that eventually entered synthetics, created a marketing machine that rivaled DuPont's. Celanese sponsored French couture shows in New York, paid for fiber promotions in department stores, and advertised heavily in print and on television. Such efforts helped to familiarize American retailers, manufacturers, and consumers with synthetics. DuPont remained the leader but had to devise new schemes to stay ahead (Blaszczyk 2007: 211–12).

The success of the Paris–New York couture program led DuPont to launch a similar Italian effort from its Geneva office. In 1958 it established a Swiss subsidiary, DuPont International SA (DISA), to manage manufacturing, marketing, and merchandising in Europe. In 1959 marketing specialist Don W. Gay transferred from the Textile Fibers Department in Wilmington to "DuPont Swiss," where he served as DISA's first merchandising manager until 1962. Under his auspices, DuPont embraced concept marketing. Fortunately for historians, Gay documented his experience in an extensive memoir that takes us behind the scenes and explains DISA's role in fashion production (Blaszczyk 2007: 213–14).

In the late 1950s, DuPont had some contact with Italian designers, whose work was attracting the attention of American department stores. As casual styles gained popularity, Gay expanded DuPont's Italian connections. In 1961 DISA sponsored its first fashion show in Milan, featuring Orlon acrylic garments to say, "Europe, we are here—DuPont comes to Europe" (Gay 1976). DuPont's first fashion show in Milan included couture apparel made by French designers under the Paris–New York program. The show impressed Italian fashion entrepreneur Beppe Modenese, who ran a modeling agency, wrote a newspaper style column, consulted with the Italian linen industry, and owned a group of boutiques. DISA hired Modenese as its major fashion consultant (Blaszczyk 2007: 214).

Modenese was an important fashion intermediary for DISA, providing an entrée into the elite world of Italian jet-set designers, who semiannually showed their couture collections, primarily knitwear, at the Palazzo Pitti in Florence. Gay recalled how Modenese used his social connections to introduce DuPont fibers to the Rome-based fashion designer Irène Galitzine (1916–2006). An exemplar of aristocratic Russian taste, Galitzine had caused a sensation with her "palazzo pajamas," wide-legged silk trousers for evening and leisure wear. The initial conversation revolved around boats, cars, food, and travel before Modenese mentioned the new collections, offering to sew up Galitzine's designs in synthetic fabrics, free of charge. Galitzine and her Italian colleagues approved of the new synthetic look, and within two years, 25 percent of the Italian couture garments on the runway at Palazzo Pitti were made from fabrics in Orlon acrylic fiber. DISA received millions of dollars in free press. DuPont purchased the Italian couture garments and assembled them into an Orlon fashion show that circulated to major European cities, where they were seen by spinners, knitters, and retailers. The DISA press release announced, "Orlon is good enough for Simonetta, Fabiani, Ava-golf, Nacci, Pucci, and Galitzine. Orlon is good enough for you" (Gay 1976). DuPont also publicized the Italian fashions in the United States, building on the growing cultural preference for casual styles (Blaszczyk 2007: 214–15).

BEYOND THE BIAS CUT: FASHION HISTORY AS BUSINESS HISTORY

The new business history offers a promising avenue for advancing our understanding of fashion production. This essay has explored aspects of the story through the lens of innovation for the American mass market, with reference to its intersections with European textiles and haute couture and the transatlantic flow of fashion information. These flows are not visible if one looks at runway shows and brand advertisements, but their vitality becomes apparent when one looks behind the scenes to business operations. In recent years, other scholars working in new business history have examined other hidden spaces of fashion production, with exciting results.

By way of example, recent issues of the *Business History Review* have included essays on the rise of Milan as a fashion center (Merlo and Polese 2006) and the different attitudes toward design piracy and the different copyright practices in the American and French fashion industries between the wars (Pouillard 2011). Several contributions in *Producing Fashion: Commerce, Culture, and Consumers* (Blaszczyk 2008b) look behind the public face of fashion to examine, among other things, the editorial practices at Russian fashion magazines, the design and marketing of aesthetic dress by the Wiener Werkstätte, and the operations of Belgian couture houses in the interwar era. In *Beauty Imagined: A History of the Global Beauty Industry* (2010), Geoffrey Jones shows how entrepreneurs shaped markets for cosmetics, toiletries, and perfumes. Most recently, the journal *Business History* has published a special issue on fashion. The articles address topics such as the internal workings of British *Vogue* (Cox and Mowatt 2012), Parisian couturiers who opened branches in the United States before World War II (Font 2012), and debates over copyright law in Sweden, France, and the United States (Dahlén 2012). In each case, scholars have pored over the business sources—the records of manufacturers, publishers, consultants, and trade associations; government archives; trade journals and trade newspapers; and oral history interviews with managers, designers, retailers, and other practitioners—to uncover a wealth of data on how fashion is produced.

One of the most promising areas of research is the production of fashion for the ordinary consumer. Rachel Worth's (2007) study of the British retailer Marks & Spencer sheds light on product development, marketing, and sales on "the high street." The extensive Marks & Spencer archive has just opened its doors to scholars in an extensive new facility at the University of Leeds in the United Kingdom. Similarly, the Centre for Business History in Stockholm has recently started to collect the archives of the global retail chain H&M and has been documenting the firm's history through recorded interviews (Giertz-Mårtenson 2012). Projects like these have the potential to open the doors onto novel interpretations of fashion production for the mass market.

The spaces for fashion promotion—the work of firms and individuals in public relations, advertising, and publishing—are often hidden from public and scholarly view. Historians should be skeptical of the media-fashion powerhouses—of the magazines, newspapers, publicists, reality TV shows, and blockbuster exhibitions—that tell us what's hot and what's not, past and present. Sociologists who study the fashion industry have begun to explore the persuasive power of the press (Rocamora 2009), but this field is ripe for analysis. Until the business records of editors, photographers, and publishers enter the public domain, scholars need to think creatively about how to access the hidden spaces of the great publicity machine that backs the fashion industry.

An example from the American scene is instructive. Fashion scholars often credit the journalist George Frazier with coining the term *peacock revolution,* based on his use of it in *Esquire* magazine in 1968. If we look into other spaces, we learn that the phrase was coined in 1966 by the motivation research consultant Ernest Dichter at a menswear conference sponsored by the DuPont Company. Dichter ran the Institute for Motivational Research in Croton-on-Hudson, New York, and he did market surveys for American companies who wanted to know more about the consumer. We don't know if Dichter knew of the press coverage on London menswear that referred to peacocks (Ross 2011), but he introduced the term *peacock revolution* to describe the American consumer's rising interest in flamboyant casual fashions made possible by the confluence of California styling, imported Italian menswear, and the easy-care synthetics revolution (Blaszczyk 2010). Here, the creative use of business sources sheds new light on an old stereotype.

Fashion production isn't simply a matter of trickle-down styles, but trendsetters like haute couturiers, pop stars, and fashion editors have been and will continue to be important. To deny the influence of elites would be, as the historian Richard Bushman noted in *The Refinement of America: Persons, Houses, Cities* (1992), to misunderstand the nature of power. Genius couturiers and great designers are very much the products of public relations efforts, and media reports and museum interpretations about them should be viewed with a critical eye.

The work of Florence Brachet Champsaur (2012) on Galeries Lafayette and Madeleine Vionnet in the interwar years is particularly instructive in this regard. Her analysis of Vionnet's business practices offers an informative counterpoint to exhibitions that have presented the couturiere as a genius who made her way in the world by making creative use of the bias cut (Golbin 2009). Brachet Champsaur shows Vionnet to be an astute businesswoman with close commercial ties to the Baders, the family that founded Galeries Lafayette in 1893. The business partnership between Vionnet and Théophile Bader was designed to float her couture house and to provide his department store with source material for its ready-to-wear collections in an era when the Chambre Syndicale prohibited French department stores from selling couture originals. By researching the corporate archives of Galeries Lafayette, Brachet Champsaur probed the hidden spaces of fashion production, introducing important information about the financing of couture houses and the design sources for confection. We now know that there was more to Vionnet than the bias cut (Brachet Champsaur 2012).

THE BODY—AND THE BUSINESS

The body, the self, and culture will always be crucial to fashion studies. More than twenty years ago, the costume historian Claudia Kidwell and the cultural historian Valerie Steele showed us that the dressing ritual is one of the most intimate spaces of fashion production (Kidwell and Steele 1989; Steele 1988, 2001). While every stylish outfit is meant to be seen in public, the ensemble is put together by the wearer in a very private moment, in conversation with her closet, her mirror, and herself, or in confidences with her dearest friends. The field of fashion studies has evolved from the desire of these pioneers to explore the role of fashion in culture and in processes of identity construction.

More recently, a new generation of business historians have started to explore the hidden economic dimensions of fashion production, looking to the spaces inhabited by entrepreneurs, designers, garment cutters, retailers, editors, and trade associations. This essay has shown how the relationships among technical innovation, product design and development, and marketing can shed light on the politics of fashion production. The spaces in which these creative interactions take place are hidden from public view, but the methods of business history can help us see them. Fashion creation owes much to tastemakers in couture houses and to street styles driven by consumers, but we cannot overlook the important role of manufacturers and marketers in defining fashion for the mass market. In the future, we hope that studies of the body, aesthetics, and high-end design will be complemented by the analysis of fashion production in the economic realm. The study of the body and the business combined will push fashion studies to new heights.

BIBLIOGRAPHY

Amnéus, Cynthia. 2003. *A Separate Sphere: Dressmakers in Cincinnati's Golden Age, 1877–1922.* Lubbock, TX: Texas Tech University Press.

Barthes, Roland. 1983. *The Fashion System.* New York: Hill and Wang.

Blaszczyk, Regina Lee. 2000. *Imagining Consumers: Design and Innovation from Wedgwood to Corning.* Baltimore: Johns Hopkins University Press.

Blaszczyk, Regina Lee. 2006. "Styling Synthetics: DuPont's Marketing of Fabrics and Fashion in Postwar America." *Business History Review* 80 (3): 485–528.

Blaszczyk, Regina Lee. 2007. "Du Pont de Nemours: Mode et révolution des textiles synthétiques." In Dominique Veillon and Michèle Ruffat (eds.), *La Mode des sixties; L'Entrée dans la modernité*, 202–19. Paris: Éditions Autrement.

Blaszczyk, Regina Lee. 2008a. "Designing Synthetics, Building Brands: Dorothy Liebes, Interior Decoration, and Post-war American Interiors." *Journal of Design History* 21 (1): 75–99.

Blaszczyk, Regina Lee (ed.). 2008b. *Producing Fashion: Commerce, Culture, and Consumers.* Philadelphia: University of Pennsylvania Press.

Blaszczyk, Regina Lee, 2009. *American Consumer Society, 1865–2005: From Hearth to HDTV.* Hoboken, NJ: Wiley-Blackwell.

Blaszczyk, Regina Lee. 2010. "Ernest Dichter and the Peacock Revolution: Motivation Research, the Menswear Market, and the DuPont Company." In Stefan Schwarzkopf and Rainer Gries (eds.), *Ernest Dichter and Motivation Research: New Perspectives on the Making of Post-war Consumer Culture*, 126–39. New York: Palgrave Macmillan.

Blaszczyk, Regina Lee. 2012. *The Color Revolution.* Cambridge, MA: MIT Press.

Blaszczyk, Regina Lee. 2011. "The Wanamakers: A History of Family and Fashion." Paper presented at the Arden Theatre Company, April 28, Philadelphia, PA.

Brachet Champsaur, Florence. 2012. "Madeleine Vionnet and Galeries Lafayette: The Unlikely Marriage of a Parisian Couture House and a French Department Store, 1922–40." *Business History* 54 (1): 48–66.

Bushman, Richard L. 1992. *The Refinement of America: Persons, Houses, Cities.* New York: Knopf.

Cox, Howard, and Simon Mowatt. 2012. "*Vogue* in Britain: Authenticity and the Creation of Competitive Advantage in the UK Magazine Industry." *Business History* 54 (1): 67–87.

Dahlén, Marianne. 2012. "Copy or Copyright Fashion? Swedish Design Protection Law in Historical and Comparative Perspective." *Business History* 54 (1): 88–107.

Fagan Affleck, Diane L. 1987. *Just New from the Mills: Printed Cottons in America.* Lowell, MA: American Textile History Museum.

Font, Lourdes M. 2012. "International Couture: The Opportunities and Challenges of Expansion, 1880–1920." *Business History* 54 (1): 30–47.

Gay, Don W. 1976. "Concept Marketing," In Joseph W. Lynch Collection, Chemical Heritage Foundation, December 15, Philadelphia, PA.

Giertz-Mårtenson, Ingrid. 2012. "H&M—Documenting the Story of One of the World's Largest Fashion Retailers." *Business History* 54 (1): 108–15.

Golbin, Pamela (ed.). 2006. *Balenciaga Paris.* London: Thames and Hudson.

Golbin, Pamela (ed.). 2009. *Madeleine Vionnet.* New York: Rizzoli.

Green, Nancy L. 1997. *Ready-to-Wear and Ready-to-Work: A Century of Industry and Immigrants in Paris and New York.* Durham, NC: Duke University Press.

Hobbs, G. D. 1952. "The Dress Industry." Box 78, Papers of the Textile Fibers Department, E.I. du Pont de Nemours and Company, Wilmington, DE.

John, Richard R. 1997. "Elaborations, Revisions, Dissents: Alfred D. Chandler Jr.'s *The Visible Hand* after Twenty Years." *Business History Review* 71 (2): 151–200.

Jones, Geoffrey. 2010. *Beauty Imagined: A History of the Global Beauty Industry.* New York: Oxford University Press.

Kidwell, Claudia B., and Margaret C. Christman. 1974. *Suiting Everyone: The Democratization of Clothing in America.* Washington, DC: Smithsonian Institution Press.

Kidwell, Claudia B., and Valerie Steele (eds.). 1989. *Men and Women: Dressing the Part.* Washington, DC: Smithsonian Institution Press.

Laird, Pamela Walker. 1998. *Advertising Progress: American Business and the Rise of Consumer Marketing.* Baltimore: Johns Hopkins University Press.

Lipartito, Kenneth. 1995. "Culture and the Practice of Business History." *Business and Economic History* 24 (2): 1–41.

Locke, Robert R. 1984. *The End of the Practical Man: Entrepreneurship and Higher Education in Germany, France, and Great Britain, 1880–1940.* Greenwich, CT: JAI Press.

McCracken, Grant. 1988. *Culture and Consumption: New Approaches to the Symbolic Character of Consumer Goods and Activities.* Bloomington: Indiana University Press.

Merlo, Elisabetta, and Francesca Polese. 2006. "Turning Fashion into Business: The Emergence of Milan as an International Fashion Hub." *Business History Review* 80 (3): 415–47.

Palmer, Alexandra. 2001. *Couture and Commerce: The Transatlantic Fashion Trade in the 1950s.* Vancouver: University of British Columbia Press.

A Perfect Fit: The Garment Industry and American Jewry, 1860–1960. 2005. New York: Yeshiva University.

Polese, Francesca, and Regina Lee Blaszczyk. 2012. "Fashion Forward: The Business History of Fashion." *Business History* 54 (1): 6–9.

Pouillard, Veronique. 2011. "Design Piracy in the Fashion Industries of Paris and New York in the Interwar Years." *Business History Review* 85 (2): 319–44.

Rantisi, Norma M. 2002. "The Local Innovation System as a Source of 'Variety': Openness and Adaptability in New York City's Garment District." *Regional Studies* 36 (6): 587–602.

Rantisi, Norma M. 2004. "The Ascendance of New York Fashion." *International Journal of Urban and Regional Research* 28 (1): 86–106.

Rocamora, Agnès. 2009. *Fashioning the City: Paris, Fashion and the Media.* London: I. B. Tauris.

Ross, Geoffrey Aquilina. 2011. *The Day of the Peacock: Style for Men, 1963–1973.* London: V&A Publishing.

Steele, Valerie. 1988. *Paris Fashion: A Cultural History.* New York: Oxford University Press.

Steele, Valerie. 2001. *The Corset: A Cultural History.* New Haven, CT: Yale University Press.

Sykas, Philip B. 2005. *The Secret Life of Textiles: Six Pattern Book Archives in North West England.* Bolton, UK: Bolton Museums, Art Gallery and Aquarium.

Worth, Rachel. 2007. *Fashion for the People: A History of Clothing at Marks & Spencer.* Oxford: Berg.

Zakim, Michael. 2003. *Ready-Made Democracy: A History of Men's Dress in the American Republic, 1760–1860.* Chicago: University of Chicago Press.

10

Fashion: More Than Cloth and Form

JOSÉ TEUNISSEN

> To us, fashion represents more than just cloth and form: it is an aura, an escape from reality. Coming from suburbia in a country where fashion doesn't really exist (i.e. Holland), fashion for us was like a glossy fairy tale world made real. Through our work, we still seek that emotion, over and over again. We turn the phenomenon of fashion into its own subject matter. We have expressed and reflected on just that position in various ways through various media, in an art context but also within the context of fashion.
>
> —Viktor & Rolf (2008)

Ever since the 1960s, avant-garde designers have radically changed essential components of fashion, and therefore also something of what fashion, and its ideal environment, represents. Rather than simply presenting a new feminine ideal, they have started using fashion as a discipline within which they can comment on the fashion system itself, bringing fashion to a more conceptual plane. The result of this new approach has been that the concept itself, and its aesthetic dimension, has become more important than presenting an ideal woman in clothes. These new fashion practices have evolved into a new communication model: catalogs, invitations, and press releases are regarded as suitable vehicles for embodying the designer's ideas beyond the clothing (Pecorari 2011: 70).

In the last decades of the twentieth century, along with this process of conceptualization we are seeing the emergence of a new platform for fashion: the museum hosting a designer's exhibition (Kamitsis 2009: 103). Moreover, for Viktor & Rolf, Hussein Chalayan, Maison Martin Margiela, and others, this would even appear to be a necessary component of the brand's communication strategy; the world of their label brand is "complete" and shown to best advantage only when it appears in the museum, in the same way that architectonic flagship stores have become key elements in a fashion house's communication strategy (Lipovetsky and Manlow 2009).

My argument is that from the 1960s on, the fashion system has undergone major changes. Instead of presenting a feminine ideal and displaying wealth, (avant-garde) fashion started to make overtly political and cultural comments on society and the fashion system itself (Lipovetsky 1994; Teunissen 2009). In this process of *conceptualization* (Martin 2009), *storytelling* (Evans 2003; Vinken 2009), and a shift toward a focus on *experience* design (Marchetti and Quinz 2009), the "performance" of fashion has changed. As a result, the classic spaces (catwalk and store) in which "ideal identity" used to be shaped have been redefined. Fashion shows have become performance hybrids with a direct relation to art and the theater (Gregg Duncan 2006), while the modern hyperstore is based on a shopping concept in which art and fashion, high and low culture, economics and culture are merged (Lipovetsky and Manlow 2009: 164). In this context of an increased focus on concept and experience (Marchetti and Quinz 2009), the museum has become an appropriate platform to present new fashion ideas.

PERFORMING IDENTITY IN SPACE

Until recently, fashion mainly functioned as the symbolic skin that served to negotiate and manage our desires: by means of clothing the wearer would display his or her identity and play the game of "look and be looked at" on the street, in the city, and in other social spaces. It now seems that this interpretation of fashion as a system of meaning and communication is changing. Avant-garde fashion is much more likely to focus on the concept behind the product and to expound on the problems of consumer identity by making its construction visible. "Today it dominates understandings of fashion, which is constructed both as an arena for the construction of identity and as a conceptual metaphor that explains the incompleteness and contingency of that effort" (Kinney 2009: 257). But what exactly is fashion, and how is it connected to space?

In the seventeenth and eighteenth centuries, the aristocrats demonstrated their status during theatrical rituals and ceremonies. These ceremonies made the king and nobility the center of attention in a carefully directed theatrical environment (Sennett 1977). However, in the early nineteenth century, fashion developed into a property allowing the wearers to simultaneously express their individuality and show affiliation with one or more social groups (Lipovetsky 1994; Simmel [1905] 2000). This major transition had an effect on the rituals and locations normally associated with fashion. Outdoor city culture, with Paris in the lead, became more and more focused on the ephemeral mundane aspects of everyday public life. Newly built boulevards and public spaces designated for the masses emerged in which people could view both the architecture and each other (Rocamora 2009; Steele 1998). All this turned anonymous city life into a public spectacle, a reality that had an "aura" and could be experienced collectively. "Through *flânerie*, spectators commanded the spectacle: they participated in it at the same time that they believed it was constructed for them. They also occupied a variety of viewing positions: both individual and socially determined" (Schwartz 1999: 203). From the very moment the fashion game started to be staged on the street, an essential part of this experience took place there. The emergence of the department store, the first mannequins strolling in the Bois de Boulogne, and the rise of the flâneur all fit in these new fashionable public spaces where fashion was performed as an aesthetics of the moment (Garelick 1998; Hollander 1975; Teunissen 2006: 209). This process of using public space as a new fashion site resulted in the invention, in 1910, of the *défilé* by Paul Poiret, Lucille, and others (Evans 2001: 271). In this way the phenomenon of the catwalk turned out to be a mix between theatrical scenery (the ideal fashion location of the seventeenth and eighteenth centuries) and the casual stroll of the street.

> The emergence of the fashion show in around 1910 therefore coincided with the radical change that had taken place in the aesthetics of women's fashion at that time. The new aesthetics of the body in motion attained its perfected and crystallized form in the fashion show. You might say that the fashion show was an artificial form of parading. The "natural" body in action was now put on a stage, and in this way the interplay between attitude, pose and clothing could be seamlessly read. Suddenly fashion could be distributed through "realistic channels" by means of fashion journals and magazine photography, since photos could now be printed in magazines for the first time. (Teunissen 2006: 209)

The fashion show turned into a fashion moment: the place where fashion took form and the ideal identity was given shape—an idealized personal identity realized through aesthetic performance.

The French philosopher Gilles Lipovetsky has explored how contemporary visual culture has come to regard personal identity in aesthetic terms. Following this argument, the *fashion person*—an aloof and mobile individual with a malleable personality and taste—is understood as the embodiment of performed identity (Lipovetsky 1994: 149). Fashion, according to Lipovetsky, is the ideal textbook. In fashion we can learn how to be flexible, mobile, and psychologically adaptive in a playful way in a contemporary media-based society, where effortlessly shifting between jobs, identities, and backgrounds has become customary practice.

FASHION AS POPULAR CULTURE: A NEW VISION, A NEW APPROACH

During the 1960s this definition of fashion as the performance of an ideal identity started to change slightly. With the emergence of youth culture, fashion became a mass-market product, something within the reach of everyone. Through happenings, music, and the rise of street fashion, it also became part of the popular visual culture in which media played an important role (Martin 2009). All of that added to the complexity of the fashion system as a whole. Next to the object, the designer, and the wearer, the social context in which fashion operated became increasingly important, while other media increased fashion's presence and visibility (Teunissen 2009: 11). Suddenly, fashion had turned into much more than the presentation of a female ideal and the display of wealth. Fashion as "the scenography of elegance" as it was developed during the nineteenth century with the culture of strolling evolved now in "a theatricality of meaning" in which the concept and idea were crucial (Lipovetsky 2002: 8). Clothes not only featured as the material expression of personal identity but also served to propagate political ideals, as the punks did, for example, with their printed T-shirts. Even now, in the twenty-first century, fashion designer Hussein Chalayan is using installations such as *Afterwords* (fall/winter 2000), *Kinship Journeys* (2003), *Readings* (2008), and *Micro Geography* (2009; Figure 10.1) to address challenging political and societal issues such as migration, alienation, and the effects of globalization on daily life.

> It is true that my work is initially always based on a concept and that in the final instance I use the body as model. I have to say that the concept is never arbitrary; it really needs to grab me or move me. Like in *Afterwords a/w 2000,* in which I presented a portable home. The division of Cyprus into Greek and Turkish areas is something I have experienced. What do you take with you when you have to abandon hearth and home? (Hussein Chalayan, quoted in Teunissen 2003: 62–80)

From the 1960s on fashion began to deliver a message. And it continues to do so. "Fashion was stirred by the transgressive, avant-garde role it assumed in the 1960s. For some twenty-five years, fashion's principal theme was its capacity to be advanced and liberal, its aesthetic propensity being slightly *outre* yet always acceptable within the principle of being radical and permissive" (Martin 2009: 41). These changes transformed fashion into a cultural phenomenon whose facets and manifestations were increasingly important. Thus, as Lipovetsky states:

> Since the 1950s and 1960s, organizational, social and cultural transformations have thoroughly disrupted the earlier structure [of fashion]; we can reasonably conclude that a new stage in the history of fashion has come into view. New centres of creation have emerged, and new criteria have been imposed. The earlier hierarchical and unitary configuration has exploded. The individual and social meanings of fashion have changed along with the tastes and behaviours of women and men. (1994: 88)

In that way, from the 1960s on fashion increasingly became an expression of ideas and concepts. The fashion avant-garde escaped the straitjacket of functional demands

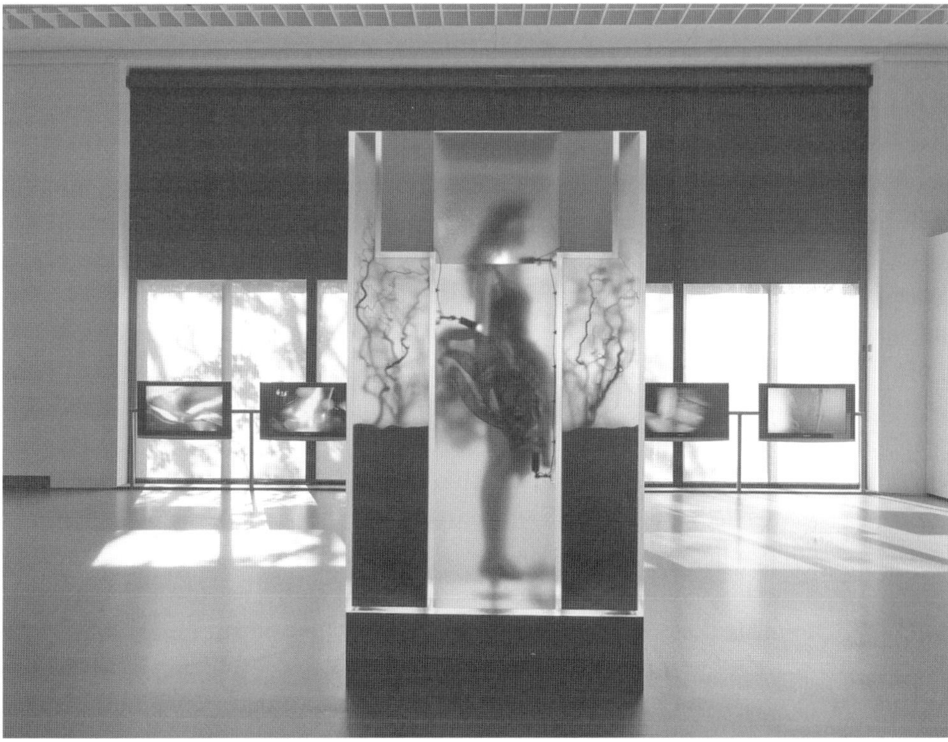

FIGURE 10.1 Hussein Chalayan, *Micro Geography*, 2010.
Credit: Museum Boijmans Van Beuningen, Rotterdam/Studio Hans Wilschut.

that the applied arts traditionally used to have: fashion became the product of a design that was "attached" to the human body but that also sought to research and explore its own relationship with the body, with identity, self-image, and the environment. In doing so, it came to strongly resemble pop art and the kind of performance art that emerged in those years (Teunissen 2009: 24). Thus Martin asks, "In forming this liaison with art and in marrying Pop Art specifically, what did contemporary fashion accomplish?" To which he answers:

> It became avant-garde in sensibility, it came under and drew from the thrall of popular culture, and it became the nexus of democratic social values and the clarifying aesthetic order of art. Fashion, like art since ca. 1960, has continued to fulfil the rich and elite, but it has taken this form from popular culture, celebrating that culture and not limiting itself to the supreme elements of *haute couture* of the most hierarchical "art." (Martin 2009: 27)

The new sensibilities (using more registers of expression) also meant that the fashion world started to explore new sites of presentation like the (art) museum or use classic locations like the store and the catwalk in new and unexpected ways.

THE CONCEPTUALIZATION OF FASHION: FASHION AS A DESIGN PROCESS

In the early 1980s Japanese designers Yohji Yamamoto and Rei Kawakubo (head designer of Comme des Garçons) brought about a minor revolution at the Paris prêt-à-porter shows. Both played with traditional forms and patterns of Western clothing while mixing them with elements of Japanese clothing styles or combining them in unorthodox ways (Fukai 2006: 291), thereby seeking and pushing the boundaries of the classic fashion garment. "There is no standard pattern which the patterners work with and adapt each time. They are expected to innovate," says Kawakubo (quoted in Sudjic 1990: 31). Like a modernist artist, Kawakubo develops her designs from a formal, if not formalistic, point of departure: for instance, she made collections using only sample-length fabric (as a primary building material). In another instance, she designed a collection of skirts whose separate parts were combined in ever-different and arbitrary ways. The same parts then led to totally different skirts. The importance of the concept in her designs is well illustrated by the now famous lace sweater from 1982 whose "seemingly random pattern of holes provided a commentary on the redundancy of handicraft in an era of machine-made perfection" (Sudjic 1990: 93). Sudjic compares Kawakubo's way of designing with the approach of an abstract painter: "just as abstraction in art usually depends on an underlying knowledge of traditional drawing skills, so pattern-making at Comme des Garçons is rooted in a thorough grounding in basic principles, which are then subverted" (31). The exceptional and innovative thing about Japanese designers such as Kawakubo, Yamamoto, or Issey Miyake was their focus on the underlying *processes* of clothing design and garment construction, which they turned into visual properties (of their designs). Comme des Garçons and Yamamoto purposely held small-scale shows where the public was allowed to sit very close to the runway, allowing them to inspect the clothes' fabric and construction. In the process they have been redefining the catwalk from a space where the ideal "identity" of the consumer is given shape into a space where the "identity/concept" of the product/label comes to expression.

Furthermore, they sought to make sure retail design and brand communication were underlying the philosophy of the designs (Blanchard 2004: 50). In the 1980s Kawakubo (in collaboration with the architect Takao Kawasaki) was one of the first designers to create retail environments where the philosophy of her clothes would be matched by a poetics of space. "A shop for her is not just a box to put clothes in: she has a strong sense of the qualities she is looking for in a space" (Sudjic 1990: 109; Figure 10.2). Sparsely furnished, the shops often had an aura of emptiness to them. Some of the garments were laid out unfolded on flat plinths to display their construction. By means of a museum- (or gallery-) like interior design, the products' material expression was given center stage, said Kawasaki.

> "There had been a shift from hard to soft. The concrete style was a barrier, you couldn't see in. Now the look is more inviting," maintains Kawasaki. "The thing to remember

is to look at her work as a piece. Sometimes you can even see direct influences on the interiors coming from the clothes. The collection in 1989 had a lot of gold and you could see gold coming up in the shops as well. She had both the spaces and the clothes in mind at the same time, she doesn't see them separate." (Sudjic 1990: 111)

Not only did Kawakubo revolutionize fashion shows and retail spaces, but she is also one of the first designers to have launched her own magazine, *Six*, which allowed her to make poetic links between fashion, photography, and the world of art. Using a variety of idioms and disciplines, the Comme des Garçons universe was given the clearest possible all-encompassing aesthetic signature form and, ultimately, even transcended the garment itself. The exhibitions and campaigns developed by Issey Miyake and Dai Fujiwara for the introduction of A-POC (A Piece of Cloth), a pattern-making and cutting technique based on a single piece of cloth/fabric, are good examples of how a clothing concept could be consistently visualized and explained by means of ingenious presentations,

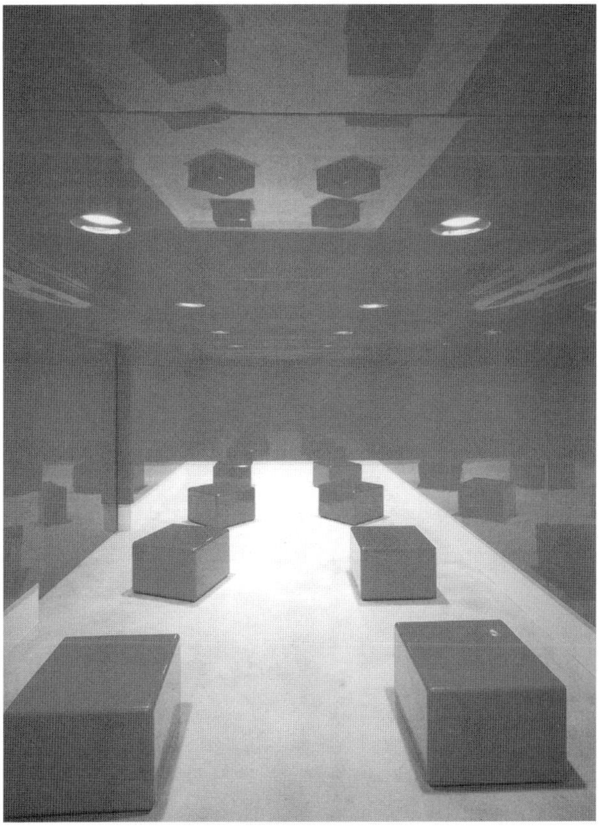

FIGURE 10.2 Comme des Garçons boutique at Rue Saint-Honoré, Paris.
Credit: Designed by Architecture & Associés, Jean-Christophe Poggioli and Pierre Beucler.

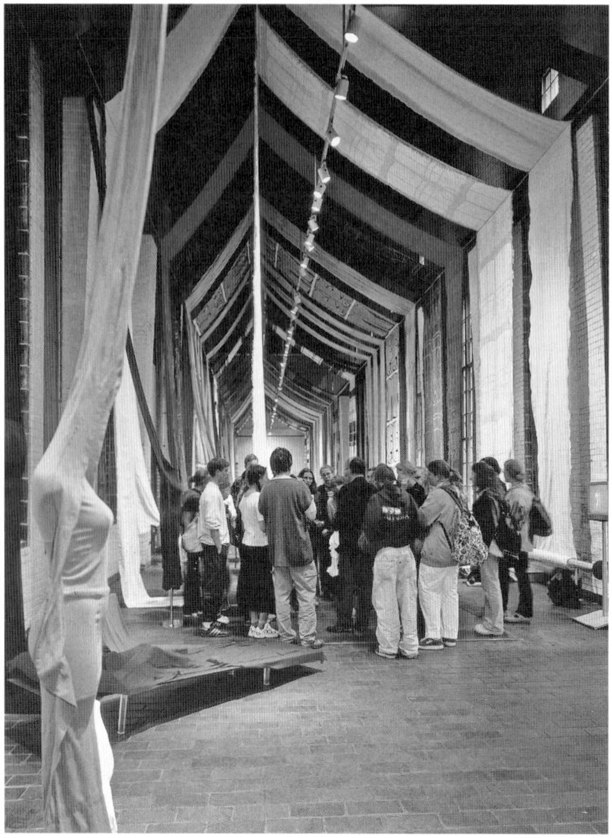

FIGURE 10.3 A-POC Exhibition, Vitra Design Museum, Berlin.
Credit: ©Vitra Design Museum. Photograph by Yasuaki Yoshinaga.

including an exhibition at Vitra Design Museum in Berlin in 2001 (Blanchard 2004: 24–29; Figure 10.3). The mark of distinction for this avant-garde generation was that they started to express themselves across a variety of disciplines. In an effort to show their work to the best advantage they often supported their work through graphic design, films, performances, and special architectural commissions.

FLAGSHIP STORES, THE NEW RETAIL EXPERIENCE

When Charles Frederick Worth opened the first couture salon in 1858, the garment itself was elevated to a piece of art. Nowadays, the garment is only one element of a (commercially driven) brand whose principal aim is to achieve high selling prices. Shops have become spaces of collaborative efforts between architects, fashion designers, artists, and product designers. The worlds of fashion and architecture, luxury and avant-garde, commerce and culture all converge here, and the result is a hyper-store based on a shopping concept in which the hybridization of art and fashion, high and low culture, economics and culture is the key element (Lipovetsky and Manlow 2009: 164). These flagship stores give the idea of a creative universe. Far from being mere points of sale, they serve as cultural and artistic meeting places. Today, a label's cachet is strengthened not only by its marketing and brand image but also by its retail environment. It is only through the combination of multiple aesthetic economies such as architecture, design, and art that a fashion label is enabled to present its myriad faces. "While contemporary art functions as a consecration-communication instrument for the major fashion brands, fashion is focused on staging contemporary art in its stores, using it as a window for creativity in motion" (Lipovetsky and Manlow 2009: 162). As a result, the actual product is becoming less and less important. The label itself has (been) turned into a spectacle. Image, show, and brand communication are important elements in tapping into new sensations and emotionally charged experiences. A good conceptual example of this development is Viktor & Rolf, who designed their website as a virtual fashion salon where visitors are encouraged to spend some time lingering and exploring the archives.

> When consumption is no longer structurally status-enhancing, distinguished by the imperative of signifying its place in the social hierarchy, there is an increase in the incessant search for hedonistic and perceptible experiences, for renewed and surprising emotions which contemporary art, amongst other things, is able to provide. That is why the act of purchasing must be rich in aesthetic and cultural emotions. (Lipovetsky and Manlow 2009: 165)

Therefore, the aesthetic and appearance of a product are no longer crucial in the label's concept. Nowadays it is the quality of the experience that counts. Shopping in the Prada epicenter in New York (opened in 2002; Figure 10.4), for example, is no longer just about the product but focuses on a process of familiarization: "approaching the object, becoming acquainted with it, and finally, possibly, buying it. The experiential commercial space is not just a showcase for the product, but rather a content generator for the brand" (Marchetti 2009: 176). The visitor is expected to go with the flow: the experiential value of a product outweighs its aesthetic cachet. As a result, the act of looking is only one facet of the total experience. Brands increasingly stage certain experiences by engaging customers, which could be achieved by affecting their senses by, for instance, using special lighting and fragrances and giving them certain memorabilia (Gilmore and Pine 1999: 15). The effects on muscles and skin, on the senses of touch and smell, are just as much part of the visitor's embedded, direct, and complete experience. To experience fashion, its visual components are no longer enough. Product experience is given more and more attention and is becoming increasingly important: consumers want to buy into unique consumption and ownership experiences (Gilmore and Pine 1999). And consultants are hired to develop and articulate the complex worlds in which a brand's virtual world—a narrative based on the values

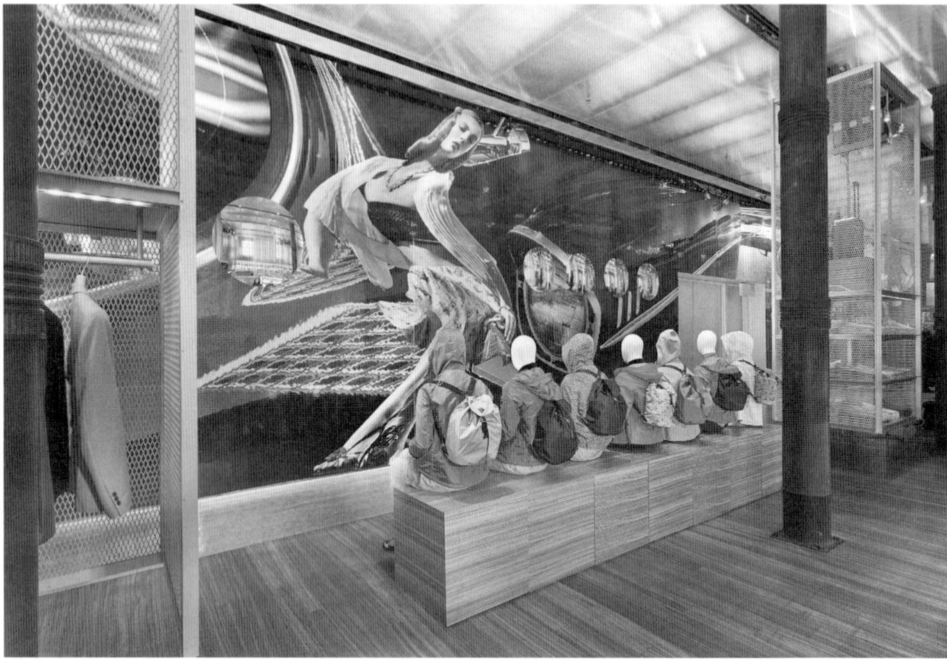

FIGURE 10.4 Prada store, New York, designed by Rem Koolhaas.
Credit: Courtesy Prada Epicenter New York.

and meanings synthesized by the brand—is brought to life and in which the consumer takes an active role (Bettiol 2013). This is so-called fun shopping, or retailment as conceived by "experiential" marketing. The participation of the public, substituting for the position of simple observer, becomes a form of performance in which what happens—the fact that the audience is sharing a space and time, is part of an event, is creating a community—is more important than the product or piece of cloth itself. "In this context clothes take on another value: they become interface" (Marchetti and Quinz 2009: 122).

> The megastore is a continuation of the innovations ushered in by the nineteenth century department store, and is devoted to transforming shopping into a pleasurable lifestyle experience. In the new store concepts, the focus is on transporting the consumer emotionally and making the retail store the cult locus for the cult brand. Even luxury sells experience in the hyperconsumer society (and no longer merely social status), blending prestige, glamour, beauty, sensation and art. This is how a hyperbrand or a *brand cult* is created. The aim is to transform consumers into "fans" of the brand itself. They must not only buy in the stores, but convince their network of friends to buy that brand's product as well. (Lipovetsky and Manlow 2009: 163)

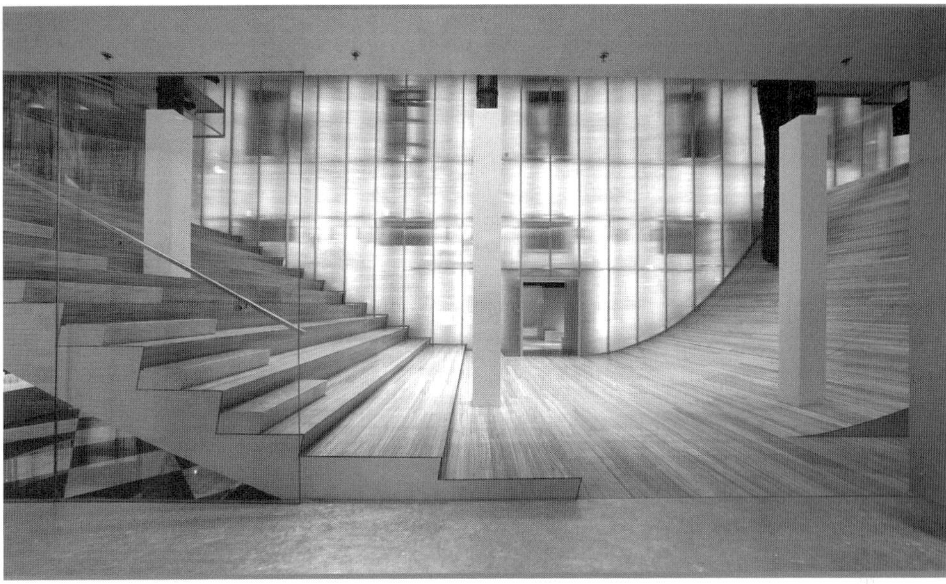

FIGURE 10.5 Prada store, New York, designed by Rem Koolhaas.
Credit: Courtesy Prada Epicenter New York.

Thus, Lev Manovich has defined Rem Koolhaas's Prada store in New York (Figure 10.5) not so much as a cult locus but as an experience related to the contemplative, serene world of the church, and it is worth quoting him at length:

> Koolhaas seems to achieve the impossible by creating a flagship store for the Prada brand—and at the same time an ironic statement about the functioning of brands as new religions. The imaginative use of electronic displays designed by Reed Kram of Kramdesign is an important part of this statement. On entering the store you discover glass cages hanging from the ceiling throughout the space. Just as a church would present the relics of saints in special displays, here the glass cages contain the new objects of worship—Prada gloves. The special status of Prada gloves is further enhanced by placing flat electronic screens throughout the store and on the horizontal shelves right among the merchandize. The gloves are equated to the ephemeral images laying on the screens, and, vice versa, the images acquire certain materiality, as though they are objects. By positioning screens showing moving images right next to gloves designers ironically refer to what everybody today knows: we buy objects not for themselves but in order to emulate certain images and narratives presented by the advertisements of these objects. (2005: 25–26)

Moreover, nowadays the modern store inherits a flux of invisible data that augment the space and can be captured at any moment with smartphones or devices that can connect via Wi-Fi or Bluetooth. In this way the information-based society is making an invisible experience as important as, if not more so than, a tangible one, so that the meaning of the object further transcends its functional dimension and its ritual value.

A CHANGING AESTHETIC: DECLINE AND MELANCHOLY/STORYTELLING

Apart from the fact that Japanese designers started to develop a multidisciplinary vocabulary for their brand, they also introduced a radically new aesthetics in their fashion designs. Yohji Yamamoto, for instance, based his autumn/winter 2001/2002 collection on images by the German photographer August Sander depicting workmen in their traditional working clothes. Yamamoto was so fascinated by the worn-out character of the clothing—elbows showing through sleeves, creases, threadbare spots—that he wanted to include these characteristics in his designs (Vinken 2006: 32). In the late 1980s this Japanese approach to design inspired the Antwerp Six and Martin Margiela to explore clothing from the tailoring perspective (33). Margiela focused on secondhand clothes, because these had, in his opinion, already had a former life and therefore were inscribed with various meanings. He created tops made of overlapping gloves or, more simply, a series of women's jackets made of men's jackets with extra padding halfway across the shoulder, in order to make them look narrower. Melancholy, decay, and aging, along with all sorts of experiments related to form, have become recurrent themes in fashion ever since the 1980s; themes, after all, that had been the privilege of the visual arts. Barbara Vinken suggests that after the 1980s avant-garde fashion no longer focused on the *new* but rather made *time* and *mortality* the dominant themes of their work:

> Its theme is the process and not the finished product—hence the many pieces that are labelled "unfinished." What is new in this fashion is that the old is not excluded or denied but is made into the material of the clothes. It is not the matter of historicism, a revival of a past epoch, but an inscribing of traces of mortality—not the animation of the dead, the erasure of the traces of time, but the marking of the traces of a death, whose carrier the living body becomes. (2009: 87)

Up to this point, fashion had been widely seen as a phenomenon that disavowed the aging process by continually offering consumers new products.

In the postmodern age an awareness of transitoriness—widely discussed in both literature and the visual arts—was no longer ignored or silenced but began to form an essential part of the dialogue of fashion. Fashion then also became a domain within which the modern subject could test its own mortality (Vinken 2009: 89). "This new look exists in time and no longer in dreams" (Vinken 2006: 32). To bring to life those "traces and emotions" through clothing, new forms of presentation were needed. Alexander McQueen became notorious for creating macabre, magical worlds that transformed his catwalk shows into theatrical happenings. In What a Merry-Go-Round (2001–2002), for example, McQueen emphasized the sinister side of childhood toys, sampling the voice of the child catcher from the film *Chitty Chitty Bang Bang.* The makeup of the models, based on the white clown, with a golden skeleton dragging at the feet, enhanced the mournful and alienating effect. According to Caroline Evans in *Fashion at the Edge,* these traces and emotions in the avant-garde fashion of the late twentieth century were referring to the idea of resisting and opposing the voice of the "civilisation process":

> On the edge of discourse of "civilisation," of speech itself, experimental fashion can act out what is hidden culturally. And, like a neurotic symptom, it can utter a kind of mute resistance to the socially productive process of constructing identity. As we produce a disciplined and controlled self, via the "technology" of manners for example, what is repressed comes back as a trace, under the weight of a cultural trauma, of which experimental fashion can function as a tell-tale memory. Seen thus, fashion is hysterical. It can be a symptom of alienation, loss, mourning, fear, of contagion and death, instability and change. Like psychoanalysis, it "investigates the domain and configuration of incoherence, discontinuity, disruption and disintegration." (2003: 6)

For almost twenty years now Maison Martin Margiela has chosen to present clothes in a manner that shows the underlying concept to best advantage; this can range from a film on instructions for use for the launch of a duvet jacket to small public performances that reveal the collection's conceptual point of departure. The analogy between the ragpicker and the poet, artist, or designer can be chased into many other urban spaces, which Margiela went on to use to pioneer a new form of fashion show:

> The earliest spaces in which he showed included an old theatre, an area of wasteland, a warehouse corridor, a disused hospital and an empty supermarket. These derelict Parisian spaces echoed the chaos and marginality of the nineteenth-century ragpickers' milieu in the *zone militaire* and beyond the *barriers,* and remind us of the ragpicker's literary provenance in texts and images of urban *derivés* and derelict spaces. (Evans 2003: 250)

The retail design, look books, and flyers all come in the firm's trademark look of white cotton and simple whitewash to suggest that the clothing had already had another, previous life (Blanchard 2004: 104).

FROM MATERIAL TO EXPERIENCE: VIKTOR & ROLF AND THE MAGIC OF THE FAIRY TALE

In 1999 Viktor & Rolf presented their Russian Doll collection in Paris (autumn/winter 1999/2000)—not as a show, but as a live performance. The show started by showing a model on a rotating platform wearing only a sackcloth petticoat and ballet shoes. As the show progressed, the model was dressed by the two couturiers, layer for layer. By the time they had reached the eighth layer the model almost disappeared in the volume. In fact, the designers had turned her into a matryoshka doll in reverse. Needless to say, the performance played with more layers and references than only this one. Viktor & Rolf were taking the role of classic couturiers here, dating from before the prêt-à-porter age, when everything had to be made to measure for each individual client. It was also a reference to the film *The Red Shoes* (Powell and Pressburger 1948). On the one hand, the designer duo tried to comment on the fashion system in general: Where are we heading? What has happened to craftsmanship? On a more prosaic level, they were simply examining the ritual of designing couture: How far can you go with layering? How do certain proportions impact on the shape of the human body? At what point do these experiments start to border on the grotesque, eclipse the natural human body? It was exactly this delicate interlayering of imagined worlds and underlying ideas and concepts that Viktor & Rolf became well known for. Unlike Kawakubo and Maison Martin Margiela, for Viktor & Rolf it was not so much about the concept behind their designs. Rather they sought to emphasize the link between the fairy-tale worlds they created and fashion design. Viktor & Rolf criticized fashion while simultaneously capitalizing on its glamorous character and creative potential to frame their commentary. The retrospective The House of Viktor & Rolf (2008) they were asked to set up for the Barbican Art Gallery in London perfectly illustrates how fashion design and the dreamscapes they create are inseparably linked (Figure 10.6).

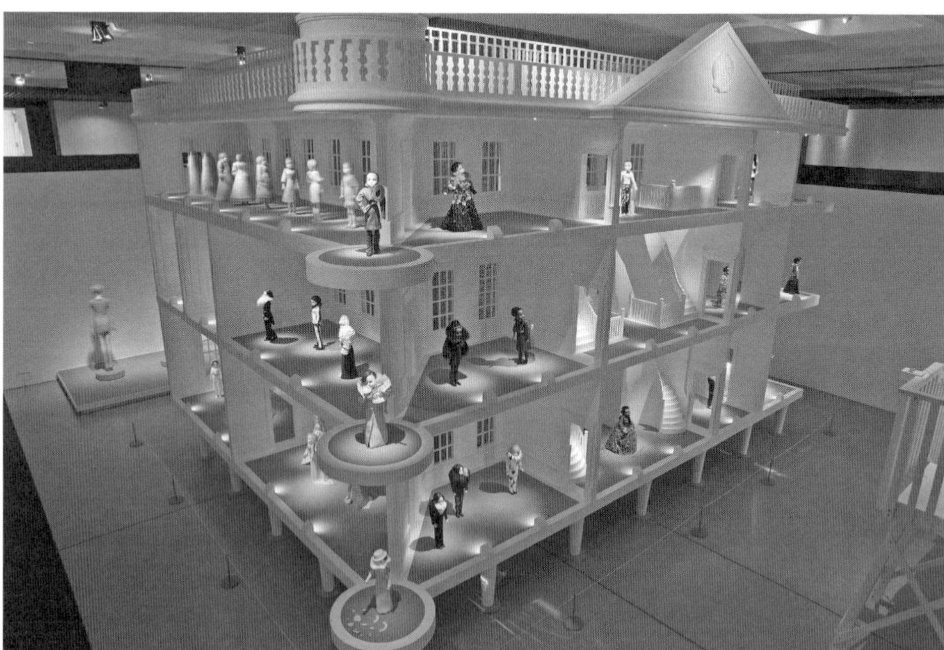

FIGURE 10.6 The House of Viktor & Rolf, Barbican Art Gallery, London, 2008.
Credit: Courtesy of Viktor & Rolf. Photograph by Andrew Lamb.

At the heart of the exhibition was a doll's house sixteen feet (five meters) in height, inside which all their collections were reproduced in miniature on classic porcelain dolls. The House of Viktor & Rolf effectively summed up their entire history as designers within the playful world of a doll's house. All their designs were scaled down with utmost precision and craftsmanship. Here, too, the duo used the fairy tale–like setting to achieve an almost uncanny effect: not only were their designs displayed in miniaturized versions, but in the adjoining rooms the original designs were displayed on life-size dolls, chubby and somewhat shapeless. The macabre aesthetic—beautifully crafted dresses on childish doll's bodies—called into question the beauty ideals of the fashion world, prompting visitors to reconsider their own conceptions of beauty.

The exhibition was a chance for the designers to reflect their unique aesthetics on different levels. As Viktor & Rolf explained in *T Magazine* (2008):

> We always have mixed feelings when it comes to fashion exhibitions because somehow, life is taken out of the subject. But a museum show is also a more democratic way of showing fashion than a catwalk presentation. It allows us to explore perspectives and ideas beyond that format. Challenged to enliven the static form of most fashion exhibitions, we created a special installation for the Barbican and conceived the entire show around it. The installation forms the heart of the exhibition and brings together our past, present and future work, creating a new reality to showcase the clothes and installations that make up our world.

The self-contained contemplative space of a museum, far away from the bustle and noise of commerce and consumption, provided the ideal setting to absorb all the elements of "the magic world" and, along with it, the ideas and background connected to Viktor & Rolf's entire oeuvre. In this way, for Viktor & Rolf the museum or gallery appeared to be a necessary component of their brand strategy: the world of the brand is shown best when it appears in the museum.

THE MUSEUM AS THE NEW FASHION SPACE

The encounter between avant-garde fashion designers and the museum is both the result of and the reason for the new exhibition practices that started in the 1990s. The rapid growth of specialized fashion and design museums in the twenty-first century has provided new platforms of expression for avant-garde fashion designers, taking them out of their professional routines.

> It is now a strategic necessity for every designer to "curate" an exhibition, whether monographic or not. To exhibit, both literally and figuratively, is to cast aside the static aspect of clothing. An exhibition may therefore legitimately be considered

> the transposition of a fashion show on a larger scale, where the obviously restrictive framework of a museum is largely offset by the possibility of putting the clothes in contact with other objects and experiences aiming to deliver a more universal message, outside the concerns of immediate commercial profitability. (Kamitsis 2009: 103)

To understand the work of avant-garde designers as well as to understand fashion as part of our contemporary visual culture, the museum, it seems, has become a new and natural partner.

CONCLUSION

From the 1960s on, then, avant-garde designers have increasingly sought to add to their product additional, less tangible dimensions (Vinken 2009). In so doing, the desired goal is to direct the viewers' attention not to the object itself but to their own relationship with it. Designers want their audience to "get to know" the material object in order to understand its underlying conceptual idea or register. It is this cognitive aspect that elicits an emotional response in the viewer, provoking ideas, memories, and stories.

Along with this process, fashion aesthetics have undergone a shift from an object-centered discourse to one driven by concepts and ideas, the creative process, and multi-dimensional product experiences.

> Everything from theatre, film and political protests, to Fluxus, Dada performances and Surrealist techniques has been incorporated into fashion productions. Regardless of the influence or motivating factors, each section illustrates a unique symptom of the phenomenon—the recent blurring of the boundaries that separate fashion and art. (Gregg Duncan 2006: 243)

Fashion has moved from the ideal body and identity to direct experiences of the body: away from its quality as a vector of meanings toward its quality as a material object or as a carrier of ideas comparable to a work of art. "Clothes become an instrument for meeting, exchanging, giving, acknowledging. And the performance is no longer defined as a show, destined for the eyes of an audience, but as a lived experience that no longer needs a witness" (Marchetti and Quinz 2009: 122). Concomitantly, the two primary venues for staging fashion—the catwalk and the store—have become hybrid locations that ever more closely resemble art destinations such as museums, galleries, and theaters, places where every form of displaying/exhibiting clothes has become possible. In this manner, in the twenty-first century the museum has become a new, vital third venue for staging fashion.

BIBLIOGRAPHY

Bettiol, Marco. 2013. "Slow Fashion: New Perspectives from the Italian Textile and Fashion Industry." In Jan Brand and José Teunissen (eds.), *A Fashion Odyssey: Progress in Fashion and Sustainability,* 130–42. Arnhem, the Netherlands: ArtEZ Press.

Blanchard, Tamsin. 2004. *Fashion and Graphic Design.* London: Laurence King.

Evans, Caroline. 2001. "The Enchanted Spectacle." *Fashion Theory: The Journal of Dress, Body and Culture* 5 (3): 271–311.

Evans, Caroline. 2003. *Fashion at the Edge: Spectacle, Modernity and Deathliness.* New Haven, CT: Yale University Press.

Fukai, Akiko. 2006. "Japan and Fashion." In Jan Brand and José Teunissen (eds.), *The Power of Fashion: On Design and Meaning,* 288–314. Arnhem, the Netherlands: Terra and ArtEZ Press.

Garelick, Rhonda. 1998. *Rising Star: Dandyism, Gender and Performance in the Fin de Siècle.* Princeton: Princeton University Press.

Gilmore, James, and Joseph Pine. 1999. *The Experience Economy.* Boston: Harvard Business School Press.

Gregg Duncan, Ginger. 2006. "The Greatest Show on Earth: A Look at Contemporary Fashion Shows and Their Relationship to Performance Art." In Jan Brand and José Teunissen (eds.), *The Power of Fashion: On Design and Meaning,* 222–48. Arnhem, the Netherlands: Terra and ArtEZ Press.

Hollander, Anne. 1975. *Seeing through Clothes.* New York: Avedon.

Kamitsis, Lydia. 2009. "An Impressionistic History of Fashion Shows since the 1960s." In Jan Brand and José Teunissen (eds.), *Fashion and Imagination,* 92–104. Arnhem, the Netherlands: d'jonge Hond and ArtEZ Press.

Kinney, Leila W. 2009. "Fashion and Fabrication in Modern Architecture." In Jan Brand and José Teunissen (eds.), *Fashion and Imagination,* 248–60. Arnhem, the Netherlands: d'jonge Hond and ArtEZ Press.

Lipovetsky, Gilles. 1994. *The Empire of Fashion: Dressing Modern Democracy.* Princeton, NJ: Princeton University Press.

Lipovetsky, Gilles. 2002. "More than Fashion." In Ulrich Lehmann and Jessica Morgan (eds.), *Chic Clicks,* 8–11. Ostfildern, Germany: Hatje Cantz.

Lipovetsky, Gilles, and Veronica Manlow. 2009. "The 'Artialization' of Luxury Stores." In Jan Brand and José Teunissen (eds.), *Fashion and Imagination,* 154–68. Arnhem, the Netherlands: d'jonge Hond and ArtEZ Press.

Manovich, Lev. 2005. "The Poetics of Augmented Space." http://www.manovich.net/articles.php (accessed October 25, 2010).

Marchetti, Luca. 2009. "From the Object to the Invisible: Retail Experience within Space, Fashion and Body." In Jan Brand and José Teunissen (eds.), *Fashion and Imagination,* 168–84. Arnhem, the Netherlands: d'jonge Hond and ArtEZ Press.

Marchetti, Luca, and Emanuelle Quinz. 2009. "Invisible Fashion: From the Interface to Re-embodiment: Experience beyond the Clothes." In Jan Brand and José Teunissen (eds.), *Fashion and Imagination,* 116–26. Arnhem, the Netherlands: d'jonge Hond and ArtEZ Press.

Martin, Richard. 2009. "Beyond Appearances and beyond Custom: The Avant-Garde Sensibility of Fashion and Art since the 1960s." In Jan Brand and José Teunissen (eds.), *Fashion and Imagination,* 26–44. Arnhem, the Netherlands: d'jonge Hond and ArtEZ Press.

Pecorari, Marco. 2011. "Zones-in-Between: The Creation of New Fashion Praxis." *Art Monthly Australian* 242 (August): 67–70.

Powell, Michael, and Emeric Pressburger. 1948. *The Red Shoes*. London: The Archers (Pressburger and Powell).

Rocamora, Agnès. 2009. *Fashioning the City: Paris, Fashion and the Media*. London: I. B. Tauris.

Schwartz, Vanessa R. 1999. *Spectacular Realities: Early Mass Culture in Fin-de-Siècle Paris*. Berkeley: University of California Press.

Sennett, Richard. 1977. *The Fall of Public Man*. London: Faber and Faber.

Simmel, Georg. [1905] 2000. *Philosophie der Mode*. Berlin: Suhrkamp.

Steele, Valerie. 1998. *Paris Fashion: A Cultural History*. New York: A&C Black.

Sudjic, Deyan. 1990. *Rei Kawakubo and Comme des Garçons*. London: Westbourne Grove.

Teunissen, José. 2003. "Hussein Chalayan." In José Teunissen, *Woman By*, 65–81. Utrecht, the Netherlands: Centraal Museum.

Teunissen, José. 2006. "From Dandy to Fashion Show: Fashion as Performance Art." In Jan Brand and José Teunissen (eds.), *The Power of Fashion: On Design and Meaning*, 194–222. Arnhem, the Netherlands: Terra and ArtEZ Press.

Teunissen, José. 2009. "Fashion and Art." In Jan Brand and José Teunissen (eds.), *Fashion and Imagination*, 10–26. Arnhem, the Netherlands: d'jonge Hond and ArtEZ Press.

Viktor & Rolf. 2008. "For the Moment | Viktor & Rolf." *T Magazine*, June 12. http://tmagazine.blogs.nytimes.com/2008/06/12/for-the-moment-viktor-rolf (accessed June 12, 2008).

Vinken, Barbara. 2006. "Eternity: A Frill on a Dress." In Jan Brand and José Teunissen (eds.), *The Power of Fashion: On Design and Meaning*, 28–42. Arnhem, the Netherlands: Terra and ArtEZ Press.

Vinken, Barbara. 2009. "Fashion: Art of Dying, Art of Living." In Jan Brand and José Teunissen (eds.), *Fashion and Imagination*, 82–92. Arnhem, the Netherlands: d'jonge Hond and ArtEZ Press.

11

Markets as Fashion Spaces

PATRIK ASPERS

INTRODUCTION

Markets have gradually become a more important form of coordination of human resources and activities and have increasingly replaced other forms, such as the reciprocal gift economy, characterized by networks, and organizations (hierarchy), in which decisions are the leading principle. Fashion, characterized by volatility and change, may not appear to have much to do with coordination. However, it takes much coordination and order to experience the "wanton vagaries" of fashion.

Fashion in markets implies space, often in physical terms, and in other cases virtual space. This chapter looks at how markets do two things simultaneously: (1) they enable free choice, which is characteristic of markets but is also essential for the logic of fashion, and (2) they send out information on choices made by people. The argument, in a nutshell, is that fashion emulation calls for the free choice of producers and consumers and that these choices are made in marketplaces—spaces of virtual and nonvirtual character. The chapter discusses the observation, diffusion, and constitution of fashion in relation to market spaces. Put in other words: space is an essential dimension of fashion, though often neglected in sociological research.[1] This work is tied to studies of the spatiality of fashion consumption (Rocamora 2009). Moreover, fashion is concerned with more than clothes; it is a profoundly social phenomenon with a very large domain of applicability.

There are obviously some elements that this text does not deal with. This chapter will not deal with the coordination of the fashion industry, a topic that has been researched by others (e.g., Aspers 2010; Hirsch 1992; Kawamura 2004). Following the antiessentialist approach of fashion, the objects themselves will be bracketed out of the analysis. Why some people prefer certain clothes to others is yet another question that is of less importance for the argument made here.

This text uses a sociological perspective and draws on existing research in two fields, fashion and markets, to analyze the role of space. I will analyze fashion spaces—predominantly related to markets—in several steps. The idea of space and spatiality is often seen as physical, but in this chapter I will also look at virtual space. First, I analyze the observation of fashion and the ways in which fashion is constituted in a social space, zooming in on the Internet. I then look at how producers and consumers of garments use market spaces, highlighting the role of choice as essential for both fashion and markets.

OBSERVING FASHION

At the beginning of the twentieth century fashion was largely diffused by means of direct observation. In order to see and learn what was in fashion, a phenomenon then most clearly associated with the upper classes, people had to observe each other, in private interaction, but of course also on the street, in cafés, and in other public spaces. Those who did not, or could not, visit these places had few means to really know what was in fashion and what was not. Prior to the distribution of visual means of information, communication was largely restricted to direct observation. Over the last 100 years, other media—first of all printed media, then television, and more recently the Internet—have provided channels of information that allow observers of fashion to also be located at a distance from the physical setting of the social interaction out of which fashion is produced.

Moving and still pictures of fashion are today important in the fashion industry, for producers and consumers alike. Today, the Internet is the most obvious way to gain access to these pictures. Let us look at an example. People in the industry are frequently surveying the Internet for ideas, to keep track of what their competitors are doing and to keep their own sites updated. Fashion blogs, run by professionals and amateurs, are additional means that cater to the same need. Catwalks, for example, can be seen on the Internet, either live or with some delay. There are several ways in which nonprofessionals and, more important, customers can also use visual means to inform themselves on trends, fashions, and what others are wearing.

Paparazzi are a type of photographers who intrude in the private sphere of celebrities to take pictures for which they get money from the press, which is eager to publish them on the Internet but, above all, in the magazines they oversee. The interaction often strengthens both the celebrity and the photographer, who makes a living by shooting these pictures.[2] However, most would say that this intrusion is a way for common people, some of whom are dedicated fans of the so-called celebrities, to have a glance into both the public and private lives of celebrities. Celebrities are often icons of fashion, and many people are interested in what these trendsetters are wearing.

It is easy to illustrate how the pictures of a celebrity matter for the diffusion and constitution of fashion (Miller 2010). Readers, for example, are told about a picture of the actress Angelina Jolie, showing what clothes she is wearing. Both the picture and the text provide detailed information the readers can use to find the clothes or look for similar ones. In addition to simply looking at pictures showing what celebrities are wearing, one can "steal the style" of a celebrity. This is facilitated by an additional feature of many Internet sites: hyperlinks. Not only is some information provided on a celebrity's outfit, but the reader is only one click away from the site where it can be purchased. Thereby the photo, taken on a specific date at a certain place where both the celebrity and the paparazzi were, is connecting the items to an electronic point of sale. The viewer can move from a "noncommercial" site to the company selling the item at another website, which may use the very same picture as an advertisement. Sites are also interactive, asking customers to help those who run them to find out what the celebrities are wearing. Among the customers who willingly provide information, it is likely that one will find representatives of the companies that are selling these items. The pictures re-present the space—the town square—where the distant viewer can observe what others are wearing. What can be learned, then, is that the photos are more directly included in the economy.[3]

There are also other means having the same effect as these "fashion peepers" in providing information on fashion. Today algorithms create spaces on the Internet. Algorithms are programmed procedures for solving problems. An algorithm can be programmed to trace what a customer is searching for or to create systems of offers that customers can be expected to use. As a result, Internet users may encounter messages like "Others who looked at this also looked at . . . " or "frequently bought together," or they may simply be offered something of interest to them, for example, ads. In this way the space around the offers is plastic and individualistic, which is to say that companies can form a virtual bubble and embed customers in it because of what the customers seem to prefer; the alternatives made available to the customer, as it were, are programmed by a customer's past behavior. The process of creating plastic spaces that embed the customer in a commercial virtual space means that differences are largely the result of the machines that interact with humans. These algorithms are indeed market devices (Callon, Millo, and Muniesa 2007), but they cannot be reduced to the intention of one single individual, not even that of the programmer, since they are programmed to evolve in interaction with humans.

CONSTITUTING FASHION

Observation of clothes and use of the Internet do not generate fashion, even if the clothes are in focus. Fashions in dress call for bodies wearing clothes, and minds reflecting on what is worn. In the fashion space of modern market economies, fashion producers make up one necessary component of buying and selling fashion, consumers the other. My point is that the interaction between buyers and sellers is crucial for constituting fashion. When known buyers—characterized as ideal-typical consumers of various types—interact with well-known sellers (e.g., brands), fashion is constituted

(Aspers 2010). Let us look closer at an empirical example to see how this is played out on the Internet.

The well-known artist Katy Perry has made headlines for her music but also for her style. She is followed by many people, and her activities are regularly reported in magazines, often using pictures. Obviously, very few would know about her whereabouts, clothes, and so on unless the media existed. It is by means of reappearing on the Web and in magazines that her style comes to be known to many people. Here are a few representative quotations from the Internet on her style and her clothes:[4] "The news that Katy Perry has become the first celebrity ambassador of the world leading hair styling brand GHD has excited many of the diva's fans just a while back."[5] She has also done some modeling for the Victoria's Secret 2010 Fashion Show, at which she also performed a song. Another piece of information for customers who want to copy her style is a picture of her in May 2011 captioned with the following words:

> Katy Perry was recently spotted out with friends at Australia's Taronga Zoo. Here she is wearing a fabulous Wheels & Dollbaby Dita Rose Embroidered Cardi in Red with Black which you can pick up online for $190.00. The cardigan comes from Wheels & Dollbaby's collaboration with burlesque model Dita von Teese. Katy's sunglasses are the white Ray-Ban Clubmaster which she also wore at JC de Castelbajac's runway show back in March.[6]

These few examples are included to show how labels can become fashionable because icons structure and order the field of fashion (Aspers 2006). Fashion is made, or, put differently, performed, in the public interaction of clothes, brands, and known wearers.

Though this is a result of interaction, and the two sides, buyers and sellers, constitute each other as well as the object, the economic principle of shortage often means that it is the icon that endows the seller (the brand) with status rather than the other way around. In short, there is only one Lady Gaga or Katy Perry, to take two fashion icons, but many brands—all of which are able to produce several garments to be offered to many customers. It is important to realize that this is not explained by the number of people involved but by the relative status of those involved. Though each person has a personal name, a unique body, and a narrative, very few are known enough to fulfill the role as one who endows the other side with status. Essentially only those whose fame reaches beyond a network can further a fashion across spaces and domains in a direct and fast way. Furthermore, if status is the ordering principle, normally one side is endowing the other side with status more than the other way around. If a well-known designer made only one item of a kind, he or she could be endowing the wearer with status. Should, in contrast, the wearer be extremely well known, his or her status will rub off on the designer. It is thus an empirical question which side is offering status to the other, and this depends on their relative status. That status is distributed in this particular case is, of course, above all because Katy Perry has gained a reputation as a singer, and it is her identity with high status in the field of music that explains her influence on fashion. This is to say that the status order in the field of music brings order to the field of fashion (cf. Aspers 2010).

CHOICE IN MARKETS AND CHOICE OF FASHION

In this section I look at the conditions of free choice needed for fashion to exist. The "free" choice is one central aspect to be discussed. It is shown that the market enables people to choose. In other words, much of what I have discussed so far is played out in a market context. There is, put differently, a similarity between fashion and the market; both imply space and choice. A central point is that fashion is not one choice but the result of very many. Fashion is an unintended consequence, and, moreover, it cannot be organized, though attempts at organization have been observed, for example, efforts to control what colors will become fashionable (Aspers 2010). Fashion is the result of many people's decisions but is not itself the result of a decision. Though many people and organizations have an interest in steering fashion, due to economic or other motives, neither a single actor nor a group of actors can control fashion, not even in a concerted way.

Fashion is often seen as being existentially and emotionally important to human beings. It is seen as a means of expression and as a way to allow individuals to construct and maintain their identities. All this presupposes that people can make choices and thereby uphold differences, which ultimately can be turned into distinctions. The coordination of fashion presupposes choices among alternatives. Fashion, however, does not presuppose markets. If people were allowed to borrow—essentially free of charge—clothes from a storage area filled with different clothes, one could observe trends in fashion. People would borrow different things, and some choices would be deemed to be "in fashion" and others "out of fashion." In this game, here illustrated as a thought experiment, people could simply borrow garments, and money would not have to be involved.

Furthermore, people making clothes for themselves is another way in which, as a first step, difference can be created, which, in a second step, can be turned into distinctions and stratification into "good" and "bad," or "nice" and "not so nice." This social game can be played among girls on a soccer team who have their hair dressed and styled in a certain way, among dog owners who train their pets to do certain things, among hunters who use a certain car model, among academics who cite a certain author, and so on. Fashion is a general phenomenon and is not restricted to clothes (Lieberson 2000). The general logic of fashion, however, is clearly the same regardless of what is subject to fashion.

Nonetheless, in most contemporary forms of social life, when fashion plays a role, money matters. This is not a surprise, since in the contemporary market society, choices are often made using money in markets. This has the consequence that economic stratification, which exists in all societies, makes it easier for some to follow fashion than for others. Before I turn to the notion of choice and the conditions for fashion, I first discuss the attempt to mimic the Western and capitalistic mode of fashion as it was unfolding behind the Iron Curtain. This is, as it were, the negative case, and it is a step to gain a better understanding of fashion and of the central role of choice.

The communist Soviet Union was the main contender for world dominance facing the capitalist system between World War II and 1989, when the fall of the Berlin Wall unleashed the forces that led to the collapse of the totalitarian regimes in the Eastern European countries. Jukka Gronow (2003) has studied the role of fashion in the Soviet system. He finds that the Communist Party wanted to show that its system could offer the citizens of the Soviet Union a life that was as good as those of people living in the capitalist West. The following quote, reported by Gronow, from the secretary of the party organization of the Leningrad clothes-printing factory in 1935, makes this clear: "but who has told [us] that we could not produce a better drawing than foreigners. Comrades, we have to produce our own beautiful drawing which could gratify the demands of a young girl, a child and a middle-aged woman alike" (2003: 97).

To understand the fashion production under the Soviet system one must look at how production was coordinated and what choices users could make. Since the economy was coordinated through the means of organization—that is, a form of social order based on decisions on, among other things, how products are made and how to behave (Ahrne and Brunsson 2011)—free choice was eliminated at several levels, in particular at the levels that concerned the decisions on what to produce. How did it actually happen that some items were produced and not others? Soviet designers launched fashion lines, and real garments were made, but it was the party members who decided what could be produced or not, reflecting the aesthetics of communism. This meant that the actual alternatives that the citizens had were relatively limited in number. The inefficient system, in addition, meant that of those garments that were to be produced only a small fraction actually reached users. In practice, only a few people in Moscow could enjoy these garments. Thus the lack of quality was not the largest problem but rather the supply of goods (Gronow 2003).

Other goods that were seen as luxury goods in the West, like champagne, were produced in abundance in the Soviet Union. The result was that these goods could not be used to make distinctions and, in effect, were not seen as luxury goods at all by the citizens of the Soviet Union. Fashion calls for choice between resources and is facilitated if these resources are scarce, or made scarce (Daoud 2011).

Though these examples are brief and simplified, it is nonetheless clear that it is not the goods themselves that create distinctions, and that alternatives, or, seen from the perspective of users, choices, must exist. Money and other economic means are not necessary conditions for fashion, but they strengthens the capacity for wealthy people to consume things, making distinctions in a conspicuous way, so that others cannot use the same things or have to copy them using other means. Fashion, hence, cannot be the result of organized coordination; it cannot be forced on people, and free choice must exist.

The idea of choice is implicit in Georg Simmel's (1971) and also Thorstein Veblen's (1945) models of fashion. Choice implies alternatives to choose from under the influence of some kind of scarcity. When selecting among alternatives in your wardrobe, you have a choice, though some of the options are not necessarily highly interesting. One may say that this is an example of choice, but there is no competition, as competition implies agency. To understand the dynamics of fashion choice today, I now look at the role of markets.

THE MARKET AS A SPACE OF CHOICE

The introduction of the market as a coordinated form of fashion implies two things: the notion of choice and the notion of space. I define markets as a social structure for the exchange of rights in which offers are evaluated and priced and compete with one another, which is shorthand for the fact that actors—individuals and firms—compete with one another via offers (Aspers 2011: 4). This definition covers the market both as a place and as a form of exchange characterized by competition.

If one analyzes the concept closer and traces the etymology of *market,* its dual meaning is seen more clearly. The Latin origin, *mercatus,* refers to trade and to place. Another notion, *forum,* should also be mentioned. It refers to a place and more specifically the marketplace. Both, however, refer to public activities. Each market normally has a name, which refers to what is being traded—for example, the market for handmade boots or the market for scarves. Some markets are associated with a certain place, such as the Petticoat Lane market in London, in which garments are traded. A marketplace must not, however, be about one good or service only. A bazaar (Geertz 1978) is a designated area for the trade of many different things. The Petticoat Lane market, however, is not only a marketplace in general but a market, much like many other London markets, with an identity tied to specific objects of trade, namely, garments. In larger shops, prices are announced on tags attached to the clothes, and bargaining is usually not possible. One may try clothes on, and there are many more "rules," some of which may vary between countries, or even market segments, that make up the culture of the market. In essence, most of these defining traits are similar to what one finds in other markets.

CHOICE AND COMPETITION IN MARKETS

I have already mentioned the central role of choice, and due to competition this is a defining trait of markets. Competition, however, takes place on both sides of the market. Not all garment-producing firms that also have an identity (brand) in the market have their own stores, but those that do not are represented in other stores or in larger department stores. The aim of producers competing with different products in markets is to reduce competition, primarily by means of product differentiation and niches. Edward Chamberlin (1948) and later Harrison White (1981) developed market theories that account for the fact that producers try to create niches in markets. By controlling the environment and creating partial monopolies, economic organizations generate identities, and market order follows because of the interaction between the organizations and their buyers. As Alfred Marshall already pointed out, brands—or, as sociologists often say, identities—are central for creating distinctions.

It is, in other words, only the rhetoric of the neoclassical market model that calls for the utterance that "we, as producers, want competition." Reduction of competition enables firms to increase profits and to use the mental space created by their identity to further control their environment. A small difference may be enough for other actors—competitors and buyers—to act on to increase the difference between themselves and to carve out unique identities and market niches. It is only in relation to other producers, all of whom share a collective identity, that firms can be clearly separated from each other and become different. Sellers try to convince potential buyers to choose their clothes. Sellers, moreover, can control what they put out on the market, and they try to convince potential buyers to choose their clothes. Control efforts are central, and advertisement, pricing, and other means can be used, most effectively by the sellers, since they are fewer in number and much more powerful than individual buyers are. The best way for producers to control the environment is to successfully perform fashion, that is, to set the agenda of what is in fashion and what is not.

Though producers can do much to try to affect consumers, it is ultimately the differences perceived by consumers that matter. Producers, put differently, are not in control of their identities. Even though the garments up for sale at any given time may look somewhat similar, it is the variation within the similarity that matters, but it is important that differences matter only in relation to the perceptions of the consumers. It is thus of utmost importance to consider consumers in order to understand how producers act. Consumers can choose from the multitude of options in the available garments. Buyers may be looking for garments that enable them to make distinctions, to comply with or defy the current fashion. Brand-new store-bought clothes, as well as used (acquired from friends or secondhand stores) and homemade clothes, can be considered as options by buyers, but the bulk is made up of new garments bought in stores.

SPATIALITY

The competitive logic of fashion, I have argued, has a clearly spatial component. Spatiality is both constituted by fashion and helps to constitute fashion. How do fashion producers use space? There is research showing that producers gather in industrial districts (e.g., Uzzi 1997). The spatial distribution of garment sellers is the visual manifestation of competition. Each type of seller tends to be concentrated in a particular spatial location. In London, as in Paris or any other large city, stores from the different market segments are located in different places: the luxury shops are concentrated in Bond Street, whereas the large retailers' stores are in Oxford Street. The difference, in terms of physical distance, can be measured in yards (or meters) and may thus be seen as marginal, but the phenomenological distance is significant. It is not uncommon for firms to wait several years to open a shop, until the "right" location becomes available. Not only is the geographic location of importance, but the presence of other stores in the area, or the style of the building of the store, can be of equal importance.

A shopping mall or a certain street may create an identity, enough to bring producers together and facilitate comparisons among producers and consumers alike. To occupy a position, that is, to have a specific store in an area, may be enough to gain an identity as a competitor to the others in the market. This is to say that fashion status, which is concerned with objects that lack a standard of evaluation, rubs off (Podolny 1993).

The consequence is that producers may do much to control the physical environment. In addition, owners of malls, shopping centers, and the like are prone to control which companies they rent space to and which they do not. This meta-control, that is, a form of organization of socioeconomic spaces, is an important way in which the meaning of fashion producers is generated and reinforced.

Carnaby Street is located in London; in reality, it is an area containing several streets that hosts smaller shops with brands with a medium to high fashion profile, including Replay, Lee, Diesel, and Miss Sixty. This "street" has its own website,[7] which shows how the marketplace is organized. Events are organized, such as catwalk shows, and there is a distinct narrative, heralded in a book titled *Carnaby Street: 1960–2010—The Book*. This, to repeat, frames the perception among the producers, creating a "we" that is organized by a private firm, Shaftesbury PLC.

It is thus clear that the public sphere in which fashion and other aspects of social life largely reside is to some extent organized. The company is open to investors about what they do: "We invest in locations close to streets traditionally regarded as prime with the aim of assembling clusters of buildings or villages where we see opportunities to create rental growth." Furthermore, there is a strategy: "An essential ingredient of this strategy is our encouragement of new trading concepts . . . in this way, our villages are a refreshing antidote to what is available elsewhere in increasingly homogenous high streets and shopping centres."[8]

Shaftesbury PLC is explicitly trying to create what I call "consumer districts" (to paraphrase Alfred Marshall's notion of industrial districts). Here is what they say:

> Shaftesbury's strategy is very clear and focused. The Group invests only in those districts within the West End [in London] which have an enduring demand from occupiers and popularity with their customers. Our investments are all close to the unique cluster of shops, restaurants, theatres, cinemas and world class galleries, museums and historic sites, which are the essence of London's West End. These districts all have excellent access to a wide choice of public transport both day and night.[9]

The orchestration of what they call an "antidote" creates homogeneity among the sellers of fashion products, who not only sit next to one another but also next to others selling other products, which nonetheless are of a similar status. The portfolios of firms in these areas are creating the spaces of commerce.[10]

It is clear that fashion sellers of different types are clustered. Stores are concentrated in shopping areas or districts, and frequently the fiercest competitors, such as H&M and

Zara, are located on either side of the same street, but it is of course not the physical layout that is the most important issue here. However, it is only through the concentration of firms with certain identities, and the corresponding status that gives them meaning, that the place becomes meaningful. The narrative of a place can help, but a commercial space is necessarily tied to what is traded. Some garment chains, such as Zara and H&M, are better known than most local areas, and they are increasingly giving meaning to places, rather than the other way around. This means that their shops partly give an identity to a mall, by either being there or not having a shop. Especially well-known brands define the socio-aesthetic status of an area. It is because of this that malls try to attract the "right" firms and labels, some of which are magnets that attract other stores to also establish themselves in the same area.

Fashion companies' stores are physical places that can be used to advertise what they are offering. In addition, billboards and other forms of public advertisement are parts of contemporary cityscapes that serve the same end. It should be mentioned that billboards and advertisements in various magazines are important strategies for firms to send out signals of who they are. However, only some firms use billboards, and from the position of the billboards, firms can transmit their messages to customers. These are attempts by competing firms to affect their environment, which includes the physical environment.

I have so far talked only about the space of stores. The Internet, with advertisements, links, Facebook pages, and other social media, provides other "spaces" where producers watch each other (White 1981). This is an important reflexive arena, easily accessible in the offices of most staff members at firms in this industry. It is simply a shorter "walking distance" to use the Internet than to enter the stores of one's competitors to see what they have coming.

COMPETITION BETWEEN CONSUMERS

I have shown that there is competition in the market between producers. This competition is economic in nature. Is there also competition between consumers? The short answer is that there is fierce competition, or at least rivalry, among consumers as well, but this is not economic competition regarding how to make profit or to avoid buying expensive items. The rivalry is about defining fashion and avoiding being seen as out of fashion, whereby some, perhaps those who do not really take part or who fail to keep up with fashion trends, become only the backdrop to those who are in fashion. The rivalry I look at is primarily of an existential nature. Rivalry among consumers in relation to fashion is about making distinctions. These distinctions can be related to economic capital, but economic capital per se is not exchangeable for fashion. Fashion is a form of symbolic capital (Bourdieu 2001). It is clear that there is no *one* fashion or *one* field of fashion. What I analyze below is the logic of fashion, without offering a full picture of the spatial positions of all consumers in the market and the multitude of different styles and groups. This means that there are in reality many fields of fashion and many fashions.

Consumers do not care how the firms from which they purchase fashion items do economically. Consumers in markets try, I argue, to get as much fashion as possible for as little as possible. This, obviously, is very different from trying to get garments for as little as possible. Fashion, in contrast to just providing bodily coverage and protection, is about making distinctions. People become something by consuming fashion. Veblen's (1953) notion of consumption resembles this; the consumption has to be seen, by necessity in public places, and it has to be known that the clothes are expensive. Place and style are intimately related, so that the spatial dimension is constituted by this. Several studies testify to how areas are primed by people spending time there (Kawamura 2006) or by those living in an area and their look (le Grand 2010).

The market here operates in favor of this practice of becoming "someone," in at least two ways. The first is that the market space is an arena of display, as was shown. You can show to others where you make purchases, but you can also show what you are wearing to others in public. These two aspects often go hand in hand. Another aspect is that the economic competition between several sellers of fashion in the market provides everyone with information on prices. In the potlatch "economy" (Mauss 2002) destruction of valuable goods was very public, to manifest the position of the head of the clan and the status of the clan itself. Today the prices of goods are public, and the price level of each different brand can be used by actors to uphold and identify distinctions. However, money and price must not per se, as in the case with the potlatch, have anything to do with fashion as a social phenomenon. Money is one aspect of fashion but not the sole reason for distinction; distinctions are culturally and aesthetically rooted. The display of economic wealth drives fashion, and to do as many humanist-oriented scholars do (Vinken 2005) and focus only on the garments is utterly wrong, if one is to understand fashion.

CONCLUSION

Markets are central coordination forms in contemporary society. Fashion can and does exist outside of markets. However, garment fashion, at least today, is intimately connected to markets. The market offers choices for consumers to define themselves. Though it is possible for consumers to make clothes, and to compete to be the first with the latest with one's own products, this comes with demands on social skills and limited choice. The spatiality of fashion markets is a condition for the observation of what people, known and less known, are wearing, but these are also arenas that offer choices to people. The main point in this chapter has been to highlight the role of spatiality for fashion markets. Markets provide an ordered social structure of sellers that enables actors to create identities using the goods from sellers of clothes. Both producers and consumers, as it were, open up the space by differentiation.

Much more can be done to continue the analysis of space, markets, and fashion. The spatiality of diffusion of fashion items, in cities, in countries, and on the Internet, would be a fascinating topic. More generally, the diffusion of fashion—in which space and time are central aspects—is still a theme that is little understood and analyzed.

NOTES

1. Economic geographers have, of course, analyzed the spatial dimension of fashion. This research, however, is often concerned with the spatial distribution of fashion industries (Scott 2000) and less often with specific markets.
2. Most people are celebrities because of what they have done, for example, musicians or actors. Some are known as celebrities only because they are children of a celebrity or because they have appeared on a reality TV show.
3. In the future it can be expected that people will mark items on the pictures, and they may then automatically get information on these items, perhaps making text unnecessary.
4. The idea is not to show where these come from but to give some idea of what type of text is communicated based on her appearances. Sites like http://www.becomegorgeous.com or http://stealherstyle.net are examples of places where one can find similar stories and where fashion is on display.
5. "Katy Perry for GHD Professional Hair Styling," Become Gorgeous, April 12, 2011, http://www.hair.becomegorgeous.com/celebrity_hair/katy_perry_for_ghd_professional_hair_styling-4291.html (accessed August 22, 2012).
6. Pearl, "Katy Perry: Embroidered Red Cardigan," Steal Her Style, May 14, 2011, http://stealherstyle.net/2011/05/14/katy-perry-embroidered-red-cardigan/ (accessed August 22, 2012).
7. Carnaby Street website, http://www.carnaby.co.uk/ (accessed December 26, 2011).
8. Ibid.
9. Shaftesbury PLC, "Shaftesbury's Strategy," http://www.shaftesbury.co.uk/about.php (accessed December 26, 2011).
10. This is not a novel thing to do. Kings and princes have always tried to organize trade and marketplaces—often within the secure realms of their fortresses, which allowed them to tax traders—to gain income.

BIBLIOGRAPHY

Ahrne, Göran, and Nils Brunsson. 2011. "Organization outside Organizations: The Significance of Partial Organization." *Organization* 18: 83–104.

Aspers, Patrik. 2006. *Markets in Fashion: A Phenomenological Approach.* London: Routledge.

Aspers, Patrik. 2010. *Orderly Fashion: A Sociology of Markets.* Princeton, NJ: Princeton University Press.

Aspers, Patrik. 2011. *Markets.* Cambridge, UK: Polity.

Bourdieu, Pierre. 2001. "The Forms of Social Capital." In Mark Granovetter and Richard Swedberg (eds.), *The Sociology of Economic Life,* 96–111. Boulder, CO: Westview.

Callon, Michel, Yuval Millo, and Fabian Muniesa. 2007. *Market Devices.* Oxford: Blackwell/ Sociological Review.

Chamberlin, Edward. 1948. *The Theory of Monopolistic Competition: A Re-orientation of the Theory of Value.* Cambridge, MA: Harvard University Press.

Daoud, Adel. 2011. *Scarcity, Abundance and Sufficiency: Contributions to Social and Economic Theory.* Göteborg, Sweden: Göteborgs Universitet.

Geertz, Clifford. 1978. "The Bazaar Economy: Information and Search in Peasant Marketing." *American Economic Review* 68: 28–32.

Gronow, Jukka. 2003. *Caviar with Champagne: Common Luxury and the Ideals of the Good Life in Stalin's Russia.* Oxford: Berg.

Hirsch, Paul. 1992. "Processing Fads and Fashions: An Organization-Set Analysis of Cultural Industry Systems." In Mark Granovetter and Richard Swedberg (eds.), *The Sociology of Economic Life,* 363–83. Boulder, CO: Westview.

Kawamura, Yuniya. 2004. *The Japanese Revolution in Paris Fashion.* Oxford: Berg.

Kawamura, Yuniya. 2006. "Japanese Teens as Producers of Street Fashion." *Current Sociology* 54: 784–801.

le Grand, Elias. 2010. *Class, Place and Identity in a Satellite Town.* Stockholm: Department of Sociology, Stockholm University.

Lieberson, Stanley. 2000. *A Matter of Taste: How Names, Fashions, and Culture Change.* New Haven, CT: Yale University Press.

Marshall, Alfred. 1920. *Industry and Trade: A Study of Industrial Technique and Business Organization; of Their Influences on the Conditions of Various Classes and Nations.* London: Macmillan.

Mauss, Marcel. 2002. *The Gift: The Form and Reason for Exchange in Archaic Societies.* London: Routledge.

Miller, Claire Cain. 2010. "Selling a Celebrity Look." *New York Times,* February 21. http://www.nytimes.com/2010/02/22/technology/internet/22celebrity.html?ref=clairecainmiller (accessed January 2, 2012).

Podolny, Joel. 1993. "A Status-Based Model of Market Competition." *American Journal of Sociology* 98: 829–72.

Rocamora, Agnès. 2009. *Fashioning the City: Paris, Fashion and the Media.* London: I. B. Tauris.

Scott, Allen J. 2000. "Economic Geography: The Great Half-Century." In Gordon L. Clark, Maryann P. Feldman, and Meric S. Gertler (eds.), *The Oxford Handbook of Economic Geography,* 18–48. Oxford: Oxford University Press.

Simmel, Georg. 1971. "Fashion." In Donald Levine (ed.), *Georg Simmel on Individuality and Social Form,* 294–323. Chicago: University of Chicago Press.

Uzzi, Brian. 1997. "Social Structure in Interfirm Networks: The Paradox of Embeddedness." *Administrative Science Quarterly* 42: 35–67.

Veblen, Thorstein. 1945. "The Economic Theory of Woman's Dress." In Leon Ardzrooni (ed.), *Essays in Our Changing Order,* 65–77. New York: Viking.

Veblen, Thorstein. 1953. *The Theory of the Leisure Class: An Economic Study of Institutions.* New York: New American Library.

Vinken, Barbara. 2005. *Fashion Zeitgeist: Trends and Cycles in the Fashion System.* Oxford: Berg.

White, Harrison. 1981. "Where Do Markets Come From?" *American Journal of Sociology* 87: 517–47.

SECTION IV

Fashion and Materiality

Introduction

AMY DE LA HAYE

> Objects hang before the eyes of the imagination, continuously re-presenting ourselves to ourselves, and telling stories of our lives in ways which would be impossible otherwise.
>
> —Susan M. Pearce, museologist (1992: 47)

This section of the *Handbook* explores how and why fashionable garments are used in object-led research foci as items around which to construct rich, multidimensional narratives within text-based, museum, and virtual environments. The *Oxford English Dictionary* definition of *materiality*—the overarching title—comprises just two words, "of material" (Allen 1991: 731). It is an object-specific word that simultaneously evokes the fabric (frequently described as *material*) from which garments are made and the infinite possibilities it holds as an embodiment of value and meaning. In his essay Philip Sykas explores concisely the trajectory and historiography of object-based fashion and dress studies, material culture analysis, and their intersections.

Sequentially, the first two contributors take fashion fabric and/or the constructed garment as the starting point for their research, which spans chronologically from the late eighteenth to the twenty-first centuries. Another, by comparison, is an anthropological perspective on the material study and collecting of dress and its recent articulations with fashion studies. At the outset, each author articulates the textiles and/or garment(s) that form the subject of their inquiry, makes explicit their research methodology (or methodologies), and proceeds to evidence it/them by presenting clear case study examples. This section of the *Handbook* is the most extensively illustrated (and three contributors campaigned for the inclusion of further images!), as visual evidence is critical to the methodology and dissemination of object-led research. The final essay explores "immateriality" and the ways in which technological advances in the twenty-first century have facilitated new ways of engaging viewers with fashion objects. While this approach can never replace experiencing "the real thing," it certainly expands curatorial possibilities, is inclusive, and safeguards the material object. What is its potential?

In the first chapter of this section, Philip A. Sykas argues eloquently that fashion studies have barely focused on "the physical substrate of garments"—the cloth used to make fashionable dress—but have instead privileged the made-up garment. Drawing initially on primary documentary sources he reveals the significance and value that eighteenth- and early nineteenth-century consumers placed on the textiles they purchased. His examination of surviving garments reveals furthermore that consumers were reluctant to alter permanently their widths of precious cloth by cutting into them and that loosely sewn stitches, rather than evidencing poor workmanship, were used deliberately to permit easy refashioning. The desire to preserve the intact fabric is one of several themes that run concurrently throughout this section.

One of Sykas's disciplinary interventions is the incorporation of nondestructive scientific methodologies, notably use of the handheld digital microscope. His research case studies are drawn from objects housed in the Gallery of Costume, Manchester, in the United Kingdom.[1] They include analysis of plain cloth, which has generally been overlooked in favor of patterned and decorated examples (another recurring theme); sewing threads and techniques, including the significance and usage of the sewing machine; and the inherent meanings and use values of small pieces of fabric. His essay concludes with a warning: while the material aspects of dress can impart valuable physical, social, cultural, and historical evidence, the uncovering of a single—in this instance, cross-cultural—reference can all too easily overturn our assumptions.

The next chapter is by Alexandra Palmer, whose objective is to illustrate "*how* a close examination of fashion objects can shift and deepen our understanding of the meanings of fashion." Palmer presents a rigorous comparative analysis of two fashionable garments, drawing in others for comparative purposes, all from the collections of the Royal Ontario Museum. The first is a chinoiserie evening dress designed by Tom Ford for the Paris house Yves Saint Laurent for fall/winter 2004–2005, which was photographed for the cover of the September 2004 issue of Australian *Vogue.* To substantiate her methodological stance, Palmer initially contrasts the evidence that can be derived from the fashion photograph (by Justin Smith) and the material garment. The other item is an English semiformal open robe made of silk embroidered in the neoclassical taste dating from 1795–1802.

We are taken on a research journey that takes in historical and contemporaneous preoccupations with orientalism as a fantasy "other" (Said 1977), nostalgia, postmodernism, and the ways in which notions of empire and nationhood are embedded within fashionable dress, past and present. An Ottoman caftan and late eighteenth-century *Turquerie* are shown to have influenced the open robe and in turn the modern fashion dress. Importantly, Palmer also considers the spaces in which fashion is performed, noting that in an English domestic context, "probably outside of the social center of London, colorful export goods underwent another level of mutation and hybridization as they were reframed and incorporated into fashionable daily life."

As we have seen in the opening paragraphs of this introduction, material culture studies has roots embedded within the discipline of anthropology. Sarah Fee, an associate curator working in the Department of World Cultures at Royal Ontario Museum, explores the recent literature on the anthropology of fashion and the ways in which, historically—even though there was substantive evidence to disprove this—many anthropologists disregarded notions of fashion and fetishized practices of consumption. She examines how reigning ideologies determined what was collected and how it was interpreted. During the 1970s, when clothing was examined, it was generally to shed light on kinship and social structures and reinforce cultural and racial stereotypes.

By the 1980s anthropologists were drawing on the same body of material culture texts as fashion historians (including Appadurai (1986) and Küchler and Miller [(1987) 2005a, 2005b]), while the boundaries between border zones, local and global fashion, were blurred (Craik 1994; Eicher 2010; Niessen 2003). Nonetheless, Fee argues that moments of Euro-American contact, colonization, and tailored garment forms were highlighted, such that the view that fashion is driven by "the West" has prevailed. Drawing on anthropologist Sandra Niessen's conviction that the study of fashion demands an exhaustive study of cross-cultural clothing systems, Fee presents two case studies drawn from the western Indian Ocean. To date, this region, along with the striped cloths she examines, has generally been overlooked. She argues persuasively, drawing evidence directly from surviving textiles and contextual evidence, for local fashion aesthetics and cycles of change.

Robyn Healy extends the analysis of objects located in museums to explore the possibilities of curating the immaterial in the twenty-first century, an era during which digital technologies and collaborative, multidisciplinary practices have transformed how fashion is communicated and presented. She considers how this has expanded the museum environment and poses the question, "How does fashion experienced across immaterial forms and conditions suggest alternate curatorial approaches from traditional exhibition experiences based primarily on physical engagement with fashion objects, particularly clothing?" To answer this she extends the debate beyond extant forms, "to test the capacity of exhibitions based on intangible or nonphysical encounters." Maintaining the care of museum objects while facilitating inclusive access to them is an ongoing curatorial preoccupation: this is embedded implicitly within this research and its practical outcomes.

Healy explores what she defines as "the expansive museum environment," which can engage innovatively with visitors though on-site and online technologies, and she presents case study examples to demonstrate how "user"-generated material has been incorporated within international museum exhibitions. The analysis is contextualized with other creative industry-led initiatives such as the pioneering interactive fashion website SHOWstudio, launched in 2000. A subsection "The Virtual Museum" considers the possibilities not only for public museums with explicit visitor remits but also for greater accessibility to the private archives annexed with fashion houses. Ultimately, Healy argues that technology can facilitate research on the fashionable garment within the broader contexts of its designing, making, marketing, and wearing, incorporating testimony from interviews and links to catwalk shows—and that the individual can tailor-make and in turn communicate their own links and networks.

Each of these authors works, or has in the past worked, in a curatorial capacity. For museum scholars working with fashion, object-led research also has important practice-based application, which is critical for the effective museological display and interpretation of fabric and the material garment. Indeed, as Palmer makes explicit, "Actual worn garments can verify the canon of fashion history, and they can also complicate what we think we know to generate new ideas that contextualize the production and wearing of fashion."

NOTE

1. Until the 2000s the fashionable dress housed within museum collections was generally referred to as *costume*. The same term was used for world dress (items that are virtually universal, such as denim jeans), fancy dress (extraordinary dress that pertains to a different period, an artifact, an animal, and so on, worn to a celebratory event), occupational dress (work wear such as agricultural smocks or high-tech firefighting uniforms), and fantastical theatrical garments worn onstage. In contrast, world clothing is usually housed in departments that collect—and are named after—specific countries or continents. As the popularity of fashion as a museum medium has burgeoned, the term *fashion* is now made more explicit—for instance, the Museum of Costume in Bath, England, was renamed the Bath Fashion Museum in 2007.

BIBLIOGRAPHY

Allen, R. E. 1991. *The Concise Oxford English Dictionary.* London: BCA.

Appadurai, Arjun. 1986. *The Social Life of Things: Commodities in Cultural Perspective.* Melbourne: Cambridge University Press.

Craik, Jennifer. 1994. *The Face of Fashion: Cultural Studies in Fashion.* London: Routledge.

Eicher, Joanne B. (ed.). 2010. *Berg Encyclopedia of World Dress and Fashion.* Vol. 10, *Global Perspectives.* Oxford: Berg.

Küchler, Susanne, and Daniel Miller. [1987] 2005a. *Material Culture and Mass Consumption.* Oxford: Blackwell.

Küchler, Susanne, and Daniel Miller (eds.). 2005b. *Clothing as Material Culture.* Oxford: Berg.

Niessen, Sandra. 2003. *Re-orienting Fashion: The Globalization of Asian Dress.* Oxford: Berg.

Pearce, Susan M. 1992. *Museums, Objects and Collections: A Cultural Study.* Washington, DC: Smithsonian Institution Press.

Said, Edward. 1977. *Orientalism.* London: Penguin.

12

Investigative Methodologies: Understanding the Fabric of Fashion

PHILIP A. SYKAS

Fashion studies has devoted little attention to the physical substrate of garments. Beginning with the structuralists, the represented garment has been the principal focus of investigation, that is, the immaterial semantic dress of signification. This chapter aims to describe the shaping of the field for object-based study of dress, offering a theoretical basis for such work and pursuing some examples that demonstrate the opportunities offered by physical analysis of surviving dresses. Far from being *mere things* that conceal meaning, physical materials offer the possibilities from which meaning is constructed and provide the chance to see beyond the consumer to the maker, merchant, manufacturer, and commodity suppliers.

During the eighteenth century and much of the nineteenth century, fashionable women bought their dresses as lengths of fabric, imagining them in the cloth, thereby engendering a relationship to cloth that later diminished when garments were purchased from made-up models. Dresses were identified by their fabric, such as Lady Mary Coke's 1767 sack, "a white striped water'd tabby" (Home [1889] 1970: 170), and dress lengths of fabric were known as *dresses,* like the "curious fine long Callico Muslins, at 13s. per dress" of a 1793 advertisement (*Observer* 1793: 1). The real dress, fulfillment of the dress envisaged in the cloth, retained the potential to return to fabric. Pioneer dress historian Anne Buck suspected that the indifferent sewing found in surviving eighteenth-century dresses ensured "the expensive material could more easily be unpicked to make up again" (1979: 160).[1] Among the better-off, social pressures enforced frequent re-making and gifting of clothing. Novelist Maria Edgeworth's late Georgian heiress Isabella Moneygawl is lauded because she "seldom or ever wore a thing twice the same way…always pulling her things to pieces, and giving them away" ([1800] 1980: 48).

This attitude toward cloth lasted even after women's dresses were no longer largely made from easily deconstructed straight widths of fabric.[2] John W. Urquhart, describing sewing machine stitches, cited the chain stitch as "pre-eminently suited to those classes of goods which ladies frequently take to pieces for reshaping or other purposes" (1881: 17–18). And a middle-class Illinois woman detailed the remakings of her garments in fabric diaries that trace a cycle from cloth to cloth in the late nineteenth century:

> Japanese silk 85 cts a yard. Bought at Field & Leiters in Chicago in 1872. . . . It was not made up however till May 1873. . . . It was always my favorite dress, as far as material and pleasant memories could make it. . . . In 1880 Sue helped me make it over. . . . Had a bonnet of the same and wore this suit when I went riding. . . . In 1884 made over again combined with striped goods. . . . Ripped [seams] in fall of 1886. (quoted in Oberly 1993: 12)

Here it is notable too that the silk was kept before its first making. Cloth was relished in its pristine state, a state of opportunity before the inevitable compromises of sartorial transformation. When a fictional heroine of 1854 acquired her much-coveted "two-dollar silk," she showed it off to her intimate friends "in the piece" (*Ladies' Cabinet* 1854: 123).

Despite the apparent importance of cloth and the process of making (and unmaking) to historical consumers, its study has been largely confined to the museum field, grounded in close observation of surviving examples. Curator Otto Thieme emphasized the importance of inspecting a wide range of actual garments "for details of construction and condition. Such first-hand knowledge is available in no other form" (1986: n.p.). The typical aim was to reveal a chronological sequence, or features common to a locality or maker, indicators of practical value in museum cataloging. Thus this research not only served a professional body eager for more information but was able to be directly evaluated without theoretical reflection.

Such undertheorized museum-based studies were largely discounted by academic historians seeking to answer wider social and cultural questions about dress. This rejection may also have been due to the implied stance of logical empiricism in the work, since conclusions were drawn through gathering and systematizing facts based on observed reality rather than socially constructed reality.

For the object-based researcher, interpretation of accumulated empirical evidence began with comparative analysis and moved toward generalization. Charles A. Lave and James G. March envisage this route as a process involving (1) abstraction from observed reality to a speculative model, (2) elaboration of the implications derived from the model, and (3) evaluation of such implications against further observations in order to modify or refine the model ([1975] 1993: 2–4). Mats Alvesson and Kaj Sköldberg define this process as *abduction*:

> In abduction, an (often surprising) single case is interpreted from a hypothetical overarching pattern, which, if it were true, explains the case in question. The interpretation should then be strengthened by new observations. . . . During the process, the

> empirical area of application is successively developed, and the theory (the proposed over-arching pattern) is also adjusted and refined. ... The research process, therefore, alternates between (previous) theory and empirical facts whereby both are successively reinterpreted in the light of each other. (2009: 4)

The abductive method underlies much object-based dress research; questions arising from initial observations spark a search for a linking pattern among similar garments and for supporting historical texts and images.

PART I: THE DEVELOPMENT OF OBJECT-BASED DRESS STUDIES

In her 1961 introduction to *Victorian Costume and Costume Accessories,* Buck proposed that "for every period there are unconscious hall-marks of decoration and construction," details such as "the way a dress fastens" that can provide more salient evidence than *style* lines (style at that time was the main focus of fashion studies; [1961] 1984: 9). She proceeded by synthesizing a range of physical measures and observations about women's dress, progressing chronologically to distinguish the features affected by materials and technology as well as cut and style. Buck reports only the findings of her masterful interpretation; the scheme for selection and the concepts employed for generalizing are not made explicit. However, she pioneered an approach that placed emphasis on the *unconscious* details of construction alongside the *conscious* structuring of style. Such unconsciously imposed physical markers derive from the inherent conservatism of craft and industrial practices, in which change is usually incremental despite radical stylistic evolution. When Buck laid out her method of cataloging, it was aimed at enabling assistant curators to record a consistent and hierarchical set of information about cut, construction, materials, ornamentation, and measurements. Specialist matters were necessarily omitted (fiber and weave identification; dyeing, printing, and finishing techniques; constructional stitching). Unfortunately, this left the detailed study of unconscious markers underdeveloped.

Janet Arnold's comparative studies of the pattern and construction of Englishwomen's dresses used individual museum examples to represent generic types (see, for example, Arnold 1972a, 1972b, 1985, 2008). She combined scale drawings of garment parts in flat patterns with extracts from contemporary dressmaking accounts and visual sources. Intended as a practical guide to making model or full-scale costumes, the implied approach is one of "triangulation" between pattern, text, and image, correlating the different forms of evidence to obtain a more complete understanding. In addition to such evidence, Arnold brought to her own interpretations tacit knowledge (developed through years of painstaking observation and construction of replicas) of how dress fabrics, garment structures, and wearers interact. In her published work, these are visually expressed in drawings showing front and rear views of each dress in the round.

The conceptual basis for Arnold's work was expanded in lectures and published studies of individual garments. Assembling diagnostic features culled from datable examples formed a core for comparative study. She noted, for instance, the tuck on the lining of the buttonhole panel of men's coats appearing as early as 1710, and from 1720 that buttonholes are "stitched long but slit only partially" (Arnold 1986). Arnold's study of women's riding dress demonstrates her complex synthesis of evidence: garment shaping along with evidence of wear is used to posit the historical alteration of a particular garment. She concludes that it originated as a youth's doublet around 1625, but "crease marks and stitching and also the shape of the back when mounted on a stand . . . curved to lie smoothly over a dome-shaped petticoat" indicate adaptation for wear by a young female. By comparison with a named diagram in a Spanish tailor's pattern book, Arnold proposes that the transformed garment would have been called a "cassock" (1999: 14). Ultimately, her method relied on tacit skills for recognizing evidence of craft practice that often went unstated.

Arnold's work is sometimes seen as similar to that of Norah Waugh (1954), who also assembled scaled patterns, contemporary text, and images. However, Waugh pursued a thesis to show that while changes in fashion detail were rapid, "changes in cut were much slower, each one evolving from the previous style" (1968: 20). A postpositivist perspective can be distinguished here in which reality is conceived as an expression of underlying structures and meanings. In pursuit of the underlying development of cut, Waugh's diagrams favor the generalized shape, often leaving out material details such as seams joining fabric widths.[3]

Also in the postpositivist realm, Dorothy Burnham's (1973) pioneering work on the cross-cultural evolution of cut in nonfashion garments put cloth back into the center of study. She worked out cutting arrangements from surviving garments to see how they were derived from the original length of cloth. Her thesis was that materials had an overriding influence on shape. She posited "two separate developments . . . cuts based on the shape of animal skins, and those dependent on the rectilinear form of loom-woven cloth" (Burnham 1973: 2). Cultures that made the transition from skin to cloth preserved earlier forms of shaping even though these were more wasteful of cloth. By contrast, weave-based cultures sometimes shunned the cutting of cloth, preferring draped garments; when sewn garments were adopted, they were cut neatly with straight edges and little wastage. Nonetheless, in a conservatism similar to that observed in skin-based cultures, cloth-based groups clung to methods based on traditional loom widths well after the introduction of materials of alternative widths. Burnham concludes that cloth widths are a fundamental aspect of the study of dress.

Recently, the work of Frances Pritchard used a similar approach to provide "an overview of the development of clothing in the first millennium AD through an empirical study of surviving dress" from Egyptian archaeological sites (2006: 11). Her study showed a wane in use of woven-to-shape tunics from the mid-seventh century and a growing tendency toward cut-and-sewn garments with gored shaping, reflecting Persian influence and the decline of classical Roman traditions (114–15). By surveying a closely linked group of garments from seventeenth-century Cologne, Johannes Pietsch

(2008: 60–62) was able to go further than describing the development of cut and workmanship, drawing attention to details indicative of localized practice and to aspects of garment fit.

Close observation of garments in museum collections links the work of these researchers; years of concentrated application were required to accumulate evidence. Contrary to expectation, these authors do not simply systemize evidence from observed reality but pursue correlations between objects, texts, and images to add weight to arguments that can indeed accommodate a social construction of reality operating beyond material matters. A weakness can be that object-based historians are guided by conventions in clothing materials and construction even when these remain poorly analyzed or expressed. Their work is distinguished from scientific investigation by its technique and the scope of questioning, while it differs from connoisseurship in general orientation and the type of verification pursued.

Scientific Analysis of Dress

Allied to the object-based approach, and sometimes used in tandem, is the scientific study of dress, often applying nondestructive techniques developed in archaeology, forensic science, and technical art history. Scientific methods of observation, measurement, and analysis can be used even when a fully scientific methodology is not endorsed. Microscopy, for example, is a powerful tool for observation available to all visual researchers.

William D. Cooke and Brenda Lomas used the scanning electron microscope (SEM) to study the form of textile fiber fractures in order to identify wear and damage in historical textiles. A fatigue break resulting from wear produces a characteristic brushlike fracture in textile fibers that is distinct from those formed by tearing or cutting. SEM observations also make it possible to distinguish a cut made with scissors from that made by a knife (Cooke and Lomas 1987: 215–26). However, much can be learned by observing clothing under low magnifications. The technique used by Cooke and Lomas involves the use of both optical microscopy and SEM; the fabric is scanned under low magnification to observe wear patterns at macro scale and thus to identify sampling zones for high-powered examination (Hearle, Lomas, and Cooke 1998: 382). Forensic examination of textiles explores similar evidence. Again, an initial overview of damage is recommended to determine the potential morphological information that might be found through microscopy. In fact, forensic specialists have found wide observation under lower magnification of more practical value than SEM (Adolf and Hearle 1998: 398). Nevertheless, SEM images such as those in Hearle and colleagues' Atlas of Fibre Fracture and Damage to *Textiles* (1998) aid understanding of what is seen at lower magnifications, like the crowns of weaving yarns flattened and damaged from wear (see Figure 12.1).[4]

Normal tests of textile mechanical properties are destructive, but studies that translate such measurable properties into the features by which we judge the handle of cloth show promise for application to historical dress. Mitsuo Matsudaira and Masao Matsui

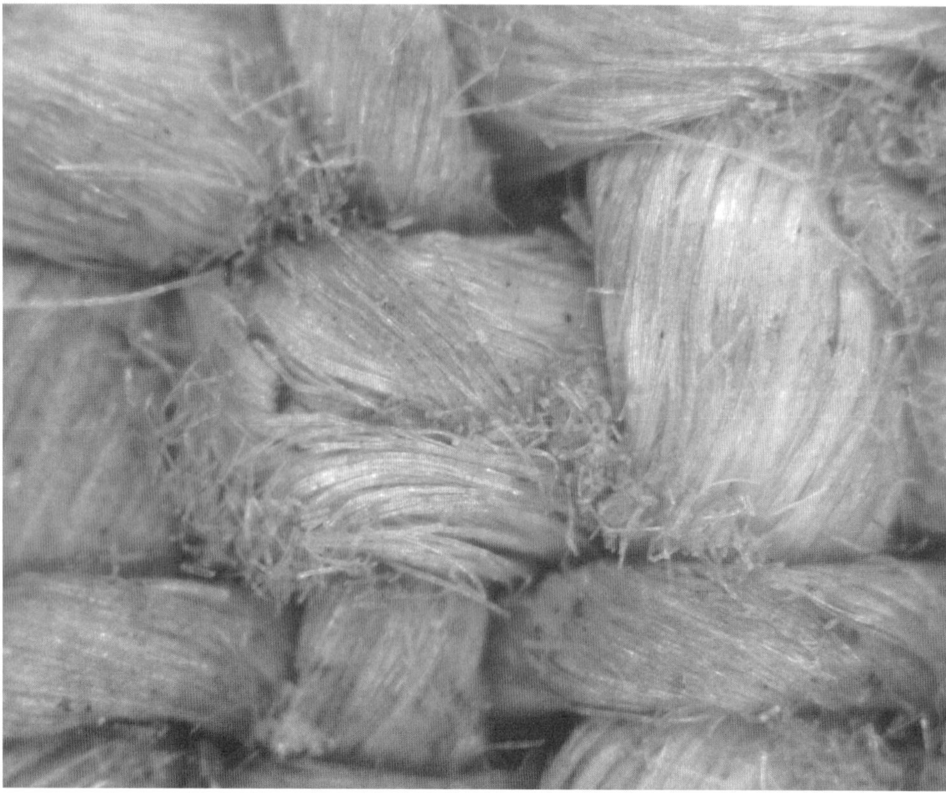

FIGURE 12.1 Photomicrograph (190x) of wear to indigo-dyed linen presenting as brushlike fiber formations to the sides of the weave crowns.
Credit: Downing Collection at Manchester Metropolitan University.

(1992: 133–43) studied six fine silk dress fabrics using an evaluation method developed by Sueo Kawabata and Masako Niwa (1989: 19–50) that converts six measurable properties to primary hand values such as crispness, smoothness, and flexibility with a soft feel. Their study demonstrated how the characteristic handle of several silks can be clearly separated according to their mechanical properties, even if some, like shantung and *habutae,* overlap to an extent. Such work may eventually enable better understanding of the physical factors involved in qualitative perceptions of handle.

The engineering of dress has received only intermittent attention. G.W.H. Stevens, an aeronautics engineer, investigated the stability and deformation of flexible structures using the crinoline skirt as a model that can be represented mathematically with greater precision than is possible in many aeronautical structures (1950, 1952). His work suggests fruitful avenues for study, not simply of hooped structures, but of the load-distribution properties of different pleating types.

Conservation science has transformed connoisseurship since the 1980s, and it is now hard to imagine discussing oil paintings in the absence of X-ray imagery, microphotography, and chemical analysis. Issues of cost and accessibility of equipment have often inhibited application of such technology to dress. Sonia A. O'Connor and Mary M. Brooks (2007) provide practical information on radiography of dress and document the shift in use from the study of nontextile substructures and metallic threads to the examination of textile elements in greater depth. Susan North and Jenny Tiramani, investigating the cut of women's seventeenth-century clothing, published X-ray imagery of two upper-body garments, demonstrating its effectiveness for recording constructional details and alterations in multilayered garments (2011: 38–39, 78–81). More active collaboration between technical art historians and dress historians may provide a fruitful direction for future object-based studies.

From the New Connoisseurship to Materiality

Connoisseurship traditionally deals with dating, attribution, and assessment of aesthetic quality. *New* connoisseurship uses the same skills to explore the context of production and consumption, as well as the creation of cultural meaning.[5] Curator Linda Baumgarten's work is representative of this school; in *What Clothes Reveal: The Language of Clothing in Colonial and Federal America* (2002), she teams her knowledge of materials and techniques with detective skills in order to gain an understanding of surviving early American garments. The new connoisseur's broadened approach encompasses plebeian as well as fine objects and accepts transformations made over time as an essential aspect of an object's historical record. While valuing information obtainable by means of microscopy and infrared photography, Baumgarten sees her study as going beyond "surface aspects" to questions of consumer choice and the cultural function of clothing.

Quilting specialist Clare Rose (2000) employed the connoisseurship approach to answer questions of dating, rarity, conformity to pattern, and caliber of execution in a study of eighteenth-century quilted garments. She analyzed evidence of constructional sewing in considering whether garments were produced as ready-to-wear or bespoke items. The results are correlated with textual evidence to suggest locality of production. This subject has also been examined from a material culture approach, in which a theoretical formulation is usually the starting point for examination of objects. Cultural historian Beverly Lemire undertook a study of ready-made clothing based on evidence from quilted petticoats. Her assessment premised that specific observable traits could be associated with workshop production: a reduced level of variety in design and fabric, evidence of speed of manufacture (use of running stitch and patterns designed to minimize stitching), and rudimentary execution (lack of outstanding needlework). On this basis she found a dozen petticoats that "showed a direct connection to the ready-made trade, with standardized elements of construction and composition" (Lemire 1994: 66).

The theoretical components of material culture research are ably consolidated in Ann Smart Martin's study of a small country shop in eighteenth-century Virginia. She sets out two basic principles. The "first holds that objects do not merely reflect culture but also are the means by which it is created. They symbolize and communicate intangible ideas, build relationships, and proffer pleasure" (Martin 2008: 9). This is possible because objects are bundled with meanings that derive from human interaction with their design, production, and marketing. The second principle is that objects are linked with values that are determined by subjective and personal perceptions of worth as well as economic forces (10). Both meanings and values are based on the mutable relations between people and material objects and are thus unstable.[6]

Anthropologist Webb Keane adds to the material culture understanding of the creation of values and meaning by the addition of a *meta* level to the understanding of how material things operate. Keane rejects the oversimplified communication model of analysis that treats objects as no more than instruments that convey meanings or identities—a tradition that sees the material aspect as something to be stripped away in order to reveal the meaning. To do so is to "privilege meaning over actions, consequences, and possibilities" (Keane 2005: 104). Keane sets out an alternative based on Charles Sanders Peirce's relationships between signs and signified objects: iconicity (resemblance of properties), indexicality (representing actual connection), and symbolism (based on cultural rules). He combines this with the concept of *semiotic ideology*—"people's background assumptions about what signs are and how they function in the world"—assumptions that predispose us to certain habits or expectations and that constrain our possible perceptions and interpretations (191).

Material things have properties that can objectify certain values. For example, the fine fabric known as muslin can be read in terms of the values of softness or lightness. Such qualities are inevitably bundled together with others (to continue the example, perhaps whiteness or semitransparency), and "the qualities bundled together in any object will shift in their relative salience, value, utility and relevance across contexts" (Keane 2005: 188). The resemblance of material properties and their social values (iconicity) offers people the potential to intuitively abstract qualities from objects in order to place them within their own social value system. On the other hand, indexical traits stem from the marks left by production, distribution, and use that disclose causation, intention, agency, and identity. Thus Indian muslin in Britain can index power and luxury (maritime prowess, control of distant markets, rarity), while in India it may index the labor of the fine spinner or the region of Bengal. Ultimately our reading of textile fabrics is based on embedded potentialities that exist whether or not they are taken up for interpretation, and they can thus give rise to new realizations in changing social, cultural, or historical contexts.

PART II: EXPLORATORY STUDIES AT THE GALLERY OF COSTUME, MANCHESTER

Textile fabrics have often been a focal point for innovation. The art historian and theorist Ernst Gombrich (1979: 60–92) sensed that novelties act in accordance with situational logic to introduce instabilities into systems of style and taste, forming a stimulus for fashion changes. Innovations may be matters of emphasis or technological changes, and sometimes both acting in tandem. Gombrich was interested in how they can bring

TABLE 12.1 ADVERTISEMENT FROM *PRESCOTT'S MANCHESTER JOURNAL*

QUILTED COATS.
The Public may be supplied at TAYLOR'S WARE- HOUSE, No. 22, Bishopsgate-street, London, with all Sorts of Sattin, Silk and Stuff QUILTED COATS, at the following reduced Prices, viz.

				S.	D.
3½ Breadths	Tammy Coats, lined with Stuff and quilted with Silk,	–	–	7	6
4 Ditto	ditto ditto	–	–	8	6
3½	Prunella,	–	–	8	6
4	ditto	–	–	9	6
3½	Fine Tammy,	–	–	9	6
4	ditto	–	–	10	6
3½	Superfine Durant,	–	–	10	6
4	ditto	–	–	11	6
7	Calamanco	–	–	12	6
8	ditto	–	–	14	0
5	Superfine Russel,	–	–	17	0
6	Ditto	–	–	20	0

Persian Coats, quilted in Border and Shells, from 16s. to 21s. Sarsnetts from 23s. to 30s. Sattins from 30s. to 3 l. 10s—Likewise a great Variety of Silk and Sattin PUCKERED COATS, puckered in the genteelest Taste and at the lowest Prices.

Ladies have not only the Advantage of buying consider- ably cheaper at this Warehouse, but also, of seeing a much greater Variety of the newest and more fashionable Patterns, than at any Shop in London, as no Article but PETTICOATS is sold at the above Warehouse.

N.B. An Allowance to Shopkeepers who take a Quantity.

Source: Taylor's Warehouse, "Quilted Coats…Taylor's Warehouse," *Prescott's Manchester Journal* 7 (314), March 22, 1777, p. 4.

about an inflationary spiral as one person exaggerates a novel trend to outdo another. When following a trend requires the choice between one camp and another, this leads to social polarization. However, innovations can simply expand the range of consumer choices, allowing these choices to be placed in a hierarchy of taste. This is seen, for example, in the progression of cheap to costly quilted petticoats enumerated by a London warehouse (Taylor's Warehouse 1777: 4; see Table 12.1). The following part of this chapter presents a deeper exploration of material properties to show how these have given rise to historical meanings, using examples gathered from exploratory research undertaken at the Gallery of Costume in Manchester.

Fabric Widths and Dress Lengths

The eighteenth- or nineteenth-century consumer of dress fabrics was attuned to material qualities and quantities because garment acquisition usually began with the purchase of a length of fabric. The length required depended on the type of dress and the fabric width. British dress fabrics came in a wide range of widths, but for each fiber type there were a number of predominant widths. The manufacturer and merchant generalized these into fractions of a yard or ell.[7] Widths of linens and cottons were often expressed in quarters of a yard: three-quarters, four-quarters (yard wide), five-quarters (ell wide), and six-quarters; however, the nominal width was often greater than the true measure, originating in allowances for shrinkage from the loom state to the finished fabric. Designations became conventional, and conventions changed from time to time. For example, most dress silks were referred to as half an ell or three-quarters of a yard wide, but a commentator in 1765 remarked of mercers that "the breadth of their goods which are in general only 19 1/2 inches–21 inches yet they sell them for 1/2 ell, that is 22 1/2 inches. The lustrings too... are only from 23 1/2 inches–24 inches which they call 3/4, that is 27 inches" (Mercator 1765, quoted in Rothstein 1987: 34). These reduced measures generally accord with those found in surviving English silks.

The French used similar fractional measures based on the French ell of about forty-three French inches, equal to approximately forty-six and a half English inches (Arnold 1972a: 5). Thus French silks were generally somewhat wider than their English counterparts, although narrow French widths overlap with wide English widths for eighteenth-century silks. With greater standardization in the nineteenth century, fabric width may be sufficient to posit national origins in certain cases. For example, mid-nineteenth-century warp-printed silks at the Gallery of Costume divide into two groups by width: those consistently around 25 1/2 inches are thought to be French, and those measuring 19 1/2 to 20 1/2 inches, probably English.

Chinese silks exported in the eighteenth century are wider than European silks. Maruta Skelton and Leanna Lee-Whitman cite British East India Company records that specify widths from 2 to 2.2 covids, the covid being about 14.1 inches; accordingly, they found extant eighteenth-century Chinese silks to "measure consistently between 28 and 31 inches" (1986: 133). When these widths are found in association with other properties such as softness imparted by calendering, contrasting selvage weaves, and characteristic temple marks, they proposed it is possible to identify eighteenth-century silks of Far Eastern origin.

In the early nineteenth century, the advent of printing with engraved copper cylinders led to the establishment of two widths of printed cloth, seven-eighths and nine-eighths, determined by the printing machinery. Calico printer William Neild surveyed the accounts of Thomas Hoyle and Sons from 1812 to 1860, noting that seven-eighths cloth was 28 inches wide at first although this was reduced to 27 inches around 1843, while nine-eighths cloth measured 36 inches wide (1861: 491). He indicated that nine-eighths was little used early in the period, while seven-eighths was phased out toward 1860. It is not yet clear why these changes arose, or how the consumer adjusted to the fact that for every four yards of the narrower cloth only three yards of the wider were needed to provide the same overall area. Excise duties on fabrics were based not on length but on area: the fabric width to the nearest hundredth multiplied by the length.

This implies that manufacturers' understanding of textile quantities involved their area. Were eighteenth- and nineteenth-century consumers also guided in this way?

When a person was purchasing a familiar type, it was possible to use a routine standard for dress lengths. Lady Mary Wortley Montagu wrote in 1723 to her sister in Paris about a commission for a nightgown: "I had rather the money was laid out in plain lutestring, if you could send me eight yards at a time of different colours" (Wharncliffe 1837: 425). In 1788 Betsy Sheridan commissioned her sister in Dublin to buy "two poplin gowns and petticoats—22 yards I think for each" (Lefanu 1986: 223). Departure from established norms could lead to uncertainty. In 1798 Jane Austen sought advice from her sister: "I believe I shall make my new gown like my robe, but the back of the latter is all in a piece with the tail, & will 7 yards enable me to copy it in that respect?" (Chapman 1932: 266).

Barbara Johnson, the eldest child of a Buckinghamshire vicar, kept an album of samples from the dresses she wore (Rothstein 1987). From 1756 she recorded, sporadically at first, not only the yardage but also the width of the material. Analysis of around seventy examples determines that the mean requirements for gentry dress types in particular date ranges are allied more closely with fabric area than with length.[8] Between 1756 and 1778, her dresses fall into two main groups, the negligee, requiring at least twelve square yards, and the nightgown, needing only seven square yards. She documents six gowns with matching petticoats between 1779 and 1795; these most commonly employ ten square yards. Between 1796 and 1808, the fabric required for a gown increased from seven to eight square yards, possibly due to increased gathering of material at the center back and the use of demi-trains. Three of Miss Johnson's dresses in the middle of this period are of a type that employed nine or more square yards; she distinguishes two of these as "round gowns." By contrast, the period from 1809 to 1815 saw a reduction in fabric for gowns to only five or six square yards, possibly fashion's response to wartime stringencies.[9] Finally, from the end of the war until 1823, dresses again grew in fabric requirements to an average of seven-and-a-half or eight square yards. This increase relates to the fashion for application of self trimmings. A letter exchanged between the Philadelphia Quakers Jane and Ann Haines in 1827 explains that four and a quarter yards of fabric will "make a plain one [dress]—but according to the present mode of trimming with the same material as the dress, it would take seven yards—as broad bias folds [flounces] reaching to the knee are indispensable" (Groff 2003: 109–10).

Consumers were probably reliant on their dressmaker to establish how much of a particular fabric was required for a dress, or they may have taken the advice of mercers and drapers, but none of these were completely impartial. More numerate consumers could calculate rough fabric equivalents by breaking widths into eighths of a yard; a dress that required 12 yards of five-eighths (half-ell) would need 10 yards of six-eighths (three-quarters), 7 1/2 yards of eight-eighths (yard), or 6 yards of ten-eighths (ell), all giving a quotient of sixty (eighths times yards), but evidence for this is lacking. In actual accounts, departure from whole-number yardages for dress lengths is uncommon.

A possible explanation is the reluctance of mercers to be left with unsalable remnants. Curator Miles Lambert cites one such occurrence in the correspondence of the Williamsons of Bedfordshire: "you desired 12 yards; now there was 13 1/2 in that piece that I sent... for the mercer would not cut the odd yard and a half off... for the yard and a half would be quite lost to him. But he said if I would take it all as it was, he would give the half yard in for nothing" (2009: 72). Extra material could be used for covering shoes, for trimmings, and for infants' clothing, but the wasteful expense of overbuying must have been strenuously avoided by most. As basic as the matter is, it remains unclear precisely how the consumer negotiated the complex reckoning of yardages. Surviving garments often incorporate small remnants or stamped ends of cloth that may have been signals that the dressmaker thriftily employed the entirety of the provided material, thus acting to reassure the uncertain client.

The Pursuit of Fineness

Plain fabrics have elicited much less notice from historians than patterned or decorated cloth. However, plains are rich in potential signification. The property of fineness—iconic of refinement and indexical of skill—is almost universally associated with the caliber of cloth. Fine spinning has always required higher-quality raw material, more exacting manipulation, and greater fiber wastage, making for greater expense and scarcity.

Egyptologist Gillian Vogelsang-Eastwood remarked that Tutankhamen's loincloths "had the same structure as those of his subjects, but the... linen in the loincloth of an ordinary Egyptian had 37 to 50 threads per inch, while the linen in Tutankhamen's loincloths had 200 threads per inch" (quoted in Fowler 1995). In the European tradition, cloth of the same structure but varying fineness is given different names. Victorian weaver George White distinguished six distinct muslin types each with the same density of warps but differing fineness of yarn: "the yarn for a cambric may be about 60s, for a jaconet, 80s, 100s for a medium, for a light jaconet 120s, for a lawn 140s, and for a book of this count of reed, perhaps 200s" (1846: 53). In modern values, these run from 10 tex through 7, 6, 5, 4, and 3 tex. Cambrics and common jaconets were also *overwefted;* that is, they had a greater count of wefts per unit length than warps, as distinguished from lawns, which had an even balance of threads. White claimed that Manchester muslins "which pass by the same names are much heavier set, and, in general, heavier wefted, than the Scotch muslins" (84). By the end of the nineteenth century, jaconets were at the top of the quality scale in English production, indicating a shift in the meaning of the term (Curtis 1928: 1290).

The difficulty of spinning fine linen yarns assured that fine linens remained expensive. However, the development of mechanized spinning of fine cotton yarns from the late 1780s appears to have fed an inflationary trend in the fashionability of fine fabrics as cottons began to compete with linens. The Scottish linen industry rose to the challenge with delicate linen lenos and lawns, sometimes spotted with cotton (see Figure 12.2).[10]

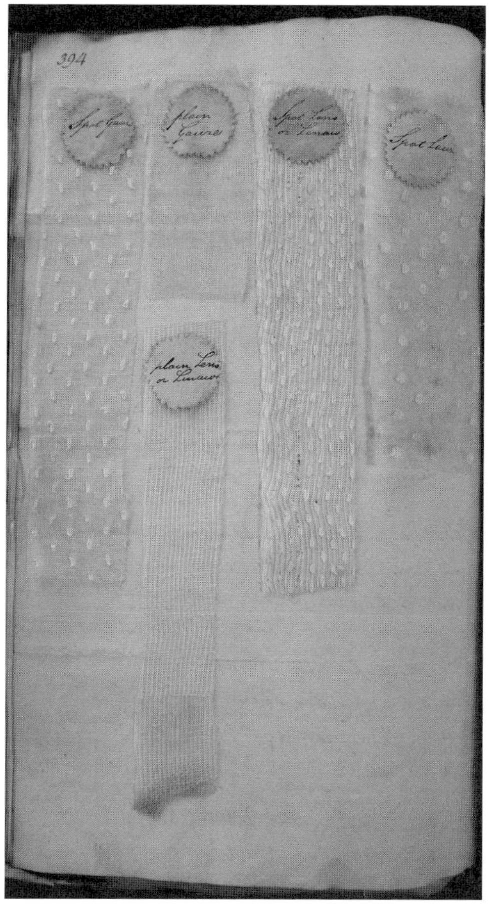

FIGURE 12.2 Samples of Scottish linen lawns, lenos, and gauzes, 1789.
Credit: National Archives BT6/244.

Linen dresses dated around 1805 to 1810 from the Cunnington Collection include a linen lawn around fifty by fifty threads per centimeter and a linen cambric of forty-nine warps by fifty-eight wefts per centimeter, evidence that fine linens maintained a place in the market.[11] But an extraordinary cotton dress of similar date having sixty warps by seventy-six wefts per centimeter outrivals these; the grain of the weave is hardly visible to the naked eye (see Figure 12.3).[12] Lancashire industrialists of the time proudly claimed to spin cotton yarns finer than three tex (over 200 count), and this dress demonstrates that, at least occasionally, such physical limits of production were realized in pursuit of fashionable fineness. Houldsworth's cotton yarn price list indicates the escalating cost for fineness, jumping more than five times for 240s over 120s, which points to a probable greater price differential for goods at retail prices (White 1846: 315; see

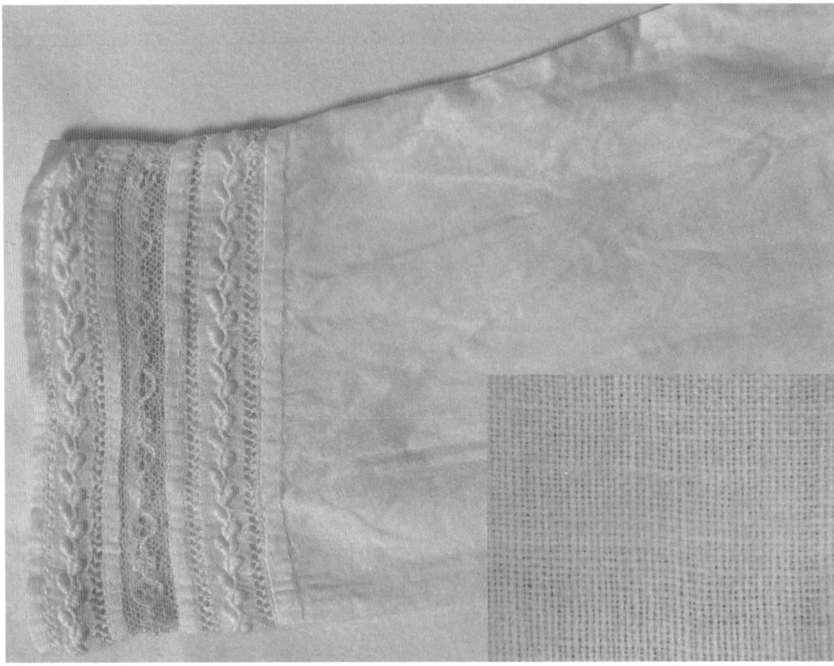

FIGURE 12.3 Detail of sleeve of dress (1950.347) made from ultrafine cotton lawn, around 1810, with inset photomicrograph of the fabric (65x). Compare the ordinary muslin used as an embroidered insertion.
Credit: Manchester City Galleries: Gallery of Costume.

Figure 12.4). Thus, fine cottons embodied values of both luxury and modernity in early nineteenth-century Britain.

Muslins

Duncan Bythell's pioneering study of handloom weavers during the Industrial Revolution exploded some of the myths about the move from hand- to power-loom production, and the changeover from putting out to factory production, clarifying that British muslins were handwoven until the 1830s (1969: 25–93). However, we still know little about the physical makeup of these fabrics and the ways in which changing spinning technologies may be manifest in surviving cloth. These are factors that would aid discrimination of muslins woven in India from those of British make. Fine muslins were hand-spun and handwoven in Bengal from early times, but fine cotton spinning in Britain became possible only with the general adoption of Crompton's spinning mule by around 1787 and the importation of long-fibered cottons (including sea island cotton from around 1789).[13] A tract of July 1789 claims that "since the improvements of last year" muslins are "greatly superior in fabric to the foreign goods of the same quality,

PRICES OF COTTON YARN.

MR. THOMAS HOULDSWORTH'S LIST,

MANCHESTER.

NET CASH PRICES.

NO.	SINGLE YARN OR TWIST.		DOUBLED YARN OR THREAD.	
	s.	*d.*	*s.*	*d.*
120	3	11	4	7
130	4	4	5	1
140	4	11	5	7
150	5	7	6	2
160	6	5	6	10
170	7	3	7	6
180	8	1	8	4
190	9	1	9	3
200	10	1	10	3
210	11	4	11	6
220	13	0	12	10
230	14	8	14	5
240	16	8	16	3
250	19	2	18	4
280	37	0	28	0
300	57	0	37	0
320			48	0
350			70	0
400			120	0
450			227	0

FIGURE 12.4 Houldsworth's cotton yarn price list (see White 1846).
Credit: Author's collection.

and since the reduction [in price] of the raw material, such goods can unquestionably be sold cheaper than it is possible to import from India" (Colquhoun 1789: 14). So this seems to mark the point at which Britain produced muslin yarns equal to Indian imports, with capacity for finer yarns increasing in the early 1790s (English 1969: 74). James Cooke Taylor dated the decline of the Dacca cotton manufacture to 1793, when British yarns effectively replaced former imports (1851: xiii).[14] However, Indian fabrics were still reputed to be softer and more durable, as noted in Jane Austen's *Northanger Abbey* (Hughes 2006: 188). Taylor states that Indian muslins continued to be exported until around 1817 (1851: xiii), so for about a quarter of a century, while muslin was at the height of fashion, British and Indian muslins competed in the marketplace. My exploration sought features that might disclose the origin of muslins found in surviving garments.

It is not possible to measure precisely the weight per unit length (yarn count) of the warps and wefts in historical garment fabrics by nondestructive methods. However, an estimate can be formed based on predictive equations established by textile technologist Frederick T. Peirce (1937: 77–80). William D. Cooke employed this method to calculate the counts of yarns in archaeological sailcloth, providing a modernized equation in metric units (Cooke, Christiansen, and Hammarlund 2002: 206–7).[15] Vitor Carvalho and colleagues (2009) provide another formula based on yarn diameter. Since British yarns attained similar counts to the Indian ones by the late 1780s, such measurements are not diagnostic but can demonstrate the range of fine yarns produced, both hand- and machine-spun.

Hand-spun cotton can be expected to be less uniform than machine-spun cotton. It is said that the usual practice of the Indian weaver was to combine yarns of "three or four assortments or degrees of quality" (J. Taylor 1851: 42). Such combinations are difficult to assess by eye but might be discoverable by computerized image analysis of the fabric surface (Bueno, Durand, and Renner 2000; Hosseini Ravandi and Toriumi 1995). Colin R. Cork, William D. Cooke, and John-Peter Wild (1996) measured mean twist angle and variability using image analysis, a technique well adapted for distinguishing the spinning "signatures" of yarns but not yet applied to the study of muslins (Wild et al. 1998). The mid-nineteenth-century commentator Taylor thought that the difference between Indian and British yarns could be judged by the simple aid of a microscope because of the degree of hairiness found in shorter-fibered Indian cottons (W. Taylor 1843: 155, quoted in J. Taylor 1851: 21). My study found such yarns only on two self-checked muslins, one of these dated to the 1780s, lending additional probability of Indian origin.[16] But their yarns appeared more loosely spun, contrary to John Forbes Watson's observations in his study of French, English, and Dacca muslins in the 1860s that Indian yarns were twisted about one and a half times more than others. He found fewer filaments per yarn, but the diameter of the filaments was larger in the Dacca yarns than in the European yarns (Watson 1867: 146). However, the quality of both British and Bengal muslins had changed in half a century. Already in 1808, a weaver from Bolton felt that the quality of British yarns had deteriorated; improved machinery meant that fine yarns could be spun from poorer-quality cotton. "It is not so level; it is full of little lumps of cotton, which should be picked out in spinning. . . . I could have taken and dressed my yarn in 1797, without any trouble of picking" (quoted in Stanley 1808: 23). Such uncertainties pose aspects for further study.

Another line of investigation is provided by the standards agreed on between manufacturers and weavers for wage purposes. White tabulated ten common widths of cotton and linen fabrics: 24, 27, 30, 33, 36, 37, 40, 46, 48, and 54 inches, qualifying shrinkage in the weaving: "a yard wide web will shrink from about half an inch to an inch" (1846: 294). Widths ranging from 25 to 51 inches were found in a sample of just eight muslin dresses dating between 1800 and 1810. The largest, nominally yard-and-a-half or six-quarters width, was a standard frequently mentioned in nineteenth-century Select Committee reports for muslins woven in Stockport and Bolton, whereas yard-wide

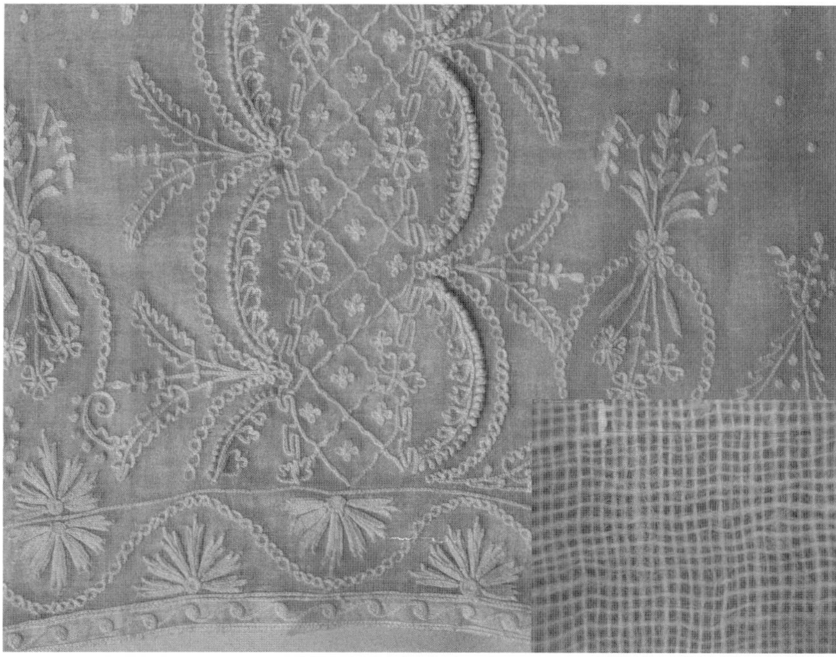

FIGURE 12.5 Hem detail of Martin-Edwards wedding dress (1951.341), 1806, made from six-quarters muslin, with inset photomicrograph of fabric (65x).
Credit: Manchester City Galleries: Gallery of Costume.

muslins were normal for Bengal imports (yard-and-a-quarter being the limit of reach for the unassisted hand weaver). Joseph Sherwin, a weaver from Stockport, wove eighty-reed, six-quarters cambric between 1798 and 1824, specifying that eighty reed meant eighty ends in each inch (Hume 1824: 419). In fact, this standard corresponds closely to a fine muslin dress worn by Charlotte Martin on her marriage to John Edwards of Ness Strange, on December 2, 1806, affirming its British origin (see Figure 12.5).[17] Wider muslins imported from the Madras Presidency are recorded in the mid-nineteenth century; T. N. Mukharji (1888: 327) describes three-handed weaving of wide muslins at Aarani, while Watson (1866: 7:43) provides one example woven two yards wide. Thus fabric widths probably distinguished domestic from imported muslins for only a limited period.

Some distinct trends based on weave specifications were found in a group of twenty printed cottons, mainly hand-block prints, in garments dated between 1775 and 1810. The majority of print grounds fell into two groups that can be called calicos and muslins (see Figure 12.6). The calicos all had Z-spun warps combined with S-spun wefts, the spin directions possibly corresponding to the use of stronger mule-spun yarn for the warp and softer jenny-spun yarn for the weft. The combination allowed the fibers of both warp and weft to slope in the same direction in the woven product, thus suiting it for prints by giving more even absorbance and reflectancy of colors. S-direction

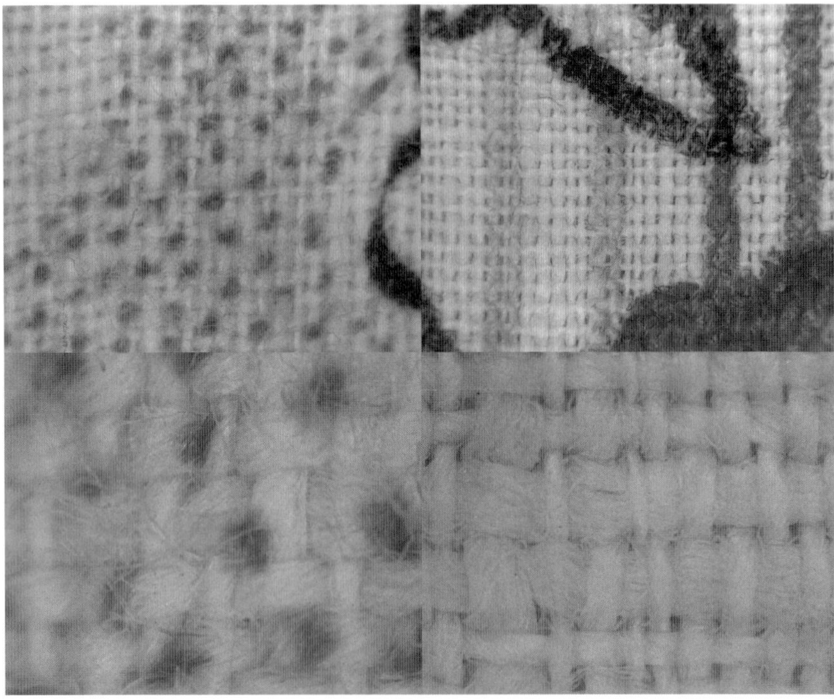

FIGURE 12.6 Photomicrographic comparison of print cloths: calico style with S-spun weft on left (1947.1607, around 1800) and muslin style with all Z-spun yarns on right (1968.70, around 1780). Magnification 65x top and 190x below.
Credit: Manchester City Galleries: Gallery of Costume.

spinning was not practiced in India; thus such calicos would have been home-produced. The calico group had medium weave density, with thread counts in the range of eighteen to twenty-seven per centimeter. The muslin group, made with Z-spun yarns (either mule-spun or hand-spun), averaged twenty-nine to forty threads per centimeter. A trend was observed for muslins under yard wide to have higher weft counts than warp counts, while wider fabrics displayed the opposite trend. The overwefted and underwefted types suggest different production centers, perhaps Manchester versus Glasgow (see White 1846). While this study of muslins did not produce definitive diagnostic features, it shows the abductive method used to question textual and physical fact-finding, and the refining of theory undertaken as study proceeds.

A Splice-Spun Bast Fiber Gown

Alvesson and Sköldberg found abductive modeling often arises out of a single surprising case. As survival in museum collections favors the exceptional over the typical, dress historians are often faced with remarkable garments. A trained Regency gown with neoclassical embroidery provides an example whose material is the key to its origin.[18] The dress is made from muslin with an unusual light and translucent character. Low-power microscopy showed that it was woven from a bast fiber but that the yarns had been splice-spun. Splice-spun linen is associated with royal garments from ancient Egypt, where the technique enabled production of ultrafine yarns from filaments peeled off dry stalks of flax. Technologists William D. Cooke, Mohamed El-Gamal, and Angela Brennan demonstrated the viability of splice-spinning, obtaining yarns with a smooth profile free from hairs as in ancient examples; they asserted that "fabrics produced from them would be light, smooth and semitransparent" (1991: 22).

It was first conjectured that the dress material might derive from a workshop preserving the ancient technique. However, although archaeologist Elizabeth Crowfoot (2011) found splice-spun linen in a medieval context, modern examples are not reported.[19] Also, the ancients laid their peeled fibers side by side using adhesive, whereas the splices in the dress are made with a weaver's twist knot of the type used to join warps (Cooke, El-Gamal, and Brennan 1991: 21). In addition, the pattern of the embroidery, its technique, and the materials are in keeping with mainstream European fashion (see Figure 12.7).

A literature search revealed that dry preparation of bast fibers had been reinvented in England by James Lee of Enfield, who patented a process in 1812 and established a

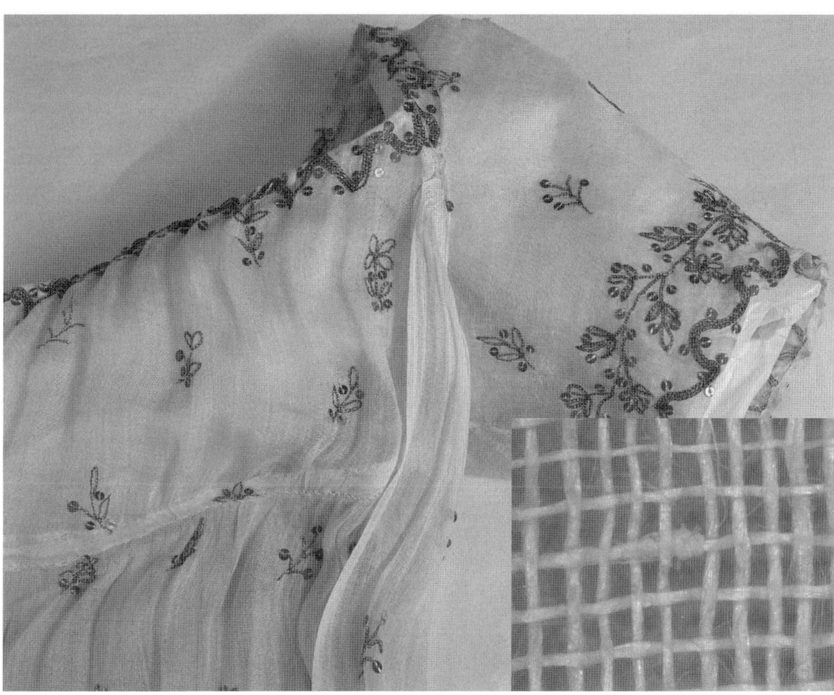

FIGURE 12.7 Detail of dress (1947.1738) made from splice-spun fabric, around 1810, with inset photomicrograph of fabric showing a weft splice.
Credit: Manchester City Galleries: Gallery of Costume.

factory at Old Bow on the River Lea by 1815, as noted in the *Repertory of Arts* (1817: 364–65). Since the flax was mechanically stripped off its chaff rather than retted, it did not require bleaching, only washing, to become white. Thomas Gill claimed that "the fibres so treated were mistaken for silk by the dealers in the latter article, from the splendour and glossiness of them" (1836: 359). A few years later Samuel Hill and William Bundy began production using a similar method deemed not to infringe the patent, and large orders were reportedly received from Messrs. Benyon and Co. at Leeds (*Repertory of Arts* 1817: 367). However, Andrew Ure noted in 1839, "This promising improvement has apparently come to nought, having been many years abandoned by the patentee himself" (141). Gill explained that the process was "too expensive to come into general use" (1836: 359). Since the dress has been stylistically dated to 1805 to 1810, it may slightly predate the Lee patent, although that does not rule out a possible association.

A series of correspondence among Board of Trade papers of 1789 showed that Reverend J. Hutchinson, residing in France, also perfected a dry preparation process but applied it to hemp fiber. The stripped filaments were left at their full length and could be "carried to any degree of whiteness and fineness that may be desired," even fit for making lace (National Archives BT 6/244: 256). By the early 1800s, Hutchinson induced Sir Brook Watson to bring a bill into parliament to promote the cultivation of hemp in England (Hutchinson 1808: 484). Thus, if the dress fabric is made of hemp, it might have been produced by Hutchinson's process. Fine bast fiber fabrics such as ramie could also have been imported from East Asia at this period (Hamilton and Milgram 2007). An accurate fiber identification appears to hold the key to the history of this dress and its interpretation—an Eastern novelty, an agricultural improvement, or a new invention.

Sewing and Sewing Threads

Respected practitioners of object-based dress studies have often used observations of the character of sewing in their assessments of authenticity and alterations to dress. However, little attempt has been made to define diagnostic traits by which sewing can be classified. The sewing of the eighteenth century has been particularly disparaged as crude, and machine sewing seldom receives mention. In the 1990s, my research tried to rectify this gap, although it is only possible to present here a brief summary (Sykas 2000: 123–35). The production of sewing thread in Europe in the hand-spinning era was generally limited to two-ply constructions of silk or linen with the ply in the S direction. Sewing threads used in garment seams in the 1700s are generally of a coarser character than modern ones, and there is seldom an effort to match the color of thread and fabric apart from the general aspect of white, neutral, or dark. Original stitching of this era can be described as workmanlike, matching stitch length to need and not pursuing regularity as an object in itself. However, the sewing observed in extant eighteenth-century garments is more often a later alteration of the garment where speed was valued above quality, and such rough stitching has been taken as general. Proof that fine work was achievable when needed can be found in the careful piecing of small bits of fabric often seen in eighteenth-century silk dresses. Such piecing uses minute and regular rentering stitches in fine silk, a technique coming from men's tailoring where piecing allowed more efficient use of material. Mantua makers ostensibly emulated the process for the same reason, but it is possible that this was a demonstrative form of economizing to mark the mantua maker's thrift or her client's purported disdain of extravagance.

Two-ply yarns have a ribbonlike character and tend to spread and cinch the cloth within the stitch, thus making seams resistant to pulling; this quality is largely exploited in tailoring. Fine dressmaking techniques that became widespread in the 1820s produced a demand for rounder three-ply yarns suited to gathering and close stitching. This decade also saw a general switch from linen to cotton sewing thread, which was by then produced in assorted colors to allow matching of thread to fabric. Cotton thread had been introduced, probably in the late 1790s, but seems to have found a market for lace making before sewing. It was not until much later, with the introduction of combed cotton in the 1850s, that manufacturers could produce a superior thread able to surpass silk and linen. Machine sewing made strenuous demands on sewing thread, which for dressmaking could at first only be met by silk.[20] A suitable cotton thread for machine sewing required the introduction of a six-cord construction[21] made up from fine yarns of strong sea island cotton. Six-cord plied constructions were made by the mid-1830s, but their spread awaited demand and the right economic conditions; with the rise of the sewing machine, they became widely available in the 1860s. A report of 1890 places an attempt of the Sagamore Company of Portsmouth, New Hampshire, to imitate six-cord thread imported from Scotland "not long before 1850" (Census Office 1894: 180). This implies that six-cord cotton threads were available from the early years of machine sewing but took a decade to gain wide consumer approval.

The expense of sewing threads was such that nineteenth-century dressmakers conserved on requirements by using cheaper threads for the hidden underthread in lockstitch or double chain-stitch sewing. In lockstitch work, where the strain on the needle thread was greater than on the bobbin thread, the underthread chosen was usually finer or softer (see Figure 12.8). This progression of developments in constructional sewing can be taken into consideration when evaluating surviving garments, giving additional evidence for amateur or professional work, economies of production, and the intended caliber of garment.

The Introduction of Machine Sewing into Dressmaking

The sewing machine was first conceived as an industrial tool but was to become "one of the first mechanical consumer durables" (Godley 1996: 59). Already in 1856, Singer introduced a machine aimed at the domestic market. However, Andrew Godley has shown that in Britain, the majority of machines were sold to tailors, dressmakers, and outworkers to manufacture clothing for resale rather than personal consumption (65). Certainly factory use of machines developed quickly within the ready-made clothing sector. George Holloway & Co. of Stroud were said to have been the first to "sew by

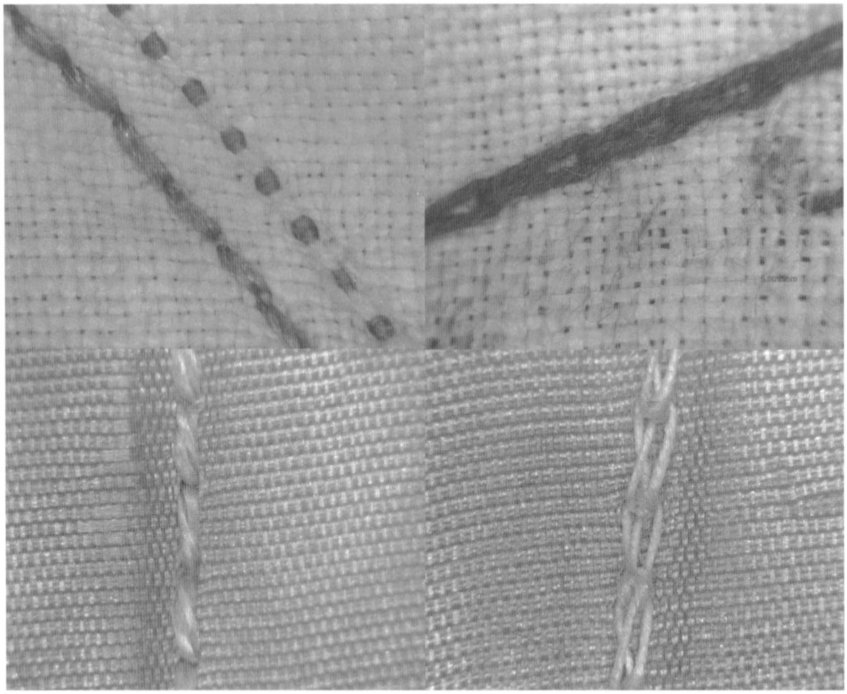

FIGURE 12.8 Machine sewing stitches (clockwise from upper left): lockstitch both sides (1947.2428), single chain-stitch underside (1947.2418), double chain-stitch underside, and double chain-stitch face (1947.506).
Credit: Manchester City Galleries: Gallery of Costume.

steam," seen in an 1854 engraving, when twenty machines were each capable of producing 150 pairs of men's trousers per week (*Illustrated London News* 1854: 624; Chaloner and Musson 1963: fig. 212; see Figure 12.9). The female operatives stand at their machines, while ancillary handworkers (cutting, tacking, and dealing with buttons and buttonholes) seem more fortunate in being able to work seated, along with the male manager. The depicted conditions are far better than in the sweated trades, but it may be the intention of the article to extol the new technology.

Karin Hausen asserts that with the adoption of domestic-model machines at the end of the 1850s, an era began in which "female labour cannot be included in the usual economic categories, which tend to separate consumption from production, [and] productive from unproductive labour" (1985: 260). She found that domestic and industrial machine sewing tended to divide along the lines of linen goods (undergarments, shirts, collars) produced by outworkers in the home, and a ready-made clothing industry in competition with professional dressmakers and tailors. By the end of the 1860s, machine sewing was an essential requirement for profitability in both sectors of the market (*Vierteljahresschrift für höhere Töchterschulen* 3, 1869, cited in Hausen 1985: 271, 276).[22] Machine sewing of dresses was probably still the province of professional dressmakers at

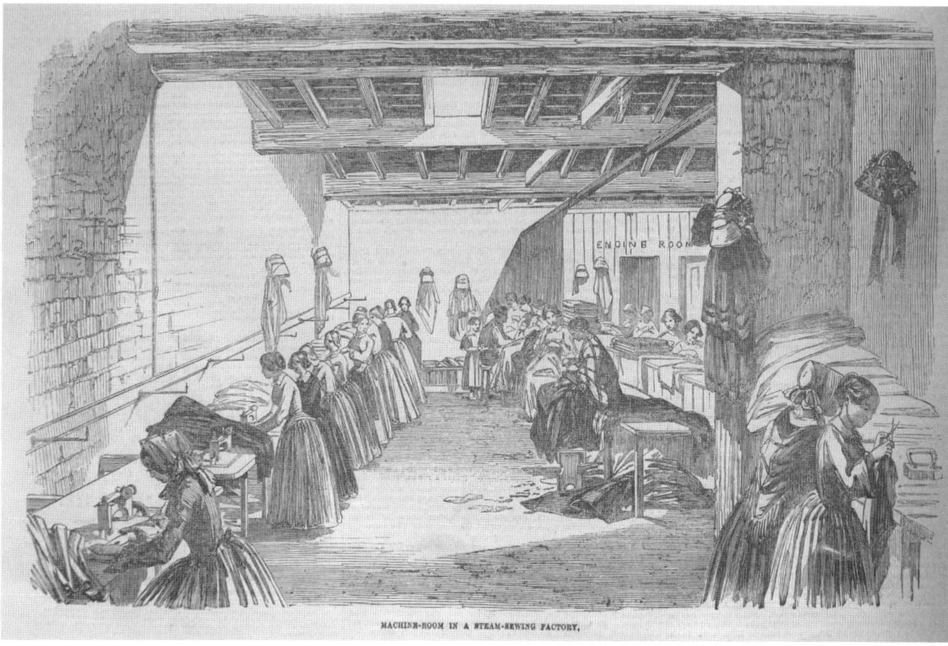

FIGURE 12.9 Holloway and Co. machine sewing workshop, from the *Illustrated London News*, December 16, 1854.
Credit: Manchester Metropolitan University Libraries.

this time. Writing of the 1860s, Joan Severa notes, "The difference between a dressmaker and a seamstress was considered to lie mainly in the ability to achieve a smooth, perfect fit in a garment. Personal records of many women still tell of having bodices fitted and made by a skilled dressmaker, while they themselves made up the skirts at home" (1995: 191).

This study looked at how the earliest machine-sewn dresses in the Gallery of Costume collection mapped onto historical studies, and what might be revealed by the choice of machine sewing over handwork. The earliest dress in the collection that is sewn by machine is a wedding dress of 1861.[23] The lack of 1850s machine sewing among surviving dresses is in keeping with the reported use of machines for ready-to-wear garments, mainly undergarments and men's clothing, during that decade. However, the wedding dress suggests that opting for machine sewing may have had other meanings. It was worn by Elizabeth Goodier (b. 1828) at her marriage to Abraham Haworth on September 5, 1861, at Eccles Congregational Church. This union must have been momentous for Elizabeth, as upon marriage before a priest she would have been disowned by her Quaker meeting. Attitudes were softening at this period as reflected in the Marriage (Society of Friends) Act 1860, but it was not until 1872 that marriages between Quakers and non-Quakers were fully legalized. Haworth was a prosperous commission agent in the cotton yarn trade, and the marriage lifted Elizabeth from dependence on her

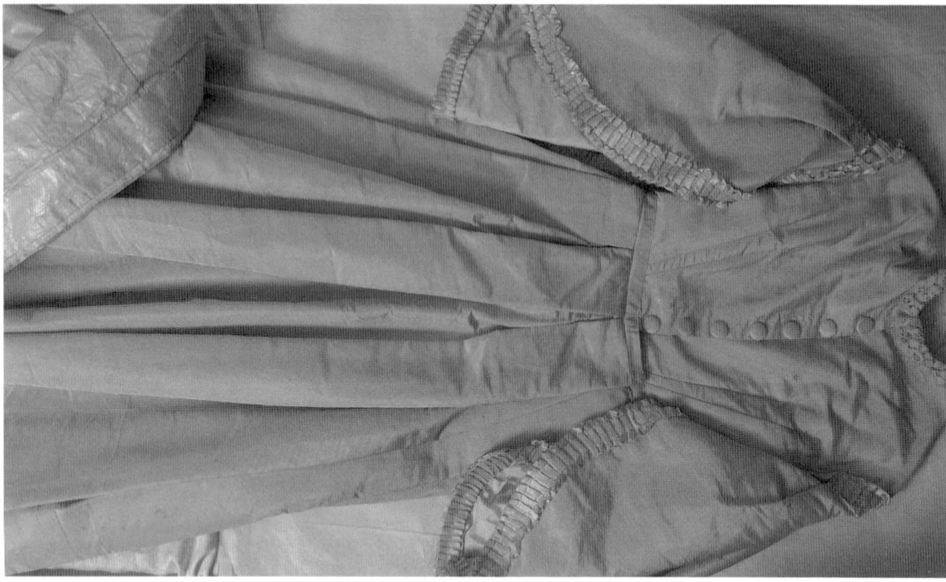

FIGURE 12.10 Goodier-Haworth wedding dress, 1861, showing glazed cotton lining at upper left (1952.160).
Credit: Manchester City Galleries: Gallery of Costume.

brother, who had been supporting his five sisters since the death of their parents. It is not surprising that the dress seems to represent Elizabeth's difficult moral reconciliation of her former self with her future life.

She chose a ribbed ivory silk with a soft sheen, the uniformity of the weave suited to Quaker concepts of simplicity and plainness of dress (see Figure 12.10). But in keeping with her husband's status, Elizabeth opted for a fashionable, although still low-key, pleated ribbon to decorate the bodice. A row of seven false buttons at the front are a concession to extravagance, but these involved less work than real buttonholes. And the dressmaker-made bodice was machine sewn in lockstitch, balancing fashionable fit with another time-saving gesture. The hand-stitched skirt may have been assembled at home, and a glazed cotton lining was used rather than the usual stiffened muslin. The Goodier family had been in the calendering trade for nearly a century, and with the glazed cotton, the bride showed that on the inside she still held onto her family values, despite a new fashionable exterior. It can be seen here how material properties have potential for signification that can be realized within a personal as well as a cultural context.

Patchy Memories

The cloth-centered stance to clothing can also be manifested in the use of small pieces of fabric to represent, or carry the memory of, a larger whole. Seen widely in devotional practice, a fragment of a saint's robe was able to embody power to intercede with the deity. In secular life, faith was also required for the merchanting system that used a sample to represent the nature of goods able to be supplied, thus allowing goods to be ordered in advance of their ready availability.[24] However, sale contracts were not made absolute until the goods were presented, and it took some time before dealing based on samples shed its appearance of speculation. Charlotte Luetkens asserted that "it was only with the improvement of postal service and transport towards the end of the seventeenth century that the volume of trade based on samples increased" (1939: 677).

By the eighteenth century, the system of selling based on samples was familiar in the retail trade. Lambert cites patterns of silk requested by an Edinburgh merchant in 1710, followed by a complaint: "The patterns were no way answerable to what I wrote for, being old fashioned, too light and flowered. . . . I am sure you had not my letter by you when swatches were cutt" (2009: 76). Likewise, Samuel Richardson's heroine Pamela chooses her new genteel wardrobe through patterns of fashionable silks sent from a London mercer for her consideration (Buck 1992: 29).

In the Illinois diaries referred to above, it is significant that swatches of material were chosen to memorialize garments, rather than photographs or sketches. It seems that the sensuous qualities offered by fabric, even in a fragmentary sample, are able to stir memory beyond descriptions of form, whether visual or textual. Victor Hugo preserved a small souvenir of printed dress fabric, framed beneath the painted portrait of his eleven-year-old daughter Léopoldine, that sharply brings into focus values that are only suggested in the picture.[25] Likewise, a printed cotton sample preserved alongside an American daguerrotype from around 1850 vivifies the photographic evidence beyond the mere addition of color and scale (Severa 2005: 113). John Styles explored samples resulting from the system of child identification used at the Foundling Hospital in London in the eighteenth century, employing a match piece of fabric that was split between the institution and the mother. Here the fabric piece conveyed not simply a cherished garment but a maternal relationship, severed but retained (2007: 114–22). Such examples make apparent that there is a significance held by the materiality of textiles that is not conveyed by visual representations.

Recent times have seen the adoption of printed skeleton motifs in fashion, projecting a countercultural message by reference to the memento mori, emblems of the transience of the material world normally catered to by fashion. A *Punch* cartoon of 1853 lampoons a similar novelty in shirts observed at that time, when skeletons and skulls were ostensibly added to the usual sporting vocabulary of men's printed shirtings (*Punch* 1853: 31). One could be tempted to take this as the artist Leech's exaggeration were it not for the survival of samples from proof prints in the archive of the Crayford calico printer Charles Swaisland, showing just such motifs (see Figure 12.11). A colorist's notebook from the archive indicates that these were still being printed in May 1860 when an order for two pieces (28-yard lengths) was filled. Thus the style was not merely a passing fad. The fresh face of Leech's wearer suggests this is a youth fashion, possibly suited to medical students

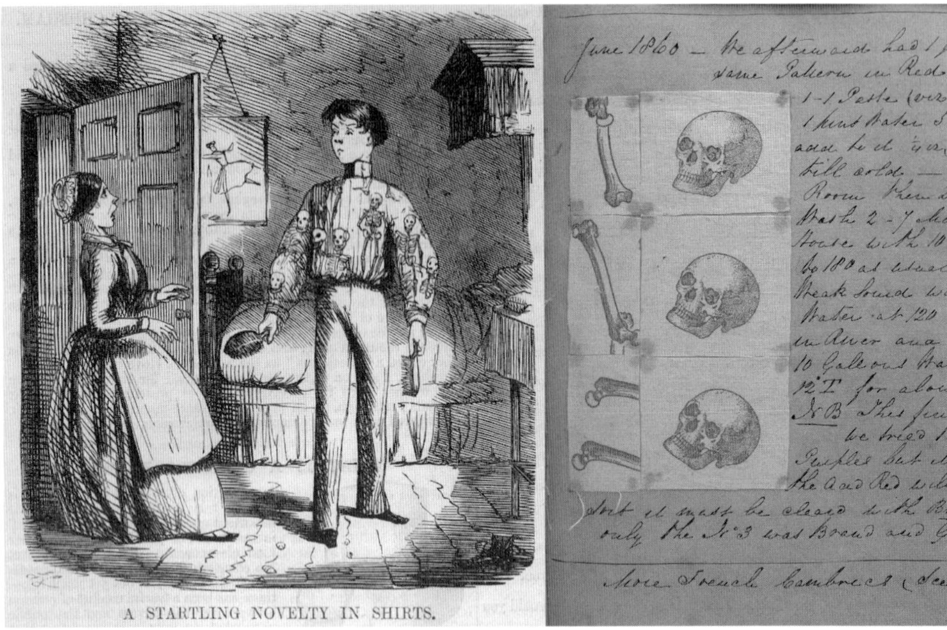

FIGURE 12.11 *Punch* cartoon, 1853, alongside samples from the notebook of Thomas Royle, Swaisland Print Works, 1860 (Inv. 106).
Credit: G.P. & J. Baker Archives.

or a similar confraternity.[26] In this case, surviving swatches corroborate the existence of a little-known fashion that might otherwise be interpreted as imaginative.

CONCLUSION

The work of Charles Dickens points to a changing attitude toward dress arising by the mid-nineteenth century. Rather than fragile assemblies on the verge of return to their material origins, garments are perceived as entities with power of their own, both collaborative and subversive. In *Little Dorrit,* the shady Mr. Merdle wears "a somewhat uneasy expression about his coat-cuffs, as if they were in his confidence, and had reasons for being anxious to hide his hands" (Dickens [1857] 1982: 247). Clothes are transformed into samples of their past wearers: when people wore cast-off clothes, they were "made up of patches and pieces of other people's individuality, and had no sartorial existence of their own proper" (91). The ascendancy of clothing over cloth may be an underlying source of the neglect of materiality in dress studies. It is perhaps natural that anthropologists have led in the rehabilitation of this study. The work of Daniel Miller and his co-essayists (1987, 2005, 2010) helps to provide a theoretical grounding for the direction in which object-led and connoisseurship-based museum studies have evolved.

The material aspect of dress affords access to information imparted consciously or unconsciously by makers and merchants, whether or not this was understood, sensed, or ignored by users and contemporary observers. Materiality interprets such information in its social, cultural, and historical dimensions. In the light of such factors, values and meanings of material properties are easily overturned, as Elizabeth Fenton found as an Irishwoman in India in 1827: "it is, I must tell you, the extremity of bad taste to appear in anything of Indian manufacture—neither muslin, silk, flowers, or even ornaments, however beautiful. This at first amazed me; when I wanted to purchase one of those fine-wrought Dacca muslins I was assured I must not be seen in it as none but half-castes *ever* wore them. These dresses sell in London as high as £7 or £10. . . . So much for the variations in taste" (Fenton 1901: 82).

NOTES

The research on which this essay was based was made possible through the generous collaboration of Dr. Miles Lambert, senior curator, Gallery of Costume, Manchester.

1. The mediocre stitching is often evidence of remaking rather than of original construction.
2. Men's tailored garments did not easily allow return to fabric and were consequently worn longer and not cast off so readily.
3. Waugh recognized that changes in cut "were influenced to a great extent by new textures in materials" (1968: 20), which makes it more surprising that she did not record the materials.
4. The clarity and value of the information observable in museum garments are diminished by prior washing.
5. The epithet "new" may be taken to represent a reemergence. John Nevinson was a pioneer in relating the physical aspects of surviving dress to contemporary comments about acquisition and wearing (see Nevinson 1949).
6. Martin suggests organizing the analysis of material culture around five basic cultural choices: "whether to replicate, differentiate, simplify, exaggerate, or hybridize stylistic ideas in the world of goods." She speaks of "looking for larger patterns by *quantifying the quotidian*" to describe her process of sifting biographical meaning from the account books that form her raw evidence (see Martin 2008: 108).
7. Divisions were ultimately based on the nail, which was one-sixteenth of a yard, or two and a quarter inches.
8. The published version of the album was used for this analysis (see Rothstein 1987). The assumption was made that some plain silks were three-quarters width as commonly found, although this was not always specified.
9. In 1811 Miss Johnson's brother gave her a French sarcenet that she made into a pelisse using slightly more than five square yards. Along with a gift of French satin she received in 1795, this fabric may have come from French merchant vessels captured as prizes by the British Navy and could thus be both fashionable and patriotic.
10. National Archives BT6/244: 393–97.
11. Manchester City Galleries, Gallery of Costume 1947.1740 and 1947.1739, respectively. Each linen is approximately yard wide.
12. Manchester City Galleries, Gallery of Costume 1950.347. Dress presented by the Hon. Rachel Kay-Shuttleworth, philanthropist and needlewoman. The cotton is roughly a yard wide.

13. Philipp Andreas Nemnich observed that Georgia cotton is "scarcely good enough to spin beyond 100 or 110," and "to spin higher numbers, it is necessary to employ the so-called East India, that is, Bourbon cotton; and such may be spun to about No. 300" (see Nemnich 1799).
14. The firm of McConnel and Kennedy produced fine counts (above 100 English cotton count, around six tex) from its start in 1795 (see Lee 1972: 25).
15. $K = (t/\mathrm{cm} \times \mathrm{tex}^{1/2})/9.572$, where K is the cover factor and t/cm is the number of warps or wefts per centimeter accordingly.
16. Manchester City Galleries, Gallery of Costume 1947.1608 (printed muslin dress, 1780–1790) and 1974.28 (printed muslin dress, 1795–1800); the muslins are 38- and 40-inch widths respectively.
17. Manchester City Galleries, Gallery of Costume 1951.341. Charlotte Martin was the daughter of Lady Mary Murray, who married the Reverend George Martin; she was the granddaughter of John Murray, 3rd Duke of Atholl (see Mosley 1998: 139). The marriage was announced in the *Lancaster Gazette and General Advertiser...* on Saturday, December, 13, 1806.
18. Manchester City Galleries, Gallery of Costume 1947.1738 (embroidered dress, ca. 1805–1810, Cunnington Collection no. A15. C.). Willett and Phillis Cunnington deliberately masked the provenance of their collection to divorce dress history from personal associations. The selvage width is thirty-two and a half inches.
19. Thanks to John Peter Wild for calling my attention to Crowfoot 2011.
20. Machine sewing silk had a three-ply construction with the ply in the S direction during the mid-nineteenth century.
21. Six-cord can be defined as a three-ply thread made up from doubled yarns, thus having six constituent elements. The spinning direction is reversed each time, from spun single to doubled yarn to final ply.
22. An unplanned outcome of the influx of untrained labor into machine sewing was probably an expansion of innovation as workers sought to speed up piecework uninhibited by the edicts of the craft tradition.
23. Manchester City Galleries, Gallery of Costume 1952.160 (wedding dress, 1861).
24. Gérard Gayot identified the date 1407 as the time by which the term *échantillon* (sample) took on its modern meaning: a small quantity of merchandise shown in order to make known the quality of the whole (see Gayot 2000). Charlotte Luetkens cites an early instance: "in 1318, a Canterbury cloth-merchant requested the weaver who supplied him to send patterns of cloth, adding that when he had seen patterns and prices he would send a man to select the cloths and bring them to Canterbury" (1939: 677).
25. Auguste De Chatillon, *Portrait de Léopoldine au livre d'heures,* 1835, in the collection of the Maison de Victor Hugo, Musées de la Ville de Paris.
26. Estimating four yards in a shirt, two pieces would have provided enough material for fourteen shirts.

BIBLIOGRAPHY

Adolf, Franz-Peter, and John W. S. Hearle. 1998. "Textile Damage in Forensic Investigations." In John W. S. Hearle, Brenda Lomas, and William D. Cooke (eds.), *Atlas of Fibre Fracture and Damage to Textiles,* 397–401. 2nd ed. Cambridge, UK: Woodhead.

Alvesson, Mats, and Kaj Sköldberg. 2009. *Reflexive Methodology: New Vistas for Qualitative Research.* 2nd ed. Los Angeles: Sage.

Arnold, Janet. 1972a. *Patterns of Fashion 1: Englishwomen's Dresses and Their Construction c.1660–1860.* London: Macmillan.

Arnold, Janet. 1972b. *Patterns of Fashion 2: Englishwomen's Dresses and Their Construction c.1860–1940.* London: Macmillan.

Arnold, Janet. 1985. *Patterns of Fashion: The Cut and Construction of Clothes for Men and Women c.1560–1620.* London: Macmillan.

Arnold, Janet. 1986. "Costume in Hogarth and Devis." Paper presented at Costume Society Symposium "Fashion Framed," London, March 15.

Arnold, Janet. 1999. "Dashing Amazons: The Development of Women's Riding Dress, c.1500–1900." In Amy de la Haye and Elizabeth Wilson (eds.), *Defining Dress: Dress as Object, Meaning and Identity,* 10–29. Manchester: Manchester University Press.

Arnold, Janet. 2008. *Patterns of Fashion 4: The Cut and Construction of Linen Shirts, Smocks, Neckwear, Headwear and Accessories for Men and Women c.1540–1660.* Completed by Jenny Tiramani and Santina M. Levey. London: Macmillan.

Baumgarten, Linda. 2002. *What Clothes Reveal: The Language of Clothing in Colonial and Federal America.* Williamsburg, VA: Colonial Williamsburg Foundation and Yale University Press.

Buck, Anne. [1961] 1984. *Victorian Costume and Costume Accessories.* Bedford, UK: Ruth Bean.

Buck, Anne. 1979. *Dress in Eighteenth-Century England.* London: B. T. Batsford.

Buck, Anne. 1992. "Pamela's Clothes." *Costume: The Journal of the Costume Society* 26: 21–31.

Bueno, Marie-Ange, Bernard Durand, and Marc Renner. 2000. "Optical Characterisation of the State of Fabric Surfaces." *Optical Engineering* 39 (6): 1697–1703.

Burnham, Dorothy K. 1973. *Cut My Cote.* Toronto: Royal Ontario Museum.

Bythell, Duncan. 1969. *The Handloom Weavers: A Study in the English Cotton Industry during the Industrial Revolution.* Cambridge: Cambridge University Press.

Carvalho, Vitor, Rosa M. Vasconcelos, Filomena O. Soares, and Michael Belsley. 2009. "Yarn Diameter and Linear Mass Correlation." *Journal of Nondestructive Evaluation* 28: 49–54.

Census Office, U.S. Department of the Interior. 1894. *Report on Manufacturing Industries in the United States at the Eleventh Census: 1890.* Washington, DC: Government Printing Office.

Chaloner, William Henry, and Albert Edward Musson (eds.). 1963. *Industry and Technology: A Visual History of Modern Britain.* London: Vista Books.

Chapman, Robert William. (ed.). 1932. *Jane Austen's Letters to Her Sister Cassandra and Others.* Vol. 1, *1796–1809.* Oxford: Clarendon.

[Colquhoun, Patrick]. 1789. *A Representation of Facts Relative to the Rise and Progress of the Cotton Manufacture in Great Britain.* London: H. Reynell, July 16.

Cooke, William D., and Brenda Lomas. 1987. "The Evidence of Wear and Damage in Ancient Textiles." In Penelope Walton and John-Peter Wild (eds.), *Textiles in Northern Archaeology,* 215–26. London: Archetype.

Cooke, William D., Mohamed El-Gamal, and Angela Brennan. 1991. "The Hand-Spinning of Ultra-fine Yarn. Part 2, The Spinning of Flax." *CIETA Bulletin* 69: 17–23.

Cooke, William D., Carol Christiansen, and Lena Hammarlund. 2002. "Viking Wooden Square-Sails and Fabric Cover Factor." *International Journal of Nautical Archaeology* 31 (2): 202–10.

Cork, Colin R., William D. Cooke, and John-Peter Wild. 1996. "The Measurement of Twist Angle Using Image Analysis." *Archaeometry* 38 (2): 337–45.

Crowfoot, Elizabeth. 2011. *Qasr Ibrim: The Textiles from the Cathedral Cemetery.* London: Egypt Exploration Society.

Curtis, Harry P. 1928. "Manchester Piece Goods: Lesson XVIII." *Textile Educator* 27: 1290.

Dickens, Charles. [1857] 1982. *Little Dorrit.* Oxford: Oxford University Press.

Edgeworth, Maria. [1800] 1980. *Castle Rackrent.* Ed. George Watson. World Classics Edition. Oxford: Oxford University Press.

English, Walter. 1969. *The Textile Industry: An Account of the Early Inventions of Spinning, Weaving, and Knitting Machines.* London: Longmans, Green.

Fenton, Elizabeth S. 1901. *The Journal of Mrs. Fenton: A Narrative of Her Life in India, the Isle of France (Mauritius), and Tasmania during the Years 1826–1830.* London: Edward Arnold.

Fowler, Brenda. 1995. "Forgotten Riches of King Tut: His Wardrobe." *New York Times,* July 25.

Gayot, Gerard. 2000. "Different Uses of Cloth Samples in the Manufactures of Elbeuf, Sedan and Verviers in the Eighteenth Century." Paper presented at the Centre for the History of Textiles and Dress Conference "Textile Sample Books Reassessed," Winchester College of Art, June 30.

Gill, Thomas. 1836. "On Bleaching Tarred Ropes and Sail Cloth, Coarse Rags and Other Vegetable Fibres…" *The Literary Gazette and Journal of the Belles Lettres, Arts, Sciences, &c.* 20 (June 4): 359–60.

Godley, Andrew. 1996. "Singer in Britain: The Diffusion of Sewing Machine Technology and Its Impact on the Clothing Industry in the United Kingdom, 1860–1905." *Textile History* 27 (1): 59–76.

Gombrich, Ernst Hans. 1979. "The Logic of Vanity Fair: Alternatives to Historicism in the Study of Fashions, Style and Taste." In Ernst Hans Gombrich, *Ideals and Idols: Essays on Values in History and in Art,* 60–92. Oxford: Phaidon.

Groff, John M. 2003. "'All That Makes a Man's Mind More Active': Jane and Reuben Haines at Wyck, 1812–1831." In Emma J. Lapsansky and Anne A. Verplanck (eds.), *Quaker Aesthetics: Reflections on a Quaker Ethic in American Design and Consumption, 1720–1920,* 90–121. Philadelphia: University of Pennsylvania Press.

Hamilton, Roy W., and B. Lynne Milgram. 2007. *Material Choices: Refashioning Bast and Leaf Fibers in Asia and the Pacific.* Los Angeles: Fowler Museum at the University of California Los Angeles.

Hausen, Karin. 1985. "Technical Progress and Women's Labour in the Nineteenth Century: The Social History of the Sewing Machine." In Georg Iggers (ed.), *The Social History of Politics: Critical Perspectives in West German Historical Writing since 1945,* 259–81. Leamington Spa, UK: Berg.

Hearle, John W. S., Brenda Lomas, and William D. Cooke. 1998. *Atlas of Fibre Fracture and Damage to Textiles.* 2nd ed. Cambridge, UK: Woodhead.

Home, James Archibald (ed.). [1889] 1970. *The Letters and Journals of Lady Mary Coke.* Vol. 1. Bath, UK: Kingsmead Reprints.

Hosseini Ravandi, S. Abdolkarim, and K. Toriumi. 1995. "Fourier Transform Analyses of Plain Weave Fabric Appearance." *Textile Research Journal* 65: 676–83.

Hughes, Clair. 2006. "Talk about Muslin: Jane Austen's *Northanger Abbey.*" *Textile: The Journal of Cloth and Culture* 4 (2): 184–97.

Hume, Joseph (chair). 1824. *First Report from Select Committee on Artizans and Machinery.* Paper 51. London: Her Majesty's Stationery Office.

Hutchinson, J. 1808. "On the Cultivation of Hemp." *Retrospect of Philosophical, Mechanical, Chemical and Agricultural Discoveries* 13 (January-March): 484–85.

Illustrated London News. 1854. "Sewing by Steam." December 16, 624–25.

Kawabata, Sueo, and Masako Niwa. 1989. "Fabric Performance in Clothing Manufacture." *Journal of the Textile Institute* 80 (1): 19–50.

Keane, Webb. 2005. "Signs Are Not the Garb of Meaning: On the Social Analysis of Material Things." In Daniel Miller (ed.), *Materiality,* 183–205. Durham, NC: Duke University Press.

Ladies' Cabinet. 1854. "Mrs. Murden's Two-Dollar Silk." August, 122–26.

Lambert, Miles. 2009. "'Sent from Town': Commissioning Clothing in Britain during the Long Eighteenth Century." *Costume: The Journal of the Costume Society* 43: 66–84.

Lave, Charles A., and James G. March. [1975] 1993. *Introduction to Models in the Social Sciences.* Lanham, MD: University Press of America.

Lee, Clive Howard. 1972. *A Cotton Enterprise 1795–1840: A History of McConnel & Kennedy Fine Cotton Spinners.* Manchester: Manchester University Press.

Lefanu, Elizabeth Sheridan. 1986. *Betsy Sheridan's Journal.* Oxford: Oxford University Press.

Lemire, Beverly. 1994. "Redressing the History of the Clothing Trade in England: Ready-Made Clothing, Guilds and Women Workers, 1650–1800." *Dress* 21: 62–74.

Luetkens, Charlotte. 1939. "The Development of the Exchange." *Ciba Review* 19 (March): 672–80.

Martin, Ann Smart. 2008. *Buying into the World of Goods: Early Consumers in Backcountry Virginia.* Baltimore: John Hopkins University Press.

Matsudaira, Mitsuo, and Masao Matsui. 1992. "Features of Mechanical Properties and Fabric Handle of Silk Weaves." *Journal of the Textile Institute* 83 (1): 133–43.

Mercator [pseud.]. 1765. *Gazette and New Daily Advertiser,* February 5.

Miller, Daniel. 1987. *Material Culture and Mass Consumption.* Oxford: Basil Blackwell.

Miller, Daniel (ed.). 2005. *Materiality.* Durham, NC: Duke University Press.

Miller, Daniel. 2010. *Stuff.* Cambridge, UK: Polity.

Mosley, Charles (ed.). 1998. *Burke's Peerage and Baronetage.* Vol. 1. 106th ed. London: Fitzroy Dearborn.

Mukharji, T. N. 1888. *Art-Manufactures of India.* Calcutta: Government Printing Office.

Neild, William. 1861. "An Account of the Prices of Printing Cloth and Upland Cotton, from 1812 to 1860." *Journal of the Statistical Society of London* 24 (4): 491–97.

Nemnich, Philipp Andreas. 1799. *Beschreibung einer im Sommer 1799 von Hamburg nach und durch England geschehenen Reise.* Tübingen, Germany: J. G. Cotta'schen Buchhandlung.

Nevinson, John L. 1949. "A New Suit." *The Connoisseur* 123 (512): 99–101.

North, Susan, and Jenny Tiramani (eds.). 2011. *Seventeenth-Century Women's Dress Patterns: Book One.* London: V&A Publishing.

Oberly, Michelle. 1993. "The Fabric Scrapbooks of Hannah Ditzler Alspaugh." In Otto C. Thieme (ed.), *With Grace and Favour: Victorian and Edwardian Fashion in America,* 4–13. Cincinnati: Cincinnati Art Museum.

The Observer. 1793. Classified advertisements. August 25, 1.

O'Connor, Sonia A., and Mary M. Brooks. 2007. *X-radiography of Textiles, Dress and Related Objects.* Amsterdam: Elsevier Butterworth-Heinemann.

Peirce, Frederick T. 1937. "The Geometry of Cloth Structure." *Journal of the Textile Institute: Transactions* 28 (3): 43–96.

Pietsch, Johannes. 2008. "The Art of Tailoring in the Seventeenth Century." In Johannes Pietsch and Karen Stolleis, *Kölner Patrizier- und Bürgerkleidung des 17. Jahrhunderts: Translation of Chapters I–III,* 33–80. Riggisberg, Switzerland: Abegg-Stiftung.

Pritchard, Frances. 2006. *Dress in Egypt in the First Millennium AD.* Manchester: Whitworth Art Gallery.

Punch. 1853. "A Startling Novelty in Shirts." 25: 31.

The Repertory of Arts, Manufactures and Agriculture... 1817. "On the Preparation of Flax and Hemp without Steeping." 2nd ser., 31: 363–82.

Rose, Clare. 2000. "Quilting in Eighteenth-Century London: The Objects, the Evidence." *Quilt Studies: The Journal of the British Quilt Study Group* 2: 11–30.

Rothstein, Natalie (ed.). 1987. *Barbara Johnson's Album of Fashions and Fabrics.* London: Thames and Hudson.

Severa, Joan L. 1995. *Dressed for the Photographer: Ordinary Americans and Fashion, 1840–1900.* Kent, OH: Kent State University Press.

Severa, Joan L. 2005. *My Likeness Taken: Daguerreian Portraits in America.* Kent, OH: Kent State University Press.

Skelton, Maruta, and Leanna Lee-Whitman. 1986. "A Systematic Method for Differentiating between 18th Century Painted-Printed Chinese and Western Silks." In Howard L. Needles and S. Haig Zeronian (eds.), *Historic Textile and Paper Materials: Conservation and Characterization,* 131–51. Washington, DC: American Chemical Society.

Stanley, Thomas (chair). 1808. *Report from the Committee on Petitions of Several Cotton Manufacturers and Journeymen Cotton Weavers, &c.* Paper 177. London: Her Majesty's Stationery Office.

Stevens, G.W.H. 1950. "The Strength of Hooped Foundations for Gowns." *Journal of the Textile Institute: Proceedings* 41 (October): 719–24.

Stevens, G.W.H. 1952. "The Stability of a Compressed Elastic Ring and of a Flexible Heavy Structure Spread by a System of Elastic Rings." *Quarterly Journal of Mechanics and Applied Mathematics* 5 (2): 221–36.

Styles, John. 2007. *The Dress of the People: Everyday Fashion in Eighteenth-Century England.* New Haven, CT: Yale University Press.

Sykas, Philip A. 2000. "Re-threading: Notes towards a History of Sewing Thread in Britain." In Mary M. Brooks (ed.), *Textiles Revealed: Object Lessons in Historic Textile and Costume Research,* 123–35. London: Archetype Publications.

[Taylor, James Cooke]. 1851. *A Descriptive and Historical Account of the Cotton Manufactures of Dacca, in Bengal, by a Former Resident of Dacca.* London: John Mortimer.

Taylor, William Cooke. 1843. *The Hand Book of Silk, Cotton and Woollen Manufactures.* London: Richard Bentley.

Taylor's Warehouse. 1777. "Quilted Coats...Taylor's Warehouse." *Prescott's Manchester Journal* 7 (March 22): 4.

Thieme, Otto. 1986. "On Collecting Costume." *Cincinnati Art Museum Bulletin* 13 (3): n.p.

Ure, Andrew. 1839. *Dictionary of Arts, Manufactures and Mines.* London: Longman, Orme, Brown, Green & Longman.

Urquhart, John W. 1881. *Sewing Machinery, Being a Practical Manual of the Sewing Machine*... London: Crosby Lockwood.

Watson, John Forbes. 1866. *Textile Manufactures and Costumes of the People of India.* 18 vols. London: Eyre and Spottiswood for the India Office. http://tmoi.org.uk.

Watson, John Forbes. 1867. "The Textile Manufactures and the Costumes of the People of India." *Edinburgh Review or Critical Journal* 126 (July): 125–50.

Waugh, Norah. 1954. *Corsets and Crinolines.* London: B. T. Batsford.

Waugh, Norah. 1968. *The Cut of Women's Clothes: 1600–1930.* London: Faber and Faber.

Wharncliffe, Lord (ed.). 1837. *The Letters and Works of Lady Mary Wortley Montagu.* Vol. 2. London: Richard Bentley.

White, George. 1846. *A Practical Treatise on Weaving by Hand and Power Looms…* Glasgow: John Niven.

Wild, John-Peter, William D. Cooke, Colin R. Cork, and L. Fang Lu. 1998. "Vindolanda: Some Results of the Leverhulme Trust Programme." In Lise Bender Jorgensen and Christina Rinaldo (eds.), *Textiles in European Archaeology,* 85–95. Göteborg, Sweden: North European Symposium for Archaeological Textiles/Nordeuropäisches Symposium für archäologische Textilien.

13

Looking at Fashion: The Material Object as Subject

ALEXANDRA PALMER

Fashion is intimately linked with concepts of beauty. But fashionable clothing that has been worn can be viewed as limp, lifeless, and unattractive, even unsanitary. On the other hand, we often see such clothing on display, elevated into examples of art—the art of two-dimensional cloth transformed into wearable sculpture or ambulant architecture. It can also be interpreted as the carrier of remnants of past lives, not only of wearers, but of makers, merchants, and buyers. Or it can be viewed, from a more distant perspective, as a record of shifting notions of fashionability and customs over time. Given these rich and complex associations it is curious that the study of museum objects through observation is a research skill that has been marginalized in fashion studies, despite the extensive interest in material culture (Palmer 1997). Material culture studies connotes the inclusion of objects as a key strand of the research, but this does not necessarily include close examination of them (Prown 1982).

The seemingly old-fashioned museum-based approach of fashion studies, which begins with a description of the object, is a complex and underutilized approach for new scholars, one that Lou Taylor identifies as a mysterious academic boundary (2002: 72). The object-based approach following an art historical model that catalogs artifacts by date, material, design, and artist has been identified as a "descriptive approach . . . over and above any analytical interpretations . . . marked . . . by a greater focus on artifact-centered study" (Taylor 2004: 4). However, analysis of objects has to begin with a descriptive approach based on close visual examination, a skill that is often assumed determined to be innate; probably because we make daily decisions about our own clothing, it is assumed that we already have the necessary critical skills to evaluate fashion, when in fact it is a research skill that is learned like any other form of scholarship. The descriptive methodology has fallen out of academic fashion as the discipline of fashion history has expanded over the last thirty years, despite the urging of scholars such as Prown, who wrote that clothing "promises to be a particularly rich vein for material culture studies, [even though] to date little has been done with it" (1982: 13).

The close study of two objects in the Royal Ontario Museum (ROM), an evening dress and matching shawl by Tom Ford for Yves Saint Laurent from the fall/winter 2004–2005 collection, and a historical English semiformal open robe, from about 1795–1799, illustrates *how* a close examination of fashion objects can shift and deepen our understanding of the meanings of fashion.[1]

OBJECT ANALYSIS 1: YVES SAINT LAURENT EVENING DRESS BY TOM FORD

The September 2004 cover of Australian *Vogue* showed sixteen-year-old Gemma Ward in bright sunlight modeling a Yves Saint Laurent, Rive Gauche, sequined evening dress designed by Tom Ford (Figure 13.1). In this, his last collection for the house, Ford paid homage to Saint Laurent's celebrated 1977 fall/winter Chinese collection that has been made an academic icon in Debora Silverman's (1986) now classic critique. Saint Laurent had a very French idea of the Orient stemming from late seventeenth- and eighteenth-century exoticism and chinoiserie, commingled with twentieth-century collecting and the display of artifacts in European interiors and museums. In a Proustian manner he explained to *Elle* magazine:

> This China that I have so often interpreted in my creations I found to be exactly as I had imagined it. All I need is a picture book for my mind to melt into a place or a landscape. . . . I don't feel any need to go there. I have dreamed about it so much. . . . In the end the most wonderful voyage is the one that one takes around one's room. (Müller, D'Alessandro, and Charbonneau 2008: 114)

Nearly thirty years later, Ford linked Saint Laurent's Chinese collection with his own imaginings. The evening dress is based on an über-sexy version of the tailored *cheong sam* (*qipao*), the modern 1920s and 1930s Chinese garment that came to symbolize the exotic and erotic Shanghai nightlife as worn by beautiful Asian Hollywood stars such as Anna May Wong (Clark 1999: 155–65; Jackson 2005). Ford fused the unique cut of the cheongsam with the iconography of woven and embroidered imperial dragon robes of the late seventeenth to nineteenth centuries with a wave border, clouds, and rising mountains. Ford even employed the yellow ground and five-clawed dragons reserved for the emperor (Vollmer 1977, 1983, 2002, 2004; Wilson 1986). Under Ford's artistic direction, the Paris fashion house of Yves Saint Laurent fluidly crossed cultural and temporal boundaries, creating a new dynamic collage of historical imperial China, early twentieth-century colonial Shanghai iconography, and 1970s Paris haute couture. The result is a newly imagined early twenty-first-century Franco-Chinese chic interpreted though American eyes. It is a rich mélange of romantic imagery culled from

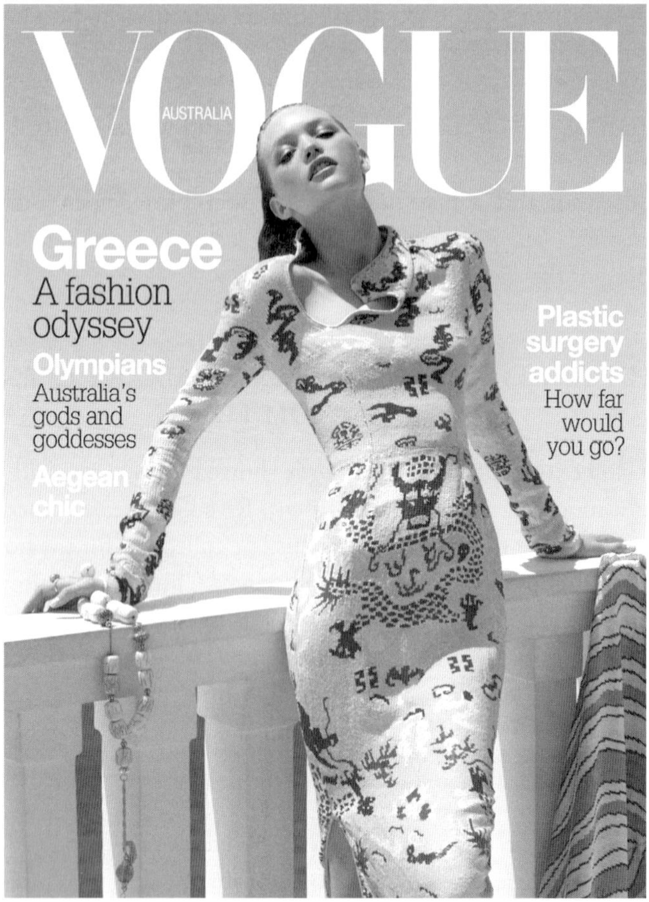

FIGURE 13.1 Yves Saint Laurent chinoiserie sequin evening dress by Tom Ford, modeled by Gemma Ward in Athens for Australian *Vogue,* September 2004 issue.
Credit: *Vogue* Australia September 2004 cover.

European art and design, 1930s Hollywood, and French haute couture traditions (Steele and Major 1999: 69–99).

This purely visual interpretation based solely on images could be described as a material culture analysis of the Saint Laurent dress. It can be greatly expanded on if the object is physically analyzed to reveal the rich details of cut, construction, and the textile itself. The singular details of the garment's construction, fabrication, and use can be set within a broader understanding of fashion and offer unique insights that are not accessible elsewhere. There are many details in this dress that are not evident in the fashion photograph. The sleeve cuffs are shaped to emulate the horsehoof cuffs of the dragon robes, thereby furthering and reiterating the historical imperial link and demonstrating that Ford understands his source material well. The surface textile pattern is created entirely in overlapping fish-scale iridescent sequins, a fact that can easily be overlooked in the photograph.[2]

The sequins are sewn to a yellow silk ground in a very controlled and shaped way. They are applied vertically on the bodice, while in the hips and hem they shift to the bias, to create a sexy and sinuous effect that is also technically more complex and expensive to produce. It is a design priority stemming from couture production, and here is applied to a high-level ready-to-wear piece. Sequins are also strongly associated with the 1920s and 1930s, and the extensive use of them in this design helps to create further the historical association of lavish couture, Shanghai, and Hollywood glamour.[3]

The dress has a white silk satin lining, which is used as a visible decorative piping at the neckline, cuffs, and hem. The lining serves as a support for the heavy sequins and makes the dress appear and feel luxurious. It eliminates the need for a slip, as the body is protected from the scratchy sequins, makes the dress comfortable to wear, and results in the dress moving smoothly across the body in a sinuous and sexy motion. It also makes it hot to wear: a fact that informs the *Vogue* photograph of it being modeled in the blazing sun. Inside the bodice there is an inner yellow silk chiffon corselette that is wired under the bust and closes with a zipper marked "YSL" on the pull. This is the support for the dress that keeps it fitting snugly to the torso. It also makes it a complete garment in the manner of haute couture production, as no bra or indeed any underwear is needed to wear this garment, allowing the wearer to feel more sensual and unencumbered by the dress.

The ROM dress has a matching shawl with a pink sequin wave border pattern. Initially this seemed to explain the pink-striped textile under Gemma Ward's left hand in the *Vogue* image; however, the credit in the magazine only describes a dress (September 2004: 20). Correspondence with Yves Saint Laurent, Paris, confirmed that that the dress was one of three units produced and that their archive does not record a shawl with this dress but that the dress had a long train.[4] This explains the pink part of the dress under Ward's hand. Saint Laurent then sent an image of the dress photographed for an unidentified Spanish fashion magazine that showed a model seated in profile on a very high block with the train cascading on the floor. It clearly showed a very long train designed in a continuation of the wave pattern in pink sequins. It is the same design as the shawl. The image also showed a five-clawed dragon that is hidden in the gathers of the ROM dress. It seems that the long train has been cut off to shorten the ROM dress and has been used to make the shawl. Close examination of the dress and shawl shows that the finishing of both pieces is the same, there is no patching in the linings, and both are piped with the same silk satin. The only trace of a change is seen in the hem of the skirt, where there are two broken blue sequins set deep in the seam between the piping and lining. When the shawl is placed at the skirt hem, the pattern does not align perfectly, indicating that there may be a narrow missing section between the hem and the shawl. This is the seam allowance needed to finish the new hem and shawl, and has been expertly altered. What can be firmly concluded is that the original design with the excessive train was not deemed practical, so Ford's design needed to be modified for actual wear. The gathers below the hip that distort a dragon motif are another alteration; they shorten the dress on the side without the slit and also make it easier to wear.

The attention-getting design with a very long dramatic train was unmanageable for the modern wearer of this expensive design, however effective it may have been on the Paris runway.

The Yves Saint Laurent dress by Tom Ford reveals how new contemporary fashion unites global historical precedents of cut, color, and form from East and West to create a modern ideal of glamour and sexy Hollywood-inspired femininity. This examination of the structure, cut, and iconography of one evening dress indicates how easily we can underestimate the value of looking closely at seemingly familiar contemporary fashion. Details are an aid to understand the production of exclusive high-end ready-to-wear in the early twenty-first century. This analysis would be helpful in directing a discussion of labor and production techniques, economics of the brand, issues around the globalization of Paris fashion in the early twenty-first century, consumption, femininity, gender, the body, and fashion photography and modeling.

LOOKING

The close study of actual objects specifically locates and extends the muddy waters of history by recording not only how designs were produced but also how designs were controlled and actually consumed. Dating and locating an object in historical time and place may appear to be a case of matching artifacts with similar published objects or those in other collections, and comparing contemporary visual sources (fashion plates, paintings, or photography). This is often not as simple as it appears. Surprisingly there is still a dearth of publications that clearly document the changing cut of historical dress.

The classic texts of sketched and measured garments in museum collections published by Janet Arnold (1964, 1966, 1985), Nancy Bradfield (1968), and Norah Waugh (1954, 1968), whose interests stemmed from theater costuming, have been supplemented by more recent ones with photographs and details of dress construction, fashion plates, paintings, and dated images (Arnold 2008; Baumgarten 2002; Landini and Niccoli 2005; Landini and Nichols 2011; North and Tiramani 2011; Pietsch 2008: 30–81; Rangstrom 2002). There are several reasons for the small number of these types of publications. Museum collections are usually understaffed, making it difficult for researchers to gain access and build up the required knowledge to assess what they are looking at, as they have not had the opportunity to examine many comparable objects. Also, when closely examined, many historical objects do not in fact fit neatly into the established chronology of fashion history or match fashion plates and other images. This may be because the garment was made and worn by someone living outside of high fashion circles; the wearer's taste may have been conservative, or age may have militated against the latest style; the garment may have been altered from its original state and even re-worn by others; or the maker may not have been technically up to date. In short, our knowledge of what was fashionable is limited and is in fact probably constrained by our desire for a neat scientific classification that gives authority to the field of fashion history.

The fashion historian's referenced "ideal" is based on and reinforces the view portrayed by two-dimensional prints and paintings, products that historically have had a higher value on the art market than clothing or textiles and that have longer academic pedigrees than fashion history. What was actually worn and what is depicted can be quite different. Lou Taylor has cautioned about the "overuse" of undocumented fashion plates and drawings that are promotional, seasonal, idealized fashions, not necessarily a social reality (2002: 134–36). In contemporary terms, most readers of *Vogue* do not expect to wear $1,000 designs (let alone look or pose like the models), but they eagerly look at the images as suggestions and indicators for personal style and perhaps purchase much less expensive versions.

The discrepancy between the surviving garments and the limited canon and scholarship of fashion history is highlighted when preparing historical fashions for display and photography. Fashion has no fixed form, so the recreation of the vacant body that the costume represents relies on contemporary interpretive judgments of the intended shape and silhouette (Flecker 2007). The responsibility for creating the body and mounting artifacts depends on the institution, but it is frequently a collaborative process between the curator and conservator or mount maker. To mount a historical garment it first has to be closely examined in order to determine a date and silhouette. The cut and construction are examined so as to begin to assess what shape and size of form is suitable, as well as what sort of understructures are required to support the garment in order to achieve the desired silhouette. The observation and measuring are very revealing, as "fastenings and decoration may suddenly make sense, the reasons for unusual cut or construction become clear and poor alterations and repairs may also show up clearly" (Heiberger 2000: 109). For example, Jean Druesedow recalled that when she was at the Costume Institute, "the dresses belonging to Queen Alexandra at the MMA indicated that she had some curvature of the spine—the center back is not straight or symmetrical, as I recall, and there was much talk about it when we did *La Belle Epoque*."[5] This information was helpful in explaining the fabrication of another dress from her wardrobe in the ROM that has an awkward mismatched back at the closure, even though it was made by a good dressmaker.[6] The requirement to look closely at seams and structure in order to display artifacts that have a malleable form is unique to textiles and dress and helps to explains why museum-based publications have tended to be so descriptive—such study is necessary to begin to understand the artifact's embodied shape. This is where the curator's time begins and where much of it is spent.

Curators have to confront the issue of how to present fashion, a perennial *bête noire* for museums. It brings into sharp focus the difference between historical and contemporary ideas of fashionable taste and style that has to be mediated, as it is impossible to be indifferent to our own time when mounting dress. Historical accuracy, as it is understood in any given period of scholarship, is required when dressing a mannequin in order to achieve fit and silhouette and to safely display the piece, but it is also important to appeal to the visitor, whose personal engagement with today's fashion will inevitably affect his or her reception of garments of other eras that have had markedly different silhouettes based on the corseted form. The choices for mounts are usually strongly dictated by display budget and staff time, over aesthetic preference. Producing fashion exhibitions that aim at historical accuracy, even the display of a singular object, is a very labor-intensive and potentially costly endeavor (Palmer 2008: 31–33). Aside from practical issues, it should be noted that it requires a great deal of dexterity, creativity, and imagination to realize the mounting of a three-dimensional costume while adhering to conservation and aesthetic standards. This intellectual and tacit knowledge is hard to measure and usually goes unaccredited and unacknowledged. Learning superior craft skills is outside the purview of academe but is an enormous asset when working with fashion artifacts so as to be able to visualize an individual form through an analysis of cut and construction. This is why a strong art school and craft background underpins the knowledge of many dress curators and technicians, particularly the pioneers in the field, who were principally women dedicated to professionalizing their area within the larger context of museum colleagues who were more easily identified as qualified because they had formal academic training.[7]

OBJECT ANALYSIS 2: AN OPEN OR DEMI-ROBE OF EMBROIDERED SILK TAFFETA (ENGLISH, 1795–1799)

The following discussion of an English embroidered open or demi-robe of plain ecru silk tabby in the neoclassical taste illustrates how and why fashion history is "a situated practice that is the result of complex social forces and individual negotiations of daily life" (Entwistle 2000: 65). The museum purchased it from an English dealer who had acquired it from Josephine Jeffery, a theatrical costumier, who said she used it for inspiration for the 1973 film *Bequest to the Nation*, starring Glenda Jackson as Lady Hamilton, and for other period costumes (Figure 13.2).

The open robe is very small and would have been worn by a young woman over a dress of fine silk or cotton. It has no fastenings or closures. It has long two-piece sleeves and a low neckline, skims the sides of the breasts, and hangs away at the side of the body. The back is fitted over the shoulders, and the skirt panels flare into a slight train. The style is characteristic of the very late eighteenth century when the earlier petticoat and overrobe were abandoned for a one-piece dress with the waistline rising to just below the bust. The 1790s were an unsettled time in Europe and North America that has been widely discussed politically and socially but relatively little in terms of dress, although swift changes in cut and silhouette were developed. One reason for this lacuna is that few objects from this period survive. Another is that fashion historians have tended to focus on fashions of the late baroque and rococo, made from luscious silks, and then skip to the early nineteenth-century classically inspired Regency or Empire fashions of lightweight silks or sheer cottons (Hughes 1913: 224–30).[8] Fashions from the 1790s are frequently ignored in favor of attention being paid to pre- and post-Revolutionary

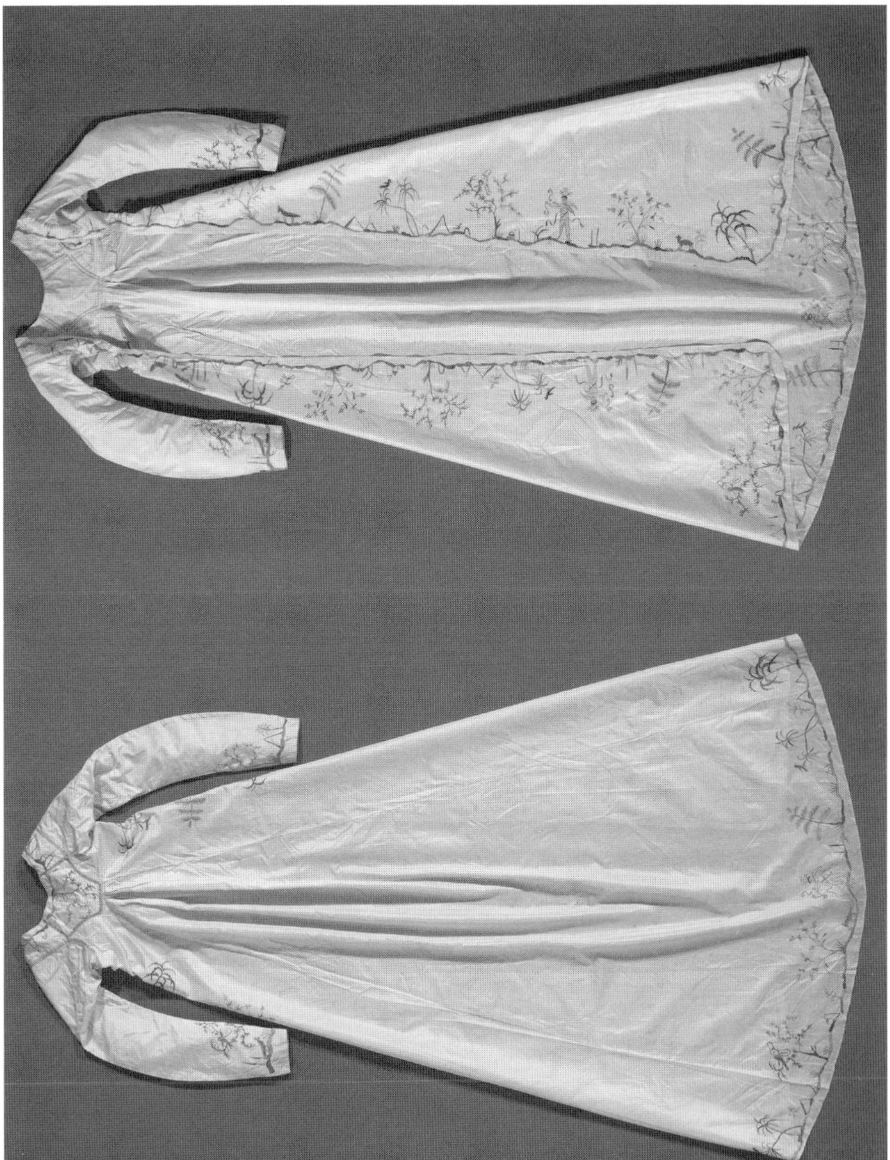

FIGURE 13.2 Front and back overview of the silk taffeta overdress embroidered in silk floss, English, ca. 1795–1799.
Credit: Royal Ontario Museum 2010.24.1.

France. They are often described as "transitional," a meaningless descriptor that could surely be applied to any moment in fashion.

The embroidered open robe is an intriguing example of late eighteenth-century fashion and dressmaking. It is cut very snug in the shoulders and back and would have been worn open or held in place with a sash or pinned. By the late 1780s and 1790s women's fashionable dress throughout Europe and North America began to combine the draped forms used in earlier fashions with more precise tailored pattern pieces, seen here in the cut of the bodice and sleeves. The mantua worn with a petticoat, which became known as the *robe à la française* (a robe open in front with released box pleats from the back neckline to the hem, worn with a petticoat), and the *robe à l'anglaise* (a robe with a closed bodice and fitted back that is released into the full skirt, which is open in front, worn with a petticoat) dominated the eighteenth century (Arnold 1964: 22–43; Diderot and d'Alembert [1751–1780] 1959: plates 12 and 15). The "transition" style of 1795–1810 was described by Norah Waugh: "the open robe of the late 1790s was usually of very thin, light, crisp silk with narrow stripes or small spotted patterns" (1968: 133), and was documented by Nancy Bradfield in actual garments in the Snowshill collection (1968: 81–90).

THE RISING WAIST

The most striking change in taste and the style of women's dress in the 1790s is the rising waist. Between 1793 and 1796 the ideal waist-length measurement (from the underarm to the hip) shortened from nine to three inches: a loss of six inches in three years (*Taylor's Complete Guide* 1796: 110). Such a radical change required a fast and complex rethinking and reworking of the cut of the bodice as women's fashion was no longer structured and fitted around a long corseted form. Instead, the bodice had to stay in place in a much-shortened torso, from the shoulder to just under the bust. The surviving dresses record the ingenuity of dressmakers, who had to invent new cuts within a few years. It was an acceleration of change in the fashionable silhouette and cut that was unprecedented. It was so radical a shift that the artist and caricaturist Isaac Cruickshank (1756–1811) skewered the new fashion in a print, *The Rage, or, Shepards I Have Lost My Waist* (1794), depicting a fashionable woman wearing a similarly shaped open robe turning away food and drink as she has sacrificed her stays (called "body"), waist, and stomach for the latest high-waisted dresses (Figure 13.3).[9]

BODICE BACK

The robe is cut with a very short bodice back in the new style seen in fashion plates and has no waist seam. The following analysis of the pattern (Figure 13.4) reveals the continuation of traditional eighteenth-century dress construction with new innovative tailoring skills. The dress has a radically new pattern piece: a small hexagonal shape, cut on the straight of the grain and inset at the center back (Figure 13.5).

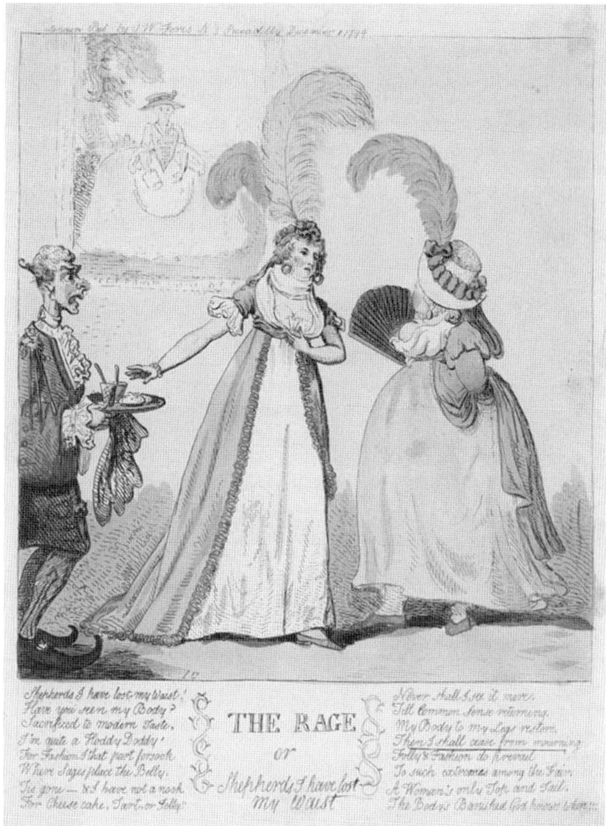
Shepherds I have lost my Waist!
Have you seen my Body?
Sacrificed to modern Taste,
THE RAGE
or
Shepherds I have lost my Waist
Never shall I see it more,
Till Common Sense returning,
My Body to my Legs restore,
Then I shall cease from mourning
Folly & Fashion do prevail
To such extremes among the Fair
A Woman's only Top and Tail.

FIGURE 13.3 Isaac Cruickshank (1756–1811), *The Rage, or Shepards I Have Lost My Waist* (1794), depicts a fashionable woman who can no longer eat or drink because she has sacrificed her stays (called "body"), waist, and stomach for the latest high-waisted dresses.
Credit: Courtesy of the Lewis Walpole Library, Yale University.

It derives from the vertical pieced, shaped, boned, and fitted back of the robe à l'anglaise, which is combined with the shaped shoulders and back pattern developed in the eighteenth century for men's coats. This was part of "a general tendency to imitate male attire . . . long coats with this character were much worn," which developed into the pelisse, a woman's coat worn over a dress, by the turn of the century (Hughes 1913: 224–30). The top of the hexagon forms the back neckline. The sloping sides attach (3C-B) to an extension of the side-front panel (4) that runs under the arm along the side of the breast to wrap over the shoulder. It also forms the neckline (4C-E). The top of the side panel (2A-B) is joined to the back. There is no waist seam that would assist in fitting the front around the bust. The two-piece sleeve (5) unites the front side (2) and the front extension (3). The bottom of the hexagon attaches to the back skirt panel (3A-G to 1A-G).

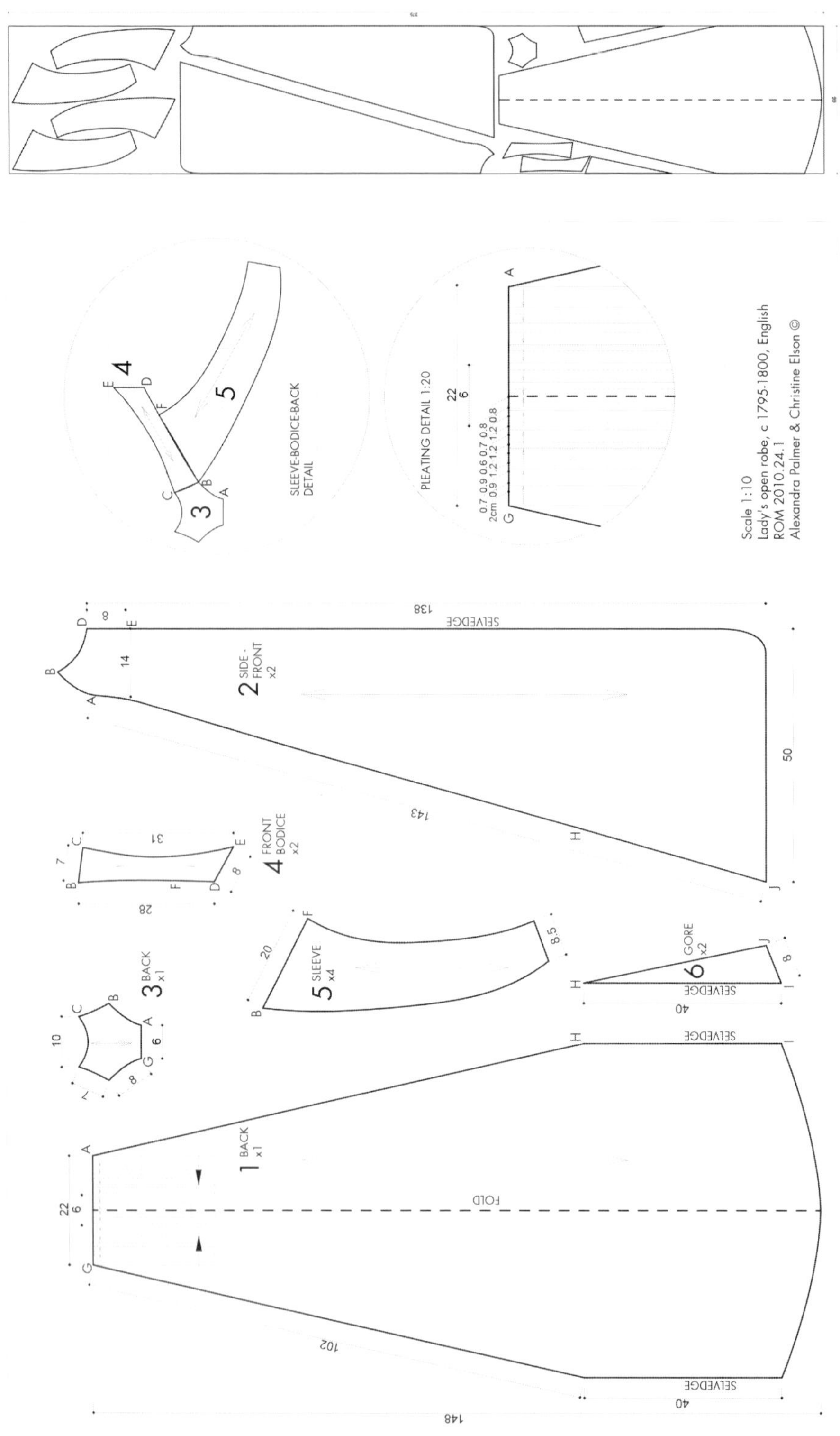

FIGURE 13.4 Pattern draft and possible layout of the English embroidered open robe, ca. 1795–1799.
Credit: Courtesy Alexandra Palmer.

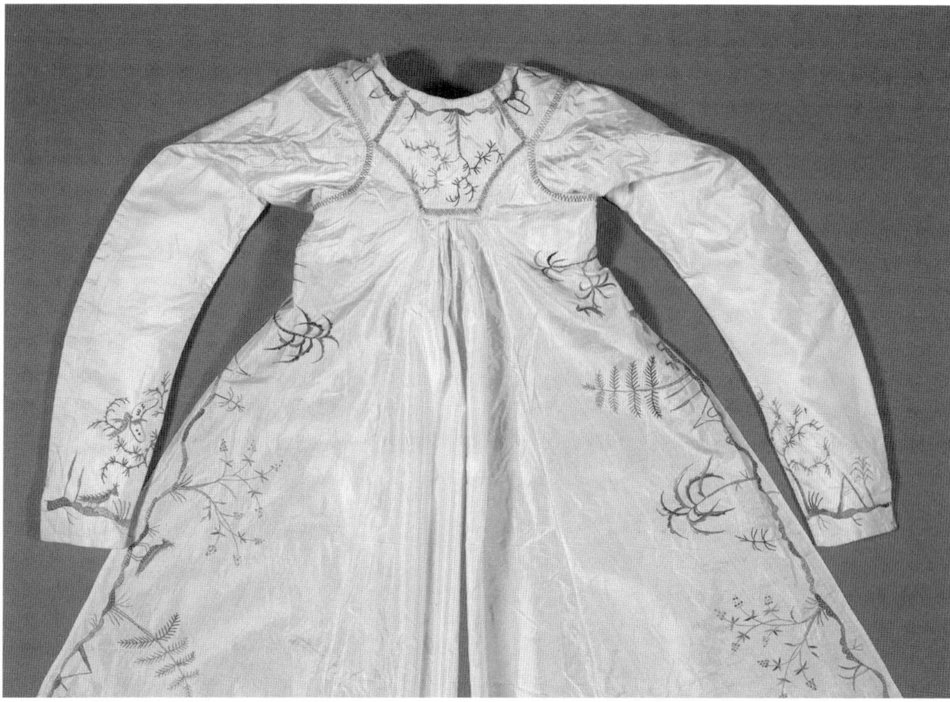

FIGURE 13.5 The back bodice hexagon (pattern piece 3) is embroidered with an upside-down tree. The deeply inset two-piece sleeve is outlined in cross-stitch. The back dress panel (pattern piece 1) is finely pleated into the center back.
Credit: Royal Ontario Museum 2010.24.1.

The hexagonal back pattern piece (3, Figure 13.5) creates a new proportion and fit that continued to be modified in the nineteenth century. Many fashion plates from about 1797–1805 were drawn to show the back or three-quarters view of dresses so that readers could understand how to make the new designs. This was an important view, as the back was the technical crux of the dress, and the new method of construction had to be understood in order to be successfully copied. A plate from *Costume Parisien* even went as far as to include a close-up detail of the back with the hexagonal pattern piece and inset of the sleeves clearly drawn for the reader to emulate (Figure 13.6). The shaped piece draws attention to the nape of the neck and accentuates a narrow back, creating a new eroticism. The focus on the small back is further exaggerated by decorative herringbone stitches around the shoulder seams that function, visually, to attract the eye to this area. The structural stitches are small back stitches. The tiny back, assisted by newly shaped stays, created a posture that opened up the sternum, held the bust up, and set the shoulders blades deep into the center back (Salen 2008: 26–33; Steele 2001: 30; Waugh 1954: 71). Thus, new methods of cut and construction changed not only the look but the wearing of fashion, which reinforced a tall, slender neoclassical ideal both visually and physically (Arnold 1970).

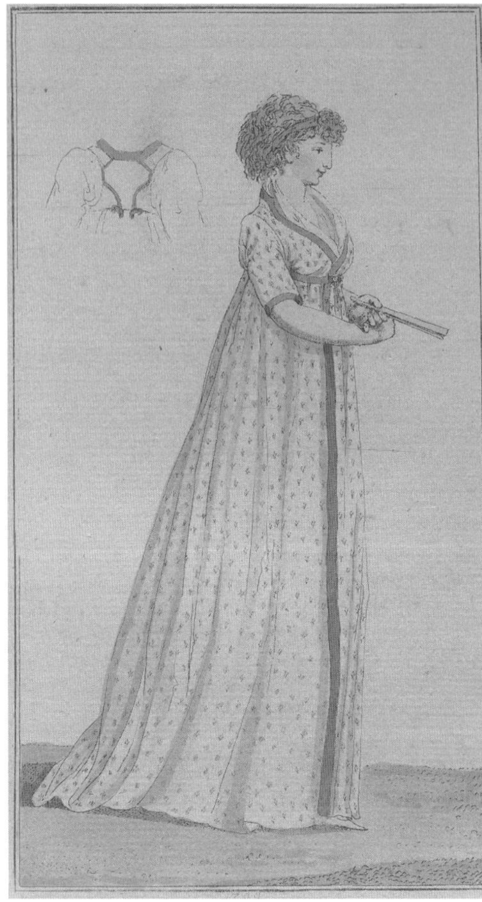

FIGURE 13.6 A 1799 *Costume Parisien* fashion plate depicts a short-waisted robe that closes in the front. It includes a detail of the center back construction. The plate is bound with other fashion plates from 1789 to 1804. The text was not included; only the images were deemed important.
Credit: Royal Ontario Museum Library and Archives, RB GT 887.C67 1789–1804.

The new cut of the bodice back is combined with pre-established dressmaking techniques. The single center-back panel runs from selvage to selvage at the train and is tapered at the top (1), in a modification of cut from earlier dresses that were used selvage to selvage from neck to hem. The back is pleasted symmetrical, miniaturized inverted "Watteau" pleats seen in the robe *à la française,* which compressed two or more full loom widths of silk into the back neck, where they were released to beautifully display the large and costly silk patterns. A similar pleating technique is carried over into the open robe in a new vestigial version compressing the full width of the top of the pattern piece (thirty-two centimeters) into a narrow width through a series of very small pleats (six centimeters; see Figure 13.4 for a detail of the pleating). The pleated back panel is then sewn to the bottom of the back bodice (1G-A to 3G-A). The released pleats permitted the dressmaker to achieve a full hem and keep the upper back flat and fitted. The side (2) and back panel (1) are joined and inset with a triangular gore (6) at the hem to allow the train to flare and move elegantly.

A comparison with other dresses helps to better understand the development of dressmaking and tailoring knowledge at this time as women worked to find unique

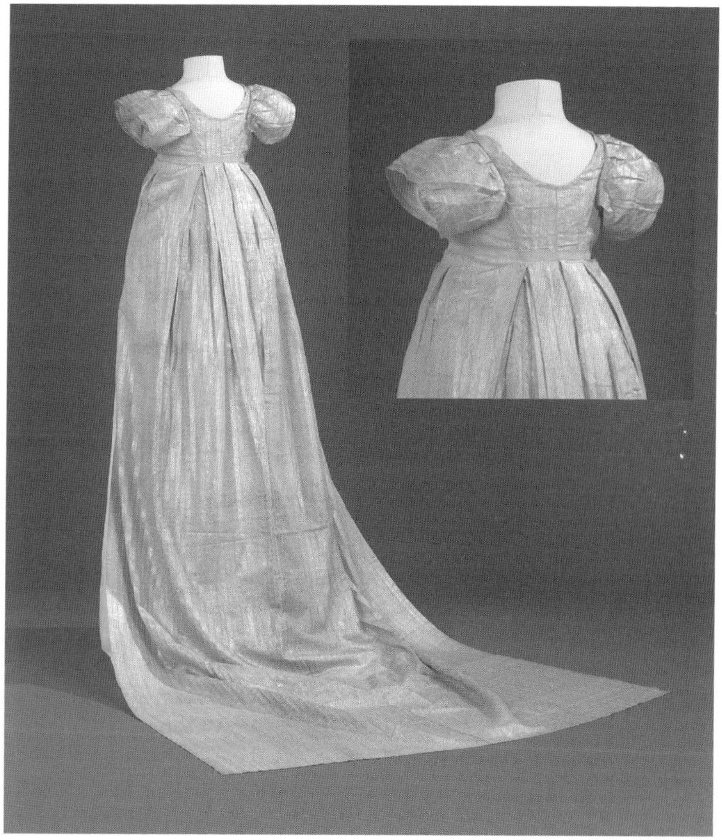

FIGURE 13.7 Overview and detail (inset) of an English overdress, 1801–1802, made from Egyptian silk tabby brocaded in chevron stripes of gold and silver *filé* given as a gift to John Hely-Hutchinson (1757–1832), second Earl of Donoughmore.
Credit: Royal Ontario Museum 2004.33.1. This acquisition was made possible by the generous support of the Louise Hawley Stone Charitable Trust.

solutions to achieve the new desirable fashionable cut. A French silk gauze dress from about 1795–1800 has the same hexagonal piece inset at the back and in the delicate overvest.[10] Another open robe is particularly useful because its provenance allows it to be closely dated to 1801–1802 (Figure 13.7). It is made of an Egyptian lightweight silk tabby brocaded in chevron stripes of gold and silver *filé*. The textile was given to John Hely-Hutchinson (1757–1832), second Earl of Donoughmore, Ireland, who fought under General Sir Ralph Abercromby in Egypt against Napoleon's troops in 1801. Upon the general's death, the British troops were placed under Hely-Hutchinson's command. He received the Egyptian textile as a diplomatic gift of appreciation from Yusuf Ziyaud-din Pasha, the Ottoman Grand Vizier, for his part in the peace negotiations. In England his distinguished service was rewarded with a peerage, the Baronetcy of Alexandria and Knocklofty, and £2,000 per annum. It is probable that the dress was made and worn by a family member for the formal ceremonies or festivities around this occasion in December 1801 or January 1802.[11]

This dress is draped directly on the body and is a less structured garment than the embroidered open robe. It has no lining nor any traces of ever having had one. It is made so that the textile is minimally "damaged" in its transformation into an open robe. The textile was cut into two lengths and sewn together at the selvages to make a center-back seam. The only other cutting and shaping of the textile is in the side back in order to create a double box pleat (in the style of the *robe à la française*) that is folded to the center back. The pleats begin at the upper back, not the neckline as in the embroidered open robe, in order to achieve a smooth, fitted back, without bulk in the pleats, and fullness in the skirt. The shape is similar to that seen in the hexagonal back of the embroidered open robe, but here it is cut in one piece with the skirt. This "Egyptian" dress has been manipulated to minimize any cutting of the cloth, even to the exclusion of shaping the train. It records the reluctance of the wearer and dressmaker to permanently alter the cloth. It also reveals the reliance on the accumulation of cultural and technical knowledge needed to cut and sew a flat textile into a sculptural form that suited the aesthetic of the moment.

Dorothy Burnham succinctly identified and explained the long history of clothing construction in *Cut My Cote* (1973) by clearly distinguishing the origins of cloth-based loom-woven cultures that developed straight-cut and draped garments from tailoring traditions developed by skin-wearing cultures. The owner of the Egyptian textile transformed it into a fashionable dress that is so minimally cut that the precious textile is 90 percent intact and ready to be reused should fashion require. It documents a straight cutting tradition that understands and recognizes the economic and sociocultural value of the cloth. In fact, it is remarkable that this textile has not been reused. Interestingly, when the dress was offered to the museum it was described as an "Egyptian textile," not as a garment, because that is how it was identified and valued within the family. Similarly, the embroidered robe has also been economically laid out on the cloth to ensure minimum waste (Figure 13.4).

The cut of the fashions at the end of the eighteenth century reveals the experiments made by dressmakers who were already skilled in draping and straight cutting, to learn and apply new and complex tailoring skills to make the newest fashions. Artifacts are an exceptional resource of information to trace this history, particularly, as Clare Haru Crowston has pointed out, because scholars have paid scant attention "to the manner in which needleworkers actually performed their work" so we know "little about how eighteenth-or nineteenth-century seamstresses made garments, the organization of production in their workshops, the range of techniques they employed" (2001: 114).

SLEEVE

The embroidered open robe has a semifitted, curved sleeve cut in two nearly identical pieces that taper to the wrist and require the inner seam to be left open as a slit for the hand. It is not flared over the knuckles, as was the fashion at the turn of the century. The fashion for long sleeves created new challenges for dressmakers, who had previously not had to fit a dress sleeve to accommodate the full length of the arm. The new difficulty was to cut and sew a long, fitted sleeve that would permit the entire arm and shoulder to move and not stress and rip the textile. This explains the curved shape of the two-piece sleeve, borrowed from menswear, but was exaggerated in women's wear as "ladies through custom have a manner of holding their arms more upon the bend than men, which requires the sleeves to be cut more crooked and bent" (*Taylor's Complete Guide* 1796: 119). Evidence of dressmakers' problem-solving abilities is seen in the outer seam, which had to be taken in for a snugger fit after it was made up.

Dressmakers would have likely learned how to make fitted garments and insert a sleeve by studying menswear, as well as women's wear made by tailors, in particular, the cut and shapes of stays and riding habits. The two-piece sleeve is a radical departure from the earlier dress sleeve of the eighteenth century, which was made from a sausage-like rectangle roughly draped and sewn around the shoulder, then hidden under the robings and back folds of the *robe à la française*. The shoulder of the sleeve is inset far into the back (Figure 13.8).[12] The sleeve head and sleeve began to be modified by the late 1770s

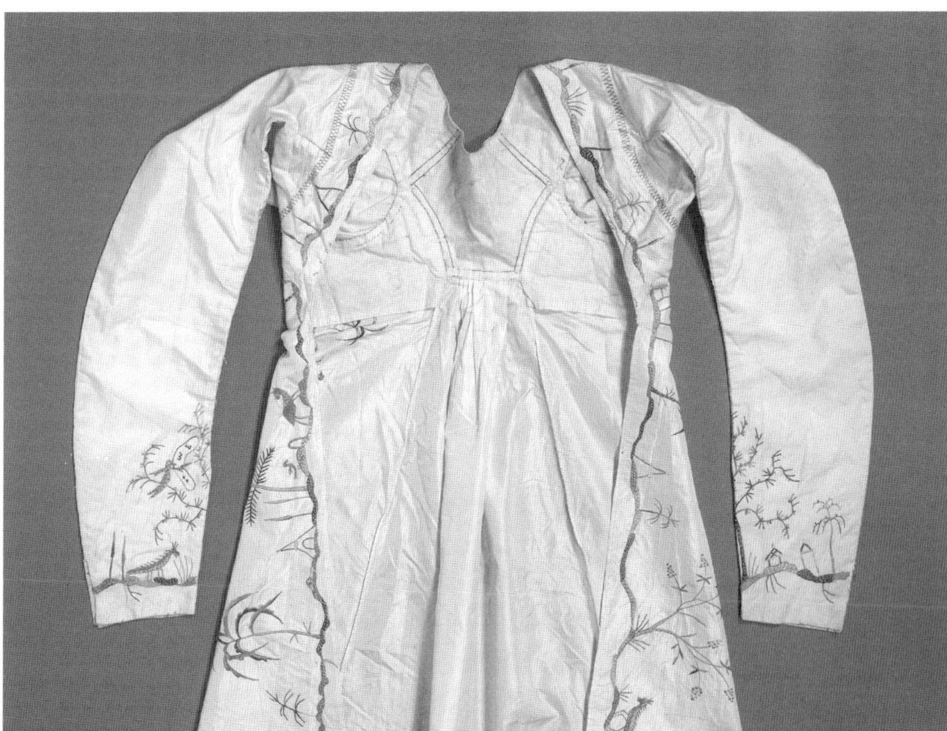

FIGURE 13.8 The cotton lining of the fitted bodice and sleeves has been used to perfect the pattern of the overdress before cutting into the more costly silk and alleviates stress on the delicate silk. The embroidered grasshopper on the sleeve cuff is a bizarre fusion of European and East and South Asian animal and insect.
Credit: Royal Ontario Museum 2010.24.1.

and 1780s in the *robe à l'anglaise* because the exposed fitted back required that it be more elegantly arranged. The hexagonal back of the open robe has a large sleeve head that covers the shoulder blade and forms part of the dress back. *The Taylor's Complete Guide* explained that careful insertion of the sleeve to the front side bodice was required in order to eliminate the "friction of the arm against the stays [that] soon wears them out" [the sides of the dress under the arm] (1796: 120). This manual was written for male tailors who had to adapt masculine cuts for women's riding habits. Dressmakers and clients would understand this problem better than tailors and worked out their own solutions.

LINING

Continuing established dressmaking traditions, the embroidered taffeta open robe is completely structured around the cotton lining of the bodice (Figure 13.8). The lining achieves several important things. The cut and fit were perfected in an inexpensive fabric, and then the silk was cut to match the lining and both were sewn together as one. The lining adds form and strength to the paper-thin textile, particularly in the fitted sleeves, alleviates the stress of fit, and protects the more delicate and costly silk from body moisture. Stable, strong, well-fitting linings were the key to dressmaking and became more accentuated with the new fashions at the end of the eighteenth century that combined a tight fit with a lightweight and delicate textile. Small rents in the paper-thin taffeta in the side bust record stress areas. To circumvent this problem the dressmaker would have needed to shape this area, either by cutting it on the bias, a method that uses more of the textile, or by piecing it and inserting a triangular gore that creates a natural bias. But it took time for dressmakers to accumulate this technical knowledge in order to not only foresee the problem but also find a solution. The open robe documents this development.

TEXTILE

The modern neoclassical taste guided by antique models called for lightweight textiles that posed new challenges in cut and required different sewing skills, as loose stitches and unfinished or crooked seams would show and the dress would hang irregularly. It was a radical departure from past dressmaking with stiff silks. Until the late 1770s fine sewing was not important for women's dress construction. It was reserved for linens that had to withstand hard wear, washing, and ironing, as well as decorative laces and needlework. The end of the eighteenth century was a turning point in more precise dress construction that also required more sewing time.

SEWING

The thin plain taffeta dress is carefully assembled. In the back and shoulder areas, where there is pull on the seams, a strong backstitch has been used. The bodice lining is neatly sewn together in one with the silk, with all seams inside. The inset back piece is

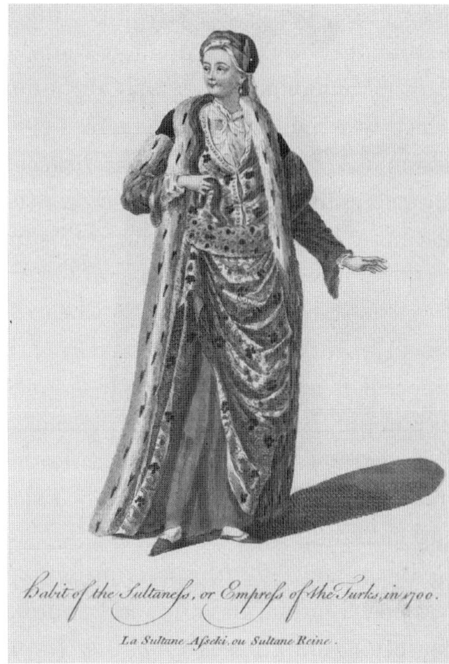

FIGURE 13.9 "Habit of the sultaness, or empress of the Turks in 1700. La sultane Asseki ou Sultane reine," from *A collection of the dresses of different nations, antient [sic] and modern,* published in 1752–1772.
Credit: Art and Architecture Collection, Miriam and Ira D. Wallach Division of Art, Prints and Photographs, the New York Public Library, Astor, Lenox and Tilden Foundations.

firmly sewn down with small, neat running stitches (Figure 13.5). The sleeves are cut on the straight of grain, fully lined and tidily finished. A strong looped thread (chain stitch) functions as piping around the neckline to the bust, strengthening this area and leaving a clean edge. The unlined back and side skirt panels are neatly sewn together with a small French seam, as are the inset gores, except where the selvage is used as a self finish to eliminate bulk and unnecessary sewing[13] (Figure 13.4).

The majority of the embroidery on the robe is silk floss except for the cross-stitch along the shoulder. The edges of the fronts and the hem are turned and caught with a rudimentary running stitch. All around the edge of the robe are traces of a brown silk Z-twist thread and stitch holes. Conservator Shirley Ellis concluded that the loose threads are original as she took samples of silk from the proper right of the upper dress opening and one from the proper left of the sleeve hem. They both appear to be a similar weight.[14] Thus it is reasonable to surmise that the open robe originally had a trim at the edges, possibly fur or fringe that would weight the very light taffeta and keep it in place on the underdress. Comparison with fashion plates of the period, discussed later, supports this theory.

TURQUERIE

The Ottoman caftan may well be the principal influence on the style of the open robe. Middle Eastern dress was "well known to upper levels of society in the West before the 15th century" (Rodenbeck 2001: 68), and European artists, such as the Venetian Giovanni Bellini (ca. 1430–1516), visited Istanbul and painted oriental costumes in great detail. By the eighteenth century *Turquerie* or Turkmania influenced music, literature, the theater, the decorative arts, and fashion. Prints based on paintings by Jean-Batiste Vanmours, *Recueil de Cent Estampes representant differentes Nations du Levant,* which were published in Paris in 1714, were circulated in England as a masquerade album in 1757 (*Collection of the Dresses of Different Nations*) and helped to feed the craze for balls and masquerades *à la Turque* (Figure 13.9). Visitors to Istanbul commissioned albums of local costume in the late eighteenth century and also returned with imported textiles and costumes (Arcangeli 2007: 137–38; Baines 1981: 162; Inal 2011; Morris 1996; Raby 2007: 113–15; Ribeiro 1979; Rodenbeck 2001: 65–100; Scarce 1987: 38–112). Turkish influence was part of the general interest in exoticism and was quickly reported on in the new fashion magazines that began to circulate throughout elite circles in Europe. The use of them for personal dress is wonderfully illustrated in *Barbara Johnson's Album of Fashions and Fabrics* (Rothstein 1987). They regularly featured oriental inspirations and undoubtedly provided ideas for the design of the embroidered open robe, and indeed the Egyptian dress.

By the late 1790s the descriptions repeatedly evoked exotic origins, and Turkmania was no exception. In Paris and London, dresses were repeatedly identified with Turkish inspiration, such as a *robe à la Turque (Gallery of Fashion,* June 1, 1798: fig. 184), a *robe en Demi-Turque* (*Costume Parisien* 8 [1800]: plate 205), or a sable-trimmed robe described as *Mamelouc (Gallery of Fashion,* February 1, 1800: fig. 208).[15] Many of the designs are trimmed with beads, fringe, or fur that seems to be missing from the embroidered overdress. Even in 1803 *La Belle Assemblée* informed its readers that "the prevailing colours are Egyptian brown, green, crimson and amber" (February 1803: 38), a description reflecting the interest in Napoleon's campaign. Interestingly, it is also the same color palette as the embroidery of the open robe, which may well have been influenced by earlier exotic descriptions, as Aileen Ribeiro notes that "at the end of the eighteenth century 'Sultane' and 'circassian' were very popular names for British dresses based on the original Turkish kaftan" (1979: 20; Pietsch 2011).

Fashion was also inspired by more factually based descriptions of Eastern customs and dress. The letters written by Lady Mary Wortley Montagu (1689–1762), wife of the British ambassador to Istanbul, which were published in 1763, were widely read, and the paintings of her wearing authentic Turkish or Turkish-inspired fashion were also known. In 1717 she carefully described her own "admirably becoming" Turkish ensemble, a "Caftan, of the same stuff as my drawers, is a robe exactly fitted to my shape and reaching to my feet, with very long straight falling sleeves" ([1763] 1800: 149).[16] The Turkish fashions described in print and images share the same features: a fitted, rounded bust and a long, open robe, and they are frequently trimmed with a fringe or fur that completed the dress. The fitted bodice of the embroidered open robe skims closely around the breast, recalling the bustline of the Turkish *anteri* or the *gomlek.* The robe also has a similar flat pattern construction with a one-piece back and triangular gores inset at the hem and long sleeves (Scarce 1987: 58, 71, 93). The design of the open robe is clearly based on the latest lexicon of images and taste of the moment, whether deliberately imitating a Turkish style or, more simply, the Turkish- and exotic-influenced fashions of the day.[17]

EMBROIDERY

The robe is a rare example of pictorial embroidery worked on fashion at the end of the eighteenth century. It is competent domestic work in an original fanciful design. By the end of the century the elaborate and often floral needlework found on silk aprons, bodices, and dresses that is typical of the first half of the eighteenth century was replaced with more delicate embroidered borders of flowers, bows, swags, and garlands or overall dotted or sprigged designs, as well as a fashion for whitework and tambour (hook) work (Kendrick 1967: 166–67; Thunder 2006). Embroidery was a clear marker of femininity, even worthy of admiring press reports about the royal princesses embroidering their own dresses (Morris 1966: 522; Parker 1984). This robe clearly signifies the creative design and embroidery skills of its maker and wearer.

The garment was sewn up before it was embroidered so that the pattern flows fluidly over the seams around the entire robe from neck to hem, and around the cuffs of the sleeves (Figure 13.2 and 13.8). A simple long-and-short satin stitch is used throughout and is animated by smaller vertical running stitches that secure the longer threads and add texture, depth, and color. One color of light brown has deteriorated wherever it has been used, indicating that something in the dye is causing it to degrade. Satin stitch was the dominant technique for needlework pictures of the period, creating "silky and smart" pictorial two-dimensional effects copied from prints (Kendrick 1967: 168–69; Synge 2001: 218–21).

ICONOGRAPHY

The iconography on the open robe is derived from a fusion of traditional European motifs seen in fine and decorative art with sources taken from Eastern export goods. The embroidered motifs are drawn from old and new prints and books published with the intention of being "useful" for gardening, painting, needlework, or japanning, as well as from details in furnishing textiles, laces, porcelains, silver, furniture, or architectural details in plaster or woodwork: all artifacts displayed and used within upper- and upper-middle-class homes (Synge 2001: 194–98). Thus, sources to inspire embroidery were readily at hand for the young woman to draw on and only required some imagination and ingenuity to adapt them to the dress pattern.

The education of young women in needlework, documented so clearly in samplers, included not only techniques of stitchery but also the skill of how to draw and transfer motifs to create new work. The embroiderer herself probably accomplished the design and transfer of the pattern, which would explain the lack of consistent scale and naive rendering, as a professional pattern drawer would have produced a more traditional or harmonious work (Kendrick 1967: 167–69; Synge 2001: 195–97; Thunder 2006). The

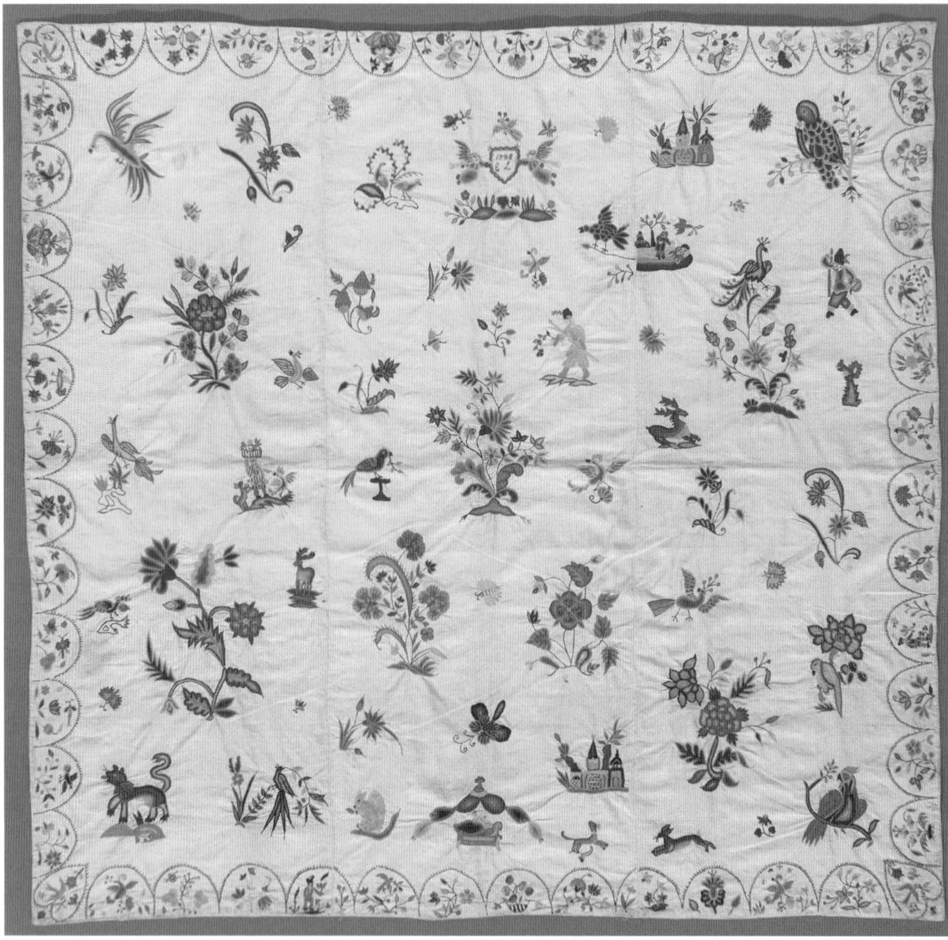

FIGURE 13.10 A child's English coverlet, dated 1728, shares a similar disregard for scale. Twill with linen warp and cotton weft embroidered in wool threads in chain, buttonhole, stem, French knot, and hollie stitches with classical and chinoiserie flora and fauna taken from seventeenth-century patterns (slips) and motifs recorded in samplers.
Credit: Royal Ontario Museum 970.128. Given in memory of Gerard Brett, M.C., M.A., director of the Royal Ontario Museum of Archaeology, by Mr. and Mrs. Edgar J. Stone.

ink outline is still clearly visible in one area under the proper right arm that is not embroidered. The motifs are repeated but not in a clear order; rather, they follow a fluid, fanciful, and continuous trail around the edge of the garment to the center back, where the tree is upside down (Figures 13.2 and 13.5). This is not a mistake but a design decision because having the tree upside down is the simplest solution to continue the pattern and keep the direction of the overall design consistent. The same tree is worked right side up at the cuffs. This circular format around the edge of the robe recalls the painted borders of plates, as will be discussed.

ENGLISH DOMESTIC EMBROIDERY

The motifs of hillocks, trees, and animated animals and birds were part of a well-known design vocabulary in the late eighteenth century. The seemingly incongruous relationship between the differing scales of the trees, animals, and cherub is seen in an earlier example of English domestic needlework. A child's coverlet is embroidered in wool with classical and chinoiserie forms of flora and fauna taken from seventeenth-century patterns (slips) and motifs recorded in earlier samplers (Figure 13.10). These have been freely adapted from English crewel work (wool embroidery) hangings that were, in turn, influenced by imported Indian chintz. The inconsistent scale of the images and the naive rendering in the child's bedcover are similar to the domestic patterning skills of the embroiderer of the open robe. The mother who may have made this coverlet is depicted in the canopied bed at the centre bottom. At the center top, a cartouche inscribed "1728 EL" probably records the initials and date of birth of the child for whom the coverlet was made. It is held up by two trumpeting angels with halos similar to those on the three winged angels or cherubs embroidered on the robe. An angel embroidered on a sampler in the City of Bristol Museum and Art Gallery (TA1459), dated 1790, worked by a twelve-year-old at Mrs. Rouches School, has similar putti with bow and arrow (Walton 1983: fig. 27). The three angels on the open robe are a fusion of Christian angels with wings and halos and naked classical putti or cherubs holding what could be heart-shaped bows, harps, or lyres (it is not clear which), and are designs sourced from girls' learned examples on samplers or other household needlework.

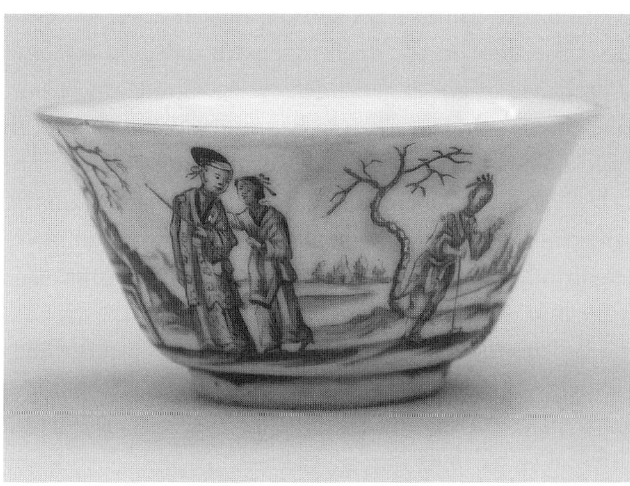

FIGURE 13.11 Chinese porcelain tea bowl, ca. 1700, later decorated with a chinoiserie scene in black enamel and gold in Breslau or Vienna in the late 1730s. The trees on the bowl and the dress are both influenced by Chinese export wares.
Credit: Tea bowl with chinoiseries, China, ca. 1700. Decorated in Breslau, ca. 1730. Porcelain, black enamel, and gold, 3.2 x 7.2 cm. Collection of the Gardiner Museum, gift of George and Helen Gardiner [G83.1.828].

CHINOISERIE

By the end of the eighteenth century, the mélange of flora, fauna, insects, and animals embroidered on the open robe was part of an established rendition of exotic images assimilated from luxury Asian export wares that decorated domestic surroundings. *The Ladies Amusement; or, Whole Art of Japanning Made Easy* explained how to do this:

> With Indian or Chinese subjects greater liberties may be taken, because luxuriance of fancy recommends their productions more than propriety, for in them is often seen a butterfly supporting an elephant, or things equally absurd; yet from their gay colouring and airy disposition seldom fail to please. ([1762] 1959: n.p.)

The embroiderer of this robe looked around her surroundings and creatively interpreted what she saw, without concern for distinctions between English, Chinese, Persian, and Indian motifs. The figures, architecture, birds, animals, and nature are playfully mixed and rendered to express an overall exoticism that today may seem incongruous but brought the "delights of arcadia, the out-of-doors inside" (Synge 2001: 194). The influence of Asian luxury goods in Europe had been felt since the seventeenth century, and by the early eighteenth century, the Dutch East India Company had imported 43 million pieces of porcelain, and the English, French, Swedish, and Danish companies another 30 million (Berg 2003: 236–37). The resultant effect on the mercantile systems created new "imitative processes" and products designed in Europe, for Europeans, based on imports from China, Japan, and India (239–40). The embroidered robe is an example of an object created in this cross-cultural mileau.

A comparison of the trees on the open robe with those on ceramics illustrates the long history and exchange of goods and imagery. A white Chinese porcelain tea bowl (ca. 1700) was later decorated (ca. 1730s) in Breslau or Vienna with a chinoiserie scene in black enamel and gold, and the tree bears a strong similarity to the one on the open robe (Figure 13.11).[18] The striking creatures in the border pattern on the open robe can be compared to the chinoiserie of Meissen's pattern of fabulous animals (*fabeltiere*) that was inspired by mythical beasts on Chinese *famille verte* porcelains. One version in the style associated with A.F. von Lowenfinck is bordered on a plate with a continuous chinoiserie scene of a sun above an oriental landscape.[19] This layout of the design and the tree itself are strikingly similar to the embroidery, indicating that imported and European porcelain patterns could well have been used as a design source for the embroidery because "Oriental styles were a breath of fresh air, and so easily mixed with other designs, and were so adaptable to innovation as to produce a new chinoiserie... le goût moderne" (Berg 2003: 231).

INDO-PERSIA

Exported luxury Indian chintz hangings (palampores) printed and painted with the tree of life, undulating grounds, rich foliage, flowers, animals, and birds that fused

Indian, Persian, Chinese, and European design traditions were widespread decorations in the interiors of the elite and could well have been another design source for the embroidery (Figure 13.12). Designing for specialized and varied markets was an expertise of Indian manufacturers and ensured their goods, particularly chintz, were available to a wide range of customers. This is reflected in a letter sent from The Hague on August 5, 1716, by Lady Mary Wortley Montagu. She apologizes for not buying her correspondent the lace she had requested because it cost as much as in London. But, in amends, she says, "If you want any India goods, here are a great variety of penny-worths, and I shall follow your orders with great pleasure and exactness" ([1763] 1800: 5).

The embroidered trees, animals, exotic creatures, and birds, as well as the hillocks and floating islands with animals, also bear strong similarities to those seen in Indian export palampores. An embroidered deer with its head turned and a dappled back recalls similarly awkwardly drawn ones on palampores (Figures 13.8 and 13.13).[20] The grasshopper is a bizarre fusion of East and South East Asian animal and

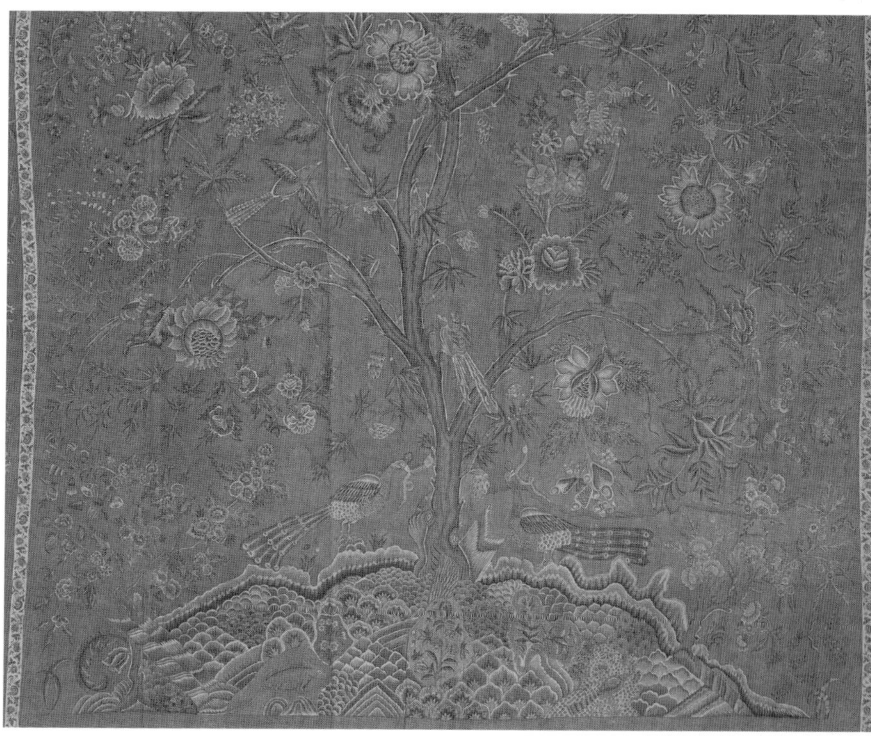

FIGURE 13.12 Motifs in the open robe bear strong similarities to those seen in the details of Indian palampores with flying and sitting birds and a peacock holding a twisting snake on a hillock with a rabbit(?). India, Coromandel Coast, for the European (Dutch?) market, first half of the eighteenth century.
Credit: Royal Ontario Museum 2011.27.1. This acquisition was made possible with the generous support of the Louise Hawley Stone Charitable Trust.

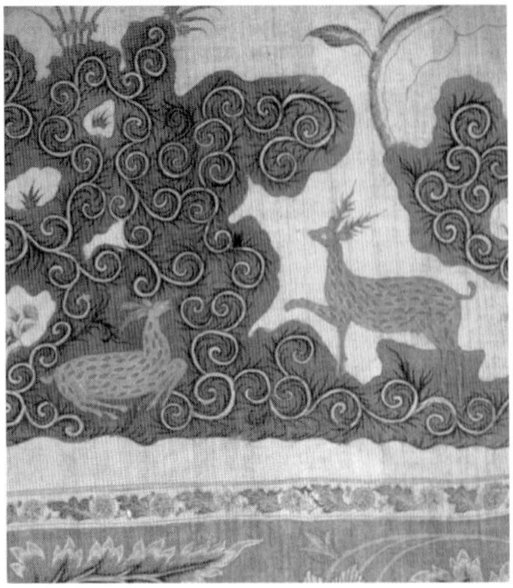

FIGURE 13.13 The rich details of a painted and dyed palmapore depicts chinoiserie rockery with deer and floral border. The embroiderer was likely influenced by similar Indian exports. India, Coromandel Coast, for the European market, second half of the eighteenth century. *Credit*: Royal Ontario Museum 934.4.6. Gift of Mrs. Harry Wearne.

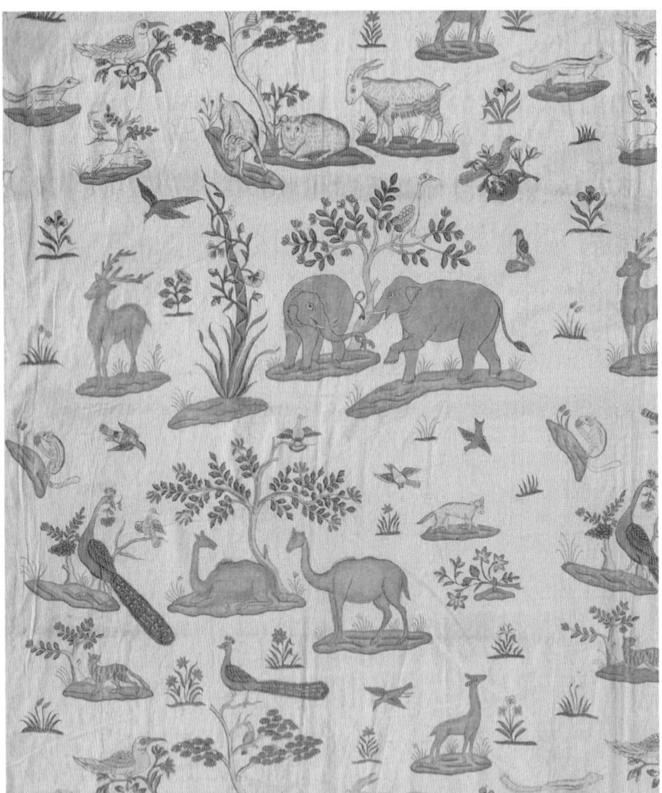

FIGURE 13.14 An Indian export block-printed and painted chintz has a repeat pattern of floating grounds with animals, flowering trees, plants, and flying and perched birds that has stylistic affinities with the embroidery motifs on the dress and is typical of the rich decorative imagery that was circulating in luxury goods across Europe. India, Coromandel Coast, for the European market, late eighteenth century.
Credit: Royal Ontario Museum 2009.125.12. This acquisition was made possible with the generous support of the Louise Hawley Stone Charitable Trust.

insect (Figure 13.8). An Indian export block-printed and painted chintz made for the European furnishing market is composed of a repeat pattern of animals, birds, and trees in the Persian and Moghul pictorial tradition (Figure 13.14). There are stylistic affinities with the embroidery on the open robe; for instance, the floating grounds, and the flowering tree behind the giraffes with the bird flying toward it, are echoed in the embroidered lilac bush and bird flying away from the pine tree or sitting in the palm tree (Figure 13.15).

The foliate borders of palampores often had inscriptions that are difficult to decipher placed in cartouches that marked the artisan, the location where it was made, or words from the Koran (Jacqué and Nicolas 2008: 98). This may account for the word or bird song "SI MOO"(?) held by the bird in the tree, which may also be derived from birds holding twisting snakes in their beaks, a motif frequently seen in chintz palampores (Figure 13.12). The "S" is rendered backward consistently three times and may be a mistake in the transfer of the word to the textile, or an interpretation of the exotic Indian marks written on the chintz by the dyers (Figure 13.16). Even Anglo-Indian ivory,

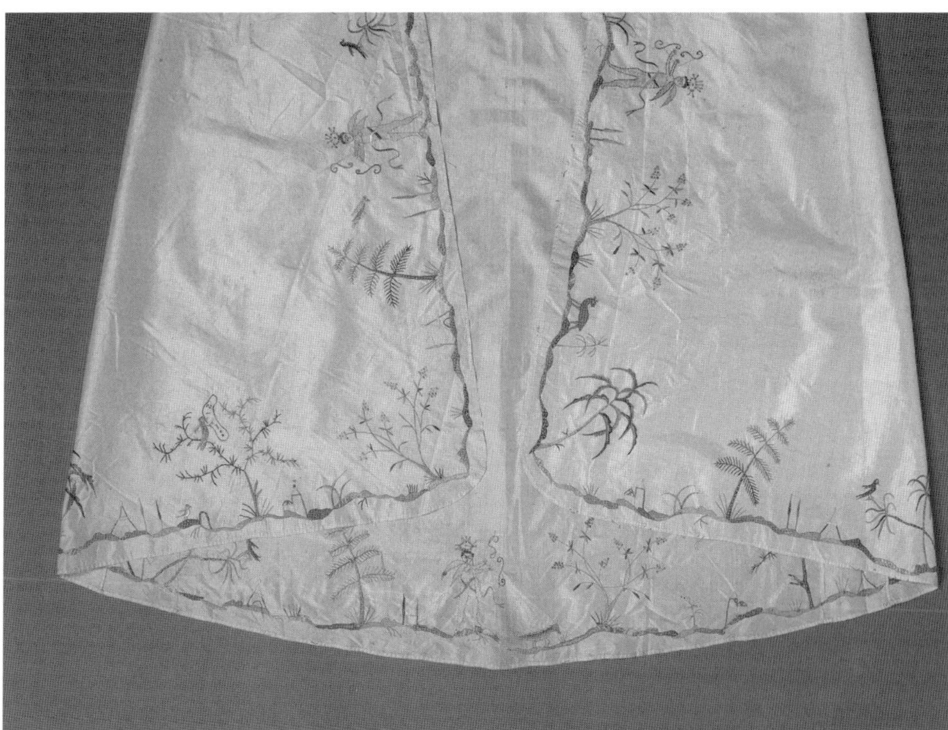

FIGURE 13.15 The border of the open robe is embroidered in a continuous landscape of rolling hillocks, trees, and shrubs including banana, palm, and pine trees and a flowering lilac bush amid structures of tents or pagoda-like forms populated by birds and animals, inspired by motifs seen on Indian export goods, as well as a cupid or angel with a bow and arrow (or lyre?) and a sparkling halo. *Credit*: Royal Ontario Museum 2010.24.1.

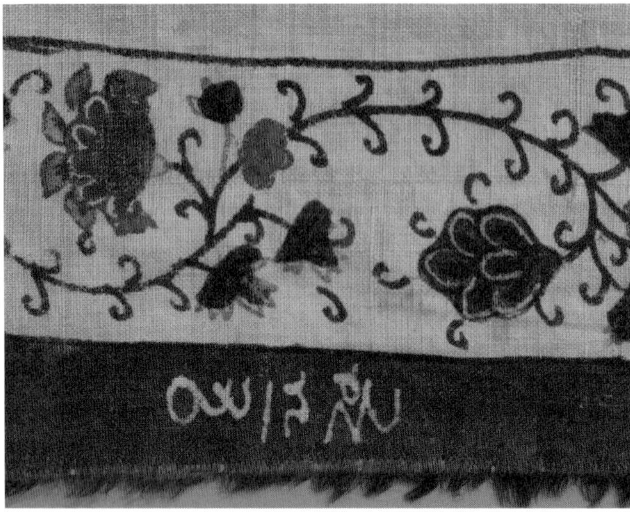

FIGURE 13.16 The source for the bird's exotic "song" may be taken from marks made by the Indian artisans or manufacturers to track orders on export goods. India, Coromandel Coast, for the European market, dated 1764.
Credit: Royal Ontario Museum 934.4.4.

veneered and etched furniture of the late eighteenth century from Vizagapatam of the same period, shares a similar neoclassical clarity of space and narrative design that can be compared to the ivory ground of the robe that is almost "etched" with the embroidery (Jaffer 2001: 172–208).[21]

SUMMARY

The dress documents the collaboration of the dressmaker and wearer to create a new overdress. It records dressmakers' changing craft skills at the end of the eighteenth century, when neoclassical taste required innovative and more complex pattern making in order to make the new fashions, which required a high waist, a tight fit over the shoulder and upper back, and long fitted sleeves. The dressmaker had to develop her existing draping skills and combine them with experimental dressmaking adapted from tailored patterns observed from menswear. It required the wearer to undergo new postural and sensual experiences to accommodate the high waist and narrow pulled-back shoulders, and even to manage the train; as Doris Langley Moore has noted, "The trailing back had to be picked up from behind and carried, a gesture as piquant as lifting the skirt a hundred years earlier" (1971: 45). A close examination of the cut reveals a sense of the physical and emotional excitement of wearing a new style that is such an important and ephemeral aspect of fashion. The feel of fashion, not only the look, makes it new, and both are central to styles becoming outdated. The open robe was made in the very latest fashionable silhouette and documents *how* fashion plates and writings were interpreted into actual three-dimensional clothes influenced by Turquerie and Ottoman dress.

The cut had to be solved, and the dress assembled, before the embroidery design was drawn and worked. The motifs were inspired and adapted from trade goods such as Indian export chintz, European and East Asian porcelain, lacquer, and earlier domestic sources such as European samplers and pattern books. The embroidery pattern and the cut show the cross-cultural links between the Ottoman Empire and Asia and the way they extended to create a new world of fashionable European domestic luxury goods. The robe illustrates how, in an English domestic context, probably outside of the social center of London, colorful export goods underwent another level of mutation and hybridization as they were reframed and incorporated into fashionable daily life. The open robe required a great deal of planning and time for each stage and conjures up a rich picture of the surroundings, influences, inspiration, and aspiration for the dressmaker and young woman who embroidered and wore this garment.

CONCLUSIONS FROM LOOKING AT FASHION

This analysis of the 1790s embroidered open robe and the Yves Saint Laurent evening dress highlights the importance of object analysis as a unique source for stimulating research in both well-documented and under-documented areas. The careful study of fashion and textiles, examining construction, style, and decoration, enlarges our understanding of historical and modern fashion and offers a unique insight into interpreting the documentary evidence in art and text. Actual worn garments can verify the canon of fashion history, and they can also complicate what we think we know and generate new ideas that contextualize the production and wearing of fashion. It is for these reasons that object analysis offers such a rich, multifaceted, and often unexpected history of dressmakers, consumers, fashion imagery, fashion writing, politics, and taste. It is evidence of the circulation, interpretation, and transformation of goods. Looking closely at physical objects helps us to understand fashion as "wearers and viewers might have ascribed... for the feelings they may have promoted, and the resonances and connections that they might suggest. Above all, our explanations must not be reductive." Extant garments encapsulate the complexity of fashion in time and make evident the "playfulness of fashion itself" (Vincent 2009: xvi).

NOTES

The author would like to thank Kristiina Lahde, Karla G. Livingston, Susan Charbonneau, Claire Lewarne, and Shirley Ellis for their tireless and careful assistance with artifacts, as well as Christine Elson for her immeasurable assistance with the pattern. Appreciation is also extended to colleagues Deepali Dewan, Patti Proctor, Karin Ruedenz, Sarah Fee, and Anu Liivandi at the Royal Ontario Museum, who have offered insights, as well as to Meg Andrews, Michele Majer, Johannes Pietsch, Peter McNeil, Giorgio Riello, Philip Sykas, Laura Thornley, and Amy de la Haye.

1. ROM 2011.59.1.1–2 and ROM 2010.24.1. This acquisition was made possible with the generous support of the Louise Hawley Stone Charitable Trust.
2. *Vogue*, Australia, September 2004.

3. Unfortunately, and interestingly, Yves Saint Laurent did not permit reproduction of a detail of the sequins for this publication. The company holds the copyright for this dress as it falls under the "useful article" relating to the production of fewer than fifty pieces under Canadian copyright law.
4. Under Canadian copyright law the museum has to secure permission (exhibition and photography rights) for use of any design that is produced in fewer than fifty units. The company did not permit the author to include a photograph of the ROM dress in this chapter as they determined it was a commercial use.
5. Jean Druesedow, e-mail correspondence with Veronika Jervers, Research Fellow Kate Strasdin, November 2, 2011 (copied to author).
6. A two-piece formal dress by Morin-Blossier of pale yellow satin applied with a design of mauve orchids, inserts of chiffon, sequins, diamante, and beads (ca. 1903, French; ROM 942.12.3.AB; gift of Lieutenant-Colonel James W. Flanagan).
7. At the ROM the final presentation of fashion and textiles is the result of a continual dialogue between the conservator, curators, and textile department technicians Karla Livingston and Kristiina Lahde, both of whom have art school and collections management training. Dorothy K. Burnham (1911–2004) joined the staff in 1929 as a second assistant draftsman and became the first curator of textiles in 1939. Katherine B. Brett attended art school and joined the ROM with Mrs. Burnham. Dr. Adrienne Hood was a weaver when she began under Mrs. Burnham.
8. Talbot Hughes (1913: 226) wrote one of the better descriptions of this period: "about 1780 we find a change of style appearing in a shorter waist. . . . About 1790 the mode again began to change to a classic style, still higher in the waist, with a short tight sleeve, at times puffed in the upper part, or an outer and under sleeve. . . . The fronts of this type of bodice were mostly buttoned or pinned up to the shoulders over a tight underfront, the skirt opening about 18 inches at the sides, thus saving a fastening at the back. . . . The sleeves were very long and were rucked on the arm."
9. The full text of the Cruickshank print reads: "Shepards I have lost my waist, Have you seen my body? Sacrificed to Modern Taste, I'm quite a Hoddy Doddy. For Fashion I that part forsook, Where Sages place the Belly, 'Tis gone—and I have not a nook, For Cheese cake, Tart or Jelly. Never shall I see it more, Till Common Sense Returning, My Body to My Legs restore. Then, I shall cease from mourning; Folly & Fashion do prevail, To Such extremes among the Fair, A Woman's only Fop and Tail, The Body's Banished God knows where!!!" It is likely that "body" also refers to the stays that were shortened or discarded for the new high-waisted fashion as well as the torso.
10. Formal evening or ball dress with spencer and fichu of linen tabby embroidered with gilt filé and sequins, European, possibly French, 1795–1800 (ROM 968.335.15.A-D, gift of Susan Carrier Meek).
11. Family history records that it is an Egyptian textile given to John Hely-Hutchinson (1757–1832), second Earl of Donoughmore, Ireland, who entered the eighteenth Dragoons in 1774 and rose through the ranks to become a full general by 1813. The *London Times* published his dispatches from Egypt describing the united British and Turkish campaign that ended in the capture of Cairo and Alexandria and the surrender of the French. The letter discussing the history of the textile is dated May 24, 1931. Rita Brown has generously drafted

a pattern of this dress (ROM 2004.33.1. This acquisition was made possible by the generous support of the Louise Hawley Stone Charitable Trust.).

12. The inset of the sleeve can be compared to a spencer (ROM 969.178.1) and a Scottish dress from 1800–1802 made from block-printed Indian silk (ROM 983.32.1, gift of Horst Dantz).
13. A French seam is a seam that is sewn twice, first with the right sides of the textile outward, and then on the wrong side to enclose the raw edges within the new seam.
14. The analysis of silk thread was conducted by Shirley Ellis, ROM textile conservator, January 12, 2012.
15. For the *robe à la Turque*, see the *Gallery of Fashion*, June 1, 1798: fig. 184; for the *robe en Demi-Turque*, see *Costume Parisien* 8 (1800): plate 205; and for the *Mamelouc*, see *Gallery of Fashion*, February 1, 1800: fig. 208. By the early 1800s it seems that *mameluck* frequently meant some kind of overdress, open in front and often with an uneven hem, and usually fur trimmed. Later it also referred to costumes with overlong puckered-up sleeves. See *Mameluck a pointe de fichu* (*Costume Parisien* 12 [1803]: plate 548), *Mameluck bordé en mousseline Turque* (*Costume Parisien* 12 [1804]: plate 572), *Jupon et Mameluck garni de Torsal (Costume Parisien* 13 [1805]: plate 594; *Turban à pointe Mameluck à garniture crevée* (*Costume Parisien* 13 [1805]: plate 596), and *manches a la mameluck (Costume Parisien* [1810]: plate 1051). Johannes Pietsch (2011) has discussed the complicated and interesting use of Circassian nomenclature at the end of the eighteenth century.
16. Lady Wortley Montagu also describes a woman wearing a caftan "of gold brocade, flowered with silver, very well fitted to her shape and showing to admiration the beauty of her bosom" ([1763] 1790: 193–94).
17. This is possibly prefigured in the *lévite* of the 1780s; see, for example, the portrait of the Duchess de Polignac by Vigée Le Brun (Musée national des chateaux de Versailles et de Trianon, MV 8971). Thanks to Philip Sykas.
18. Deep cup with figure in a boat, ca. 1550–1590, porcelain, underglaze cobalt blue. China, Jingdezhen. Gift of Ann Walker Bell, G01.2.27 in the Gardiner Museum, Toronto, Ontario, Canada.
19. Meissen "Fabeltier" and chinoiserie plate from the gold-and-black-striped service, in the style associated with A. F. von Lowenfinck. G83.1.649–650, Gardiner Museum, Toronto, Ontario, Canada.
20. For instance, ROM 934.4.6.
21. Thanks to Deepali Dewan.

BIBLIOGRAPHY

Arcangeli, Catarina Schmidt. 2007. "'Orientalist" Painting in Venice, 15th to 17th Centuries." In Stefano Carboni (ed.), *Venice and the Islamic World, 828–1797,* 120–39. New York: Metropolitan Museum of Art; New Haven, CT: Yale University Press.

Arnold, Janet. 1964. *Patterns of Fashion 1: Englishwomen's Dresses and Their Construction c.1660–1860.* London: Wace.

Arnold, Janet. 1966. *Patterns of Fashion 2: Englishwomen's Dresses and Their Construction c.1860–1940.* London: Wace.

Arnold, Janet. 1970. "The Classical Influence on the Cut, Construction and Decoration of Women's Dress c. 1785–1820." *Costume* 7: 17–32.

Arnold, Janet. 1985. *Patterns of Fashion 3: The Cut and Construction of Clothes for Men and Women c. 1560–1620.* London: Macmillan; New York: Drama Book.

Arnold, Janet. 2008. *Patterns of Fashion 4: The Cut and Construction of Linen Shirts, Smocks, Neckwear, Headwear and Accessories for Men and Women c.1540–1660.* With Jenny Tiramani and Santina M. Levey. London: Macmillan.

Baines, Barbara B. 1981. *Fashion Revivals: From the Elizabethan Age to the Present Day.* London: B. T. Batsford; New York: Drama Book.

Baumgarten, Linda. 2002. *What Clothes Reveal: The Language of Clothing in Colonial and Federal America: The Colonial Williamsburg Collection.* Williamsburg, VA: Colonial Williamsburg Foundation and Yale University Press.

Berg, Maxine. 2003. "Asian Luxuries and the Making of the European Consumer Revolution." In Maxine Berg and Elizabeth Eger (eds.), *Luxury in the Eighteenth Century: Debates, Desires and Delectable Goods,* 228–44. Basingstoke, UK: Palgrave Macmillan.

Bradfield, Nancy. 1968. *Costume in Detail: Women's Dress, 1730–1930.* London: Harrap.

Brett, Katherine B. 1966. *Women's Costume in Early Ontario.* Toronto: Royal Ontario Museum, University of Toronto.

Brett, Katherine B. 1967. *Modesty to Mod: Dress and Underdress in Canada, 1780–1967.* Toronto: Royal Ontario Museum, University of Toronto.

Brett, Katherine B. 1972. *English Embroidery: Sixteenth to Eighteenth Centuries Collections of the Royal Ontario Museum.* Toronto: Royal Ontario Museum.

Burnham, Dorothy K. 1973. *Cut My Cote.* Toronto: Royal Ontario Museum.

Clark, Hazel. 1999. "The Cheung Sam." In Valerie Steele and John S. Major (eds.), *China Chic: East Meets West,* 155–65. New Haven, CT: Yale University Press.

A collection of the dresses of different nations, ancient and modern. Particularly old English dresses. After the designs of Holbein, Vandyke, Hollar, and others. With an account of the authorities, … and some short historical remarks … To which are added the habits of the principal characters on the English stage. 1757–1772. London: Thomas Jefferys.

Crowston, Clare Haru. 2001. *Fabricating Women: The Seamstresses of Old Regime France, 1675–1791.* Durham, NC: Duke University Press.

Diderot, Denis, and Jean d'Alembert (eds.). [1751–1780] 1959. *L'Encyclopédie, ou Dictionnaire raisonné des sciences, des arts des métiers.* New York: Dover.

Entwistle, Joanne. 2000. *The Fashioned Body: Fashion, Dress and Modern Social Theory.* Cambridge, UK: Polity.

Flecker, Lara. 2007. *A Practical Guide to Costume Mounting.* Oxford: Butterworth-Heinemann.

Heiberger, Barbara. 2000. "Looking at Costume." In Mary Brooks (ed.), *Textiles Revealed: Object Lessons in Historic Textile and Costume Research,* 109–10. London: Archetype.

Hughes, Talbot. 1913. *Dress Design: An Account of Costume for Artists and Dressmakers.* London: J. Hogg.

Inal, Onur. 2011. "Women's Fashions in Transition: Ottoman Borderlands and the Anglo-Ottoman Exchange of Costumes." *Journal of World History* 22 (2): 243–76.

Irwin, John, and Katherine B. Brett. 1970. *Origins of Chintz: With a Catalogue of Indo-European Cotton-Paintings in the Victoria and Albert Museum, London, and the Royal Ontario Museum, Toronto.* London: Her Majesty's Stationery Office.

Jackson, Beverley. 2005. *Shanghai Girl Gets All Dressed Up*. Berkeley, CA: Ten Speed Press.

Jacqué, Jacqueline, and Brigitte Nicolas. 2008. *Féerie indienne: des rivages de l'Inde au royaume de France.* Paris: Somogy Editions.

Jaffer, Amin. 2001. *Furniture from British India and Ceylon: A Catalogue of the Collections in the Victoria and Albert Museum and the Peabody Essex Museum.* London: V&A Publications in association with the Peabody Essex Museum.

Kendrick, Albert Frank. 1967. *English Needlework.* London: Black.

The Ladies Amusement; or, Whole Art of Japanning Made Easy. [1762] 1959. Newport, UK: Ceramic Books.

Landini, Roberta Oris, and Bruna Niccoli. 2005. *Moda a Firenze 1540–1580: Lo stile di Eleonora di Toledo e la sua influenza.* Firenze, Italy: Pagliai Polistampa.

Landini, Roberta Oris, and Thessy Schoenholzer Nichols. 2011. *Moda a Firenze 1540–1580: lo stile di Cosimo de' Medici.* Firenze, Italy: M. Pagliai.

Montagu, Lady Mary Wortley. [1763] 1800. *Letters of the Right Honourable Lady M_y W_y M_e.* Vol. 1. London: T. Cadell, J. Murray, R. Baldwin.

Moore, Doris Langley. 1971. *Fashion through Fashion Plates, 1771–1970.* London: Ward Lock.

Morris, Marilyn. 1996. "The Royal Family and Family Values in Late Eighteenth-Century England." *Journal of Family History* 21 (4): 519–32.

Müller, Florence, Jill D'Alessandro, and Diane Charbonneau. 2008. *Yves Saint Laurent Style.* Trans. Josephine Bacon. New York: Harry N. Abrams.

North, Susan, and Jenny Tiramani (eds.). 2011. *Seventeenth-Century Women's Dress Patterns: Book One.* London: V&A Publications.

Palmer, Alexandra. 1997. "New Directions: Fashion History Studies and Research in North America and England." *Fashion Theory: The Journal of Dress, Body and Culture* 1 (3): 297–312.

Palmer, Alexandra. 2008. "Untouchable: Creating Desire and Knowledge in Museum Costume and Textile Exhibitions." *Fashion Theory: The Journal of Dress, Body and Culture* 12 (1): 31–64.

Parker, Rozsika. 1984. *The Subversive Stitch: Embroidery and the Making of the Feminine.* New York: Routledge.

Pietsch, Johannes. 2008. "The Art of Tailoring in the Seventeenth Century." In Johannes Pietsch and Karen Stolleis, *Kölner Patrizier- und Bürgerkleidung des 17. Jahrhunderts. Die Kostümsammlung Hüpsch im Hessischen Landesmuseum Darmstadt: Translation of Chapters I–III,* 33–80. Riggisberg, Switzerland: Abegg-Stiftung.

Pietsch, Johannes. 2011. "Robes à la Polonaise, à la Turque, à la Circassienne: Eastern Influences on French Fashion in the Late Eighteenth Century," unpublished paper presented at International Council of Museums Costume Committee meeting, Belgrade, Serbia, September 25–30.

Prown, Jules David. 1982. "Mind in Matter: An Introduction to Material Culture Theory and Method." *Winterthur Portfolio* 17 (1): 1–19.

Raby, Julian. 2007. "The Serenissima and the Sublime Porte: Art in the Art of Diplomacy 1453–1600." In Stefano Carboni (ed.), *Venice and the Islamic World, 828–1797,* 90–119. New York: Metropolitan Museum of Art; New Haven, CT: Yale University Press.

Rangstrom, Lena. 2002. *Lions of Fashion: Male Fashion of the 16th, 17th, 18th Centuries.* Stockholm: Livrustkammaren.

Ribeiro, Aileen. 1979. "Turquerie, Turkish Dress and English Fashion in the 18th Century." *Connoisseur* 201 (807): 16–23.

Rodenbeck, John. 2001. "Dressing Native." In Paul Starkey and Janet Starkey (eds.), *Unfolding the Orient: Travellers in Egypt and the Near East,* 61–100. Reading: Ithaca Press.

Rothstein, Natalie. 1987. *Barbara Johnson's Album of Fashions and Fabrics.* London: Thames and Hudson.

Salen, Jill. 2008. *Corsets: Historic Patterns and Techniques.* Hollywood, CA: Costume and Fashion Press.

Scarce, Jennifer. 1987. *Women's Costume of the Near and Middle East.* London: Unwin Hyman.

Silverman, Debora. 1986. *Selling Culture: Bloomingdale's, Diana Vreeland, and the New Aristocracy of Taste in Reagan's America.* New York: Pantheon Books.

Steele, Valerie. 2001. *The Corset: A Cultural History.* New Haven, CT: Yale University Press.

Steele, Valerie, and John S. Major (eds.). 1999. *China Chic: East Meets West.* New Haven, CT: Yale University Press.

Synge, Lanto. 2001. *Art of Embroidery: History of Style and Technique.* Woodbridge, UK: Antique Collectors' Club.

Taylor, Lou. 2002. *The Study of Dress History.* Manchester: Manchester University Press.

Taylor, Lou. 2004. *Establishing Dress History.* Manchester: Manchester University Press.

The Taylor's Complete Guide, or a Comprehensive Analysis of Beauty and Elegance in Dress. Containing rules for cutting out garments of every kind and fitting any person with the greatest accuracy and precision, adapted to all sizes, pointing out in the clearest manner the former errors in the profession and the method of rectifying what may have been done amiss. Rendered plain and easy to the meanest capacity. 1796. London: printed for Allen and West, 15, Paternoster-Row.

Thunder, Moira. 2006. "Object Lesson: Designs and Clients for Embroidered Dress, 1782–94." *Textile History* 37 (1): 82–90.

Vincent, Susan J. 2009. *The Anatomy of Fashion: Dressing the Body from the Renaissance to Today.* London: Berg.

Vollmer, John E. 1977. *In the Presence of the Dragon Throne: Ch'ing Dynasty Costume (1644–1911) in the Royal Ontario Museum.* Toronto: Royal Ontario Museum.

Vollmer, John E. 1983. *Decoding Dragons: Status Garments in Ch'ing Dynasty China.* Eugene: Museum of Art, University of Oregon.

Vollmer, John E. 2002. *Ruling from the Dragon Throne: Costume of the Qing Dynasty (1644–1911).* Berkeley, CA: Ten Speed Press.

Vollmer, John E. 2004. *Silks for Thrones and Altars: Chinese Costumes and Textiles.* Berkeley, CA: Ten Speed Press; Enfield: Airlift.

Vollmer, John E., Edward John Keall, and Evelyn Nagai-Berthrong (eds.). 1983. *Silk Roads, China Ships.* Toronto: Royal Ontario Museum.

Walton, Karin-Marina. 1983. *Samplers: Catalogue of the Collection of Samplers in the City of Bristol Museum and Art Gallery.* Bristol, UK: City of Bristol Museum and Art Gallery.

Waugh, Norah. 1954. *Corsets and Crinolines.* London: B. T. Batsford.

Waugh, Norah. 1968. *The Cut of Women's Clothes: 1600–1930.* New York: Theatre Arts Books.

Wilson, Verity. 1986. *Chinese Dress.* London: Victoria and Albert Museum.

14

Anthropology and Materiality

SARAH FEE

The renowned French social anthropologist Marcel Mauss (1967) marveled that some Australian Aborigines walked 400 miles (600 kilometers) in order to obtain ochre, a red pigment used for painting bodies. Ethnographic studies from around the globe have revealed the great human drive to enhance or alter the body, which may be variously—or simultaneously—linked to aesthetics, religion, politics, economy, and identity, making dress, in Mauss's term, a "total social fact." And yet, for most of the twentieth century, few anthropologists studied dress. Many rejected the notion of "fashion" for peoples outside the West, contributing in no small part to the stereotype of sartorial isolation and stasis, a stance that many current practitioners now seek to rectify. This essay examines anthropology's varied engagement with the study and collecting of dress, the methodological and theoretical stances that have abetted or hindered it, and some of its most recent articulations with fashion studies. To conclude, the article features two case studies from the western Indian Ocean, a globalized trading space from at least the first century C.E. They illustrate the benefits of the growing pan-disciplinary approach to dress and fashion, while stressing the value of placing the material nature of objects at the forefront of the inquiry, which, in these instances, reveals undocumented fashions in precolonial handwoven dress.

ANTHROPOLOGY AND THE CREATION OF "TRADITIONAL" DRESS

In her review of the recent literature on the anthropology of fashion, Karen Tranberg Hansen (2004: 372) notes that a general "anti-fashion tendency" historically prevailed in the discipline. Subject to the intellectual prejudices of their own society, anthropologists discounted fashion as frivolous. But this stance was also built into the methodologies and theories of the discipline itself. A brief review shows how as part of its "stock in trade" to underscore difference, the non-Western serving as a (utopian) foil to the West and to modernity, anthropology created the idea of traditional and unchanging dress outside the West, or, alternatively, argued that its religious or ritual significance put it above "mere fashion." It is little wonder that historians and fashion scholars have conventionally treated non-Western dress as the "non-fashion foil" (Niessen 2003: 244). In this essay, I employ Joanne Eicher and Mary Ellen Roach-Higgins's (1992: 15) expansive definition of dress as "an assemblage of body modifications and/or supplements."

Several studies have surveyed the history of anthropology's on-again, off-again interest in dress and fashion (Barnes 1992; Eicher 2000; Eicher and Roach-Higgins 1992; Hansen 2004; Schneider 1987, 2006; Schwarz 1979; Tarlo 1996; Taylor 2002).[1] American anthropologist Joanne Eicher usefully begins with anthropology's emergence as a distinct discipline in the late nineteenth century, when scholars remained in the metropolis, culling the reports of missionaries and travelers for data to create or bolster their theories. The reigning theories of the time were evolutionism and diffusionism, the former preoccupied with arranging cultures into hierarchies of progress, the second with showing historic links between societies through the diffusion of cultural traits through contact. Dress was central to both, contributing to James Frazer's theories on the origins of adornment, among others. More generally, efforts to make anthropology a distinct discipline, a science with credentials akin to natural history, led scholars to an overriding preoccupation with taxonomy and classification of peoples (Tarlo 1996). Clothing emerged as a way to reinforce cultural and racial types, to distance the colonial subject or the "primitive." These originally anthropological perspectives were spread and fixed in the popular imagination through postcards, world's fairs, and long-running museum displays (Figure 14.1).

In anglophone anthropology, the requisites and guidelines for documenting dress were dictated by the 1874 publication *Notes and Queries on Anthropology* (British Association for the Advancement of Science 1874). At first intended to guide the amateur traveler or missionary, it soon evolved into a handbook employed by anthropologists themselves (Urry 1972). In the 1892 second edition, dress was placed as the number-one query in ethnology, followed immediately by categories for personal ornaments, body painting, and tattooing. The subquestions are surprisingly sophisticated and in line with contemporary concerns, treating, in addition to materials and construction, dress's social meanings: its variation according to gender ("sex"), rank, ethnicity ("tribe"), and season; its roles in ritual; and the question "Is there anything which corresponds to what we term 'fashion'?" Since 1949, Yale University's Human Relations Area Files has compiled similar data on societies for cross-cultural comparison, with rubrics devoted to "Leather, Textiles, and Fabrics," "Clothing," and "Adornment." While today offering valuable historical information, these sources artificially separated dress and cloth making and isolated both from social life.

Emerging from sociology, early French anthropology was more sensitive to the local roles, categories, and conceptions of the body and adornment. Robert Hertz (1909)

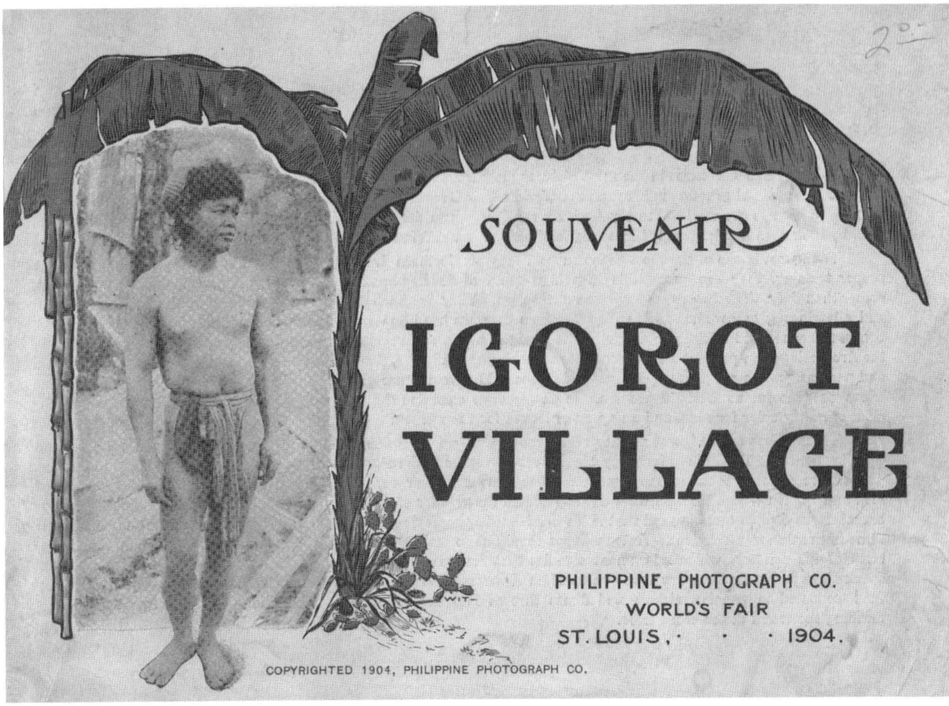

FIGURE 14.1 The large Philippines display at the 1904 World's Fair in St. Louis, Missouri, was arranged to contrast the "primitiveness" of the loincloth-clad Ifugao ("Igorot") of the highlands against the "progress" of lowland groups as evidenced by their Western dress. After public complaints of nudity, the Ifugao were temporarily clothed in American dress before returning to the loincloth. *Souvenir Igorot Village,* St. Louis: Philippine Photograph Co., 1904.
Credit: Special Collections, University of Delaware Library, Newark, Delaware.

explored the body as a symbolizing and categorizing system for social phenomena. Arnold Van Gennep (1909), also studying traits within their cultural context, found universal patterns in rites of passage. Foreshadowing recent interest in practice, performance, and the body, he documented dozens of examples from around the world showing the instrumentality of dress in ending, suspending, and creating new states and identities.

In the early decades of the twentieth century, the shift in anthropology's methodology and theoretical concerns opened potential vistas for the study of dress and fashion but closed many important ones, too. Rather than rely on reports from amateurs, or verbal statements alone, anthropologists developed a methodological hallmark, fieldwork: they themselves traveled to reside with a community, learn the local language, and observe and participate in daily life and rituals to supplement verbal reports. The new theoretical emphasis was on sociological studies of the parts of society and their interconnections. Everywhere, the belief that nonindustrial societies were fast disappearing before the face of progress led to so-called salvage ethnology: seeking the most "untouched" community and factoring out European contact. In place of sweeping cross-cultural comparisons, the end product was now a monograph that described a single "culture" in minute detail, typically based on one village or group, at a fixed point in time. In thus presenting societies in an imagined "ethnographic present," as bounded and closed, isolated from trade networks and larger political entities—notably the colonial state or nation-state—monographs greatly contributed to the myth of the traditional, that is, of non-Western peoples and their material culture as fixed and unchanging.

Anthropology's preoccupation with political systems, kinship, ritual, law, and economics in the 1950s and 1960s made little space for material culture of any type (Miller 1998). If dress appears in these studies, it is merely as an illustration or reflection of "society or social relations, as though these things exist above or prior to their own materiality" (Miller 2005: 2). In the 1960s and 1970s, semiotics, semiology, and structuralism, based on linguistic models, brought some interest in dress as systems of communication, in reading textiles as "texts" and relating garment construction or design to social categories (cf. Schwarz 1979). In this vein, Terrence Turner's 1980 landmark essay "The Social Skin" interpreted the body adornment of the Kayapo Indians of Brazil as a symbolic medium linked to social structure, the socialization of the body, and the binary oppositions of nature/culture, male/female, and so on. Marxist anthropology, meanwhile, generally disdained consumption, at best viewing objects as part of the superstructure, at worst as fetishized goods.

Several of the major criticisms that would be leveled against these paradigms—namely ahistoricity, lack of attention to agency and individual praxis, and a false division between Western and non-Western—were instrumental in returning dress and, ultimately, introducing fashion to anthropology's mainstream.

ANTHROPOLOGISTS COLLECTING DRESS

Fashion historians have remarked on the early and prolific collecting of ethnographic dress as compared to articles of Western clothing (Taylor 2004). Rather than the result of the prescience of a few individuals, or the gender or personal tastes of collectors, the assembling of ethnographic textiles and dress was built into the institutional origins of anthropology, guided by many of the same theoretical paradigms outlined above. This naturally had consequences for the types of objects collected.

Until 1920, anthropologists were typically based not in the university but in the museum, often the natural history museum. Physical objects provided the equivalent of scientific specimens. *Notes and Queries* devoted an entire section to advising on the collecting and packing of such "specimens," including dress.[2]

At the museum, they were studied and displayed to illustrate evolutionary stages or to demonstrate the diffusion of cultural traits through historical contact. Thus, in 1923, anthropologist Ralph Linton collected for the Field Museum of Chicago over 500 pieces of dress from the island of Madagascar in the hopes of tracing the origins of the inhabitants, who live near the African coast but speak an Asian language. The museum phase of anthropology ended for the anglophone world in the 1920s but continued in France and other European countries for several decades. There, it was not uncommon for anthropologists to assemble and sell collections to museums as a way of funding fieldwork. With this motive, Alfred Métraux gathered significant holdings of material, including dress, from the Gran Chaco area of South America for several large museums.[3]

Reigning ideologies had consequences for the types of things collected. Both French and British manuals advised the gathering of the daily and usual, a "tin can," over "sumptuous jewelry" (Leiris 1931). Yet collectors often preferred decorated items over the unadorned. As Lou Taylor (2004) has noted, notions of authenticity were likewise influential. The handmade was preferred over dress incorporating imported fabrics, much as Edward Curtis famously airbrushed Western items from his photographic portraits of Native Americans. Thus Linton's collection of dress from Madagascar is limited nearly entirely to handwoven garments, even though at the time of collecting many Malagasy were dressing in some form of industrial fabric. Likewise, natural dyes were preferred over synthetics. As a consequence, large gaps exist for the modern era. Beyond the aesthetic, collectors were also attracted to garments of ritual or religious significance, often the most conservative in nature. It is thus not surprising that the early fashion theorist Georg Simmel (1904: 136) concluded that the foreign "is often regarded by primitive [sic] races as an evil." Most recently, the inclusion of textiles in the canon of world art—part of the ongoing reclassification of ethnographic "specimens"—has increasingly brought international dress into art museums. Here, the "Western-aesthetic perspective" defines "museum-quality" pieces as pre-twentieth century, in good condition, with strong graphic qualities, and typically exemplars of the known "canon" (Niessen 1999: 176). The emphasis on stasis and tradition continues.

Partial as they may be, when used critically museum collections offer novel information for studying dress in a given era or its change over time. Outside royal repositories, in Africa, Asia, and most parts of the Americas, few historic textiles survive in situ: they were often used until worn out, were buried with their owners, or otherwise did not survive, especially in tropical climates. Visual and textual sources likewise tend to be partial, authored by outsiders, and plagued with many gaps. Museum collections thus emerge as an essential archive for the study of dress and fashion (Allman 2004). And yet these vast quantities of ethnographic dress amassed by museums in the first half of the twentieth century were subsequently ignored by anthropologists as they moved into university departments.

In the growing literature on the anthropology of dress, the use of dress by anthropologists themselves deserves closer attention, revealing as it is of various power relations. Anthropological fieldwork is a delicate balance of integration that seeks close relationships, but also autonomy and access, to a wide range of peoples. Dress can play a pivotal role in shaping these essential encounters. As part of the Bureau of American Ethnology's first expedition to the Southwest in 1879, Frank Hamilton Cushing (Figure 14.2) took up residence among his Zuñi hosts and adopted local dress, finding it facilitated relations (Auerbach 2008). His rival, Matilda Stevenson, stuck to full Victorian garb for her visits to the pueblos, condemning Cushing's tactics; as a woman struggling to prove her scientific credentials, she likely enjoyed less latitude.[4] In British

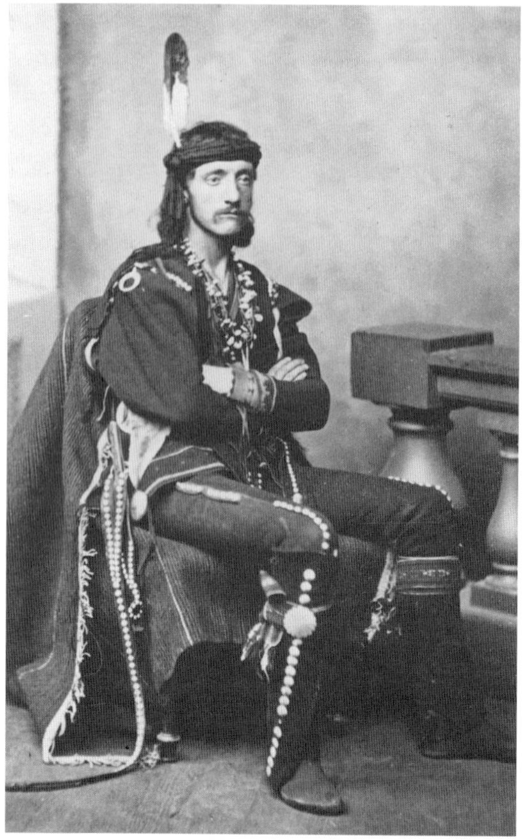

FIGURE 14.2 Pioneering field anthropologist Frank Hamilton Cushing in his Zuñi dress on a trip to Washington, D.C., in 1882.
Credit: Photograph by James Wallace Black. Courtesy of the Palace of the Governors Photo Archives (NMHM/DCA), 009147.

anthropology, often carried out in colonial possessions, dress was highly politicized, requiring full evening wear for the field, although here, too, the range of choices—and their results—were highly variable (Schumaker 2001). Many decades later, in the 1980s, the dilemma of "what to wear in the field" prompted Emma Tarlo (1996) to reorient her entire study to examining sartorial choices in India, one of several major works to begin (re-)establishing dress as a legitimate topic of inquiry.

ANTHROPOLOGY AND FASHION, 1980 TO THE PRESENT

Feminism and the rising interest in women's work and gender were instrumental in bringing textiles back into anthropology's sights. Annette Weiner's work (1976) on Trobriand women's cloth making—ignored by her famous male predecessor Bronislaw Malinowski—was followed by her seminal coedited volume, *Cloth and Human*

Experience (Weiner and Schneider 1989). The essays were concerned mainly with cloth's role as gift, tribute, or symbol, but dress soon came to the fore through the rising influence of cultural studies and postcolonial, poststructuralist, and postmodern theorists. According to Hansen (2004), three general trends in the discipline made dress of supreme interest: (1) a reorientation away from social structure and toward agency, practice, and performance; (2) a rising interest in identity, particularly ethnic and gendered; and (3) a new focus on the interconnecting forces of the global, the transnational, and the diaspora, resulting in multisited fieldwork. Rather than dress forms, anthropologists now studied the act of dressing the body, clothing's role in creating and performing identity, and garments' function as instruments of social reproduction, protest, or change. The result over the past thirty years has been an outpouring of studies from points around the globe by scholars of increasingly varied disciplines.

Where anthropology arguably made its original and lasting contribution to the field was in the realm of the cultural dimension of consumption and commodities. Particularly influential has been Arjun Appadurai's 1988 concept of "the social life of things," which emphasizes how commodities shift roles and meanings as they move over space and time and between actors; and Daniel Miller's (1998) work on meaning making in the mass-produced. Eicher's notion of cultural authentication—alternatively termed translation, indigenization, hybridization, or domestication—argues against the flattening effects of contact and globalization, demonstrating that peoples select imported items of dress as a function of preexisting patterns and adapt and make them their own. Others found evidence for the appropriation and subversion of mass-produced, foreign dress, even in asymmetrical power relations (Allman 2004; Comaroff 1996). "Non-Western consumers . . . are active agents in the construction of their own histories, even when adopting the very fashion of those they seek to resist" (Schneider 2006: 212). Adopting foreign forms of dress may offer a "technology of change," akin to railroads or the telegraph (Thomas 2003). It may enter into claims to participate in modernity and its promises of prosperity and well-being (Cole 2008; Ferguson 2002; Gott and Loughran 2010). Another body of literature emphasizes the false dichotomy of Western versus non-Western objects and peoples: the two worlds have been intertwined for many centuries, including the far reaches of Oceania (Colchester 2003; Küchler and Miller 2005; Thomas 1991) and Africa (Allman 2004; Kriger 2006; Rovine 2009a). Materiality theorists—some inspired by new smart textiles that connect the fabric directly to the impulses of the human brain and body (Küchler 2005)—have more radically argued for putting "things" at the center of anthropological inquiry and dissolving the dichotomies of mind/body and object/subject.

Concerning dress specifically, in the early twenty-first century the liveliest debates focus on fashion. Guiding most scholarship of fashion studies and history has been the assumption that it is a Western phenomenon, "an explicit manifestation of the rise of capitalism and Western modernity" (Allman 2004: 2). Anthropologists—and other scholars working in the global South—now challenge this as Eurocentric, claiming both fashion *and* modernity for Africa, Asia, Latin America, and indigenous peoples (Craik

1993; Finane 2008; Lemire 2010; Maynard 2004; Niessen 2003). Definitions of fashion continue to be varied and debated, but all share an emphasis on change (Tortora 2010). Rather than dwell on definitions, however, formerly divided disciplines and "camps" are building bridges through inclusive works on dress. In the twenty-first century it is standard for textbooks, readers, and collective volumes on fashion to include one or several chapters treating groups and designers outside Europe and North America (Clark and Palmer 2004; Lemire 2010; Paulicelli and Clark 2009; Welters and Lillethun 2007; to name a few). Since its founding, the journal *Fashion Theory* regularly features articles or entire issues on societies of the global South, while the monumental 2010 *Berg Encyclopedia of World Dress and Fashion* devoted volumes to Asia, Africa, and Latin America (Eicher 2010a). Collective and single-authored works focusing on the latter two areas are notably on the rise (Gott and Loughran 2010; Hansen 2000; Jennings 2011; Roces and Edwards 2007; Root 2005, 2010; Rovine 2009a).

The growing literature on world dress and fashion, meanwhile, highlights border zones and blurred boundaries (Brand and Teunissen 2005; Brydon and Niessen 1998; Craik 1993, 2009; Eicher 2010b; Maynard 2004). Production today occurs on all continents; designers and consumers everywhere create hybrid styles drawing inspiration from the streets of numerous locales; diaspora communities transport, adapt, and spread their dress; and "global" fashion is generally becoming "an array of competing and intermeshing systems cutting across western and non-western cultures" (Craik 1993: 5). These studies have helped to challenge the notions of the hegemony of Western fashion and a related trickle-down theory of emulation. Disciplinary methodologies, too, have become widely shared, with participant observation now a tool in cultural and fashion studies, and anthropologists increasingly historicizing their work and studying the fashion systems of European and settler societies.

Notwithstanding its opening of conceptual and disciplinary boundaries, this new scholarship largely limits its analytical framework and methodology to what Lise Skov and Marie Riegels Melchior (2010: 15) term a "culture based approach," which studies "dress and fashion as…something like a cultural formation of the visible identity." A complementary approach Skov and Melchior describe is object based; that is, it begins with the material artifacts themselves. Until recently this approach was negatively associated with "positivist" collection-bound museum curators with narrow antiquarian interests. Today scholars from many disciplines use the new material culture approaches to address contemporary theoretical interests. Their works demonstrate the great value of the physical object in divulging social and temporal aspects of fashionable dress otherwise invisible in visual or textual sources. For instance, historical specimens show that sumptuary laws were routinely flouted in societies from ancient China to eighteenth-century Africa (Kriger 2010; Steele and Major 1999: 25). As Canadian textile historian Dorothy Burnham (1973) demonstrated long ago, construction is the most conservative element of dress; fabrics, trim, and surface ornamentation are more susceptible to change. Although the untutored, outside gaze habitually overlooks such detail, local audiences—and the ethnographically informed analyst—may appreciate it as radical.

Numerous studies have argued this point in regards to Chinese dress, often held up as the iconic foil to the West's "dynamism" (Finane 2008; Steele and Major 1999; Wilson 1986). Noting continual change in the striping patterns of *mashru* cloth in Southwest Asia, A. Yusuf Ali wryly concluded in the early 1900s, "The difference is small to a casual observer; but taste and fashion account small and subtle differences to be the very criteria by which to distinguish the circle of the elite from the vulgar crowd" (quoted in Crill 1998: 145).

So, too, current scholarship betrays an overriding tendency to examine fashion within nineteenth-century modernity or, more often, the most recent phase of globalization.[5] Despite claims to reject "the West" as the motor of change, still, by insisting on moments of European contact or colonization, on industrial fabrics or tailored dress forms, or on current articulations with Western fashion styles and systems, these studies create the impression that only Western-inflected dress is fashionable.[6] It thus feeds into continuing claims from some areas of fashion studies for a unilinear trajectory, that "fashion was born in Europe" and then "spread to all the places that Europeans colonized," existing *alongside* "regional dress" (Welters and Lillethun 2007: xx–xxi). In a similar manner, most current writing celebrates the hybrid—a mixing of influences in a single dress item or an assemblage of dress forms—as a contemporary phenomenon. All too often, works retain the (opposing) categories "Western fashion" and "traditional (or ethnic) dress" rather than recognizing in the latter local fashion.

Arguably then, in several important ways the literature continues to take its cues from Euro-American systems, time lines, and concerns. Offering alternative narratives is the western Indian Ocean, a millennia-old interconnected trading space where Asian fabrics and merchants dominated the trade until the last decades of the nineteenth century.

ENGAGING MATERIAL: TWO CASE STUDIES FROM THE WESTERN INDIAN OCEAN

Canadian anthropologist Sandra Niessen (2003: 247) has forcefully observed that to be ethnographically responsible the study of fashion requires "the evidence of exhaustive cross-cultural study of non-Western clothing systems." A relatively overlooked area is the western Indian Ocean. Since at least the first century C.E. monsoon winds encouraged the exchange of peoples and goods along its shores lining East Africa, southern Arabia, and India, as well as to the Red Sea, Persian Gulf, and South China Sea. While numerous studies exist on the rich textile trade of this region, they rarely pause to consider the material properties of this cloth or its local consumption as dress. The two case studies from this region presented below use objects as their starting point to further the emerging body of literature exploring fashion cycles of fiber and surface for the most "traditional" of dress, the uncut handwoven body wrapper (Banerjee and Miller 2003: 5).

Akotifahana: *A Dynamic Nineteenth-Century Wrapper Fashion of Highland Madagascar*

The first case study comes from Madagascar, an island roughly the size of France lying off Mozambique. Notwithstanding its proximity to the African coast, it was originally settled in the early centuries of the first millennium by immigrants from Southeast Asia, who founded the core of Malagasy language and culture. Into the twentieth century, dress in the island consisted mainly in rectangular wrappers, typically woven by women using local fibers and dyes. The largest and most prestigious wrapper was the shoulder mantle (*lamba*), worn by the high ranking and well-to-do, as cover in the austral winter and for ceremonial dress. Measuring about one and a half by two yards (one and a half by two meters), it has a subdued design that characteristically featured warp striping in brick red, black, and natural shades, with twining or beadwork running weftwise at the two ends.

Departing from this classic model is the *akotifahana* mantle (Figure 14.3). Its warp stripes come in bright shades of peacock blue, magenta, green, and orange; even more unusual are its patterned figures, which run lengthwise along the cloth, sometimes covering much of its surface (Figure 14.4). For this great visual appeal, the akotifahana—which

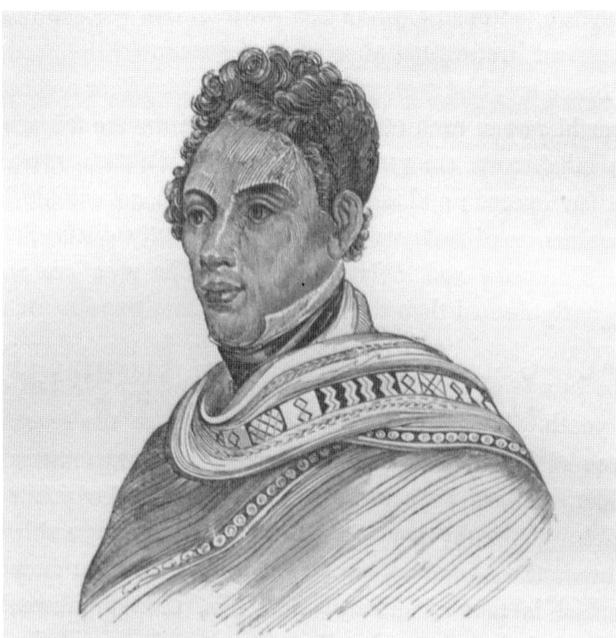

FIGURE 14.3 Andrianatsitohaiana, high-ranking Merina nobleman and civil servant, wearing a shoulder mantle with supplementary weft motifs while on a diplomatic mission to England in 1836. Engraving from a sketch from life by J. W. Sperling. From William Ellis, *History of Madagascar* (London: Fisher, 1838), vol. 1. *Credit*: George Baxter Collection, Victoria University Library (Toronto).

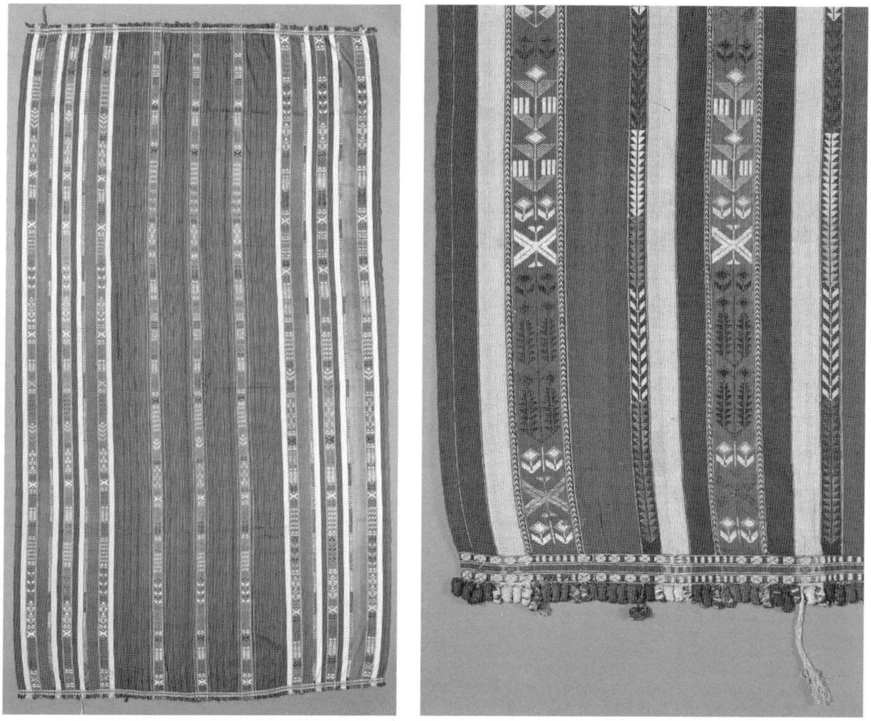

FIGURE 14.4 Overview and detail of a Merina brocaded silk cloth, ca. third quarter of the nineteenth century. *Bombyx* silk, natural dyes, supplementary wefts, warp floats, transverse selvage. 128 by 78 inches (281 by 171 centimeters). Royal Ontario Museum 2010.27.2. *Credit*: With permission of the Royal Ontario Museum. © Royal Ontario Museum.

accounts for less than 1 percent of the historical loom output—has been favored in Western publications, collections, and museum displays of Malagasy handwoven dress.

Following the general anthropological approach to dress sketched above, in the early twentieth century, authors presented the akotifahana as evidence for either the diffusion of cultural traits from Southeast Asia or the racial superiority of its weavers, the Merina people of the central highlands, perceived to be more "Asian" than their "African" coastal neighbors. From the 1980s came symbolic readings of color and motifs or, more frequently, of their communicative power as markers of sociopolitical identity. The few existing nineteenth-century accounts of the cloth indicate it was worn by noblewomen and noblemen. Various authors have thus argued that the cloth's colors or motifs encoded aristocratic or political rank, with one further claiming it as royal apparel (Mack 1989, 1993; Peers 2002, 2004; Philadelphia Museums 1906). There have been suggestions that British or French interventions encouraged or undermined the art form, but the general impression is of a timeless, sacred mantle reserved for religious, political, or ritual purposes, one far removed from external influences, market forces, and trading networks.

Examining a large number of specimens together with visual, linguistic, and textual sources, however, reveals that the akotifahana shoulder wrap was a short-lived secular aristocratic fashion. Increasing foreign trade, changing consumer demand, and professional weavers' agile responses to new fibers and dyes fueled its rise. It probably appeared early in the nineteenth century, knew regular and systematic change over time, and was abandoned as fashionable dress in the late nineteenth century, long before French colonization in 1896. Indeed, rather than from Europe, early inspiration for color, fiber, and pattern came mainly from Asia and the Arabian Peninsula.

Several physical aspects of the cloth point to recent origins and sources of stylistic influence. First are its supplementary wefts (Figure 14.5). Late eighteenth- and early nineteenth-century European descriptions of Merina handweaving—extremely detailed due to hopes to commercialize it—make no mention of this technique. Further, linguistic analysis of the term *akotifahana* suggests supplementary wefts originated as a simulation of a patterned Indian silk named *acoutis* imported into Madagascar in the late eighteenth century (Fee 2011b). The fiber likewise provides important clues. Most akotifahana were made entirely of "Chinese" silk (from *Bombyx mori*). Neither the worms nor mulberry bushes are indigenous to the island (Peers 2004). *Bombyx* floss was first made available to weavers in highland Madagascar by Arab traders, specifically by merchants from Oman, who at this time controlled the rich Persian Gulf supplies of silk

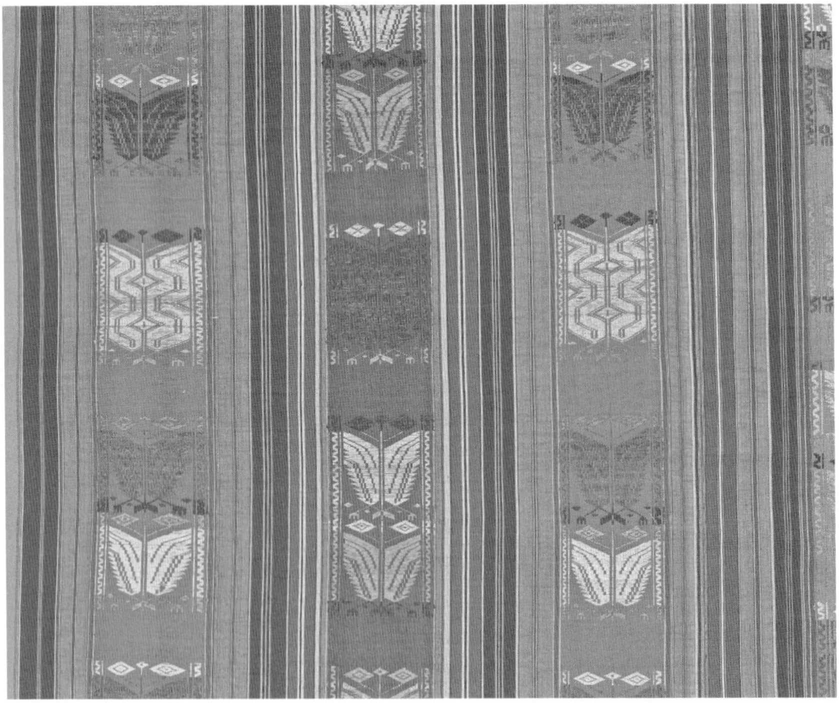

FIGURE 14.5 Detail of supplementary weft motifs (*akotifahana*). *Bombyx* silk, natural and synthetic dyes, supplementary wefts. 105 by 82 inches (231 by 180 centimeters). The presence of aniline green dates this piece to post 1877. Royal Ontario Museum 2010.75.1. *Credit*: With permission of the Royal Ontario Museum © Royal Ontario Museum.

and had radically expanded their trade to East Africa. The floss appears to have arrived predyed, in colors fashionable in Oman, or to have been colored by Merina weavers with substances provided by the same traders. This may help account for the new color schemes of light blue, purple, and magenta that broke with the past. From the 1840s, sericulture developed in earnest within the island itself. Simon Peers (2004) conjectures that the novel physical properties of mulberry silk—its combined strength and suppleness—inspired the making of supplementary wefts, being better suited to the task than local fibers. What museum specimens tell us is that by the mid-nineteenth century at least, Merina weavers were experimenting widely with *Bombyx* silk, creating novel striping patterns, or combining it with indigenous *Borocera* silk.

Such innovations in Merina handweaving can be pegged to rising local wealth and demand combined with sociopolitical shifts. As Niessen (1999: 175) has noted for the Batak weavers of Sumatra, so too in historical Madagascar "the market drives . . . textile inventions just as it drives the global fashion business, though on a different scale." Beverly Lemire (2010: 16) observes that "commercial vigour based on trade, as well as urban dynamism appear to be essential requisites, where change and distinction (however contentious) featured in the selection of possessions and diffusion of styles." These very conditions had taken root in highland Madagascar in the late eighteenth century. At this time, one chief seized control of international trade, strengthened weekly markets, and welcomed foreign traders, bringing great wealth and rapid expansion to his capital, Antananarivo. From 1820, his royal successors transferred sumptuary laws to European dress, fabrics, and accessories, using these—rather than local fibers or wrapper forms—to denote grades in a new sociopolitical hierarchy, based on schooling and rising through the state civil or military order. For noblemen and noblewomen—many stripped of past privileges—shoulder mantles of novel color, fiber, and pattern, and of personalized design, asserted distinction and fashionability.

A study of fringes—an overlooked detail of Malagasy handwoven dress—strongly suggests the akotifahana changed systematically over time. Merina silk weavings from the first half of the nineteenth century tend to have the warp ends finished with a woven end band and braided and balled fringe. These bands—a time-honored feature of southern Arabian weaving—were likely also of Omani inspiration. Around 1875, this warp finishing largely ceded to an elongated latticed fringe, the influence of "Chinese" shawls. Using these markers it can be seen that akotifahana motifs changed noticeably over time. Geometric figures—Xs, hexagons, waves, and so on—limited to one or two stripes near the selvages of the cloth gave way to naturalistic elongated plant forms that in turn ceded to more abstract and wider figures of serrated leaves with erect flowers. Motifs grew in size—from just a half inch (two centimeters) in height to some five inches (ten centimeters)—occupying an ever-increasing amount of surface at the expense of warp stripes.

Malagasy sources—both historical Merina-authored texts and interviews with contemporary akotifahana weavers—unequivocally establish the secular nature of the motifs and the dress itself (Athenor n.d.; Domenichini-Andrianina 1988; Fee forthcoming; Giambrone 1970). All concur that supplementary weft designs were "embellishment" (*haingo*), usually added to preexisting striped textile types. Nineteenth-century akotifahana motif names are usually descriptive and reference quotidian goods. The motif that scholars have variously interpreted as birds, trees of life, or butterflies in fact references a generic plant form. A source from 1870 specifies that the motifs were idiosyncratic, made in "whatever colour and shape" the weaver or patron desired, some designs taken from imported porcelains (Giambrone 1970: 267). Another romantic notion, that the akotifahana was in some way royal, directly patronized or worn by the royal court, is not supported by the historical record, including inventories of royal wardrobes (Fee forthcoming). Although high-ranking Malagasy did occasionally receive akotifahana as gifts from the royal court, it appears that as frequently the cloths were purchased at market by consumers or directly commissioned from weavers.

Confirming that the cloth's colors were not codified but rather prone to fashion and open to innovation are chemical analyses of the dyes themselves. Recent testing carried out on select pieces of the Royal Ontario Museum's (ROM) collection of akotifahana reveals that color schemes shifted over time, adapting to the new possibilities offered by synthetic colorants. Early akotifahana are distinctive for their palette of blue, magenta, pink, black, and golden yellow, which the ROM pieces reveal to be of natural sources, with the exception of the magenta, which is likely safflower imported from Arabia or India (see Figure 14.4). From 1870, while several natural shades were retained, synthetic orange, green, grape purple, and scarlet red emerged as the main color choices (see Figure 14.5).

In island Southeast Asia generally, a cloth's name is based on its striping pattern; a few patterns endure over time, while a great many others know short-lived phases of fashionability (Lewis 1994; Milgram 1999; Niessen 1999). It is not surprising, then, to find this same phenomenon in Madagascar and in the akotifahana. Studying the cloth's striping reveals that most historical examples have at the center a series of narrow blue and black stripes. Historical texts identify this striping pattern as the *arosy*, the most expensive cloth sold at market at the time (Fee forthcoming). In essence, what scholars and museums have labeled as akotifahana are in fact embellished arosy: supplementary weft motifs have merely been added to the secondary stripes (see Figure 14.4). From the 1880s, the striped colored mantle in general, including those embellished with supplementary wefts, increasingly fell from fashion as the elite of Madagascar's highlands definitively turned to European dress to demonstrate status, style, and sophistication.[7]

Yet fashion demands continued to sustain *Bombyx* brocade weaving. Eschewing the bright shades of the nineteenth century, urban Merina women developed a new taste for subtle white-on-white damask *Bombyx* shoulder mantles, of ever more diminutive size, their motifs changing regularly to reflect modern tastes for naturalistic roses, tulips, grapevines, or crowns.

"Muscat Cloth": Fashionable Stripes in East Africa

Taking stripes seriously reveals the existence of another wrapper fashion of the eighteenth and nineteenth centuries in the western Indian Ocean: the striped and checked cotton and silk blends made in the port towns of the southern Arabian nation of Oman. They were known to European traders as "Muscat cloth" for the name of Oman's largest port. My ongoing research shows that, unlike akotifahana, Muscat cloth was a mass phenomenon spread among diverse classes and groups far and wide—from Madagascar through the Comoros, from the Horn of Africa down the Swahili coast and into Central Africa. So popular was the cloth from about 1840 to 1880 that it became a critical factor in driving the area's ivory and slave trade. Muscat cloth created a western Indian Ocean fashion sensation that has gone largely unnoticed in the extensive literature on the textile trades of the western Indian Ocean. A major obstacle has been a disinterest in the physical attributes of these trade textiles—Oman's in particular—compounded by analysts' ongoing insistence on the "authentic" and "noncommercial."

The study of Muscat cloth represents a rather different research challenge from that of the akotifahana. Here, historical specimens are exceedingly scarce, with few to be located in private or public collections (Figure 14.6). This gap stems partly from collectors' preference for the figurative—notably the bright printed *kanga* wrappers of the region—over striped fabric, and, second, from the cloth's questionable authenticity. In Oman, weaving Muscat cloth was a commercial activity, concentrated in the port towns and hinterland of the coastal band lining the Arabian Sea (Richardson and Dorr 2003).[8] Using primarily imported cotton and silk, men worked at pit looms, usually in workshops, producing rectangular turbans, hip wraps, and mantles, with much of the cloth destined for export. Stripes, bands, and checks were the main decorative effects, with blues, reds, yellow, and black predominating. At the point of consumption, too, in East

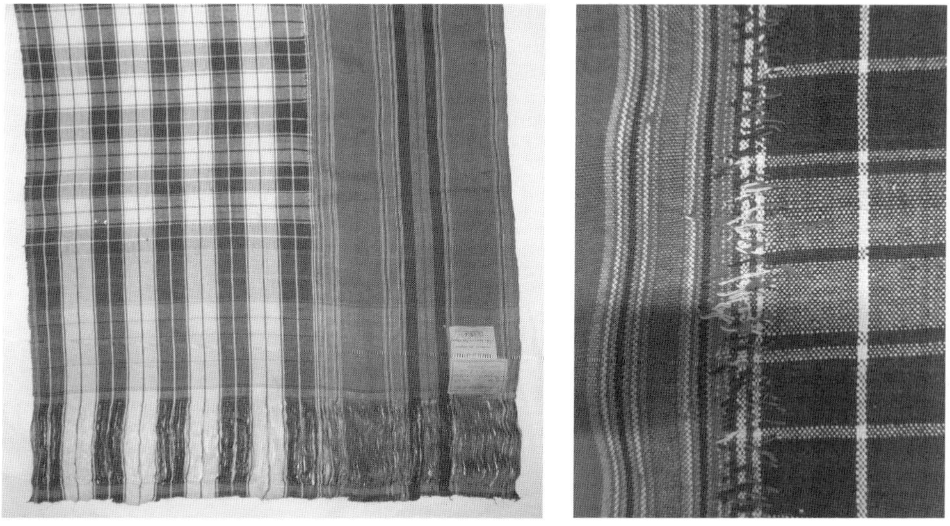

FIGURE 14.6 Overview and reverse detail of one panel of the *barwazi,* a cloth type made in Oman for the East African market, particularly favored by women. This example was sent by the French consulate of Muscat to Paris, with the hope of inspiring French industrial imitations. Silk and cotton, ca. 1900. 12153.
Credit: © Musée d'Histoire Naturelle de Lille.

Africa, the cloth was not "indigenous" and so was largely overlooked by collectors and scholars. In place of historical pieces, however, there is pictorial, linguistic, and archival evidence. Above all, it is fieldwork with contemporary Omani pit-loom weavers that confirms the existence and contours of the Muscat cloth wrapper mode.

Lexical and archival information provides the first essential clues. Trade records, dictionaries, and travelers' reports frequently make mention of, but do not describe, imported cloths called *debuani, subaya, somaili,* and *sohary.* An exception was British explorer Sir Richard Francis Burton, who, hoping to encourage British industrial imitation, identified their origin in Oman and described each type, focusing on selvage stripes and end bands. Images of Omani pit-loom weavings became available to scholars only in 2003, in the landmark study by Neil Richardson and Marcia Dorr; they illustrate a wide variety of striping patterns but do not identify them by name. Field research I carried out with Omani pit-loom weavers in 2011 revealed that the subaya, somaili, sohary, and several other wrapper types of the nineteenth century are still being made. Rather than the selvage stripes, as Burton believed, it is the center field that is the defining feature. The somaili is distinctive for its alternating very narrow stripes across the width of its center field. The *sabouni,* meanwhile, breaks up the narrow stripes with regularly placed stripes of medium width (Figure 14.7A and 14.7B). These center-field patterns remained stable over time, while the fiber types and textures, colors for the ground, selvage stripes, and end bands knew changing modes.

With this visual knowledge, turning to nineteenth-century photographs of East Africa, one can identify Muscat cloth in numerous settings (Figures 14.8 and 14.9). These images confirm scattered observations that the cloth was desired and worn by many sectors of society. Some was destined for use by the resident Omani population, who lived not only in the port towns but also far into the African interior. In the eighteenth century, having routed the Portuguese, Omani merchant-rulers established themselves as rulers in port towns from Mogadishu to the Zambezi River. In 1832 the sultan of

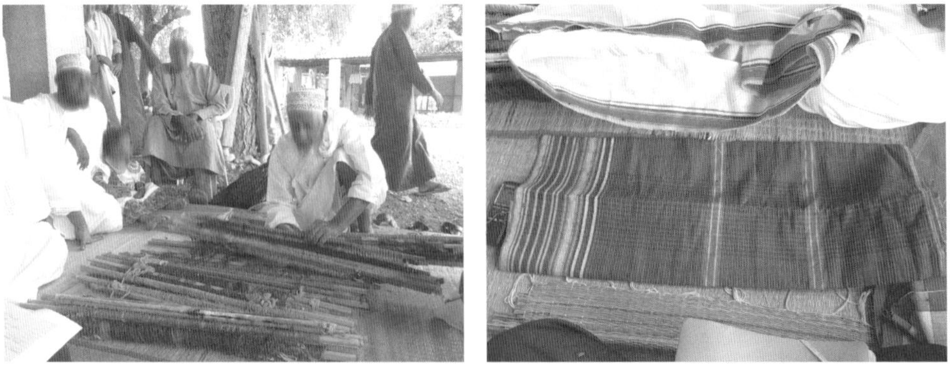

FIGURE 14.7 (A) Pit-loom weaver of Oman, showing his "archive" of loom heddles that encode the striping patterns of Muscat cloth, including the (B) *sabouni.* Quriyat, Oman, 2012.
Credit: Author's own collection.

Oman moved his court from Muscat to Zanzibar, placing governors in key ports. These governors, and other elites, had the right to wear the royal turban, also distinguished by its striping pattern. According to Burton, the most expensive type of Muscat cloth, the *masnafu,* with gold thread, was likewise reserved for this group. The vast majority of Muscat cloth, however, was sold to African consumers, from chiefs to commoners to slaves, from Mogadishu and down along the Swahili coast, to as far into the interior as Uganda. Some 100,000 cloths were imported into East Africa annually for a population estimated at 1,000,000. One French merchant observed in 1860, "To own a turban, belt and hip wrap from Muscat is the ambition of every person on the coast. Even the lowliest of slaves works in order to dress in this clothing that is so greatly desired."[9]

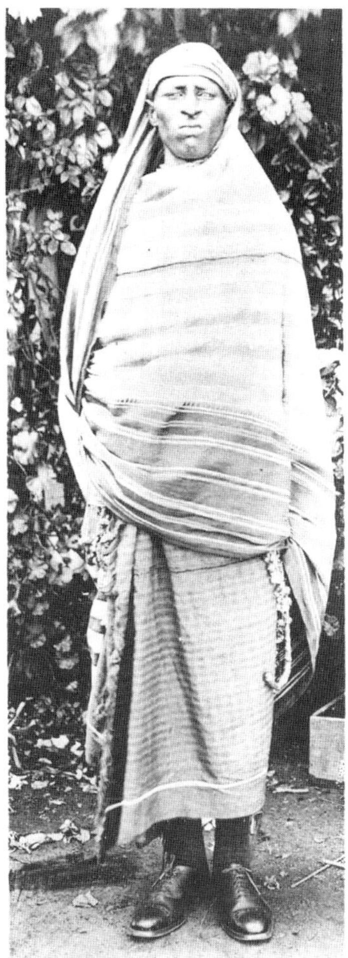

Copyright. Somali, Nairobi, B. E. A. 10.

FIGURE 14.8 Urban Somali man dressed in Muscat cloth, probably the *ismaili* pattern as a hip wrapper and *subaya* as a shoulder wrapper, ca. 1900.
Credit: Postcard, private collection. Author's own collection.

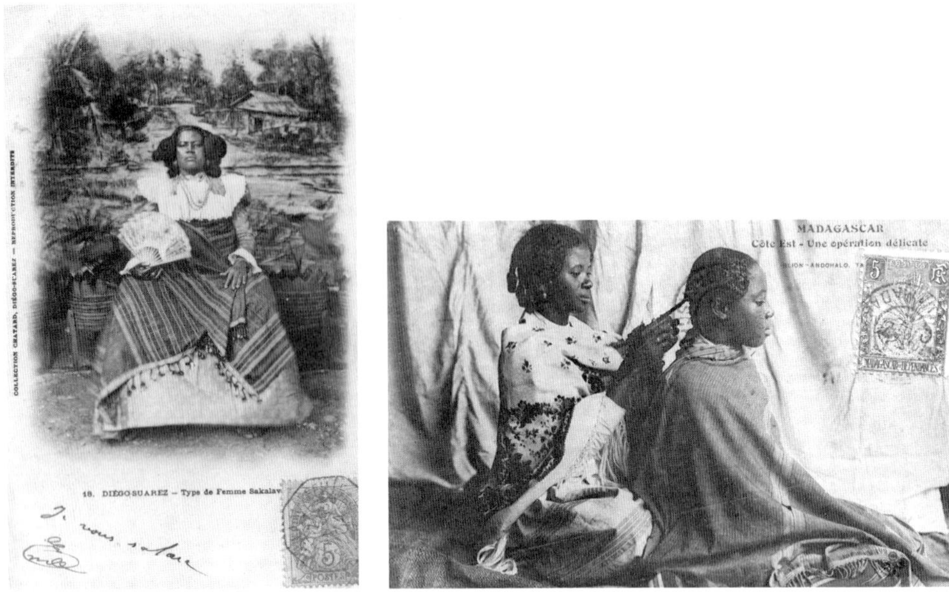

(a) (b)

FIGURE 14.9 With its wide range of qualities, Muscat cloth met the desires of both urban elites (A) and rural dwellers (woman to the right, B). Madagascar, ca. 1900. Figure 14.9B shows the two major fringe types emulated by Merina brocade weavers: the "Chinese shawl" tiered style to the left and the woven end band and heavy fringe to the right.
Credit: Postcards, author's own collection.

How does one account for this great desirability and fashionability of Muscat cloth, especially given the stiff competition from a wide variety of Indian, British, and American imports? Certainly political-economic factors cannot be discounted. While there were no preferential or protectionist measures favoring Omani cloth imports, Omanis, as the rulers of Swahili and Somali port towns, did provide the model of cultivated elegance (Fair 2004; Prestholdt 2008). Some items of tailored dress were indeed adopted by Swahili port elites. But among the majority of the population and in the interior, it was Muscat's rectangular wrappers, corresponding to preexisting dress forms, that were avidly desired.

Beyond emulation, sources reveal that several material properties of the wrappers fueled their popularity. First were the fibers. The cotton thread was said to be superior in quality and durability to that of India, and the thick weave was especially valued. Silk has long held an ambiguous status in the Muslim world: on the one hand, it was proscribed by the Prophet for the dress of men; on the other, it is believed to hold medicinal properties and was tolerated, even valued, in certain times and places. Various accommodations to silk's ambiguous status included lining it with cotton, using a satin-weave structure to place cotton against the skin and silk to the exterior, or using only small portions of silk as narrow stripes or fringes. This last was the accommodation of Muscat cloth. In hinterland East Africa and Madagascar, where such strictures did not apply, the use of small amounts of silk both made it highly attractive and kept it affordable. Dyes too contributed to the popularity of Muscat cloth, particularly a certain colorfast shade of red. Reports hint as well at a unique sheen and texture derived from Arabic gums. Fourth was the tapestry decoration of the selvages, facilitated by the pit-loom fly shuttle. Finally, and of supreme significance, was the woven band at the cloths' ends, a narrow edging made by a specialist using a separate braid loom (Figure 14.9). Difficult to imitate industrially, this bit of extra weaving seems to have served as a label for the authentic Muscat brand.[10] More generally, a key to fashion success was Omani weavers' catering to niche markets and budgets: they made the same striping patterns in a range of sizes, yarn qualities, and thread counts and left the warp ends unworked, thus allowing the consumers to add a fringe according to their budget and personal preference. India, Germany, Great Britain, Belgium, Switzerland, and Japan all attempted, with limited degrees of success, to imitate Muscat cloth.

Several factors further complicate the idea of emulation or a unidirectional core-periphery flow to Muscat cloth's fashionability. Cultural authentication occurred in that East African women wore as hip wrappers textile types such as the subaya that were made at their Omani source for use as male shoulder cloths or turbans or women's mantles. In Madagascar the subaya is reserved as the dress for mediums of royal spirits and their servants. Moreover, fashion spread in both directions, producing regional

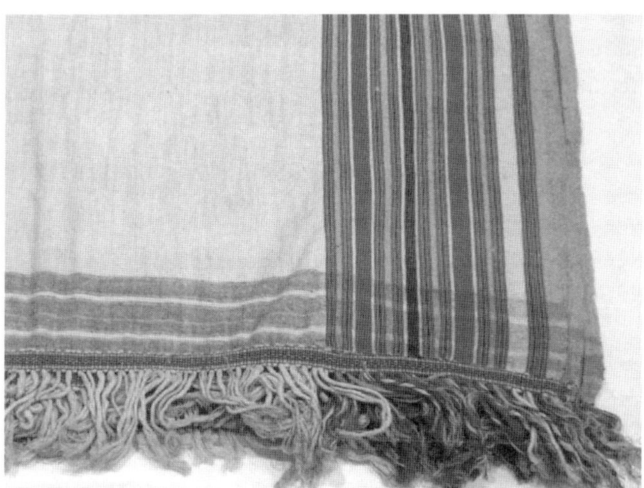

FIGURE 14.10 Material features that contributed to the popularity of Muscat cloth included the bold selvage stripes, colored bands, and woven end band (transverse selvage). Although purchased from the Madagascar section of the 1900 Paris Exposition, this piece was likely an import from Oman. Cotton, silk, dyes, ca. 1900. University of Pennsylvania Museum of Archaeology and Anthropology #2003–65–106.
Credit: Photo used with permission of Penn Museum.

hybrid forms. Dress items such as the embroidered men's skullcap (*kuma, kofia*), forms of women's cloaks (*abayeh booy booy*), and the printed kanga cloth, all likely originating in Africa, became fashions in Oman (Al-Zadjali 2010). All these testify to what Jeremy Prestholdt (2004: 755) has termed the "mutual determination and plural causality" of commercial and cultural relations in the western Indian Ocean.

Even if statistically smaller than imports from India, the impact of Muscat cloth in East Africa was significant and enduring. It greatly influenced handweaving within Africa, notably Somalia, where weavers appear to have attempted to imitate and undercut it (Fee 2011a). Long after Muscat cloth fell from fashion as daily apparel, certain types have been retained to the present day as ritual dress. Although now made in South Asian factories, these cloths must still cater to local demands for specific striping types, color combinations, and the woven end band.

CONCLUSION

Anthropologist Nicholas Thomas (2003) has reiterated the obvious point that objects do not speak for themselves. Rather, they require the analyst's interpretation. And this will vary depending on reigning interests, theories, and ideologies. This is why commercially made striped wrappers in Oman and East Africa might go uncollected and unremarked, masking a mass dress fashion that spanned a wide geographic and social space. This also explains why, alternatively, the bright figured brocaded silks of highland Madagascar might attract great interest, their motifs read as religious or sociopolitical badges rather than as a short-lived secular fashion. In both instances, however, the objects become the critical starting point for tracking and revealing local fashion aesthetics and related changes and cycles.

NOTES

I wish to express my enduring gratitude to the many colleagues, weavers, archivists, and librarians in Canada, the United States, Madagascar, Oman, France, and Britain who made this study possible. Among them I especially acknowledge Bako Rasoarifetra, Neil Richardson, Julia Al-Zadjali, and Saif al Hajri. I thank Edgar Krebs and Lynne Milgram for suggesting sources, and Alexandra Palmer, Jan-Lodewijk Grootaers, Amy de la Haye, and Silvia Forni for their comments on and discussion of earlier drafts of this work.

1. Hansen provides an excellent overview of works from 1980 to 2004.
2. Amateur collectors—missionaries, colonial administrators, and so on—might follow the guidelines of *Notes and Queries* (Barnes 1992).
3. The quality of collectors' documentation varied wildly, however, severely limiting in some instances the value of the pieces for study today.
4. Stevenson's own monograph on Pueblo dress was rejected for publication by the Bureau of American Ethnology.
5. Margaret Maynard (2004), for instance, takes 1970 as her starting point for globalization.
6. A major exception is the growing body of literature on Islamic fashionable dress, which may react against the West or look elsewhere for inspiration.

7. Large colored cloths, including akotifahana, continued to be made and used, however, to wrap the dead for first burial and rewrap them at bone-turning ceremonies.
8. By contrast, scholars and collectors embraced the woven products of Oman's interior, made by Bedouin women using local wool for domestic usages.
9. "Marchandises d'importation propres au commerce de la côte de Zanguébar," ca. 1840, Océan Indien 5/23 No. 7, Centre des Archives d'Outre-Mer, Aix-en-Provence, France.
10. Into the 1990s, the woven braid remained a vital part of dress in Oman, affixed to industrial cloth, including printed kanga wrappers.

BIBLIOGRAPHY

Allman, Jean (ed.). 2004. *Fashioning Power: Clothing, Politics and African Identities.* Bloomington: Indiana University Press.

Al-Zadjali, Julia M. 2010. "Omani Dress." In Gillian Vogelsang (ed.), *Berg Encyclopedia of World Dress and Fashion,* vol. 5, *Central and Southwest Asia,* 238–44. Oxford: Berg.

Appadurai, Arjun (ed.). 1988. *The Social Life of Things: Commodities in Cultural Perspective.* Cambridge: Cambridge University Press.

Athenor, Christine. n.d. *Malagasy Textile Collections in Europe and Madagascar.* Unpublished manuscript.

Auerbach, Jerold. 2008. *Explorers in Eden: Pueblo Indians and the Promised Land.* Albuquerque: University of New Mexico Press.

Banerjee, Mukulika, and Daniel Miller. 2003. *The Sari.* Oxford: Berg.

Barnes, Ruth. 1992. "Women as Headhunters: The Making and Meaning of Textiles in a Southeast Asian Context." In Ruth Barnes and Joanne B. Eicher (eds.), *Dress and Gender: Making and Meaning,* 29–43. Oxford: Berg.

Brand, Jan, and José Teunissen (eds.). 2005. *Global Fashion/Local Tradition: On the Globalisation of Fashion.* Arnhem, the Netherlands: Terra.

British Association for the Advancement of Science. 1874. *Notes and Queries on Anthropology.* London: Edward Stanton.

Brydon, Anne, and Sandra Niessen (eds.). 1998. *Consuming Fashion: Adorning the Transnational Body.* Oxford: Berg.

Burnham, Dorothy. 1973. *Cut My Cote.* Toronto: Royal Ontario Museum.

Clark, Hazel, and Alexandra Palmer. 2004. *Old Clothes, New Looks: Second Hand Fashion.* Oxford: Berg.

Colchester, Chloë (ed.). 2003. *Clothing the Pacific.* Oxford: Berg.

Cole, Jennifer. 2008. "Fashioning Distinction: Youth and Consumerism in Urban Madagascar." In Jennifer Cole and Deborah Durham (eds.), *Figuring the Future: Globalization and the Temporalities of Children and Youth,* 99–124. Santa Fe, NM: School for Advanced Research Press.

Comaroff, Jean. 1996. "The Empire's Old Clothes: Fashioning the Colonial Subject." In David Howes (ed.), *Cross-cultural Consumption: Global Markets, Local Realities,* 19–38. London: Routledge.

Craik, Jennifer. 1993. *The Face of Fashion: Cultural Studies in Fashion.* London: Routledge.

Craik, Jennifer. 2009. *Fashion: The Key Concepts.* Oxford: Berg.

Crill, Rosemary. 1998. *Indian Ikat Textiles.* London: V&A Publications.

Domenichini-Andrianina, Mireille. 1988. "Le Travail de la Soie sur les Hautes Terres de Madagascar, une approche technologique." Master's thesis, Université de Paris X-Nanterre.

Eicher, Joanne B. 2000. "The Anthropology of Dress." *Dress* 27: 59–70.

Eicher, Joanne B. (ed.). 2010a. *Berg Encyclopedia of World Dress and Fashion.* 10 vols. Oxford: Berg.

Eicher, Joanne B. (ed.). 2010b. *Berg Encyclopedia of World Dress and Fashion.* Vol. 10, *Global Perspectives.* Oxford: Berg.

Eicher, Joanne B., and Mary Ellen Roach-Higgins. 1992. "Definition and Classification of Dress: Implications for Analysis of Gender Roles." In Ruth Barnes and Joanne B. Eicher (eds.), *Dress and Gender: Making and Meaning,* 8–28. Oxford: Berg.

Ellis, William. 1838. *History of Madagascar.* Vol. 1. London: Fisher.

Fair, Laura. 2004. "Remaking Fashion in the Paris of the Indian Ocean: Dress, Performance and the Cultural Construction of a Cosmopolitan Zanzibari Identity." In Jean Allman (ed.), *Fashioning Power: Clothing, Politics and African Identities,* 13–30. Bloomington: Indiana University Press.

Fee, Sarah. 2011a. "*Futa Benadir:* A Somali Tradition within the Folds of the Western Indian Ocean." In Susan Cooksey (ed.), *Africa Interweave: Textile Diasporas,* 120–27. Gainesville: University of Florida Harn Art Museum.

Fee, Sarah. 2011b. "The Political Economy of an Art Form: The *Akotifahana* Cloth of Madagascar and Trade Networks in the Southwest Indian Ocean." In Walter Little and Patricia Macaulney (eds.), *Weaving across Space and Time,* 77–97. Lanham, MD: Altamira.

Fee, Sarah. Forthcoming. "The Shape of Fashion: The Historic Silk Brocades (*Akotifahana*) of Highland Madagascar." *African Arts* 46 (3): 26–39.

Ferguson, James G. 2002. "Of Mimicry and Membership: Africans and the 'New World Society.'" *Cultural Anthropology* 17 (4): 551–69.

Finane, Antonia. 2008. *Changing Clothes in China: Fashion, History, Nation.* New York: Columbia University Press.

Giambrone, Jean (ed.). 1970. *Le Manuscrit de l'Ombiasy de Ranavalona I (suite et fin).* Fianarantsoa, Madagascar: Ambozontany.

Gott, Suzanne, and Krystyne Loughran (eds.). 2010. *Contemporary African Fashion.* Bloomington: Indiana University Press.

Hansen, Karen Tranberg. 2000. *Salaula: The World of Secondhand Clothing and Zambia.* Chicago: University of Chicago Press.

Hansen, Karen Tranberg. 2004. "The World in Dress: Anthropological Perspectives on Clothing, Fashion and Culture." *Annual Review of Anthropology* 33: 369–92.

Hertz, Robert. 1909. "La prééminence de la main droite. Etude sur la polarité religieuse." *Revue philosophique* 34 (7): 553–80.

Jennings, Helen. 2011. *New African Fashion.* Munich: Prestel.

Kriger, Colleen E. 2006. *Cloth in West African History.* Lanham, MD: Altamira.

Kriger, Colleen E. 2010. "Silk and Sartorial Politics in the Sokoto Caliphate (Nigeria), 1804–1903." In Beverly Lemire (ed.), *The Force of Fashion in Politics and Society: Global Perspectives from Early Modern to Contemporary Times,* 143–65. Burlington, VT: Ashgate.

Küchler, Susanne. 2005. "Materiality and Cognition: The Changing Faces of Things." In Daniel Miller (ed.), *Materiality,* 206–30. Durham, NC: Duke University Press.

Küchler, Susanne, and Daniel Miller (eds.). 2005. *Clothing as Material Culture.* Oxford: Berg.

Leiris, Michel. 1931. *Instructions sommaires pour les collecteurs d'objets ethnographiques.* Paris: Musée d'ethnographie (Museum national d'histoire naturelle).

Lemire, Beverly (ed.). 2010. *The Force of Fashion in Politics and Society: Global Perspectives from Early Modern to Contemporary Times.* Burlington, VT: Ashgate.

Lewis, E. D. 1994. "Sikkar Regency." In Roy Hamilton (ed.), *Gift of the Cotton Maiden: Textiles of Flores and the Solor Islands,* 148–69. Los Angeles: Fowler Museum of Cultural History.

Mack, John. 1989. *Malagasy Textiles.* London: Shire.

Mack, John. 1993. "Sub-Saharan Africa and the Offshore Islands." In Jennifer Harris (ed.), *5,000 Years of Textiles,* 295–305. London: British Museum.

Mauss, Marcel. 1967. *Manuel d'Ethnographie.* Paris: Payot.

Maynard, Margaret. 2004. *Dress and Globalisation.* Manchester: Manchester University Press.

Milgram, Lynne. 1999. "Locating 'Tradition' in the Striped Textiles of Banaue, Ifugao." *Museum Anthropology* 23 (1): 3–20.

Miller, Daniel (ed.). 1998. *Material Cultures: Why Some Things Matter.* Chicago: University of Chicago Press.

Miller, Daniel. 2005. "Introduction." In Susanne Küchler and Daniel Miller (eds.), *Clothing as Material Culture,* 1–20. Oxford: Berg.

Niessen, Sandra A. 1999. "Threads of Tradition, Threads of Invention: Unraveling Toba Batak Women's Expressions of Social Change." In Ruth Philipps and Chris Steiner (eds.), *Unpacking Culture: Art and Commodity in Colonial and Postcolonial Worlds,* 162–77. Berkeley: University of California Press.

Niessen, Sandra A. 2003. "Afterword: Re-orienting Fashion Theory." In Sandra Niessen, Ann Marie Leshkowich, and Carla Jones (eds.), *Re-orienting Fashion: The Globalization of Asian Dress,* 243–66. Oxford: Berg.

Paulicelli, Eugenia, and Hazel Clark. 2009. *The Fabric of Culture: Fashion, Identity, and Globalization.* London: Routledge.

Peers, Simon. 2002. *Silk Weaving from Madagascar.* London: Francesca Galloway.

Peers, Simon. 2004. "Aspects of Hand-Loom Weaving in the Highlands of Madagascar: History and Revival." In Chaprukha Kusimba, Judy Odland, and Bennet Bronson (eds.), *Unwrapping the Textile Traditions of Madagascar,* 144–54. Los Angeles: University of California Los Angeles, Fowler Museum of Cultural History.

Philadelphia Museums. 1906. *Notes on the Madagascar Collection.* Philadelphia: The Commercial Museum.

Prestholdt, Jeremy. 2004. "On the Global Repercussions of East African Consumerism." *American Historical Review* 109 (3): 755–81.

Prestholdt, Jeremy. 2008. *Domesticating the World: African Consumerism and the Genealogies of Globalization.* Berkeley: University of California Press.

Richardson, Neil, and Marcia Dorr. 2003. *The Craft Heritage of Oman.* 2 vols. Dubai: Motivate.

Roces, Mina, and Louise P. Edwards. 2007. *The Politics of Dress in Asia and the Americas.* Brighton: Sussex Academic Press.

Root, Regina A. (ed.). 2005. *The Latin American Fashion Reader.* Oxford: Berg.

Root, Regina A. 2010. *Couture and Consensus: Fashion and Politics in Postcolonial Argentina.* Minneapolis: University of Minnesota Press.

Rovine, Victoria L. (ed.). 2009a. "African Fashion/African Style." Special issue, *Fashion Theory: The Journal of Dress, Body and Culture* 13 (2).

Schneider, Jane. 1987. "The Anthropology of Cloth." *Annual Review of Anthropology* 16: 409–48.

Schneider, Jane. 2006. "Cloth and Clothing." In Christopher Tilley, Webb Keane, Susanne Küchler, Mike Rowlands, and Patricia Spyer (eds.), *Handbook of Material Culture,* 203–20. London: Sage.

Schumaker, Lyn. 2001. *Africanizing Anthropology: Fieldwork, Networks and the Making of Cultural Knowledge in Central Africa.* Durham, NC: Duke University Press.

Schwarz, Ronald A. 1979. "Uncovering the Secret Vice: Toward an Anthropology of Clothing and Adornment." In Justine M. Cordwell and Ronald A. Schwarz (eds.), *The Fabrics of Culture: The Anthropology of Clothing and Adornment,* 23–47. The Hague: Mouton.

Simmel, Georg. 1904. "Fashion." *International Quarterly* 10: 130–55.

Skov, Lise, and Marie Riegels Melchior. 2010. "Research Approaches." In Joanne B. Eicher (ed.), *Berg Encyclopedia of World Dress and Fashion,* vol. 10, *Global Perspectives,* 11–16. Oxford: Berg.

Steele, Valerie, and John S. Major. 1999. "Decoding Dragons: Clothing and Chinese Identity." In Valerie Steele and John Major (eds.), *China Chic: East Meets West,* 13–36. New Haven, CT: Yale University Press.

Tarlo, Emma. 1996. *Clothing Matters: Dress and Identity in India.* Chicago: University of Chicago Press.

Taylor, Lou. 2002. *The Study of Dress History.* Manchester: Manchester University Press.

Taylor, Lou. 2004. *Establishing Dress History.* Manchester: Manchester University Press.

Thomas, Nicholas. 1991. *Entangled Objects: Exchange, Material Culture and Colonialism in the Pacific.* Cambridge, MA: Harvard University Press.

Thomas, Nicholas. 2003. "The Case of the Misplaced Ponchos: Speculations Concerning the History of Cloth in Polynesia." In Chloë Colchester (ed.), *Clothing the Pacific,* 79–96. Oxford: Berg.

Tortora, Phyllis G. 2010. "History and Development of Fashion." In Joanne B. Eicher (ed.), *Berg Encyclopedia of World Dress and Fashion,* vol. 1, *Global Perspectives,* 159–70. Oxford: Berg.

Turner, Terrence. 1980. "The Social Skin." In Catherine B. Burroughs and Jeffrey Ehrenreich (eds.), *Reading the Social Body,* 15–39. Iowa City: University of Iowa Press.

Urry, James. 1972. "Notes and Queries on Anthropology and the Development of Field Methods in British Anthropology, 1870–1920." *Proceedings of the Royal Anthropological Institute* (1972): 45–57.

Van Gennep, Arnold. 1909. *Les Rites de Passage.* Paris: Emile Nourry.

Weiner, Annette. 1976. *Women of Value, Men of Renown: New Perspectives in Trobriand Exchange.* Austin: University of Texas Press.

Weiner, Annette, and Jane Schneider (eds.). 1989. *Cloth and Human Experience.* Washington, DC: Smithsonian Institution Press.

Welters, Linda, and Abby Lillethun. 2007. *The Fashion Reader.* Oxford: Berg.

Wilson, Verity. 1986. *Chinese Dress.* London: Victoria and Albert Museum.

15

Immateriality

ROBYN HEALY

The changing conditions of the museum in the twenty-first century have provided new models for curatorial practices in relation to fashion and the nature of cultural production. Over the last twenty-five years, the increased presence of fashion in museums worldwide has generated debate about curatorial modes and the understanding of fashion projected by these modes. For fashion is not a simple collection or exhibition experience. The idea of fashion itself is an immaterial object, disseminated through material objects such as clothing (Kawamura 2005), which makes for a challenging curatorial proposition.

For the experience of fashion conveyed through the exhibition mode creates curious tensions between image and reality, spectacle and use, fetishism and worldliness, material and immaterial conditions. Curators experiment with the exhibition genre to test the potential of objects to elicit different meanings and experiences; they study the nature of representational form to produce new knowledge. In the collection and display of fashion there has been ambiguity and irony in the representation of the ephemeral (Debo 2002; Palmer 2008) and in the ways in which the dynamic of constant change and the "dated" is encountered. Customary approaches to fashion exhibitions (historical survey, single designer/retrospective, design practices, personal collection or wardrobe, cross-disciplinary practices between fashion and art, fashion and decorative art, fashion and architecture, commissioned thematic work, conceptual, and survey), staged in the static gallery space, construct experiences intended to immerse the community in the ideas of fashion suggested by the physical arrangement of clothes. With regard to the museum response to fashion, there are complex relationships operating in an exhibition, which is not exclusively about the clothing object and is produced by representation of design practices, states of embodiment, appearance, circulation, and consumption cycles.

However, what new models of curatorial practice are needed to take into account the emergence of digital technologies and collaborative, multidisciplinary practices (Krysa 2006b: 9), which have shifted the way fashion is communicated and presented? How does fashion experienced across immaterial forms and conditions suggest alternate curatorial approaches from traditional exhibition experiences based primarily on physical engagement with fashion objects, particularly clothing?

Curating immaterial forms and/or conditions has opened up ways to disseminate fashion knowledge broadly and test alternate fashion spaces of display. For contemporary fashion practices extend beyond the clothing form; communication is spread across a spectrum of multimedia and multidisciplinary practices (Bugg 2009). Engagement with the fashion object, clothing, or other artifact representations is a mixture of diverse forms of collaborative and social interaction.

CONDITIONS OF IMMATERIALITY

This chapter explores new relations in the field of thinking about curation of fashion in an expanded museum environment. To understand the shifts in practice it is necessary to establish the role of the museum, the context and circulation of the fashion exhibition, and the subsequent engagement with the fashion object. In these relations there are complex issues surrounding the "voice of the object" (Griffin 2011) and the ways in which knowledge about collections and exhibitions is assembled and dispersed.

The particular characteristics of a collection or exhibition are assembled via museum selection processes, motions of rejecting or collecting, preserving or letting material fade away. Sharon McDonald writes that the museum collection is a series of relations:

> Collecting is a set of distinctive—though also variable and changing—practices that not only produces knowledge about objects but also configures particular ways of knowing and perceiving. It is a culturally recognized way of "doing"—or rehearsing—certain relations between things and people. (2006: 94–95)

In the traditional environment of the museum, criticisms about relations operating within customary fashion exhibitions have targeted the dilemma of static display, exclusivity and somewhat inflexible environments, and underrepresentation of certain types of clothing such as everyday fashion (Black 2007). Yet an expanded museum environment suggests a new set of relations proposed by immaterial conditions, as an exhibition of fashion is then no longer contained within the physical site of the museum, and the form of the exhibition would be neither fixed nor static.

The increasing interface with digital forms both in the museum environment and in communication of design practices has created different conditions for curating exhibitions. Physical barriers of location or time no longer confine display and production spaces; digital formats have facilitated opportunities for more inclusive and participatory interactions. This evolving state of immateriality, curator Joasia Krysa has argued, is associated with "new conditions of artistic and cultural practices" (2006b: 9), a state where "software and digitised data are replacing the traditional physical states" (Lillemose 2006: 113). Consequently, representations of the fashion object, clothing, or other artifact forms are expanded, experienced in varied forms of individual, collective, and social interaction. The expression of fashion is articulated using new methods of display, blurring the traditional gallery space, to produce environments with an affinity to retail, catwalk, or social media spaces (Bugg 2009).

In the expansive environment of the museum, the fashion exhibition and collection are encountered in multiple and varied conditions. Objects customarily experienced in close physical proximity in museum spaces are either explored in multidisciplinary contexts or discovered through online media. Therefore, curatorial practices consider the fashion object in material and immaterial conditions, testing the capacity of objects to elicit varied meanings and experiences across different environments and representational states. This capacity has been accelerated by emergent technologies, which have shifted the nature and outcomes of fashion design practice with the application of highly digital interfaces for the development, creation, and broadcasting of work.

Social media have amplified the community's ability to interact with and access collections, which in turn has activated participatory practices through which an individual can customize the museum experience and explore diverse understandings of fashion. In these immaterial conditions, the fashion exhibition has the potential to expand beyond the standard museum environment and suggest diverse and innovative encounters.

In the evolving form of the museum, both the composition and the understanding of the fashion exhibition have changed with the exploration of new media and design practices. The increasing interface with immaterial states has challenged the conditions and representations of what a fashion exhibition should embrace in tackling practices that do not rely on customary curatorial relationships with objects or use conventional dress display techniques. The community's fluency with online communication and media devices has developed opportunities for curation outside the conventional space of the gallery and customary representational forms. Peter McNeil (2008) has observed the potential of new types of exhibitions as the community (particularly the Net Generation[1]) becomes more conversant with digital technologies, sharing the ability to read imagery through digital immersion, gleaning knowledge from multiple sources.

The essay focuses on curating the immaterial object or condition, studying the communication of fashion through the experience of fashion objects, which has extended well beyond the confines of simply engaging with physical objects and interacting with extant clothing forms, to test the capacity of exhibitions based on intangible or non-physical encounters. A discussion of curating fashion in immaterial conditions or forms, the essay studies the function of the museum as a repository and exhibition site, and the ways in which increased community access to these rich repositories has facilitated new forms of curation and experiences with the fashion object.

THE EXPANSIVE MUSEUM ENVIRONMENT

Major museum developments around the world have witnessed the rising complexity and conspicuousness of the museum design (Barker 1999) and the rapid expansion of the fashion environment. The increasing interface with digital forms has created different conditions for exhibitions. No longer does the museum provide a quiet contemplative encounter. The fashion exhibition is regularly a saturated multimedia event: the expanded museum environment relates to the community/visitors through on-site and online technologies. Design practices include a diversity of multimedia and multidisciplinary outcomes.

> PARIS—The mouth of the sculpted figure opens in precise time with that of the Turkish performer Sertab Erener, singing a song of love and loss on a giant screen. This multimedia face-off, with a digital projection creating the sculpture's moving lips, is symbolic of a 21st-century fashion exhibit and of the complexity of thought from its subject, the designer Hussein Chalayan. (Menkes 2011)

The exhibition Hussein Chalayan: Fashion Narratives (2011), at the Musée des Arts Décoratifs, represented the production of a designer working in a multidisciplinary manner, articulating his work through experimental and conceptual investigations. The exhibition, curated by Pamela Golbin, sought to let the community into the creative workings of design through an idea-generation and design process. Multimedia was integrated into the narrative of the clothes as an intrinsic part of the design process. In the exhibition multimedia is not placed as supplementary material: video conceived by the designer himself represented a holistic vision around the collection, made up of complex interrelated parts. Uptake of emergent technologies has shifted both the diversity of design practices involving digital interfaces and the representation of fashion by nonclothing products. The Endless Garment: The New Craft of Machine Knitting (2010), staged at the Royal Melbourne Institute of Technology Gallery in Melbourne, curated the shifts in design practices, highlighting designers working with integrated design systems, displayed computer software programs, and machinery that creates garments with limited hand-to-hand contact (Bigolin and Healy 2010; Figure 15.1).

In the museum augmented-reality technologies include interactive touch-screen kiosks, CD-ROMS, video walls, and downloadable podcasts. Meanwhile, online, museums are becoming progressively complex in their use of the Web. Websites are portals to information data, generative media, and social media. Links flow between different media networks like blogs, wikis, Facebook, Twitter, Flickr, YouTube, Google+, and foursquare. Connections, which break down standard hierarchies of authority and customary experiences with fashion objects, facilitate sharing of information, which evenly communicates both trivial and serious accounts (Griffin 2011). Therefore, the fashion exhibition has the potential to extend across the museum environment, communicated through diverse encounters.

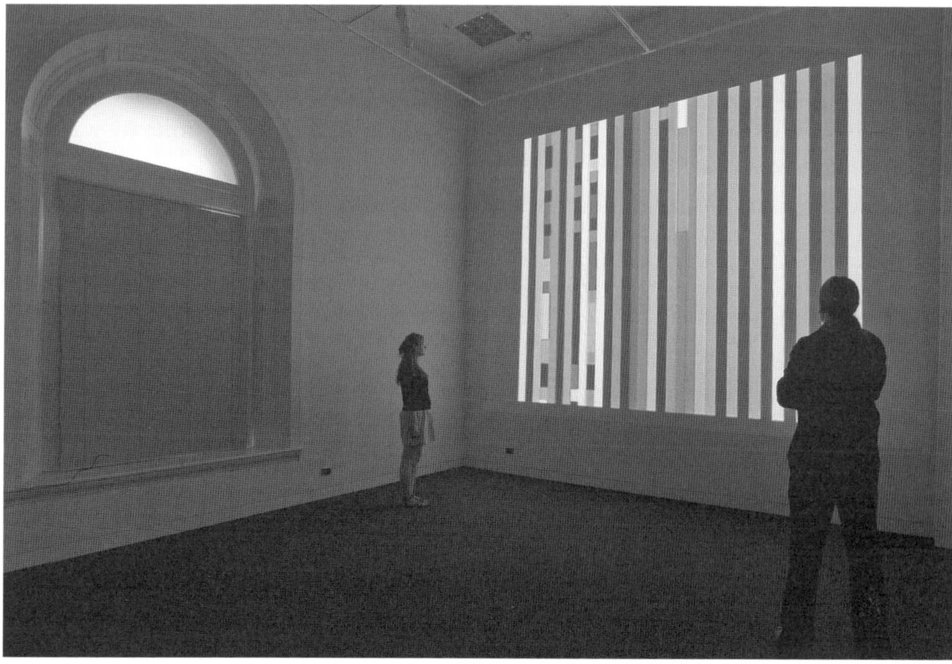

FIGURE 15.1 Computer-generated pattern for knitwear, part of the exhibition The Endless Garment: The New Craft of Machine Knitting, 2010.
Credit: Photograph by Mark Ashkanasy. Courtesy of RMIT Gallery, Melbourne.

GENERATIVE MEDIA

The increasing capacity of the museum to expand the physical experience of an object into the virtual world of the Web establishes different community relations, proposing new experiences and interactions with objects that were previously not envisaged. Curating exhibitions in an inclusive environment on the Web has encouraged the development of participatory practices and collective generation of new material.

London's Victoria and Albert (V&A) Museum developed some of the most creative Web applications, activities specifically curated to extend community relations with the physical fashion exhibition. These participatory experiences tapped into collective knowledge. Shared personal memories, opinions about curation and design practices, and creative projects became part of the exhibition composition. For example, the exhibition Ossie Clark, staged at the V&A in 2004, looked at simple ways for the community to add content. The website called for contributions that would be published and read in association with the exhibition. People were requested to e-mail their recollections about wearing Ossie Clark clothes and to scan clothing images. Although the uptake was not overwhelming, with only twenty-five responses (Durbin 2004), the entries captured a sense of everydayness, demonstrated the vital part clothes play in an individual's life. Susan posted, "I was lucky enough to find an Ossie Clark dress on sale in a shop in Oxford Street, I think. It was in a huge pile on the floor with other clothes and cost $2.50! All it needed was a dry-clean. The year was 1975 and I wore it for my 18th birthday. A few of us ended up in the Fountain in Trafalgar Square (it was New Years Eve) so it got a bit wet."[2] Comments gathered from wearers made emotional connections to the clothes and designer, contextualized the exhibition in an intimate way, and delivered another perspective to supplement the exhibition's didactic labels.

However, for the V&A's exhibition Vivienne Westwood, the website was launched six to eight weeks in advance of the physical exhibition (Durbin 2004). "Questions Answered" was programmed to prompt an open dialogue with designer Vivienne Westwood for curious members of the community. Via e-mail, curator Claire Wilcox and designer Vivienne Westwood were sent questions inquiring about either intricacies of the exhibition or design practices.[3] Another form of participatory practice intended to stimulate originality and "doing" was explored in the V&A's online activities for The Golden Age of Couture (2007), with "Create a Couture Inspired Dress."[4] A dress pattern was made available for participants to download. After construction, participants were encouraged to upload video footage of their completed dress onto the website.[5] Hats: An Anthology by Stephen Jones (2009) shared the design for making a paper hat, using newspaper sheets from the *Guardian,* in the project "My Beautiful Paper Hat." And the exhibition Postmodernism opened up awareness about the making of an exhibition in "behind the scenes," linked to the head of graduate studies and deputy head of research Glen Adamson's blog, *From Sketch to Product.* The blog presented insights into aspects of research about the mannequin design, which was based on poses from original fashion photographs.

The exhibition blog.mode: addressing fashion, held in the Costume Institute of the Metropolitan Museum of Art in 2007, experimented with a type of open-access curating. The community was invited to contribute to the exhibition commentary; participants visiting the exhibition could either log on to computer terminals in the gallery or remotely access the blog on the exhibition website. The blog proposed a type of exhibition participation in a spontaneous manner, which accumulated diverse dialogues over time. From December 18, 2007, to April 13, 2008, curators Harold Koda and Andrew Bolton wrote on the exhibition blog and gathered contributions from contemporary designers and members of the community.[6] This platform solicited subjective dialogue about specific objects and commentaries on aesthetics, personal taste, dressing style, display techniques, and curatorial selection. Individual responses worked in tandem with the customary didactic and interpretative material curated by the museum. The result was an enthralling yet sometimes jarring dialogue, which expressed diverse readings of the exhibition. For example, Hussein Chalayan's Remote Control Dress broke with standard understandings of design and attracted quite polarized reflections, from debates by bloggers on the possibilities of painful wearer experiences to admiration of the garment's futuristic expression. blog.mode built a cooperative dialogue, expressing a wide range of interpretations of fashion objects. Exhibitions from the V&A and the Metropolitan Museum of Art show the increasing capacity for exhibitions to include user-generated material. The participatory construction of these exhibitions produced "differences of experiences" that assisted crossovers of influence between the community and the museum, a relationship Andrea Witcomb describes as interactivity (2006: 353).

FASHION NETWORKING

Consumption of fashion is enabled by both material and immaterial conditions, accelerated instant access to design activities, creative processes, and participatory practices expanding the fashion community. New forms of curatorial practice are evolving to absorb new relations between producer and consumer to embrace ideas of "productive cooperation" (Krysa 2006) and inclusive creative process. The Web has provided a space where fashion followers without official invitations or buyer accreditation are able to freely experience a live catwalk parade, enter the design studio of their favorite designer, and virtually attend opening events or access museum collections. Instant access aids interested parties to become part of a broader fashion community. Consequently, formerly exclusive aspects of high fashion are transformed, and restricted experiences usually populated by industry heavyweights or affluent clothing clients are opened up to become collective experiences without limitations. The Web increasingly is shifting industry mechanisms, commercially and aesthetically, enabling fashion designers to directly engage with their peers and followers and to share their design ideas with the rest of the world. Driving innovative ways to curate fashion online and create a vibrant fashion community is the pioneering fashion website SHOWstudio.

Alice Beard has championed SHOWstudio, launched in 2000, as an example of the emergent technologies that have networked the fashion community and curated an inclusive creative process (2008: 182). SHOWstudio, under the direction of Nick Knight, is a platform for image making, "to deliver fashion live."[7] Knight was concerned with new forms of communication to represent fashion in the digital age, to open up the process and performance behind the moving images "because people can understand it more and take ownership of it. And the Internet, with its forums and chatrooms, allows people to say straight away whether they love or hate it" (Smyth 2009). The website supports a network of fashion film, performance, and participatory activities accessed by a large community of fashion creators and followers. The website features online streaming and real-time reporting methods, from blogging to tweeting. SHOWstudio is a rich repository of contemporary design projects and events, operating like an open studio of speculative and provocative creative practices. Penny Martin, former editor of SHOWstudio.com, described the website as a creative portal for generating new material:

> Whereas a magazine is essentially an intelligent container designed to periodically repeat itself in order to house new material, a good website has the potential to be that new material. Free from the fixed structures dictated by page numbers and universal categories of print cultures (news, features, shoots), a fashion website is a fluid and changeable thing. (2010: 366)

The device of image making or cinematic/video media has given fashion designers and curators the possibility to construct atmospheric environments and has facilitated interdisciplinary practices. In this context clothes are presented as part of a larger composition or image signifying the fashion idea. Film either is used to archive past exhibitions and continue their presence online or is itself the creative means used to curate an exhibition. In seeking different ways to curate traditional museum collections in a virtual form, the Austrian Museum of Applied Arts/Contemporary Art, Vienna (MAK) Design Information Pool considered how a website can build an archive of design practice that is more appealing to contemporary audiences and concerns. In contrast to traditional archives presented as an assemblage of physical objects, this new kind of repository delves deeper into the ideas underpinning design practice. This special design project of the museum, devised to build up representation of contemporary design, focused on "outstanding contemporary designers of Austrian origin, i.e. innovators pursuing design strategies against the shortcomings of time, civilization and society and thus having a certain exemplary function."[8]

On the MAK website the work of Austrian fashion designer Carol Christian Poell is encountered through a range of themes, from analysis of dressing codes and questioning of the fashion system to characteristics of the flawed and strange, representations of collection images, and film presentations. The design of the website is dark and foreboding, parallel to similar atmospheric and aesthetic qualities in her designs. This accumulative archive documents Poell's collections; the user can observe the growth of the collection, plus mechanisms to dissect the work, facilitated by a team of international critics and commentators (Figure 15.2).

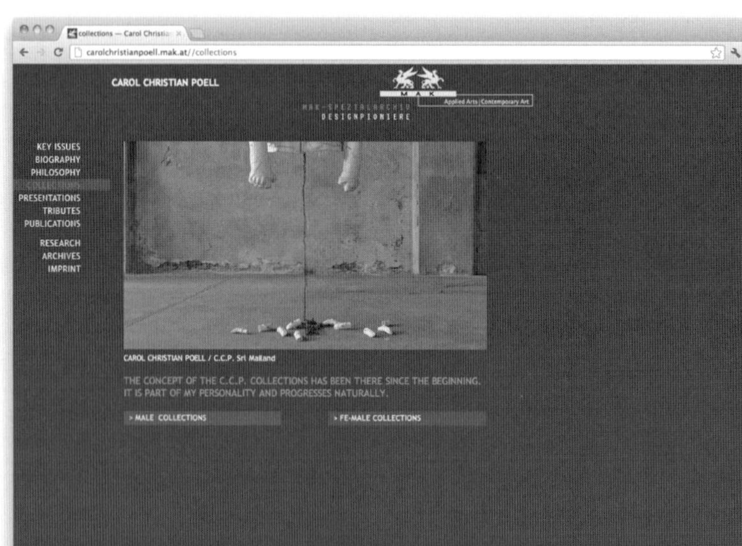

FIGURE 15.2 Screenshot, Carol Christian Poell archive.
Credit: Courtesy of MAK (Austrian Museum of Applied Arts/Contemporary Art), Vienna.

REINVIGORATING THE ARCHIVE

Designers working collaboratively with curators on museum exhibitions have grappled with concerns related to representation of contemporary design practices, as well as the powerful tool of the exhibition medium as an extension of practice. For example, the 2011 retrospective Walter Van Beirendonck—Dream the World Awake, at Antwerp's ModeMuseum (Fashion Museum) was drawn from the designer's comprehensive personal archive and aimed to create an experience of the designer's world; it was curated by Kaat Debo in collaboration with the designer (Debo 2011).

The archive revealed the forward-looking practices of Van Beirendonck in the expression of fashion, showing collaborations across diverse communication platforms, including his early uptake of and experimentation with digital media. During the 1990s, for instance, Van Beirendonck initiated new understandings of fashion by eliciting innovative experiences of real and virtual garments through complex narratives and use of cyberspace (Quinn 2009: 3). Van Beirendonck's label W.&L.T. was the first fashion brand to use CD-ROMS and Internet platforms to disseminate fashion ideas. New media were the platform to establish dynamics across diverse fashion media to integrate clothing design with music, film, images, and text. Later, Van Beirendonck addressed how to touch more extensive audiences, moving beyond the limited capacity provided by digital data stored on discs. More flexible and immediate interactions were made possible by Web communication. The establishment of a W.&L.T. website activated an ongoing dialogue with a vast community of global users. Images from Believe, autumn/winter 1998–1999, for example, were broadcast live. Activation of immediate access to the latest designs and catwalk shows transformed the exclusive nature of the fashion system, connecting fashion beyond the confines of physical or geographic space. The viewing of collections online provided an individual experience requiring only access to a computer terminal (Healy 2011).

It is therefore not surprising that Van Beirendonck's retrospective grapples with concerns about museum representation and the authority of information sources. In Dream the World Awake the role of the archive in representation and documentation of a designer's corpus is reconfigured. Jacques Derrida argued that "the question of the archive is not a question of the past. It is not the question of a concept dealing with the past that might already be at our disposal. But a question of the future..." (1996: 36). In this rethinking and sharing of the designer archive, systematic ordering of fashion objects was abandoned. Instead, the archive generated renewal of Van Beirendonck's oeuvre. The collaboration between Van Beirendonck, Nick Knight from SHOWstudio, and stylist Simon Foxton retrieved garments from different collections and decades, generating contemporary looks for menswear through a remixing process. This new arrangement was then captured in a forty-one-model photographic frieze and fashion film, displayed as the centerpiece of the exhibition and broadcast on SHOWstudio (Figure 15.3). This approach dismissed the customary chronological assemblage of garments, curated to present a historical mapping of collections. The frieze became a device of new design,

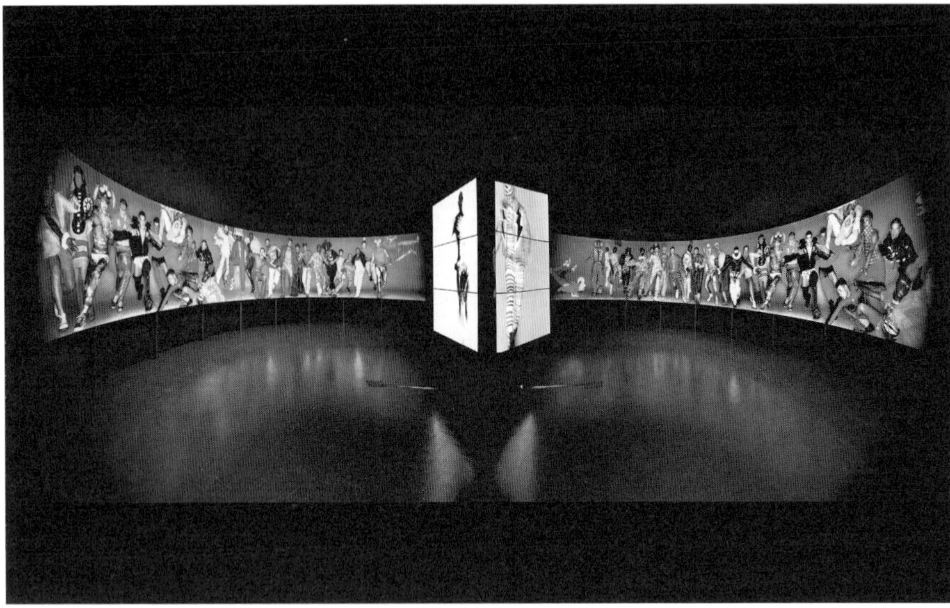

FIGURE 15.3 *Walters' Wild Knights*, from the exhibition Walter Van Beirendonck—Dream the World Awake (September 14, 2011–February 19, 2012).
Credit: Courtesy of ModeMuseum (MoMu), Antwerp. Photograph by Ronald Stoops.

generating new collections and interpretations. The depth of the archive was progressively shared on the museum's website. MoMu released video footage it had on hand from over three decades of Van Beirendonck's collections, to be uploaded over the course of the exhibition. Two videos were posted each week, which interested parties could view or download. In this manner, the museum facilitated open access to a major repository of fashion and extended the exhibition space into the virtual.

EXHIBITIONS CAPTURED ONLINE

Whether one is curating specific online material related to a particular physical exhibition or archiving a past exhibition online, both activities prolong and regenerate new experiences of fashion objects and ideas. In the case of special projects, like The Concise Dictionary of Dress, curated by Judith Clark and Phillip Adams at the V&A's Blythe House, London, in 2010, the exhibition is represented on the Artangel website, major supporters of the project.[9] The online exhibition presentation is conveyed across a range of media and networking sites, demonstrating the diversity of experiences that can be curated online and the networking reach of such a project.

New material was commissioned for the online exhibition, which suggested another expression of this exhibition built around innovative responses and creative development associated with the project. This combination of video, text, and interviews covered a range of perspectives. The online activities suggested subtle qualities and nuances.

"Slideshow: The Installations, the Definitions" presented an evocative expression of elements of the installation. "Adam Phillips: Interactive Interview" prompted a conversation, proposed by a series of questions, with the user selecting specific questions to activate Phillip's answers. Short essays by a range of writers like V&A curator Claire Wilcox shared varied textual responses. Podcasts of interviews with curators could be downloaded from the site. On the Artangel site, connections to video-sharing and networking sites like Vimeo and YouTube show the potential to access larger video files. Further links to the project from website followers are fostered through the social networking sites Facebook and Twitter.

The Concise Dictionary of Dress showed the capacity of an exhibition to work across varied platforms and reach broad audiences in a multifaceted experience. Further curatorial explorations are anticipated as independent London-based curator Judith Clark is working on an experimental space[10] dedicated to setting up exhibitions specifically to be exhibited online, a site that has the potential, like SHOWstudio, to become a hub for experimentation with fashion curation and to activate further discussion and projects in the field.

FRAGILE OBJECTS

Exhibitions of fashion, particularly of clothing and textiles, face issues related to display of fragile and historical items, such as overexposure of certain garments, especially the rigors placed on material shown for extended periods of time or displayed repeatedly. Therefore, when one is discussing museum collections and the ephemeral nature and vulnerability of the actual fashion objects, it is necessary to address the perhaps obvious questions of selection and survival: "what is preserved and what can be preserved" (Roche 1994: 7). In a public fashion collection, standard custodial actions respond to criteria informed by processes of selection, arrangement, and preservation. Conservation ethics and principles,[11] for instance, establish particular conditions for curating fashion objects in museums. Guidelines established to address the preservation of objects relate to the physical state and appearance, authenticity, and integrity, conditions that determine the exhibition status of an object. Yet preserving the appearance of a historical used garment is an onerous duty (Palmer 2008; Taylor 2002); items in deteriorating condition require intensive conservation treatments to slow down the effects of temporal and spatial change and revitalize the garment.

Criticism of the museum repository has targeted restrictive practices implied by conservation management, controlled access to collections, and potentially limited public contact with key works, which are not readily available in either permanent displays or storage. Curation of fragile historical materials is a problematic exhibition proposition. In the exhibition Fashion and Fancy Dress: The Messel Family Dress Collection 1865–2005, at the Brighton Museum and Gallery, disintegrating garments too fragile to be placed on mannequins were displayed, and the curators noted this quite unique encounter was "an experience savoured by curator, conservator and private collector, but is all too often denied to the museum visitor" (de la Haye, Taylor, and Thompson 2005: 12). Spectres: When

Fashion Looks Back[12] and Noble Rot: An Alternate View of Fashion[13] exhibited transformative states of fashion objects, bringing attention to items customarily hidden from view. When objects in the museum are recontextualized, new relationships are formed with other objects (McDonald 2006). In the exhibition translation, the museum aesthetic and containment processes filter the appearance of the object's form. The customary exhibition narrative shows fragile materials exhibited in a dimly lit museum gallery, viewed through the glass showcase lens. This exhibition genre emphasized the idea of "strangeness," "rarity," or "preciousness." However, in these circumstances small objects can be overwhelmed by the display infrastructure, potentially stifling subtle aesthetic or material qualities. Certain types of fashion objects are particularly vulnerable: historical items degraded by age, natural materials like feathers, articulated devices such as fans, or minutiae like trims. Consequently, curating historical fashion confronts obvious tensions between the community experience, conservation controls, and aesthetic surrounds.

Online exhibitions therefore create an alternate dialogue for experiencing fashion without standard conservation concerns in relation to temporal, spatial, or environmental conditions, for example, in an exhibition of small, fragile fashion objects curated to elucidate close observation. The online exhibition Accessorize![14] from Amsterdam's Rijksmuseum, winner of the Dutch design award in 2008, demonstrated how virtual presentation of fashion can enhance the experience of fragile and rarely viewed objects (Figures 15.4, 15.5, and 15.6). The exhibition profiled 250 items from the museum's accessory collection spanning 1550 to 1950. It featured a diversity of fashion objects from more familiar to obscure items, exhibiting items from across the spectrum

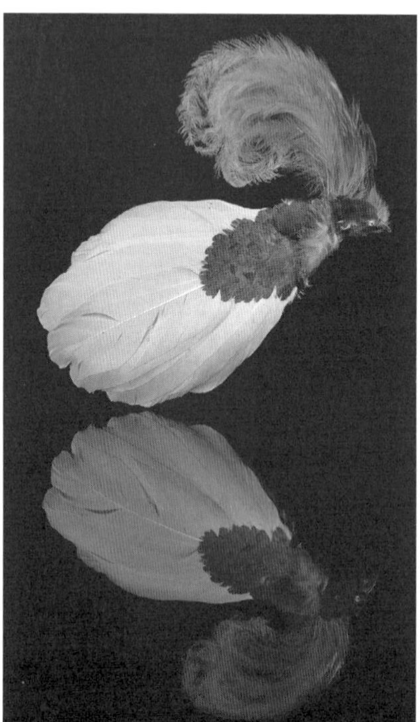

FIGURE 15.4 Corsage, ca. 1910–1915. Flamingo tail feathers, head of a glossy starling, nando feathers, paint. *Credit*: Courtesy of Rijksmuseum, Amsterdam, http://www.rijksmuseum.nl.

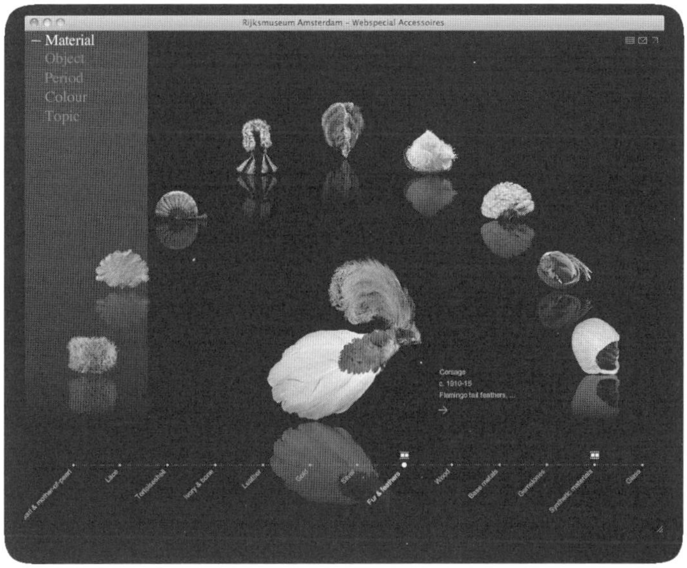

FIGURE 15.5 Screenshot of corsage and other accessories from the online exhibition Accessorize!
Credit: Courtesy of Rijksmuseum, Amsterdam, http://www.rijksmuseum.nl.

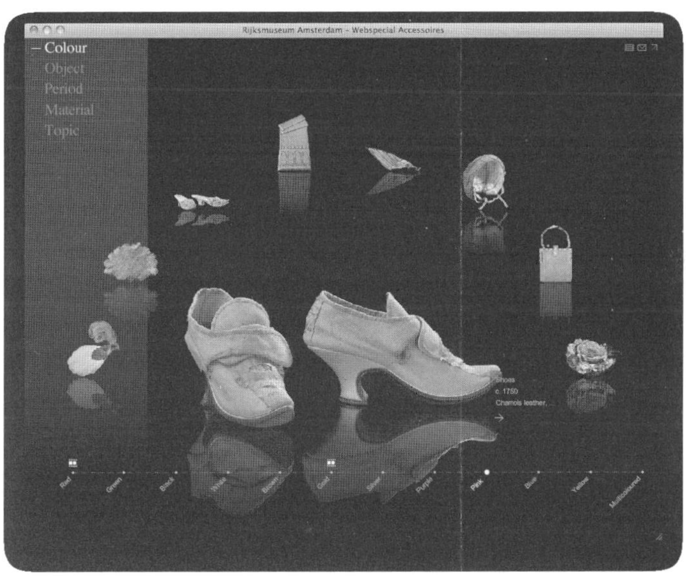

FIGURE 15.6 Screenshot of accessories from the online exhibition Accessorize!
Credit: Courtesy of Rijksmuseum, Amsterdam, http://www.rijksmuseum.nl.

of accoutrements, from hats to tassels. The exhibition navigated through interactive animations and facilitated an intimate scrutiny of and familiarity with chosen objects. Detailed inspection of each accessory was heightened when the object was zoomed in, guided by individualized selection of and enjoyment in viewing each item. Objects staged for intense observation are set in an open space on a black-mirrored surface, devoid of display infrastructure. Reflection from the ground suggested another perspective on the object, allowing the accessory item to be observed from underneath. The glossy environment accentuated the object experience, drawing attention in particular to the less conspicuous, obscure, or small-scale items. Researcher Martijn Stevens commented about the exhibition's impact: "you could never get that close at a real exhibition. Exhibits like these are almost always shown in display cases" (quoted in Gollin 2010). Different pathways for individual selections were curated through themes of materials, types of objects, color, period, and topic, building up layers of information depending on the participant's interest. The exhibition site's lush imagery of each object is supported by text, the narrative positioned not to disturb the framing of each object.

THE VIRTUAL MUSEUM

Focus on a single designer or design house has been a popular style of exhibition making, an ambitious enterprise of comprehensively reviewing and curating the design directions and creative projects of a designer or design house. This type of exhibition is large in scale and resource heavy, and key garments are exposed over long periods, particularly when the exhibition tours. The compelling experience moves design house archives outside the fashion industry into the public domain. For example, the retrospective Valentino: Themes and Variations, exhibited at the Musée des Arts Décoratifs, Paris, in 2008, later exhibited under the title Valentino Retrospective—Past, Present, Future, at the Gallery of Modern Art (GOMA) in Brisbane, Australia, in 2010, was drawn from the extensive archive of the designer, presenting a set of ideals about luxury fashion expressed through an extensive repository of fashion. The exhibition illuminated and exposed specialized fashion knowledge captured by close scrutiny of haute couture garments. The curator, Pamela Golbin, sought to engage with defining garment characteristics. Her curatorial approach dissected various elements that informed Valentino designs. In this endeavor Golbin analyzed clothing structure and aesthetic choices through the application of ornamentation and the use of volume, surface, and line (Golbin 2008). In Australia the exhibition attracted 202,000 visitors over three months.[15]

The repository of a design house, sitting outside the auspices of the museum, is a key independent source of fashion knowledge. However, archives are onerous and expensive resources to manage. The extensive archive of Yves Saint Laurent, for instance, managed by the Foundation of Pierre Bergé,[16] has established an organization and venue devoted to the management of over 5,000 haute couture garments and related materials, involving conservation, promotion, and curation of exhibitions from the archive. The archive is available to researchers and continues to generate exhibitions like Yves Saint Laurent: The Retrospective (2010), curated by Florence Müller and Farid Chenoune. However, given the limits of extensively touring retrospective exhibitions, what are other ways to curate a retrospective or travel through the designer archive?

Following the success of the Valentino retrospective and the increased interest in studying his collections, the idea of a Valentino Museum, like the Yves Saint Laurent model, was mooted. However, the model of a physical repository was abandoned for a virtual one. The potential of an online retrospective is the enormous capacity to convey the entire scope of a designer or design house's repertoire, without compromising the physical condition of the works or being limited by space or finances. The Valentino Garavarni virtual museum was launched in 2011 as a free downloadable software application, or app.[17] Described as a free desktop exhibition (Wilson 2011), the collection is experienced in a simulated museum. Set in an all-white space, within seven animated galleries, garments are presented on mannequins stationed on plinths. In the press the magnitude of this enterprise was translated in physical terms as covering the equivalent of "107,500 square-feet of exhibition space" (West 2011). As the user wanders through the extensive gallery spaces, individual garments can be selectively activated for a 360-degree point of view, actualized in real-time rendering.[18] Particular garments can be zoomed in to show close-ups of design features. However, the main attraction of the virtual museum is access to layers of information and customized pathways. The software activates a multilayered experience. The virtual exhibition goes beyond a curated arrangement of fashion garments. Specific garments are linked to other activities related to garment experiences/relationships, interviews, videos of past exhibitions and events, insights into design practices (such as sharing a master class with Valentino), and a media library with 5,000 images, including dresses, photos, drawings, and 180 fashion show videos. In launching this extensive online exhibition and fashion repository the designer Valentino commented:

> I see it as part of my legacy. I am happy that thousands of students, young designers and fashion people will be able to see and study my work in every aspect of it and in a manner easy and accessible for the younger generations. But it is also important to remember things of the past, to review the fashion that has shaped our lives. I would call it Future Memory. (West 2011)

The Valentino virtual museum provided a model that perhaps other design houses will follow, but it also suggests renewal of the retrospective exhibition and consideration of other ways to provide insight on and gain knowledge about a designer's complete oeuvre.

NETWORKING THE OBJECT

Fashion historian Giorgio Riello argued that the fashion exhibition represents only a small sampling of the museum repository. Limitations imposed by cost and location can limit the scope of an exhibition, resulting in "distillation and often a simplification" (2011). For example, the Powerhouse Museum in Sydney, Australia,[19] exhibits about 3 percent of its collection at any one time (Cameron and Mengler 2011). Traditionally the exhibition has been the main communication mode of the museum. The authority of the museum was invested in the custodianship of object collections and their storage, display, and interpretation (Schweibenz 2011).

Obviously, delivering access to the collection database is a key conduit to open participation with the museum, which potentially addresses issues of exclusive scholarship and perceived inaccessibility of collections. Digitization has made collections simply available on the Web. The Powerhouse Museum, although exhibiting a fraction of its holdings, has a database of over 99,000 objects available for interested parties to access at any time.[20] In 2006 the museum launched the browser "folksonomies," where users can search the collection with ordinary "tag" words instead of applying curatorial or technical terminology (Griffin 2011).

Users can explore the catalog in multiple ways, delving into curatorial worksheets and reading the object's history and any additional information gathered by the museum curator. The *Object of the Week* blog highlights a particular work from the repository to convey the scope of the collection in a more random way. Digitization of objects has enhanced the capacity of the user to research fashion across collection databases and has created the potential for individuals to curate their own fashion experiences. An individual has the means to compare particular works, create different object sequences, and contextualize an object further by linking with other media networks.

FUTURE DIRECTIONS AND DEBATE

New models of fashion curation have emerged to express a diversity of fashion experiences across the museum and the Web. Curating immaterial forms and conditions of fashion has spawned diverse and innovative interactions with the community. Access to and participation in exhibition and museum processes have shifted how people engage with fashion objects and experiences. Actions of navigation, retrieval, generation, and viewing create new relations of consumption, production, and distribution between the museum, curator, and community.

Collaborative multimedia formats have increased the potential for devising exhibitions as compositions accessed exclusively on the Web. Running parallel to these curatorial activities are the increasing explorations in the physical space, and the crossovers that can occur. Online curation has introduced diverse ways to present and network fashion for new and growing audiences. In online exhibitions, innovative ways are tested to complement and expand physical exhibitions, present emergent design practices, or curate independent experiences.

NOTES

1. *Net Generation* refers to people who have grown up in a world of computers and are familiar with digital ways of communicating.
2. "Your Ossie Clark Memories," Ossie Clark exhibition website, Victoria and Albert Museum, London, 2003, http://www.vam.ac.uk/vastatic/microsites/1250_ossieclark/memories/ (accessed December 22, 2011).

3. Claire Wilcox, "Questions Answered," Vivienne Westwood exhibition website, 2004, http://www.vam.ac.uk/vastatic/microsites/1231_vivienne_westwood/answers.html (accessed December 22, 2011).
4. "Create a Couture Inspired Dress," The Golden Age of Couture: Paris and London 1947–1957 exhibition website, Victoria and Albert Museum, London, 2007, http://www.vam.ac.uk/vastatic/microsites/1486_couture/create.php (accessed December 22, 2011).
5. "Your Elegant Dress Videos," The Golden Age of Couture: Paris and London 1947–1957 exhibition website, Victoria and Albert Museum, London, 2007, http://www.vam.ac.uk/vastatic/microsites/1486_couture/yourElegantDressTC.php (accessed December 22, 2011).
6. *blog.mode: Addressing Fashion,* Metropolitan Museum of Art, 2008, http://blog.metmuseum.org/blogmode/about/ (accessed December 1, 2011).
7 "Frequently Asked Questions," SHOWstudio, http://showstudio.com/faqs (accessed December 11, 2011).
8. "Research and Development," Carol Christian Poell, MAK (Austrian Museum of Applied Arts/Contemporary Art) Special Archive, http://carolchristianpoell.mak.at/research (accessed December 15, 2011).
9. Artangel, http://www.artangel.org.uk/.
10. This will be an extension to Clark's website: a workshop that will address specific online content rather than document past projects. Judith Clark Costume website, 2002–2011, http://judithclarkcostume.com/gallery/child-of-costume-gallery-1/ (accessed December 21, 2011).
11. The International Council of Museums (ICOM) "sets minimum standards of professional practice and performance of museums and staff" (http://icom.museum/ethics.html). Guidelines formulated by the Costume Committee offer basic standards of care and display ethics that are adopted by museums worldwide. The intention of the document is to assist curators and museum management in dealing with fragile garments.
12. Originally titled Malign Muses: When Fashion Turns Back (ModeMuseum [MoMu], Antwerp, September 18, 2004, to January 30, 2005), the exhibition was retitled Spectres: When Fashion Turns Back when shown at the Victoria and Albert Museum, London, February 24 to May 8, 2005, curated by Judith Clark. The exhibition researched "restaging" the relationship between contemporary fashion and its history. A section devoted to worn-out garments was entitled the "New Distress."
13. Noble Rot: An Alternate View of Fashion, National Trust of Australia (Victoria), February 18 to July 18, 2006, curated by Robyn Healy. The exhibition experimented with representational forms for conveying the circulation of fashion, documenting its demise by studying transformative and dilapidated states.
14. Accessorize! was launched on January 20, 2008, curated by Bianca du Mortier and Ninke Bloemberg, with interactive design and development by Cristina Garcia Martin and Joost van Grinsven. Accessorize! Online Exhibition, Rijksmuseum, https://www.rijksmuseum.nl/formats/accessoires/ (accessed December 1, 2011).
15. Curation of a fashion designer's archives often implies a relaxation of practices as designers wish their collections to be experienced outside of glass showcases and standard museum conditions, allowing gallery visitors/participants to touch or view garments in close proximity.

16. Fondation Pierre Bergé Yves Saint Laurent, http://www.fondation-pb-ysl.net/en.
17. *App* is an abbreviation for application. It refers to a software program that runs on electronic devices such as computers and mobile phones.
18. Real-time rendering provides opportunity for the user to interact with a virtual environment, showing an image fast enough to show realistic motion.
19. The Powerhouse Museum is the major branch of the Museum of Applied Arts and Sciences in Sydney, Australia. The collection contains a diverse range of objects covering history, science, technology, design, industry, the decorative arts, music, transport, and space exploration.
20. "Search the Powerhouse Museum Collection," Powerhouse Museum, http://www.powerhousemuseum.com/collection/database/ (accessed December 21, 2011).

BIBLIOGRAPHY

Barker, Emma (ed.). 1999. *Contemporary Cultures of Display.* New Haven, CT: Yale University Press.

Beard, Alice. 2008. "Show and Tell: An Interview with Penny Martin, Editor in Chief of SHOWstudio." *Fashion Theory: The Journal of Dress, Body and Culture* 12 (2): 181–96.

Bigolin, Ricarda, and Robyn Healy. 2010. *The Endless Garment: The New Craft of Machine Knitting.* Melbourne: Royal Melbourne Institute of Technology Gallery.

Black, Sandy. 2007. "Interrogating Fashion: Practice Process and Presentation. New Paradigms for Fashion Design in the 21st Century." In Tom Inns (ed.), *Designing for the 21st Century: Interdisciplinary Questions and Insights,* 299–314. Aldershot, UK: Gower.

Bugg, Jessica. 2009. "Fashion at the Interface: Designer-Wearer-Viewer." *Fashion Practice: The Journal of Design, Creative Process and the Fashion Industry* 1 (1): 9–32.

Cameron, Fiona, and Sarah Mengler. 2011. "Activating the Networked Object for a Complex World." In Georgios Styliaras, Dimitrios Koukopoulos, and Fotis Lazarinis (eds.), *Handbook of Research on Technologies and Cultural Heritage: Applications and Environments,* 166–87. New York: Information Science Reference.

Debo, Kaat. 2002. "The Fashion Museum Backstage." In Kaat Debo (ed.), *The Fashion Museum: Backstage,* 11–19. Ghent, Belgium: Ludion.

Debo, Kaat. 2011. "Introduction." In Kaat Debo (ed.), *Dream the World Awake, Walter Van Beirendonck,* 5. Tielt, Belgium: Lanoo.

de la Haye, Amy, Lou Taylor, and Emma Thompson. 2005. *A Family of Fashion: The Messels: Six Generations of Dress.* London: Philip Wilson.

Derrida, Jacques. 1996. *Archive Fever: A Freudian Impression.* Chicago: University of Chicago Press.

Durbin, Gail. 2004. "Learning from Amazon and eBay: User-Generated Material for Museum Web Sites." *Museums and the Web.* http://museumsandtheweb.com/mw2004/papers/durbin/durbin.html (accessed December 22, 2011).

Golbin, Pamela. 2008. *Valentino: Themes and Variations.* New York: Rizzoli.

Gollin, Rob. 2010. "Fine Art of Virtual Museums." *De Volkskrant* (Amsterdam), January 29. http://www.presseurop.eu/en/content/article/179611-fine-art-virtual-museums (accessed December 1, 2011).

Griffin, Des. 2011. "Digitisation to Social Media." In Des Griffin and Leon Parossien (eds.), *Understanding Museums: Australian Museums and Museology.* Canberra: National Museum of

Australia. http://nma.gov.au/research/understanding-museums/DGriffin_2011.html (accessed December 1, 2011).

Healy, Robyn. 2011. "Loving the Alien." In Kaat Debo (ed.), *Dream the World Awake, Walter van Beirendonck,* 47–57. Tielt, Belgium: Lanoo.

Kawamura, Yuniya. 2005. *Fashion-ology: An Introduction to Fashion Studies.* Oxford: Berg.

Krysa, Joasia. 2006b. "Introduction." In Joasia Krysa (ed.), *Curating Immateriality: The Work of the Curator in the Age of Network Systems,* 7–25. Brooklyn, NY: Autonomedia.

Lillemose, Jacob. 2006. "Conceptual Transformation of Art: From Dematerialisation of the Object to Immateriality in Networks." In Joasia Krysa (ed.), *Curating Immateriality: The Work of the Curator in the Age of Network Systems,* 117–39. Brooklyn, NY: Autonomedia.

Martin, Penny. 2010. "SHOWstudio.com." In José Teunissen (ed.), *Fashion and Imagination: About Clothes and Art,* 366–74. Arnhem, the Netherlands: ArtEZ Press.

McDonald, Sharon. 2006. "Collecting Practices." In Sharon McDonald (ed.), *A Companion to Museum Studies,* 81–97. Oxford: Blackwell.

McNeil, Peter. 2008. "'We're Not in the Fashion Business': Fashion in the Museum and Academy." *Fashion Theory: The Journal of Dress, Body and Culture* 12 (1): 65–82.

Menkes, Suzy. 2011. "Gone Global: Fashion as Art?" *New York Times,* July 4. http://www.nytimes.com/2011/07/05/fashion/is-fashion-really-museum-art.html (accessed December 2, 2011).

Palmer, Alexandra. 2008. "Untouchable: Creating Desire and Knowledge in Museum Costume and Textile Exhibitions." *Fashion Theory: The Journal of Dress, Body and Culture* 12 (1): 31–63.

Quinn, Bradley. 2009. *Textile Futures: Fashion, Design and Technology.* Oxford: Berg.

Riello, Giorgio. 2011. "The Object of Fashion: Methodological Approaches to the History of Fashion." *Journal of Aesthetics and Culture* 3. http://www.aestheticsandculture.net/index.php/jac/article/view/8865/12789 (accessed December 11, 2011).

Roche, Daniel. 1994. *The Culture of Clothing: Dress and Fashion in the Ancien Régime.* Trans. Jean Birrell. Cambridge: Cambridge University Press.

Schweibenz, Werner. 2011. "Museums and Web 2.0: Some Thoughts about Authority, Communication, Participation and Trust." In Georgios Styliaras, Dimitrios Koukopoulos, and Fotis Lazarinis (eds.), *Handbook on Research Technologies and Cultural Heritage: Applications and Environments,* 1–15. New York: Information Science Reference.

Smyth, Diane. 2009. "Nick Knight: Showman." *Aperture,* no. 197 (Winter): 68–75. http://www.dazeddigital.com/fashion/article/11272/1/20-qas-gareth-pugh (accessed December 5, 2011)

Taylor, Lou. 2002. *The Study of Dress History.* Manchester: Manchester University Press.

West, Hattie. 2011. "Valentino's Virtual Museum." *British Vogue,* November 27. http://www.vogue.co.uk/news/2011/11/21/valentino-launches-online-museum (accessed December 5, 2011).

Wilson, Eric. 2011. "Touring Valentino's Museum, Virtually." *New York Times,* December 5. http://runway.blogs.nytimes.com/2011/12/05/touring-valentinos-museum-virtually/ (accessed December 5, 2011).

Witcomb, Andrea. 2006. "Interactivity: Thinking Beyond." In Sharon MacDonald (ed.), *A Companion to Museum Studies,* 353–61. Oxford: Blackwell.

SECTION V

Fashion, Agency, and Policy

Introduction

REGINA A. ROOT

When scholars analyze dress and fashion through the lens of human engagement and cultural history, they inevitably find themselves at a juncture not insignificant to the field. Social and political forces shape culture; fashion is no exception. How, then, does one decenter fashion studies and understand more fully the contents of its scope? Given fashion's symbolic role as a cultural "happening" and a growing interest in fashion as a source of creative expression, scholars are literally in the process of piecing together the fragments of global fashion history and theorizing its content. While this long-term recovery project will surely yield many fresh insights, it also brings up important questions about fashion studies as shaped by Western discourses of power and privilege. For this reason, scholars logically question the construction of fashion as a Western phenomenon and have repositioned contemporary studies of fashion within the framework of agency, policy, and global phenomena (Barnes and Eicher 1992; Craik 1993; Hansen 2004; Niessen, Leshkowich, and Jones 2003). Yet others examine the legacies of colonial and postcolonial narratives that have altered or shaped the very fashionable constructs we seek to unlock and understand (McClintock 1995; Root 2010).

Fashion is a powerful cultural tool that conveys meaning. It rearticulates the past, inspires creative expression, enacts change, and produces meaning through the agency of its wearer. Policies governing the use of fashion, whether in the form of sumptuary laws that ultimately promote the emergence of fashion or the link to citizenship and collective identities, further impact its practices and performances. While scholars generally agree that "worn fashion generates meaning" (Evans and Thornton 1991) and that fashion constitutes part of a larger cultural process, we have already seen that its definition and meaning generate less consensus. If fashion emerged alongside European-style democracy and modernity (Lipovetsky 1994; Wilson 1985), such terms of engagement would appear to ascribe static characteristics to non-Western styles. To further complicate matters, what constitutes Western and non-Western is in itself an artificial construct. While traditional scholarly assessments can be a useful point of departure to ascertain cross-cultural registers (Ribeiro 2002, for example) and to document the development of taste and social distinction (Bourdieu [1979] 1984), the recovery project underway in global fashion studies centers on the relationship of fashion to its cultural, economic, political, and social contexts. Within the framework of colonialism and, later, contemporary globalization, matters related to appropriation and consumption become particularly complicated, as fashion represents the inevitable negotiations that unite the local to the global and tradition to modernity (Maynard 2004; Roces and Edwards 2007; Ross 2008).

Scholars have traditionally defined the terms of fashion as "a historically and geographically specific system for the production and organization of dress" (Entwistle 2000: 44) or, through Michel Foucault, as "the dominant system governing dress in the West" (Entwistle 2001: 39). One recent definition defines fashion as "changing styles of dress and appearance that are adopted by a group of people at any given time and place," only to later associate it exclusively with the emergence of capitalism in western Europe. And "fashion innovation follows power and money," the essay continues (Welters and Lillethun 2011: 5). As a matter of taste, even something called "post-fashion" now has "all the power of seduction of a moody sovereign, certain of conquering" (Vinken 2005: 3). Recent work asserts that fashion as "a characteristic of non-Western cultures remains debatable," in part because some criteria give or deny "fashionable value" through textual and visual representation (Tortora 2010: 167–68). Such tendencies to associate fashion with interpretive power marginalize the creative expressions of those cultures subjected to colonial invasions and the exploitative practices of cultural appropriation in contemporary globalization, all topics of critical significance for the field.

Volumes dedicated to the dress and fashions of entire world culture regions that were traditionally underrepresented or previously unrepresented now offer a more holistic view of the field at large. *The Greenwood Encyclopedia of World Popular Culture* (Hoppenstand 2007) covered the subject of "fashion and appearance" across world culture regions, and the *Berg Encyclopedia of World Dress and Fashion* (Eicher 2010) has documented the foundations of global fashion history through archival documents, the study of museum objects, and fieldwork and continues to be updated digitally as more information becomes available. While such substantive studies have made inroads, these works are far from complete. Scholars are in the process of piecing together the fragments in spite of the scant resources available for fashion studies research, a reality that has slowed down the process and made cross-cultural comparisons difficult. Linguistic barriers have also created issues, with the lack of fashion studies translations into English giving some scholars the false impression that theory is not produced outside Europe and the United States. As scholars engage disciplinary and interdisciplinary approaches to recover cultural memory, they will need to build on existing frameworks thoughtfully and with an eye for the kind of substantive data that can move the field along expediently.

Fashion has long been a tool for change, and yet understanding change as a series of negotiations and a process has proved remarkably challenging due to the lack of cultural connections made. For example, in the early part of the twenty-first century, one finds the ancient roots of fashion from many world culture regions represented on the catwalks that herald future styles. International luxury brands have appropriated and reinvented the free-fitting and classic shape of the Latin American poncho, for example, without ever recognizing that the style predates the arrival of Europeans, its messages and meanings altered throughout the colonial and postcolonial periods, and that it now serves as a garment evoking cultural identity and utopian possibilities. Argentine textile artists Mechi Martínez and Marián Breccia take unwanted clothing now sold by the dozen, much of it discarded U.S. clothing from the 1970s, 1980s, and 1990s, and refashion its fragments into various designs, including youth-inspired ponchos with an urban edge. With a label that evokes *los chicos del 12NA* (referring to young people who buy unwanted used clothing on sale, often for sale in units by the dozen), the artists deconstruct existing garments into new textile units, reconstructing them to communicate new meanings, cross borders, and build bridges (between the artists, artisans, and local customs central to the process of fashioning something new). In this way, the designers claim to not only reinvent classics but unite time. While the luxury brands appropriate designs without acknowledging their origins or cultural roots, los chicos del 12NA assumes a very different outlook and projects for the wearer a different type of agency in the era of contemporary globalization. Creating one-of-a-kind pieces from the very real fragments of fashion's past, ones dumped by the powerful and privileged (whether or not they see themselves as such is perhaps insignificant), these Argentine textile artists connect networks of consumer citizenship to a larger ecology of the multinational supply chain. To engage the poncho is not enough; piecing together the fragments to create an icon of South American identity implies a time-layered approach. One might argue that such an exercise in the constructedness of a garment brought together by los chicos del 12NA parallels some of the scholarly work in this section, as scholars have deconstructed various facets of fashion history and theory in order to cross borders, make connections, and reconstruct meaning as a globalized phenomenon.

While the use of fashion has traditionally been circumscribed by geography, such as the localized examinations of hand-me-downs or national styles of dress, agency takes place these days on the global stage. The way people are agents vis-à-vis fashion has changed dramatically, writes Jennifer Craik, and nothing perhaps exemplifies this more than the fashion tourist, whose gaze for fashion has expanded exponentially. Her chapter, "Fashion, Tourism, and Global Culture," reveals how luxury brands and goods acquire an almost sacred status, especially when the designer-brand version of a local appropriation means more than its homegrown original. Craik links fashion and tourism to the nineteenth-century fashion-conscious traveler to whom iconic brands like Louis Vuitton originally marketed their handmade products. Department store displays further stimulated consumption with "exotic goods from faraway places." Luxury, she writes, became "the essence of modern fashion and the motivating force behind fashion tourism." Scholars will find of great interest the proliferation of fashion shows, trade expos, and fashion weeks, which play important roles in the economic development and promotion of national cultural industries: "some fashion weeks are government funded as a way to promote the culture of a place and with the hope of attracting attention to the local fashion industry and attracting investment or boosting exports." Her analysis exposes a shift in fashion flows from north to south and west to east, with the fashion tourist emerging as "the new figure of consumerism in global culture."

The flows of international tourism and globalization have made it important for design to be relevant to the communities it represents and serves. Mary A. Littrell and Judy Frater's chapter, "Artisan Enterprise: Development, Cultural Property, and the Global Market," examines artisan enterprises through development research, integrated field notes, and personal experiences with two Indian artisan enterprises operating in the global fashion market, Kala Raksha Trust and MarketPlace: Handwork of India. While heritage designs are recognized as a cultural asset, these are not always assigned commercial value. For the many artisans employed by the global marketplace, affiliations to cultural identity in design, once clear to the workers, get devalued when designers and design firms opt for "faster, cheaper, and more uniform" models of production and manipulate art forms like embroidery. Littrell and Frater reveal how artisan enterprises grounded in an educational and human rights framework have helped workers to regain pride in their skills, become active interpreters in matters of heritage or intellectual property, create textile libraries that preserve cultural memory and provide inspiration for new designs, and learn how to reach markets that value their products. Linking artisan groups to the goals of economic empowerment and social action, the authors explain, emphasizes the agency of workers, their autonomy, and the well-being of the communities in which they live.

Latin American fashion design and history has traditionally been overlooked despite its vibrancy and significance to mass-market ranges throughout the world. "Mapping Latin American Fashion," the next chapter, situates this world culture region's dress in the context of overlapping sociohistorical influences. When *The Latin American Fashion Reader* appeared in 2005, its pages integrated the study of the region's dress into the workings of culture, identity formation, and social change (Root 2005). At a time when digital images circulate in a flash and many lament the loss of cultural heritage throughout the Americas, contemporary design professionals have begun to reassess fashions past on their own terms. This chapter provides a brief overview of the issues that have shaped Latin American fashion history and that often get referenced by the region's multiple fashion weeks and the media. Emphasizing the links between dress practices and the nineteenth-century nation-building process, a topic of great significance as nations embark on a third century of independence, this chapter provides new archival evidence from the River Plate region that demonstrates how dress served as a tool for creative agency following the retreat of Spanish colonialism.

Karen Tranberg Hansen's chapter, "Secondhand Clothing and Africa: Global Fashion Influences, Local Dress Agency, and Policy Issues," argues that secondhand clothing should be a central, not marginalized, topic of research due to its place in the global marketplace. "Our notion of fashion has changed its focus from an upscale property of the West's rapidly shifting style innovations to everyday preoccupations with multidirectional style shifts across the globe," she writes. While one may find secondhand clothing in vintage boutiques on high streets or in "open-air markets in the developing world," the latter have often been portrayed as a charitable process linking the local to the West rather than the beginning of refashioned cultural expressions. Through agency and policy, Hansen describes the international secondhand market, examines supply and demand in African clothing markets, and offers insights into how wearers in Zambia interpret style and fashion "new looks" through "clothing competence," or strategic innovations that convey cultural norms and status on Zambian terms. Consumers in Zambia, she concludes, "are arbiters of stylistic innovations that are contributing to the breakdown of fashion's Western hegemony."

Global fashion studies continue to unravel the complexities of self-fashioning and style appropriations, competing discourses and pockets of resistance, crises and disruptions, among other sociocultural issues. This section aims to lay the groundwork for new connections that will foster a more inclusive fashion studies.

BIBLIOGRAPHY

Barnes, Ruth, and Joanne B. Eicher (eds.). 1992. *Dress and Gender: Making and Meaning.* Oxford: Berg.

Bourdieu, Pierre. [1979] 1984. *Distinction: A Social Critique of the Judgement of Taste.* Trans. Richard Nice. Cambridge, MA: Harvard University Press.

Craik, Jennifer. 1993. *The Face of Fashion.* London: Routledge.

Eicher, Joanne B. (ed.). 2010. *Berg Encyclopedia of World Dress and Fashion.* 10 vols. Oxford: Berg.

Entwistle, Joanne. 2000. *The Fashioned Body: Fashion, Dress and Modern Social Theory.* Cambridge, UK: Polity.

Entwistle, Joanne. 2001. "The Dressed Body." In Joanne Entwistle and Elizabeth Wilson (eds.), *Body Dressing,* 33–58. Oxford: Berg.

Evans, Caroline, and Minna Thornton. 1991. "Fashion, Representation, Femininity." *Feminist Review* 38: 48–66.

Hansen, Karen Tranberg. 2004. "The World in Dress: Anthropological Perspectives on Clothing, Fashion, and Culture." *Annual Review of Anthropology* 22: 369–92.

Hoppenstand, Gary (ed.). 2007. *The Greenwood Encyclopedia of World Popular Culture.* 6 vols. Westport, CT: Greenwood.

Lipovetsky, Gilles. 1994. *The Empire of Fashion.* Princeton, NJ: Princeton University Press.

Maynard, Margaret. 2004. *Dress and Globalisation.* Manchester: Manchester University Press.

McClintock, Anne. 1995. *Imperial Leather: Race, Gender and Sexuality in the Colonial Contest.* New York: Routledge.

Niessen, Sandra, Ann Marie Leshkowich, and Carla Jones (eds.). 2003. *Re-orienting Fashion: The Globalization of Asian Dress.* Oxford: Berg.

Ribeiro, Aileen. 2002. *Dress in Eighteenth-Century Europe, 1751–1789.* Rev. ed. New Haven, CT: Yale University Press.

Roces, Mina, and Louise Edwards (eds.). 2007. *The Politics of Dress in Asia and the Americas.* Brighton, UK: Sussex Academic.

Root, Regina A. 2005. *The Latin American Fashion Reader.* Oxford: Berg.

Root, Regina A. 2010. *Couture and Consensus: Fashion and Politics in Postcolonial Argentina.* Minneapolis: University of Minnesota Press.

Ross, Robert. 2008. *Clothing: A Global History; or, The Imperialist's New Clothes.* Cambridge, UK: Polity.

Tortora, Phyllis. 2010. "History and Development of Fashion." In Joanne B. Eicher (ed.), *Berg Encyclopedia of World Dress and Fashion,* vol. 10, *Global Perspectives,* 159–70. Oxford: Berg.

Vinken, Barbara. 2005. *Fashion Zeitgeist: Trends and Cycles in the Fashion System.* Oxford: Berg.

Welters, Linda, and Abby Lillethun (eds.). 2011. *The Fashion Reader.* 2nd ed. Oxford: Berg.

Wilson, Elizabeth. 1985. *Adorned in Dreams: Fashion and Modernity.* London: Virago.

16

Fashion, Tourism, and Global Culture

JENNIFER CRAIK

INTRODUCTION: THE GLOBAL FACE OF FASHION

Fashion is the face of the global village. In fact, fashion has a number of faces that overlap, conflict, and mesh simultaneously. Different messages are conveyed—about cultural identity and distinctiveness, global brands, local inflections, shared knowledge about fashion systems, the universality of style, cultural sophistication, authenticity, cultural tradition, handcrafted versus mass produced, branded versus generic, and so on. As consumers—and as tourists—we absorb these messages almost unconsciously and make decisions based on how we process these messages. The result is that the world of fashion *converges* with the world of tourism (Jansson and Power 2010: 898–99), and increasingly the niche genre of *fashion tourism* has become part and parcel of the tourist industry just as tourism has become an adjunct to the fashion industry. Both fashion and tourism create dreams and images of otherness and made-up identities where consumers can "buy into/'travel to' this dream place" (Polhemus 2005: 87). Fashion tourism is the logical refinement of dream weaving. Here I briefly explore the links between fashion and tourism historically, illustrate this through the example of Louis Vuitton, and finally look at the role of fashion weeks in the contemporary development of fashion tourism.

However, it is a complex phenomenon. There are many examples showing how fashion exists within tourism, including the following:

1. Ethnic, customary, and national dress as fashion (or adopted as fashion by tourists) (e.g., saris, *shalwar kamiz,* headwraps, batik shirts, Breton shirts, etc.)
2. Souvenir fashion (e.g., logo T-shirts, hats, and accessories)

3. Tourist fashion (sports shoes, T-shirts, polo shirts, casual "easy-to-wear" pants, parka-style jackets, etc.), often mixed with the everyday dress of locals (e.g., sarongs in Bali, hibiscus board shorts at beach resorts)
4. Adoption of niche fashion of the destination (e.g., resort wear, clubbing fashion, surfwear, safari fashion)
5. Stylistic and aesthetic trends that morph into new fashion trends (e.g., kimono, *kuffiya,* mirrored and hand-embroidered blouses)
6. Local boutique and designer fashion (e.g., local specialist high-end fashion designs and brands)
7. Global designer-brand fashion (Gucci, Burberry, Louis Vuitton)
8. Global high fashion worn by fashion journalists, stylists, and celebrities who travel worldwide to attend fashion weeks and special fashion events
9. Fashion stores, designer headquarters, fashion-focused shopping malls, and fashion precincts that become tourist attractions rivaling conventional tourist sites and promoted as catering for "shopping tourism"
10. The centrality of the marketing of specialist clothes for adventure tourism and sports-related tourism using high-profile celebrities who appeal to fashion-conscious urban consumers (e.g., surfwear as streetwear, modified extreme sportswear as fashion, leisure fashion made from high-tech fibers and fabrics)

We can recognize some or all of these as forms of *fashion tourism,* suggesting that the term covers broad and diverse phenomena, some of which are more fashion oriented than others, which are generic. This paper is mostly referring to the last four types of tourism-related fashion. While these types refer to contemporary fashion tourism, there is also a close historical relationship between the development of tourism and the development of modern Western fashion. Both are characterized by the impulse for consumerism, spectacle, the exotic, the new, and the search for imaginary identities. Even the earliest shopping malls and department stores established in the nineteenth century, such as Bon Marché (1838/1852, regarded as the world's first department store),[1] were promoted as bigger and more spectacular than contemporary tourist attractions in their respective locations. In other words, from the outset, the world of fashion was part of the scope of tourism.

However, there have been few studies of fashion and tourism, as ecotourism analyst Ralph Buckley notes:

> There seems to be some strong links between the commercial travel sector and the clothing, fashion and entertainment (CFE) industries. . . . [Furthermore,] commercial practice in the CFE sectors makes use of adventure activities, professionals and imagery, but it is perhaps unlikely that the CFE sectors have any specific interest in tourism, even adventure tourism. (2003: 126)

However, Buckley's analysis of adventure tourism shows there are

> quite strong and mutually reinforcing business links... between adventure tour operators, clothing manufacturers, and the entertainment industry [that are] essentially mediated by fashion, rather than any fundamental business links, so in the longer term they may well prove ephemeral. Currently, however, they are strong enough to have quite significant financial implications for the adventure tourism sector. (129)

He illustrates this argument with reference to the promotion of snowboarding to sell casual winter clothing and the recruitment of professional basketballers to sell sports shoes as "mainstream urban streetwear" (130). On the pro surfing circuit individual surfers are sponsored by surf clothing and equipment manufacturers, who also promote the world championships, competitions, and events. These celebrity surfers sell the brands to the surf tourism sector and wider sports-aware but nonsurfing consumers. While the focus is on the star surfers, the "big money... is in selling surf-branded clothing and accessories to non-surfers" by conveying four messages: "surf clothing is cool; particular brands are coolest; here's what you need; here's how to get it" (131). As Buckley observes:

> This is very much a fashion message, and indeed, the big surfwear companies [like Billabong] see themselves in the "fashion apparel business." Note that while selling surfwear to actual surfers certainly involves an element of fashion, it does also require underlying functionality: boardshorts whose pockets are streamlined for paddling, wetsuits which keep you warm with minimum restriction, reef booties which save you from coral cuts but still let your feet feel the board, bags which let you carry your gear and your board on your bicycle or airplane. For the urban streetwear market, none of this matters—clothing can be identical to no-name equivalents, and the brand alone makes for many times the mark-up. (131)

Indeed, the streetwear version may instead need pockets for mobile phones, iPods, purses, wallets, credit cards, and car keys! The huge growth in global surfwear brands and their international market penetration have occurred because of their success in creating a generic "fashion market for surf clothing and accessories as urban streetwear, for both women and men who do not surf and live far from the ocean" and who are more "brand conscious" and buy more items than the surfers themselves (Buckley 2003: 132). Increasingly, surf brands have been promoted using images and slogans drawn from urban dreams and myths rather than surfing, making them indistinguishable from mainstream brands. Paradoxically, this may have contributed to recent falls in profits for surfwear companies and takeover bids from mainstream apparel companies. In short, their success may have also sown the seeds of their declining market share as fashion brands.

This example illustrates the interconnections between fashion and tourism as industries as well as the links between the activities and sensibilities of postmodern consumer culture. Yet they are rarely analyzed together. As Chris Rojek and John Urry have argued, tourism studies typically ignore

> the important issues of social and cultural practice and only consider tourism as a set of economic activities. Questions of taste, fashion and identity would thus be viewed as exogenous to the system. Tourism on this account is treated as a set of economic factors, and individuals are viewed as bundles of given preferences. (1997: 2)

CONSUMERISM, ADVERTISING, AND THE MEANING OF GOODS: THE MAGIC OF FASHION AND TOURISM

Some analysts have explored the passion for fashion by drawing on anthropological accounts of how possessions and rituals function as magic, the imaginary allure of qualities that can transcend the mundane experiences of the everyday. As Russell Belk argues:

> The contemporary world has been increasingly shorn of its myths, rituals, and mysteries as we have accepted that there is a rational explanation for the workings of the world we experience. In the face of this rationality, possessions have retained, if not enlarged, their role as magical vessels. (1991: 42)

This belief in magic has been enhanced by the qualities of consumer culture, especially advertising and "the cathedrals of department stores and shopping malls" (42). Luxury fashion brands have become the epitome of fashion magic where the use value of an "It" Hermès Birkin handbag or Louis Vuitton monogrammed suitcase is far exceeded by the symbolic value of its magical qualities—taste, tradition, status, and affluence. Such items are imbued with fetishistic qualities by their owners and admirers as totems of fashion, success, rarity, and the extraordinary. The irony is that despite global proliferation of luxury brands and their products and stores worldwide, luxury fashion has succeeded in retaining its cachet, yet as Belk observes:

> It may seem contradictory that the desire for rare and mysterious possessions could result in the veneration of branded consumer goods, but there is evidence that brands can sometimes be as sacred as more singular possessions. (33)

Even more bizarrely, fake or counterfeit versions of branded goods can be almost as highly valued as originals, perhaps because of the proliferation of pseudohistory, hyperreality, and pseudoauthenticity in so many contemporary consumer products, attractions, and events (Belk 1991: 33). Designers, brands, and labels are divided as to whether they should vigorously fight against the counterfeit industry—perhaps more lucrative than the legitimate one—or regard it as free advertising that ironically spurs demand and increases sales and brand awareness. Tourists often seek out fake luxury copies on their travels and proudly display them on their return home as valuable booty and symbols of their travel adventures. Once again, the worlds of fashion and tourism collide in their techniques of seduction and indulgence in the imaginary.

The vehicle for weaving consumer magic is advertising, whether it is for fashion or tourism:

> The formulas of consumer goods advertisers are not unlike those of alchemists, except that the transformation promised is in the individual who uses the product. Consumer goods become elixirs and brands become magical symbols; the advertising incantation seeks to mystify and mythologize the product. Especially when it is delivered to an audience that wants to believe, such advertising can sometimes elevate products to extraordinary status. Placing these products in the sumptuous displays of well-appointed department stores and shopping malls is a final step in successfully mystifying these goods. Thus, it is not surprising that impulse buying purchasing is often perceived as a magical synchronicity of being at the right place at the right time to indulge in the purchase of a special item. (Belk 1991: 34)

Luxury brands and goods have benefited from this phenomenon as consumers recall their travels and purchases through what they bought where, which adds to the perceived value of the item: "the Prada shirt I found on special in Milan," "the limited-edition handbag only available at Louis Vuitton headquarters in Paris," and so on. These goods serve as souvenirs of consumers' experiences as much as cherished possessions. The fusion of consumerism with modernism, urbanization, exploration, and globalization has become the marker of the new age.

Some of the most prominent luxury brands today were established from the middle of the nineteenth century targeting their products to the elite, who were also likely to be fashion-conscious travelers. Examples include Louis Vuitton (1854, selling luggage trunks), Hermès (1837, selling saddlery and leather goods and clothing), Burberry (1856, selling waterproofed gabardine trench coats), and Gucci (1921, selling luggage and leather goods). The fashion for luggage stemmed from the fashion for traveling to exotic faraway places that was at its zenith with explorers, adventurers, and voyagers taking advantage of new forms of transportation and newly colonized places, often for extended periods of time and thus requiring an extensive amount of luggage. They were not yet called "holiday makers"—their purpose was more spiritual and exotic! Luggage such as the Louis Vuitton monogram trunk "became synonymous with gracious traveling and elegant travelers."[2] This suggests that fashion and tourism were already intimately linked. So, why?

The connection between fashion and tourism was the spirit of consumerism based on creating desires that favored newness and nowness, whether that was fashions or destinations. Dating from the middle of the seventeenth century, urban life in particular became organized around conspicuous consumption and conspicuous leisure as epitomized by creating a display or spectacle, phenomena that were central to shopping and traveling. This consumerist impulse was well underway by the time department stores came along and took it to new heights (Henderson-Smith 2002; Kwass 2003). The new consumer citizen wanted to see and be seen, so shopping and traveling provided places to view and be viewed, spaces in which to promenade and be the flaneur, as well as creating a fantasy of otherness, freedom, and escape from the everyday.

Shops displayed exotic goods from faraway places that were imported as travel opened up new vistas and treasure troves of luxury, diversity, and the bizarre. Shops and travel were both "transitory spaces" (Henderson-Smith 2002: 57) in which consumers both escaped to and created new identities appropriate for these fantasy places. By stimulating desire, "fashion and travel stimulated consumption which further stimulated demand" (62). In the second half of the nineteenth century, department stores became megaspaces for consumption, the palaces of consumerism as well as of leisure and pleasure. They were also friendly places for women to visit and provided safe, well-equipped, yet alluring places for women to indulge themselves and discover the latest fashions, crazes, and trends. By placing a myriad of goods under one roof grouped into separate "departments of existence"—soft furnishings, corsetry and underwear, home furnishings, evening wear, men's suits, and so on—shoppers were introduced to unimaginable possibilities for living including imported exotica from far-flung colonies.

By the late nineteenth century, department stores were acknowledged sites of "leisure consumption," especially for women, who frequented stores appropriate to their social status. Wealthy women could buy fabric and have it made up by their dressmakers, while poorer ones purchased ready-made fashion. Catalogs and mail order made it possible to shop from home—a boon for women who lived far from a city. Promotion was all about carefree leisure and pleasure and "the 'femininity' of the shopping environment, clothed and draped with textiles" (Doy 2002: 76):

> For example, the 1880 *Au Bon Marché* catalogue showed women on a bench in the garden, women in a park, women holding parasols and fans, women painting and girls chasing butterflies. . . . The store [itself] became a machine-like woman, clothed in commodities. (76)

However, shopping was not always a benign experience. Although often interpreted as a democratizing development that dissolved class distinctions, early department stores *reinforced* social distinctions between shoppers, and between shoppers and the serving staff. Shoppers demonstrated their own pecking order of importance and fashion savvy, while staff were poorly paid and harshly treated as well as being pitted against one another due to the commission system (Doy 2002: 64). They could, however, exercise a measure of revenge by treating customers with disdain—what we now call "attitude"—if they seemed out of place. If customers had money, they were welcomed, but poorer customers hunted for bargains. Soon, those without cash took advantage of credit options that the stores thoughtfully introduced, creating a new social category of consumer debt and debtors. Customers could be ruthless and demanding, "keen to demonstrate their higher status by insulting the women sales staff" (64). The clash of fashion and consumerism produced a contested terrain.

To promote fashion in department stores, clothes were carefully displayed on mannequins in elaborate visual merchandising through scenes that told narratives about how and where clothes should be worn, thus conveying to consumers the possibility of unimagined lives and spaces to occupy. The new consumer citizen was shown

> things about which they did not know—that stimulated trade. Other elements of these displays stimulated future trade by creating wants and desires for the goods on display. The element of fantasy incorporated into the displays, for example, portrayed the types of pleasure to be gained from obtaining goods. (Henderson-Smith 2002: 61)

As Michael Miller argued:

> Fashions were the clearest example of this. It was not simply that clothing styles varied from year to year or that complete changes occurred. There were also entirely new kinds of clothing to fit entirely new wants. (1981: 185).

New fashions and goods created new desires that fanned the fashion for fashion. The desire to be fashionable and keep up with the Joneses kept the cycle of consumerism turning. This was also the period of the Great Exhibitions (London 1851, Paris 1889, Chicago 1893), which promoted amazing new inventions, technological masterpieces, exotica from the New World, and the latest in consumer goods. The world was recreated within this tangible experiential space of display and consumption, creating more wants and desires in new types of retail spaces and tourist promotion that incorporated the latest innovations and fashions.

In other words, there was a fusion of consumerism with other markers of contemporary civility—the spectacle and display, voyeurism and the flaneur, leisure and pleasure, newness and exotica, spaces and places, and fashion and fantasy. Among the retailers, "innovative merchants realised the advantages that lay in 'courting' women customers by settings that played upon fantasies of luxury" (Henderson-Smith 2002: 70). Consumerism was built on the proposition that "the commodities at the heart of capitalism display their key function—relations between people become relations between things" (Doy 2002: 77). Department stores and arcades became "public cathedrals that enhanced the mystery and sense of otherworldliness of the sacred... extravagant show places where functional and financial considerations pale in the magnificence of their grandiose display" in the service of consumer culture. Visiting these cathedrals "enlarged desires and created a sense of reverent awe for luxury and consumption" (Belk, Wallendorf, and Sherry 1989: 10). Luxury has become the essence of modern fashion and the motivating force behind fashion tourism.

LOUIS VUITTON AS EMBLEMATIC OF THE FASHION-TOURISM SYNERGY

As mentioned above, the Louis Vuitton flat suitcase covered in distinctive gray waterproof canvas became the fashionable travel luggage for those who could afford its handmade status (Thomas 2007). It was so popular that the shape and design were soon copied by other manufacturers of luggage. In those days, travelers went on long trips by slow transport, requiring much luggage, and thus a set of Louis Vuitton cases assembled together magnified their importance as the essential travel accoutrement. To retain its marketing edge, Louis Vuitton opened a store in London in 1885 (appealing to the Grand Tour clientele) and promoted its products at the Paris Exhibition of 1867 and in Chicago in 1893. Designs were produced to deter copies (thus enhancing the uniqueness and distinctiveness of the Vuitton brand). Aware of the likelihood of counterfeit—even at this stage—the so-called checkerboard Damier canvas pattern with the Louis Vuitton logo was adopted and later the brown-and-beige plaid canvas, and then the even more distinctive diamonds, stars, and flowers design interspersed with the logo with the entwined LV. All of these are still used today. Rather than confirm the uniqueness of the Louis Vuitton brand, this seemed to increase the allure (or magic) and inspire would-be copyists. In fact, Louis Vuitton is the most copied luxury brand, and the company spends considerable time filing counterfeit lawsuits.

Yet the company seemed to thrive on such niche competitiveness and—while maintaining the handcrafted quality and appeal to an exclusive clientele—continued to produce limited-edition products as well as commissioned items. It also launched a series of new products that appealed to new submarkets—such as Steamer bags, Keepall bags, and Speedy bags—that catered for the day-to-day needs of travelers. By naming each product and maintaining its finish, the company embedded the personalization of consumer goods with a name and an identity, furthering their consumer appeal to the identity and vanity of possessors of Louis Vuitton products.

During the early decades of the twentieth century, wealth and leisure were shifting from the aristocracy to the nouveau riche, and Louis Vuitton appealed to this group of social aspirants. The film industry produced celebrities who promoted the brand. The combination of advertising, new product development, and bourgeois vanity kept the company buoyant even during World War II and the occupation of Paris. In the postwar period, new materials and new product lines kept the brand au courant, although its clientele was aging and the brand was seen as old-fashioned (Thomas 2007: 34). Vuitton's cachet as elite fashion declined in the 1960s.

The firm's fortunes were reversed with the formation of the luxury brand conglomerate Louis Vuitton Moët Hennessy (LVMH) in 1987, heralding the birth of a new phase of luxury branding and high-end fashion consumerism. New products, marketing strategies, retailing approaches, art directors, collaborations with artists, stores, and product lines combined to make Louis Vuitton hip once again, especially appealing to new groups of aspiring consumers in new fashion capitals. Stores opened in Tokyo, Osaka, Taipei, Seoul,

Beijing, Marrakech, Milan, Mexico City, Yekaterinburg, São Paulo, Cancun, Johannesburg, Shanghai, and Singapore. There are now over 130 stores worldwide. Louis Vuitton is deemed to be the world's twenty-ninth most valuable brand[3] and one of the ten most powerful brands, worth US$24.3 billion.[4] Although most attention is paid to the flagship, stores in regional cities have proved more profitable (Moore and Doherty 2007: 284).

Flagship stores are often loss leaders, important as the visible symbol of the brand and useful for hosting promotional events and seducing celebrity clients but rarely financially profitable. Recent estimates suggest that 5 percent of flagship store customers account for 52 percent of sales, while 20 percent of all customers account for 60–80 percent of sales. This suggests that the vast majority of customers are "just looking." In fact, over half the income of luxury brands comes from wholesaling (Moore and Doherty 2007: 281, 283). Some markets are more profitable than others. China currently accounts for 15 percent of global sales, although most sales occur outside China on tourist trips and online. It is estimated that China's "share of the global luxury market will triple, to 44 percent, by 2020... [although analysts predict that] the wealth of China's upper-middle class has reached an inflection point" (*The Economist* 2011).

Unlike the retail sector generally, luxury brands are expanding their reach and product lines sold through brand boutiques, in-store franchises, and online. Louis Vuitton has embarked on new approaches—handmade manufacture has given way to at least some use of sewing machines, an assembly line, and possibly other mechanized processes described as "mass-produced luxury" though it still promotes its handcrafted traditions in advertising (Daily Mail Reporter 2010; Modigliani 2007: 92). It also launched a prêt-à-porter line of fashion in 1999. Celebrity endorsement is still central to promotional strategies, and recent campaigns have used popular musicians, sports stars, models, actors, and even iconic politicians.

Alongside aggressive promotional activities, Louis Vuitton has launched corporate citizen campaigns such as the Eye You See project, which displayed work commissioned from contemporary artists such as Takahashi Murakami. One project used installation artist Olafur Eliasson to create spectacular displays for its store windows to illustrate the synergies of fashion and high art marketing (Modigliani 2007).

Such ventures have been promoted as part of Vuitton's civic duty to "the greater good, its commitment to solidarity with culture, youth, and the great humanitarian causes of public health issues," with the company stating:

> Through patronage, LVMH intends to defend, and thereby redefine luxury as generous, affective, authentic, a definition to which the Group's chairman and his associates are truly committed. (LVMH website, quoted in Modigliani 2007: 92)

Yet, despite this declaration, in 2007 the company brought a case of infringement of intellectual property rights against a Danish art student who depicted a starving black child holding an LV Audra handbag with the caption "Simple Living," though she eventually won in 2011.

The example of Louis Vuitton shows that the links between fashion, global movements, travel, celebrity, and consumerism are firmly entrenched. This has set the scene for the collision of the contemporary world of fashion with trends in tourism.

THE CHANGING DYNAMICS OF TOURISM AND DEVELOPMENT OF FASHION TOURISM

The success of the modern fashion system and the tourism industry from the mid-nineteenth century rested on the development of mass markets, although both industries continued to appeal to elite consumers to launch new products, which then filter down to the mass market. Luxury goods also use extravagant advertisements to reinforce the elitism and desirability of the brand in order to lure middle-income markets.

Marketing campaigns for tourism feature new fashions, in particular promoting resort wear and sportswear. Although attention has been paid to the relationship between sports and fashion, there has been little interest in tourism and fashion. Rojek and Urry (1997: 2) argue that "a series of temporary frontiers [were] erected between what we can loosely term tourism and culture," which have only recently been challenged by the "culturalisation of society" or the merging of cultural forms. Ways of living and consuming have broken down due to the McDisneyization of postmodernity (Ritzer and Liska 1997).

Tourism and other cultural experiences are cast as *simulacra,* unreal semblances, representations, or artificial versions of the real. In tourism, this is called the "tourist bubble," where the tourist moves from one contrived and controlled space to another. While familiarity, safety, and comfort and security are central tourist packages, simulacra of hedonism, escape, and choice are structured into the tourist bubble to varying degrees.

Throughout the twentieth century tourism and mainstream fashion became increasingly more sophisticated at appealing to ordinary people—especially using the allure of Hollywood and the simulacra it created of stardom, spectacle, glamour, travel, and exoticism (Eckert 1990; Wilson 1985). Charles Eckert argued that Hollywood sparked a completely new phase and level of consumerism. Cosmetics, swimwear, leisure wear, resort wear, and lingerie were shaped by the film industry. So too were fashions in tourism. And, of course, tourists needed holiday fashions, which became a regular feature of popular media.

In the twenty-first century, this is changing as global brands position their flagship stores in luxury fashion enclaves "that are geographically and socially proximate and accessible to 'high net worth individuals,' fashion-aware consumers and international visitors/tourists" (Moore and Doherty 2007: 286). In 2011 LVMH and PPR (Pinault-Printemps-Redoute) both reported sales increases of over 20 percent (Passariello 2012). Growth is not just limited to Asia—and in particular China; Brazil and Indonesia have also been targeted as growth in sales of "men's fashion shoes and watches" joins the increasing "taste for expensive bags, perfume and champagne," with demand outstripping supply (Passariello 2012).

Equally, tourist authorities and local business organizations are aware that the majority of flagship customers are tourists and business visitors, and many cities now promote fashion tourism as a side attraction of conventions. As a result, the profits of luxury brands come from international tourists known as the "traveling luxury consumer," radically boosting profits by as much as 30 percent. According to Burberry's chief executive, Angela Ahrendts, wealthy Chinese tourists now account for 10 percent of Burberry sales:

> When Chinese consumers travel, they spend six times more than when they stay at home. . . . Saying "I bought this in London" adds further cachet. For this reason, Burberry has sunk £20m into upgrading its London flagship stores, with Regent Street on target to complete just in time for the [2012] Olympics.[5]

Chinese tourists have become big spenders on luxury goods across Europe, Asia, and North America because of the high luxury consumption tax in mainland China, which almost doubles the cost of goods. Credit Suisse analyst Grégoire Biollaz believes:

> Other attractions for Chinese tourists include art, culture, architecture and gastronomy. The trends from shopping tourism towards a cultural travelling experience still has further room to grow. . . . We believe that luxury goods companies will be the key beneficiaries of the boom in Chinese international tourism flows. (quoted in Waki 2011)

A study of fashion in Milan observed that fashion dominated the visual skyscape starting at the airport and throughout central Milan, while tourist maps were sponsored by fashion and design brands and listed fashion and design attractions (Jansson and Power 2010: 898). Milan's prime fashion shopping district, Quadrilatero d'Oro, "is oriented towards an exclusive group of consumers drawn from around the world," but fashion premises spatially distinguish between tourists and high-profile clients:

> Almost every fashion boutique in the area is divided into two sections. The ground floor houses the windows towards the street, attracting tourists and window shoppers. Away from prying eyes special showrooms cater to an exclusive cadre of high-spending and high-profile consumers. This sense of a cloistered exclusivity is reinforced by the narrow streets and the intimate scale of the establishments and stands in contrast to the scale, openness, and public spectacle seen in other prestigious retail streets such as 5th Avenue in New York or Omotesando in Tokyo. (900)

Fashion tourism epitomizes the trend for the "experience economy" (Moore and Doherty 2007: 277), which ranges from the "magic" of white-water rafting in the "wilderness" (Arnould, Price, and Otnes 1999) to "luxury consumption experiences" (Moore and Doherty 2007: 278). Meanwhile, luxury brands are populating airport stores, cruise ships, hotel lobbies, urban fashion and tourism precincts, and suburban shopping malls. Luxury brands have become household names—owned by the wealthy but desired (or reviled) by the everyday consumer.

Fashion cities have realized that they need to create a series of events and attractions to maintain global interest in their status as a fashion city, by staging—alongside fashion weeks—showcases, catwalk shows, trade fairs, media events, and events at flagships and showrooms, and inviting celebrities to select occasions. As Jansson and Power conclude, attracting outside interest and branding Milan as a fashion city are vital to maintaining its fashion magic:

> The sheer scale and scope of shops and retailers from Italy and the rest of the world means the city often feels like one gigantic dressed window on the world of fashion: a window to be looked at, but also one designed to project a multiplicity of images outwards. (2010: 901)

FASHION SHOWS AND TOURISM

The events with perhaps the greatest potential as a lure for visitors and tourists are the fashion shows, fashion trade expos, and fashion weeks. In 2012 there were more than 300 fashion weeks globally—about 120 in North America, 100 in Europe, 50 in the Asia/Pacific region, and 20 each in South/Central America and Africa/the Middle East.[6]

A cursory analysis of the proliferation of fashion weeks indicates that the dominant sphere of fashion is shifting from western Europe to North America and Asia, while many new cities are also staging fashion weeks, for example, cities in eastern Europe, South America, Africa, and the Middle East. Overall, we can conclude that fashion flows are shifting from *north to south* and *west to east.* Even lesser-known cities—ones not usually associated with fashion—are holding fashion weeks, including Qingdao (China), Malabo (Equatorial Guinea), Suva (Fiji), Minsk (Belarus), San Juan (Puerto Rico), and Dar es Salaam (Tanzania). While many cities host one or two fashion weeks, some cities are opting for numerous fashion weeks to spread the focus on fashion throughout the year (see Table 16.1). The number of fashion weeks bounces around within and between venues as other strategies influence the decision to stage such events for promotional and economic purposes. Fashion weeks are increasingly promoted as a means to kick-start the creative industries as part of economic restructuring around adding value to new industries and encouraging consumption-based activities.

The importance of fashion weeks has also been recognized in places new to Western fashion, such as Asia (for example, in India, Hong Kong, China, and Bangladesh) as well as Africa. The company African Fashion International promotes African fashion weeks as a way to put African culture and heritage on center stage through spectacular designs, colors, textiles, and textures. These appeal to Westerners who like to dress up as "Afrocentric" as well as the African diaspora who "dress this way all the time, making African attire a part of their everyday wardrobe" (Pope 2011). African fashion shows are not confined to Africa but are happening worldwide. As Pope observed:

> Fashion shows are emerging as one of the next frontiers in tourism, and talented African fashion designers are taking their valued products to the world stage. People from all

TABLE 16.1 CITIES WITH THREE OR MORE FASHION WEEKS STAGED IN 2012 (ESTIMATED)

CITY	COUNTRY	CONTINENT	NUMBER OF FASHION WEEKS
New York	United States	North America	20
Los Angeles	United States	North America	9
Milan	Italy	Europe	9
Paris	France	Europe	9
London	United Kingdom	Europe	7
Miami Beach	United States	North America	6
Stockholm	Sweden	Europe	6
Athens	Greece	Europe	4
Atlanta	United States	North America	4
Johannesburg	South Africa	Africa	4
Kiev	Ukraine	Europe	4
Madrid	Spain	Europe	4
Moscow	Russia	Europe	4
Rio de Janeiro	Brazil	South America	4
Vancouver	Canada	North America	4
Dubai	United Arab Emirates	Middle East	3
Karachi	Pakistan	Asia	3
New Orleans	United States	North America	3
New Delhi	India	Asia	3
Philadelphia	United States	North America	3
Singapore	Singapore	Asia	3
Toronto	Canada	North America	3
Washington, DC	United States	North America	3

Source: "Fashion Weeks around the Globe," Fashions.org, 2012, http://www.fashions.org/community/fashionweeks.php (accessed August 18, 2012).

> over are flocking to see the dazzling fashion shows where models showcase traditional, modern and unique African styles. African fashion shows are proving to be just as lucrative as they are entertaining in the cities where they take place. Fashion shows and events are playing an ever increasing role in boosting the profiles of tourism destinations.

There are now major fashion weeks in Cape Town, Senegal, Ghana, and Nigeria, while London staged its first African Fashion Week in 2011, featuring fifty designers from African countries, and New York staged its second African Fashion Week. Other fashion weeks, too, are incorporating an African component, such as those in Paris, Milan, and Baltimore. According to Pope:

> Because fashion events are attracting professionals from the media, entertainment, film and music industries, in addition to fashion experts, it is certainly helping to increase tourism for cities. As tourists and fashion-lovers flock to see the latest trends

and designs in African fashion, this will not only benefit the tourist industry, but also promoters, producers and designers of African fashions.

While fashion shows, tours, and weeks have been a long-term part of the industry (Evans 2011), the number of fashion weeks has mushroomed since the turn of the century due to three motivating factors. First, some fashion weeks are government funded as a way to promote the culture of a place and with the hope of attracting attention to the local fashion industry and attracting investment or boosting exports. Second, other fashion weeks are funded by the local fashion industry, usually with sponsorship from an international brand or label, to put the destination on the map and to advertise the industry's capacity. The aim is to secure global attention for the industry and, it is hoped, attract buyers by promoting local talent and industry sectors and providing opportunities for international exposure. Third, other fashion weeks are funded by tourism bodies that are keen to promote the destination and expand awareness of cultural attractions, events, and vibrancy alongside more conventional tourism sites and sights.

Sometimes—and perhaps increasingly so—these agencies jointly organize and back the hosting and sponsorship of fashion weeks. Global luxury brands such as Mercedes Benz, L'Oreal, Audi, Volvo, MasterCard, and Emirates frequently sponsor fashion weeks alongside local brands and organizations. Across all three motivations, there are underlying factors that account for the growth of the phenomenon including the search for new industries, urban development strategies, the promotion of place and identity, and desire to attract tourism (Kawamura 2005).

Fashion weeks are designed to appeal to the fashion industry (local and international), fashion media, buyers, talent spotters, and fashionistas (and celebrities) rather more than to the local community, even though star events aim to attract local media attention and public interest (Teunissen 2005). This is a multipronged strategy that sometimes does not pay off for the brand. Historically, fashion promotions were held as efficient ways of disseminating information about fashion by creating magic and myths about the glamour and spectacle of fashion. It also entailed extending the reach of fashion to new consumer groups and thereby democratizing fashion. This was the central preoccupation of the twentieth-century fashion system. Fashion as a spectacle became its god.

Nonetheless, fashion promotion has retained the hierarchical dimension that characterized the appeal to exclusive clients from the outset, although there are now hierarchies among the makers, marketers, and retailers of fashion (Entwistle and Rocamora 2006: 738). Of lower status are designers whose collections are shown, models on the catwalk, journalists and fashion editors, buyers from stores, fashion stylists, and fashion students (736). These hierarchies are actualized in the spatial arrangement of the seating for shows and through differential access to the various events and key players during fashion weeks. Trade fairs also color-code fairgoers into buyers, exhibitors, or press, which determines where visitors can go and what activities they can undertake (Skov 2006: 767).

Rather than establishing status across the fashion world as a whole, the hierarchy of fashion weeks is obsessed with the self-referential "community" that populates fashion weeks, that is, how participants appear to one another. The winners are those who score front-row seats to see and be seen, usually invited celebrities whose photos in fashion magazines do more for publicity than advertising and feature articles (Entwistle and Rocamora 2006: 737). As well as a ticketing system and discretionary invitations that create spatial divisions between participants, there are also social and cultural hierarchies established based on personal friendships and professional recognition. The pantomime of performativity at fashion shows reinforces the existing status quo of the fashion industry by the reproduction of identities and status within the field of fashion (742). Bodily performances—the clothes participants wear, the bestowing of air kisses on people recognized or deemed worthy, the play of gestures, hyperbolic greetings, and a "cool" deportment and demeanor—create a hierarchy of gazing: being gazed at and gazing at others. The bodies of fashion show participants are as much on show as the fashions themselves.

As the number of fashion weeks grows, attending becomes a matter of judging which shows have the greatest cachet or prestige for the participant. Electronic news, blogs, websites, and videos have made the visibility of fashion shows truly global, and coverage almost instantaneous. This has unsettled the hierarchy of the fashion media as fashion bloggers have created high online profiles with bands of dedicated followers, displacing well-known fashion journalists who used to be the arbiters of the next fashion sensation and denouncers of the passé and pretenders (Murray 2011). Some argue that bloggers have added to the diversity of taste making and trendsetting, while others believe bloggers add little to fashion knowledge and trends.

Moreover, although much of the rationale for such events is promotion of a destination, fashion weeks and fairs must "adapt to international standards" and promote a "cosmopolitan atmosphere," which is contrived to create an "international setting." This creates a phony reality that is the fashion version of the tourist bubble mentioned earlier:

> A world unto itself; for the short duration of the fair it can provide everything for the fairgoers. Hotels are built within easy access to exhibition centres, and full provisions are available at the fair; in fact, many fairgoers rush to eat a boxed lunch in less than half an hour. An overseas visitor who comes to Paris, Frankfurt or Hong Kong for a fair may leave the city after four days without actually spending any time outside the exhibition. (Skov 2006: 773)

Whereas doing business was the original rationale for fashion weeks and fairs, Skov concludes that they are equally—if not more—important for creating neutral spaces for encounters between the multiple players in the fashion juggernaut:

> Whereas historically trade used to be dominant, the reproductive function is now more important, at least in European fairs; yet the two are not mutually exclusive.

> Trade continues to be dominant when trade fairs are established in the new peripheries of the global clothing industry. (781)

CONCLUSION: THE POTENTIAL OF FASHION TOURISM

By charting the growth of demand for fashion luxury brands and goods and the phenomenal growth of fashion weeks across the globe, we are witnessing a major restructuring of fashion as a cultural industry that is entirely dependent on crossing borders and traveling globally (Brand and Teunissen 2005; Maynard 2004; Niessen 2005). Fashion has become a traveling show whose spectacle rivals the more familiar attractions of the tourism industry. And as the tourism industry reframes itself to incorporate and promote cultural attractions, events, and activities, there is a growing convergence between these two similar yet formerly arm's-length industries. In this process, the importance of fashion tourism can only increase, and, in this scenario, fashion weeks have the potential to orchestrate the scope and fortunes of fashion precincts and chart future trends in the consumption of fashion. In this, the fortunes of fashion and tourism have converged to become the cornerstone of identity and self in the twenty-first century. The fashion tourist is the new figure of consumerism in global culture.

NOTES

1. Other early department stores included Galeries Lafayette (1895), Samaritaine (1869), Macy's (1858), Wanamakers (1877), Marshall Field's (1881), Lord and Taylor (1826), John Lewis (1856), Harrods (1849), Selfridges (1909), Hudson's Bay Company (1821), and David Jones (1825/1887).
2. "Louis Vuitton History," 1st 4 Louis Vuitton, 2012, http://www.1st-4-louis-vuitton.com/index.php/louis-vuitton-information/louis-vuitton-history/?action=print (accessed February 27, 2012).
3. Millward Brown, *Top 100 Most Valuable Global Brands 2010,* 2010, http://www.slideshare.net/duckofdoom/millward-brown-brandz-top-2010 (accessed March 2, 2012).
4. "LuxuryDiffusion.com Highlights Louis Vuitton Most Valuable Luxury Brand for Sixth Consecutive Year," LuxuryDiffuson.com, May 9, 2011, http://www.prlog.org/11481063-luxurydiffusioncom-highlights-louis-vuitton-most-valuable-luxury-brand-for-sixth-consecutive-year.html (accessed March 2, 2012).
5. "Tourists Flood to UK for Luxury Goods," *Fashion United,* December 20, 2011, http://www.fashionunited.com/executive/management/tourists-flood-to-uk-for-luxury-goods-20112012488219 (accessed February 20, 2012).
6. "Fashion Weeks around the Globe," Fashions.org, 2012, http://www.fashions.org/community/fashionweeks.php (accessed August 18, 2012).

BIBLIOGRAPHY

Arnould, Eric, Linda Price, and Cele Otnes. 1999. "Making Magic Consumption: A Study of White-Water River Rafting." *Journal of Contemporary Ethnography* 28 (1): 33–68.

Belk, Russell. 1991. "The Ineluctable Mysteries of Possessions." *Journal of Social Behavior and Personality* 6 (6): 17–55.

Belk, Russell, Melanie Wallendorf, and John Sherry. 1989. "The Sacred and the Profane in Consumer Behavior." *Journal of Consumer Research* 16 (1): 1–38.

Brand, Jan, and José Teunissen (eds.). 2005. *Global Fashion, Local Tradition: On the Globalisation of Fashion.* Arnhem, the Netherlands: Terra.

Buckley, Ralph. 2003. "Adventure Tourism and the Clothing, Fashion and Entertainment Industries." *Journal of Ecotourism* 2 (2): 126–34.

Daily Mail Reporter. 2010. "Louis Vuitton Ads Banned after Design House Misled Customers by Suggesting Its Bags Were Hand-Stitched." *Daily Mail Online,* May 26. http://www.dailymail.co.uk/femail/article-1281443/Louis-Vuitton-ads-banned-suggesting-bags-hand-stitched.html#ixzz1nuxP9rlT (accessed March 2, 2012).

Doy, Gen. 2002. "Commodification, Cloth and Drapery." In *Drapery: Classicism and Barbarism in Visual Culture,* 58–97. London: I. B. Tauris.

Eckert, Charles. 1990. "The Carole Lombard in Macy's Window." In Jane Gaines and Charlotte Herzog (eds.), *Fabrications: Costume and the Female Body,* 100–121. London: Routledge.

The Economist. 2011. "China's Luxury Boom: The Middle Blingdom." February 17. http://www.economist.com/node/18184466 (accessed March 8, 2012).

Entwistle, Joanne, and Agnès Rocamora. 2006. "The Field of Fashion Materialized: A Study of London Fashion Week." *Sociology* 40 (4): 735–51.

Evans, Caroline. 2011. "The Origins of the Modern Fashion Show." In Giorgio Riello and Peter McNeil (eds.), *The Fashion History Reader,* 470–72. London: Routledge.

Henderson-Smith, Barbara. 2002. "From Booth to Shopping Mall: Continuities in Consumer Spaces from 1650 to 2000." PhD diss., Griffith University, Brisbane, Australia.

Jansson, Johan, and Dominic Power. 2010. "Fashioning a Global City: Global City Brand Channels in the Fashion and Design Industries." *Regional Studies* 44 (7): 889–904.

Kawamura, Yuniya. 2005. *Fashion-ology: An Introduction to Fashion Studies.* Oxford: Berg.

Kwass, Michael. 2003. "Review of *Luxury in the Eighteenth Century: Debates, Desires and Delectable Goods.*" *Reviews in History,* review no. 357, November 2009. http://www.history.ac.uk/reviews/review/357 (accessed February 27, 2012).

Maynard, Margaret. 2004. *Dress and Globalisation.* Manchester: Manchester University Press.

Miller, Michael. 1981. *The Bon Marché: Bourgeois Culture and the Department Store, 1869–1920.* London: Allen and Unwin.

Modigliani, Leah. 2007. "Louis Vuitton and the Luxury Market after the End of Art." *Art Criticism* 22 (1): 91–104.

Moore, Christopher, and Anne Marie Doherty. 2007. "The International Flagship Stores of Luxury Fashion Retailers." In Tony Haines and Margaret Bruce (eds.), *Fashion Marketing: Contemporary Issues,* 277–96. 2nd ed. Oxford: Butterworth-Heinemann.

Murray, Alex. 2011. "Fashion Week: The Ordinary People Who Stole the Show." *BBC News Magazine,* September 9. http://www.bbc.co.uk/news/magazine-14813053 (accessed September 15, 2011).

Niessen, Sandra. 2005. "The Prism of Fashion: Temptation, Resistance and Trade." In Jan Brand and José Teunissen (eds.), *Global Fashion, Local Tradition: On the Globalisation of Fashion,* 156–81. Arnhem, the Netherlands: Terra.

Passariello, Christina. 2012. "Luxury Goods Makers Are Bagging a Fortune." *The Weekend Australian,* February 18–19, p. 26.

Polhemus, Ted. 2005. "What to Wear in the Global Village?" In Jan Brand and José Teunissen (eds.), *Global Fashion, Local Tradition: On the Globalisation of Fashion,* 82–95. Arnhem, the Netherlands: Terra.

Pope, Kitty. 2011. "African Fashion Shows: An Emerging Frontier in Tourism." *African Diaspora Tourism,* August 29. http://www.africandiasporatourism.com/index.php?option=com_contentand view=article&id=652:africa-fashion-shows-an-emerging-frontier-in-tourism&catid=113:featured-4 (accessed February 20, 2012).

Ritzer, George, and Allan Liska. 1997. "'McDisneyization' and 'Post-tourism': Complementary Perspectives on Contemporary Tourism." In Chris Rojek and John Urry (eds.), *Tourism Cultures: Transformations of Travel and Theory,* 96–109. London: Routledge.

Rojek, Chris, and John Urry. 1997. "Transformations of Travel and Theory." In Chris Rojek and John Urry (eds.), *Tourism Cultures: Transformations of Travel and Theory,* 1–19. London: Routledge.

Skov, Lise. 2006. "The Role of Trade Fairs in the Global Fashion Business." *Current Sociology* 54 (5): 764–83.

Teunissen, José. 2005. "Global Fashion/Local Tradition: On the Globalisation of Fashion." In Jan Brand and José Teunissen (eds.), *Global Fashion, Local Tradition: On the Globalisation of Fashion,* 8–23. Arnhem, the Netherlands: Terra.

Thomas, Dana. 2007. *Deluxe: How Luxury Lost Its Lustre.* London: Allen Lane.

Waki, Natsuko. 2011. "The Power of Chinese International Tourists." *Global Investing,* November 8. http://blogs.reuters.com/globalinvesting/2011/11/08/the-power-of-chinese-international-tourists/ (accessed February 20, 2012).

Wilson, Elizabeth. 1985. *Adorned in Dreams: Fashion and Modernity.* London: Virago.

17

Artisan Enterprise, Cultural Property, and the Global Market

MARY A. LITTRELL AND JUDY FRATER

Artisan participation in the global fashion industry engenders debate. Ashoke Chatterjee, an internationally respected leader for craft development in India, observes that Indian politicians and international development leaders question whether craft-sector employment is a "fringe, feel-good activity unrelated to power and economic vitality" (2007: 12). In response, Chatterjee warns that "crafts offer India the only sustainable answer to its need of job opportunities for a population that has crossed one billion" (12).

Longtime craft administrators Maureen Liebl and Tirthankar Roy express concern about the potential for global appropriation of intellectual property held in artisan industries—enterprises that draw on deeply enmeshed cultural knowledge and production processes (Liebl 2005; Liebl and Roy 2004). In order to meet the demands of the constantly changing global fashion market, designers often borrow from the Indian textile design traditions of a particular region or ethnicity and then de-ethnicize and exploit the traditions. Yet as artisans lose their local markets for handcrafts to machine-produced and cheaper alternatives, income generation through participation in the global fashion market may serve as a critical precursor to cultural asset protection and continued evolution (Liebl and Roy 2004).

Nongovernmental organizations (NGOs) provide yet another perspective. NGO leaders argue that participation in artisan enterprise holds potential for human capability development as a catalyst for change. Robert Chambers (1997), an international development scholar and practitioner, identifies capability development as a core first step for development. Enhanced capabilities contribute to improved livelihoods through a dependable source of cash and food to meet basic needs and to promote eventual social, psychological, and spiritual well-being.

Artisan enterprise research is a multidisciplinary endeavor. Scholars from anthropology, development studies, economics, fashion studies, history, philosophy, and sociology have described a number of critical issues for artisan development.[1] Scholars have examined topics such as urban versus rural lifestyles; artisans' gender, ethnic, national, and global identities; enterprise organization and leadership; internally versus externally driven product development; and artisans' cultural property as they bear on the global craft market.

In this chapter we compare and contrast two Indian artisan enterprises operating in the global fashion market, both of which offer insights into development issues raised by scholars as identified above. Through a compare-and-contrast approach, we provide insights into commonalities shared by artisans in the global fashion market. At the same time the cases offer opportunity to examine the particularities of the context that contribute to differentiation in their enterprise approaches and impacts.

The first enterprise, Kala Raksha Trust (Kala Raksha), operates in a number of ethnic- and caste-distinct rural villages in the Kutch region of Gujarat. The Kala Raksha business office, the museum, a retail shop, and a production facility are in Sumrasar, a village of 7,500 people located sixteen miles (twenty-five kilometers) from Bhuj city. Members produce apparel, accessories, and household textiles that are designed within a context of long-standing traditional embroidery styles. These traditional arts serve as launching points as well as potential constraints to the artisans' participation in the global fashion market. Kala Raksha products are marketed in India and abroad.

The second group, MarketPlace: Handwork of India (MarketPlace), is an urban enterprise with workshops located in several Mumbai slums and a central office in the Santa Cruz East area of the city. Most MarketPlace artisans, upon marriage, have migrated to Mumbai from various regions across India. As is common in Mumbai slums, the artisans work together in workshops of multiple religions, ethnicities, and castes (Boo 2012). MarketPlace produces apparel, accessories, and household items exclusively for the U.S. market. In contrast to Kala Raksha, MarketPlace artisans do not bring Indian art traditions to their work. Rather, they have been taught sewing, embroidery, and business skills for producing apparel that is *India inspired* but not rooted in the textile traditions of a singular geographic region.

These groups were selected as they offered an opportunity to examine two organizations with more than twenty-year histories in the same country, yet one operates from a rural context, the other in an urban setting. Both are active in the global market. In addition, the two authors have been closely involved with the two groups. The first author's initial interaction with MarketPlace centered on marketing and design issues; her engagement eventually expanded to a three-year social audit of impacts from artisan work with MarketPlace (Littrell and Dickson 2010).[2] The second author offers day-to-day lived experience with Kala Raksha as a cofounder and collaborator/marketer with the artisans at venues in India and abroad, and as a catalyst and active leader for the design school.[3]

Scholarship that informed our analysis is presented in the next section of this chapter. This is followed by the two case studies, each of which begins with a description of a fashion show that serves as a metaphor for the organization's goals and outcomes. Discussion follows on the cultural context in which each group originated and operates, the founders' backgrounds and motivations, organizational structures and operations, and current outcomes and issues. In the final section of the chapter we compare and contrast the organizations with respect to capability acquisition and application, acquisition of cultural knowledge, organizational evolution, and future involvement in the global fashion market.

SCHOLARLY GROUNDING

Two theoretical frameworks provided insight for conceptualizing and evaluating development of the two enterprises (Robeyns 2005). The work of Amartya Sen (1980, 1993) and Martha Nussbaum (2000) proved useful in understanding the opportunities (capabilities) and outcomes (achieved functionings) of individuals in the artisan groups. In contrast, Femidy Handy and colleagues (2006) offered a framework for assessing, at an organizational level, how the enterprises have evolved in relation to their goals. These overarching frameworks allowed us to assess Kala Raksha's and MarketPlace's development in relation to many of the issues that have been described by artisan scholars.

Human Capabilities

The capability approach, pioneered by Sen and Nussbaum for comparative appraisal of development, has resulted in extensive interdisciplinary discussion (Robeyns 2005). The scholars differentiate between means and ends, or capabilities and functioning. Conceptualizing capabilities as "means," Nussbaum describes how, "instead of asking about people's satisfactions, or how much in the way of resources they are able to command, we ask, instead, about what they are actually able to do or be" (2000: 12). Capabilities are viewed as an opportunity set for achievable functioning that is influenced by the social context, including cultural norms as well as the social institutions of which individuals are a part. Functionings demonstrate the end applications or outcomes of the capabilities.

Nussbaum has proposed a list of central, interconnected human functional capabilities (see Table 17.1). She asserts that the capabilities approach not only provides an orientation for measuring quality of life but also "can serve as the foundation for constitutional guarantees to which nations should be held by their citizens" (2000: 298). Her list has not been without its challengers, who critique the value of a universal list, given cultural and societal differences. However, Nussbaum counters,

> If we agree that all citizens are worthy of concern and respect... then we ought to conclude that politics should not treat people as agents or supporters of other people,

TABLE 17.1 CENTRAL HUMAN FUNCTIONAL CAPABILITIES

CAPABILITY	DESCRIPTION (ADAPTED)
Life	Being able to live to the end of a human life of normal length
Bodily health	Being able to have good health, including reproductive health, and adequate nutrition and shelter
Bodily integrity	Being able to move freely from place to place with one's bodily boundaries treated as sovereign; having opportunity for sexual satisfaction and choice in reproduction
Senses, imagination, and thought	Being able to use the senses to imagine, think, and reason, informed by an adequate education
Emotions	Being able to have attachments to things and people, without overwhelming fear or anxiety or traumatic abuse or neglect
Practical reason	Being able to form a conception of the good and to engage in critical reflection about the planning of one's life
Affiliation	Being able to live with others, including showing concern for others, engaging in social interaction; being treated as a dignified being with worth equal to others
Other species	Being able to live with concern for animals, plants, and the world of nature
Play	Being able to laugh, play, and enjoy recreational activities
Control over one's environment	Being able to participate in political choices that govern one's life; having property rights; having the right to seek employment on an equal basis with others

> whose mission in the world is to execute someone else's plan of life. It should treat each of them as ends, as sources of agency and worth in their own right, with their own plans to make and their own lives to live, therefore as deserving of all necessary support for their equal opportunity to be such agents. (58)

High-Impact NGOs

Handy and colleagues draw from their research with twenty Indian NGOs to propose a model of high-impact all-female NGOs. High impact is reached when an NGO is

> raising women's awareness in a holistic way, so that they are not only educated, healthy, or able to run a micro-financed enterprise, but that she can eventually effectively navigate the way in the socio-cultural environment in which she functions. Such empowerment…depends largely on the development of the capacity to exercise a certain amount of control over the social, economic, and political conditions that determine her life. (2006: 130)

The researchers isolated three central concepts useful for our assessment—female leadership in a solely or largely female NGO, vertical integration, and generational activities. In high-impact NGOs, female leaders passionately promoted social justice and gender equality through collective, inclusive, and consensus-building approaches to organizational development. In vertical integration, an NGO sequentially added programs and services to complement the original core activity and, through multiplier effects, promoted holistic development by "catering to the whole woman" (162).

Generational activities referred to organizational evolution in how an NGO helped its members (Korten 1987). First generational activities provided for basic human needs, often in response to a crisis or disaster. Over time, the organization progressed into higher generational activities that fostered capacity building, advocacy, decision making, and inter-NGO networking to promote a broader social vision of human development. Such generational growth was organic in nature, evolving from grassroots participation and discussion in the field (Handy et al. 2006).

KALA RAKSHA TRUST

> The bright lights of the fashion show ramp were just dimming and the energy under the stars was high. A TV reporter zoomed in to interview a Kala Raksha founder in the wake of the fifth Kala Raksha Vidhyalaya fashion show. "But how much progress have you made?" he asked. "These artisans are still wearing their village dress up there on the stage." Little did he know that in everyday life, these artisans wore the latest local fashion. They had deliberately worn traditional dress for the show as an expression of pride in their identity. In fact, it was significant progress. (Frater's field notes, December 2011; see Figure 17.1)

The twenty-first century crashed into Kutch. In January 2001, a massive earthquake devastated this historically isolated, drought-prone district. Suddenly it was inundated with a wave of individuals and organizations intending to offer shelter, health care, and rehabilitation. Struck with the rich craft traditions, many relief workers saw opportunity and began cultural industries. Designers came for "design intervention." While designers and entrepreneurs wanted to work with traditions, the first thing they wanted to do was appropriate them.

The commercialization of craft traditions began in Kutch in the 1960s. For Kutchi women, it was a viable option. In many traditional societies, social constraints prohibit women from going out to earn through manual labor in areas such as construction, agriculture, or drought-relief work. Lack of education precluded other livelihoods. Embroidery could be integrated with essential household work. But few alternatives for earning meant little negotiating power, and embroidery usually earned less than manual labor. The social status of an artisan was commensurate.

The embroidery that many ethnic communities had stitched for centuries was never assigned commercial value. However, it was recognized as a cultural asset. Traditional embroidery was created for social exchange, as gifts to children, family, the fiancé, and in-laws. Often, embroidery was received before the bride was met by her husband and

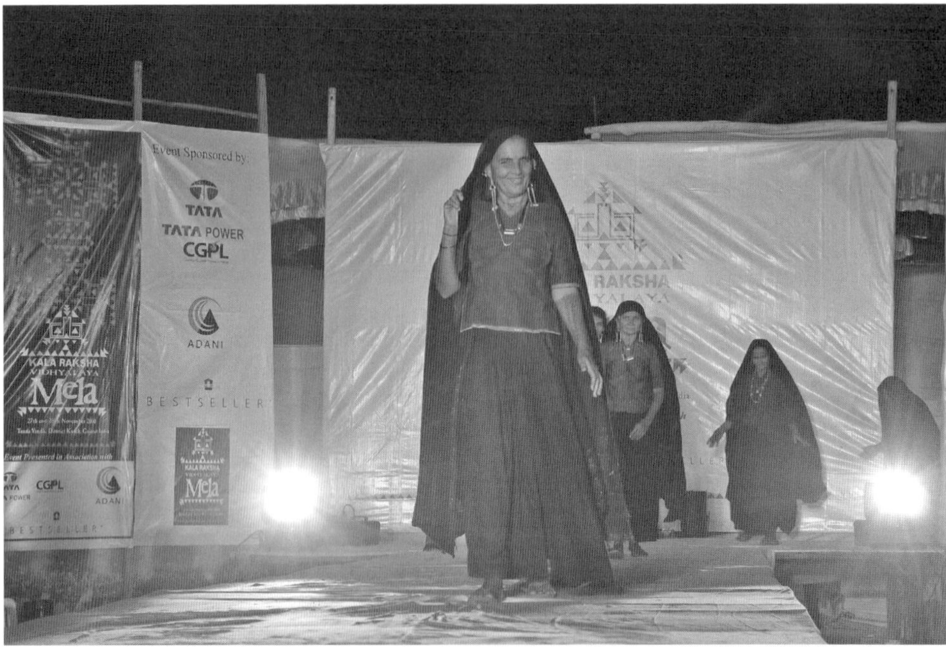

FIGURE 17.1 Kala Raksha design interns at the annual Kala Raksha Vidhyalaya fashion show in 2010. *Credit*: Photograph by Ketan Pomal, Studio LM.

in-laws, so it introduced her, demonstrating her creativity, intelligence, and love (Frater 2010). Above all, embroidery proclaimed identity.

In traditional South Asian society, a person first belongs to a region, then an ethnic community, then a family, and finally is an individual. Embroidery styles eloquently expressed this cultural identity (Frater 1995). Far more than technique, traditions were design languages comprising stitches, colors, motifs, patterns, and composition, and each was understood as cultural property. An artisan understood where and how she could vary her work. Innovation within this context breathed the essential life into a tradition.

Tradition and Fashion

Styles evolved over time. But localization of trends ensured that visual expression of group affiliation remained clear (Frater 2003). Fashion came to Kutch with the advent of synthetic fabrics, increased mobility, and spiraling inflation. Fashion's rate and extent of change, duration of trends, sphere of influence, and sense of volition were distinctly different from those of tradition.

Indirectly, commercial embroidery enabled local fashion. By the 1990s, NGOs and traders were providing work to hundreds of artisans. Women had less time for their own handwork, but they now had the power to purchase. This motivated innovations such as application of ready-made trims, machine embroidery, and the use of new materials. Each embroidery style followed a course of its own. Yet each retained cultural integrity, and the distinctions between styles remained as clear as ever.

In turn, fashion began to directly impact traditional embroidery. Commercial work targeted urban and international markets. Professional designers intervened to make embroidery "less ethnic," manipulating motifs, pattern, and colors with little knowledge of or interest in styles. Emulating the industrial model—faster, cheaper, and more uniform—designers printed patterns and had women fill them in with embroidery. Concept was separated from execution. Traditions were diluted. Personal identity and creativity were out of the question.

Deeply aware of their position in the social hierarchy, artisans were not accustomed to critiquing such situations. They were in awe of power and grateful to get work. Prakash Bhanani, cofounder of Kala Raksha, explains,

> Artisans never thought of doing work for commerce, and they had no access to the results of their work. But when they learned that traders were earning very well from their embroidery, they felt they had underpriced themselves. This taught artisans to value their traditions. Community members who understood business then tried to take advantage of traditional work too! But the concept of intellectual property had not occurred to artisans. They don't have the luxury or the perspective to think of their traditions in this way. (Frater's field notes, August 2011)

Simultaneously, commercialization insidiously eroded the artisans' sense of aesthetics and self-worth. Perfected, decorative renditions of tradition were selling as fashion. So artisans felt these were "better." Young women were beginning with commercial embroidery and did not enjoy a deep connection to traditions. Embroidery became a matter of aesthetics, and cultural identity was devalued.

Enter Kala Raksha

In 1990, when Judy Frater was researching *suf* embroidery on a Fulbright grant, Dayaben, a suf embroiderer, asked her, "Why are you studying us? Why don't you help us?" Dayaben changed Frater's perspective from concern for cultural heritage to realization that fair wages might enable traditions to continue. Dayaben, her brother Prakashbhai, and Frater all shared a vision of artisans engineering their own economic and social development through their heritage. Together they founded Kala Raksha in 1993, taking the challenge to create work with cultural integrity for the contemporary fashion market.

Kala Raksha began with $1,000 from Aid to Artisans to start a museum to serve as a resource base and RS13,000 ($433) from a Ford Foundation project. In seventeen years, the trust grew from twenty-five artisans to over a thousand and increased its sales by forty-four times. Kala Raksha's greater successes are harder to quantify. Women quietly broke social barriers as their income became significant. They traveled to cities in India to sell their work. More controversial, they went out locally, to bazaars and to the Kala Raksha center. They learned to read, sign their names, and keep accounts.

Kala Raksha used local resources as a strategy for building the organization. They established a museum of older traditional textiles and developed products by engaging artisans to innovate from its collections. They hired community members as staff and expanded using local networks. But Kala Raksha's key asset and resource was cultural heritage. The leaders understood traditions as core entities rather than means to an end. They sought to mobilize these unique aesthetic identities. This valuation of traditional knowledge and skills activated creativity. Nearly every development within the organization has come from artisan initiative. Hariyaben demanded fair payment, thus founding artisan pricing committees. Raniben fashioned tiny elephants and camels out of workshop scraps, initiating a recycled line. Pabiben sampled what has become a best-selling ribbon bag based on new Dhebaria fashion.

Fashion and Cultural Identity in the New Millennium

Meanwhile, money, exposure, and new fashion accelerated changes in cultural identity. Aware of the urban-rural divide, village girls no longer wanted to wear their traditional dress. Women replaced traditional fabrics with synthetic replicas and soon preferred ethnic-neutral polyester prints for skirts, blouses, and veils. Ethnic community differences in dress began to blur. Most significant, fashion, increased possibility, and choice—coupled with the revolution of the cell phone—altered the hierarchy of identity. The concept of the individual emerged.

Kala Raksha in the New Millennium

The earthquake of 2001 and its aftermath of cultural industries jolted Kala Raksha to reflect on its goals. Competition in the craft-production market had increased, and the labor wages of industries that had proliferated in the region lured artisans. Kala Raksha realized that despite so much effort, the wages and social status of artisans were still equated with those of manual laborers. Yet artisans' innovations within their own traditions demonstrated vibrancy and the ability to define and fulfill a design brief. The founders were clear that income could not justify the loss of cultural heritage; empowerment must be cultural as well as economic. They knew they needed to find alternatives to the industrial development model and to take into account cultural property—not only skills but also knowledge—and transfer these important assets to new arenas. They returned to the challenge of increasing value for handwork, with the understanding that the artist is the steward of tradition.

Enter Kala Raksha Vidhyalaya

In 2005 Kala Raksha founded Kala Raksha Vidhyalaya (KRV), the first design school for artisans, as a sustainable solution for the survival of craft traditions. The school's premise is that if artisans themselves design, this will ensure the thread of integrity—and raise their income and status. The venture multiplied Kala Raksha's visibility and capacity. A network of excellent contacts within and outside India grew. The trust received financial and human resource support from all over the world.

As of 2011 ninety-nine artisans have graduated from the yearlong program. Local orientation and sustained input have ensured its success. Visiting faculty and professional design educators work with local permanent faculty to utilize the Kutchi language and culture. The curriculum guides artisans to appreciate the unique aspects of their traditions in the context of the world. Artisans have expanded their cultural knowledge about the global market by learning to segment markets and to interpret and evoke trend forecasts. Each artisan makes a final collection, which is juried by craft and design professionals (see Figure 17.2) and presented in a fashion show with a public attendance in the thousands. The fashion show has highly motivated the artisans and has been an important instrument in educating the public to think about craft and artisans in other ways. In 2010 Kala Raksha launched the concept Artisan Design, a trademark to certify that a product is an artisan's own creative innovation.

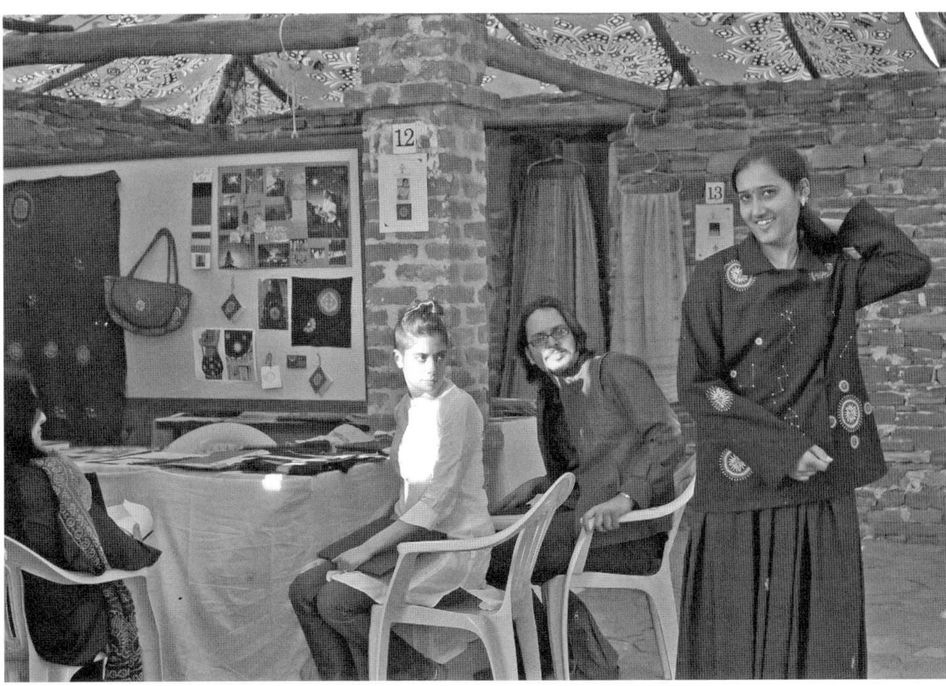

FIGURE 17.2 Monghiben Rana presents her final collection to a jury of design professionals. *Credit*: Photograph by Judy Frater.

The Impact of Kala Raksha

Working with Kala Raksha has changed artisans' attitudes. First, artisans gained pride in being an artisan, simply through earning. Pride in tradition and cultural identity followed. In interviews, artisans who had graduated from KRV described their capacity to create and their prerogative to collaborate:

> Harkhuben: "After I completed the course and participated in two Kala Raksha design workshops, I realized what I had learned. It was easy and fun to develop new designs. If we want our art to flourish, this is the way we must go!"

> Deviben: "I only went to 4th grade, but now I feel educated. I learned how to talk. I was able to correct what the Mentor wrote! We can correct each other because we have reached a level of education."

KRV's year of design exploration focuses on craft as fashion. When craft is fashion, concept and execution are reunited. Kala Raksha artisans have begun to develop their unique expressions within traditions and to own their work. When Kala Raksha receives an order for Sajnuben's embroidered ornaments, she wants to embroider them herself. Babraben says of her award-winning quilt, "No one else can do my work" (see Figure 17.3). The cultural evolution of a stronger individual identity created a space for the concept of intellectual property. The concept Artisan Design eventually accesses intellectual property to raise income and respect above the level of manual labor.

Current Issues and a Look to the Future

Whereas Kala Raksha artisans felt helpless to address appropriation of cultural heritage, the issue of protection of one's designs emerged with the concept of intellectual property. Aware of their creative input, artisans have become indignant when a new design is copied. In the realm where a new design can net important orders, authorship becomes a matter of livelihood. Value for creative work is the central issue.

Both cultural heritage and intellectual property require marketing to create awareness and value. Kala Raksha's challenges now are to reach markets that appreciate and value products with cultural integrity and to equip artisans to tap cultural heritage most appropriately.

The television reporter's question about village dress on the stage was rooted in the assumption that tradition is old-fashioned—even antifashion. The graduates of KRV consciously began the custom of wearing traditional dress on the ramp with their collections. Artisans no longer have to wear this dress. But when they have knowledge and design skills, can create from their traditions for the global market, earn a decent wage, and become recognized, they can pay respect to their cultural heritage. Taking traditional dress to the stage, they are taking a big step toward establishing a relationship between fashion and cultural identity.

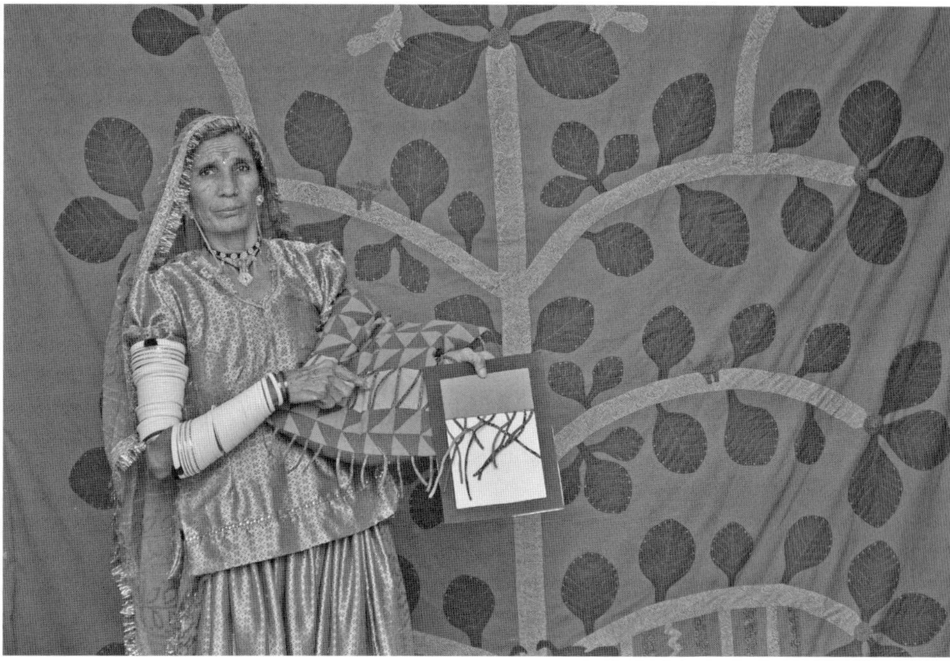

FIGURE 17.3 Babraben Moru with her award-winning quilt.
Credit: Photograph by Judy Frater.

MARKETPLACE: HANDWORK OF INDIA

Amid fashion show runway lights and before an audience of two hundred, eleven artisans adopt a model's prance as they enter on stage in MarketPlace's western attire. Some wear jeans with the garments while others add western-style blouses and accessories. The women, young and old, have combed their hair in pony tails and flowing locks, a contrast to their usual neck buns and braids. The audience enthusiastically supports their fellow artisans who are showcasing, with pride, the garments they produce on a daily basis. The occasion marks the 2011 launching of a book that chronicles the artisans' transformed lives across twenty five years as they built MarketPlace into a global enterprise that produces for the U.S. market. As the fashion show winds down, the models return to their richly embellished, special-occasion saris, garments they would not have afforded prior to their involvement with MarketPlace. (Littrell's field notes, January 2011)

Confidence, self-respect, and group affiliation—all qualities conveyed by the runway artisans—seemed far removed from women's lives in MarketPlace's early days in the 1980s. Extreme poverty, chronic family illness, malnutrition, and the determination to support and educate their young children drove the women's search for work.

In contrast, the lives of the MarketPlace founders, Pushpika Freitas and Lalita Monteiro, differed in striking ways from those of the women with whom they would initiate MarketPlace. The sisters had grown up in a Mumbai family of modest means but with parents who insisted on educating their daughters. In 1980 Pushpika returned to India from the United States with a master's degree in social work, ready to apply development strategies that encouraged women to achieve economic self-sufficiency in their lives.

Pushpika was well aware of the challenges they would face in establishing an artisan enterprise in the global fashion market. Women in the slums had limited formal education and little experience in expressing opinions or taking initiative. Many women were confined to their homes due to religious practices, or because husbands and in-laws did not believe women should be outside the home (Littrell and Dickson 2010).

Beginning with three women, the fledgling MarketPlace organization concentrated on making patchwork products and learning embroidery skills. As Pushpika elaborated,

> Hand embroidery is crucial to our mission. Most of the women, when they started had to be trained in hand embroidery. However, they needed to earn a living immediately and a long training period was out of the question. So, in the beginning the hand embroidery designs were simple but added a unique touch to the garments. (Littrell's field notes, January 2011)

Over time, the early patchwork products evolved into today's fashionable, Western-style apparel, accessories, and household items, all with aesthetic links to Indian textile traditions. Two hallmarks distinguish MarketPlace's "India-inspired" products. The base fabric incorporates hand dyeing, printing, or weaving techniques that are native to India but not necessarily to the artisans practicing them. Striking points of interest are added through embroidered embellishment (see Figure 17.4). The embroidery follows the easy-to-see lines in the fabric motifs, as many artisans embroider by single overhead lightbulbs in their homes. Products are sold in the United States through a catalog, placement in specialty stores, and the Internet.

Across its twenty-five years, MarketPlace has held steadfast to its founding objectives. While the means to reach the objectives have evolved, MarketPlace's founders remain committed that artisans are paid fair wages, have opportunities to acquire business and entrepreneurial skills that enhance their self-worth and respect, and are empowered as individuals to identify and address the social issues affecting their lives and the community around them. Essential characteristics of the MarketPlace approach include grassroots participation in business decisions and leadership development through working in groups.

Working at Home

From the beginning, MarketPlace leaders listened to the women and their needs in establishing an organizational structure. From conversations, they realized that some

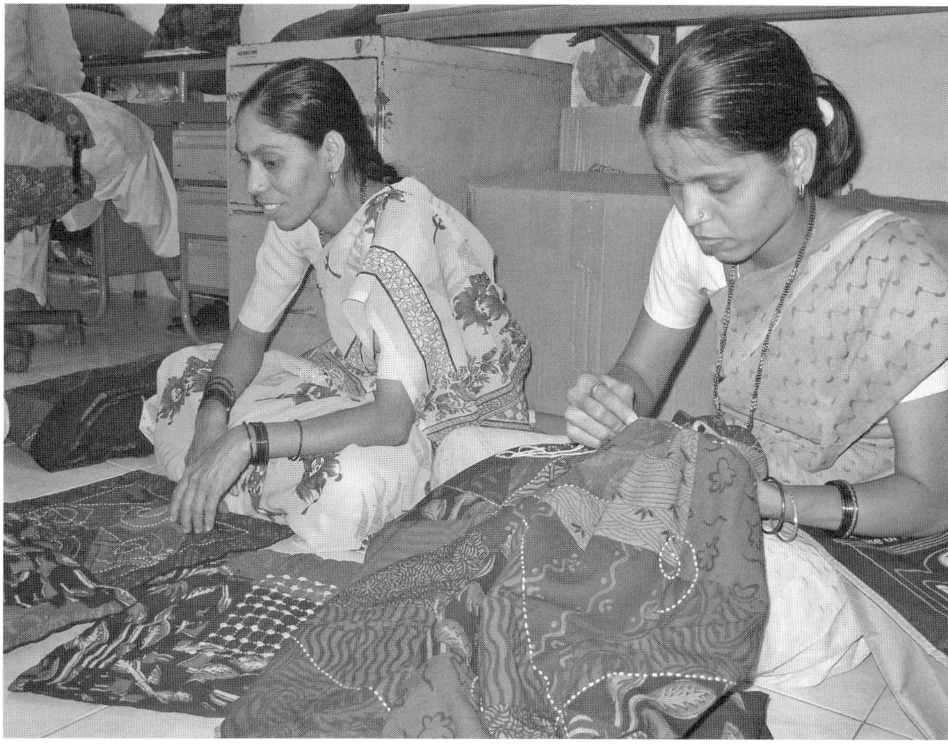

FIGURE 17.4 MarketPlace artisan embroidering on fabric motif lines.
Credit: Photograph by Mary Littrell.

women, usually those who were younger or unmarried, were able to leave their homes to work in a centralized workshop for an extended period of time. Others with significant household responsibilities needed to carry out much of their work within the home. MarketPlace's flexible work structure honors the context of the artisans' lives. Younger women assemble the garments on sewing machines that are housed at workshops in the slums. The garments are then distributed to artisans who walk to the workshops to collect the products, attend training, and participate in meetings. Returning home, the artisans embellish the surfaces while carrying out their household tasks.

A Critical Change

MarketPlace was founded as a single production unit, which served many important functions in the early days—developing systems for streamlining production and time management, working with cash flow, establishing quality and delivery standards, and developing an organizational identity (Littrell and Dickson 1999). As the organization grew to over 175 women in the mid-1990s, and as more women were capable of assuming leadership roles, MarketPlace became top-heavy with supervisors. Pushpika assessed that the organization had lost sight of its mission to help all women with business and personal decision making and leadership development. Decentralization into smaller workshops was in order. By early 2000, seven groups, scattered in several slums across Mumbai, had taken the challenge to form independent business groups that now serve as contractors with the MarketPlace central office.

With decentralization, groups bid for orders to produce the twice-yearly apparel lines. Preceding the bidding, Indian and U.S. apparel designers plan the product lines around a set of seasonal colors and garment styles. Next, the seven group leaders meet to discuss the impending order; production is contracted based on the group's size and expertise related to the season's garment features. Skills acquired through MarketPlace training come into action as artisans plan the season's production based on the number of group members, the artisans' speed in production, and the projected delivery date. Artisans source supplies at sites across Mumbai, cut fabric and sew products, conduct quality control, maintain workshop records, and deliver finished goods to the main office—often involving considerable bus and train travel across the city.

The women's new business capabilities evolved into cultural knowledge for conducting business in a Mumbai slum and in the larger city of Mumbai. Workshop leaders were becoming successful business leaders. This model of widespread artisan participation in workshop decision making promotes active engagement in leadership development. The model contrasts sharply with a system where artisans serve merely as workers as they passively fulfill garment orders directed by top-level managers.

Becoming Strong Women

As with many artisan groups worldwide, programs for economic empowerment and social capacity development are integrated. To illustrate MarketPlace's social thrust, women regularly gather at the workshops to discuss an evolving array of important issues in their lives. Health concerns dominated early dialogue. More recently, legal issues surfaced surrounding women's property rights, domestic violence, and divorce.

As the women acquired leadership skills, each group was encouraged to explore ways they could create impact in their communities by identifying a problem and brainstorming solutions. Social action projects have centered on preventive medical practices, removal of trash in the slums, and communication with teenagers. Through the group discussions and social action projects, women have gradually acquired cultural knowledge of life beyond their one-room homes in the slums. As community problems evolve, new social action projects emerge; as Pushpika describes:

> The women have decided that domestic violence is becoming an even bigger problem than it was in the past. They are writing and performing street plays to bring the problem out in the open. The plays show abused women that they are not alone and it is

not their fault. By acting out domestic abuse and violence, they are able to illustrate the first signs of abuse and the different methods used by the abuser to exert control. When acting in front of their neighbors, friends, and family, artisans may be looking at the audience and recognizing some abusers or women who are abused. Despite everything their determination remains strong.

Impacts and Challenges

While working at MarketPlace, the women acquire a broad range of new skills that range from speaking up in meetings to communicating on the telephone, using public transportation, and taking responsibility when the workshop supervisor is away. The women cite their "ability to support other women" as one of their most important new assets. Initially, many felt isolated and were unaware that other women were suffering similar problems of mental and physical abuse. Women's comments that "I can talk about anything here" or "I had no one to talk with before I came here" speak to the relief the women feel at the workshops and to the capabilities they have acquired for supporting other women in similar circumstances. As women become active in the workshops, they assist each other in communicating openly, garnering self-respect, and becoming leaders—all assets of strong women that have application both within and outside the workshops.

Within their homes, their influence as decision makers has broadened to significant involvement in deciding the number of the children they bear, the schools their children will attend, their children's activities, and their daughter's marriage age and choice of husband. In addition, the women assessed that they gained greater respect from neighbors, in-laws, and husbands.

In another application, three of the artisans have used their business and production skills to establish Indian Roots, an entrepreneurial offshoot company that uses rejected or leftover MarketPlace fabrics to produce a line of fashionable apparel for the local Indian market. As they meet and talk with their local customers, the entrepreneurs adjust styles to meet customer demand for the Indian Roots product line.

In summary, one artisan, a member of MarketPlace for nineteen years, reflects on how her life has changed. Entering an arranged marriage at age fifteen, the artisan bore her first daughter at age sixteen. Education was not a priority, and she left school after the fifth grade. The artisan assesses:

> Looking back, the most important thing I have learned through my work is independence—to think for myself, to look at all sides before making a decisions and to consider all the possible outcomes a decision could have. I recently became the production manager of my cooperative and have learned to keep accounts, pay the bills, and manage production. This has given me confidence, and my family and neighbors now see me as a different person. We (my family) are not rich, we do have problems, and there will always be challenges that will come up. But my children are educated

> and we are a strong, close family. Every day I learn more about being the manager of my cooperative.

Not surprisingly, the MarketPlace women are eager to expand their workshops, yet, as with most artisan groups worldwide, they are dependent on their leader, marketing staff, and designers for guidance in understanding the global market customer. As contractors, the artisans enter the picture only after design decisions have been made and it is time to bid with the other workshops for orders. While a few artisans have begun designing the embroidery motifs requisite to the MarketPlace look, the remainder of the design work is done by the central office. As with much of the worldwide apparel industry in the past few years, orders have not expanded at the rate the artisans would wish. To counteract this situation, MarketPlace designers have begun to develop a more fashion-forward appearance while still retaining the India-inspired look.

CONCLUSION: ARTISAN GROUPS IN THE GLOBAL FASHION MARKET

The creation and wearing of fashion are about the expression of identity. MarketPlace artisans did not begin with craft or business skills but trained as entrepreneurs and acquired skills for business leadership. For Kala Raksha artisans, fashion thrust in as a double-edged sword. It offered an opportunity to earn but posed a threat to existing craft traditions and cultural heritage. Both organizations worked in the fashion market for the dual goals of income generation and social development. Kala Raksha, in addition, had a third goal of conserving cultural heritage. It attempted to utilize cultural heritage as a primary asset to capture a more significant part of the market.

Two scholarly frameworks offered points of departure for this chapter in exploring issues raised by scholars in relation to organizational development. In reference to Nussbaum's (2000) set of core human capabilities (see Table 17.1), the two artisan groups illustrate clearly how context can shape which capabilities are developed and how identities are nurtured. Both groups expanded artisans' capabilities of imagination and thought and of practical reasoning but toward different ends.

Kala Raksha utilized artisan cultural heritage as a core strength for engaging artisans more fully. Drawing on the museum collections, Kala Raksha encouraged artisans to appreciate the design languages of their unique embroidery traditions and to realize their abilities to create and innovate, within the constraints posed by the practicalities of production and the tastes of contemporary markets. As a result, Kala Raksha artisans have acquired an identity as *designers* who are in control of their cultural property—embroidery traditions—for participation in the global fashion market.

The MarketPlace artisans acquired new knowledge in the form of a range of business skills for application in planning, management, and completion of large production orders within the Mumbai business environment. For the artisans, their evolving business and decision-making skills emerged as new cultural property. Women who previously rarely left their homes now project an identity as business leaders in producing fashion for the global fashion market.

A second scholarly framework of organizational evolution also proved useful in assessing the two enterprises' evolution. Handy and colleagues (2006) suggest that vertical integration and generational activities distinguish successful NGOs. In vertical integration and generation, organizations enlarge their programs in concert with their originating goals but in recognition of their members' expanding needs and expectations. Here again, the two enterprises illustrate how context can direct the focus for organizational generation.

With Kala Raksha, founders observed the expansion of commercial work for artisans coming into Kutch following the 2001 earthquake. They were aware that Kutch artisans were understood as *workers* who earned manual-labor wages, and they believed artisans were not accessing their most valuable creative capabilities. To offset this trend, and in concert with their originating goal of preserving cultural heritage, Kala Raksha established a design school where artisans acquired a wide range of skills in designing for the global fashion market. Artisans have completed the design course, become design interns, and participated in marketing opportunities in India and abroad. In addition to their increased income, artisans now feel respect for and pride in their ethnic identity, are rewarded for their creative capacity, and experience greater voice through expanded participation and involvement in decision making in their society.

In their organizational evolution, MarketPlace first reorganized from a single top-heavy workplace to seven decentralized workshops where decision-making skills could be more broadly honed. Organizational generation centered on expanding business skills that encourage greater autonomy for the workshops in apparel production. As MarketPlace artisans began to equate commercial participation with broader impacts on their own lives, MarketPlace responded with programs for promoting greater self-efficacy through understanding legal rights for women related to dowry, property rights, and domestic abuse, and for handling the stress of daily life. Through these generational activities, MarketPlace artisans exhibit agency for running a fashion business, positioning their own lives for individual and family decisions, and advocating for others in the community.

In looking to the future, the global fashion market presents challenges for sustainability and growth in relation to each group's unique approach to its work. Increased appropriation of design intellectual property across cultures in the global market has resulted in a generic ethnic fashion look that appeals to consumers who have limited knowledge of textile traditions. Kala Raksha's challenge is to innovate within traditions while appealing to those consumers and to tell a story that makes cultural integrity more valuable and thus marketable. Consumer demand for constant fashion change speaks to MarketPlace's need for greater cross-season design innovation that competes for customers' demand and provides the work on which the artisans depend. For both groups, the world's fluctuating economic market impacts consumption patterns that directly affect the sales potential for artisan groups who view the fashion market as an avenue toward economic self-sufficiency and social development.

Kala Raksha and MarketPlace illustrate how their respective sociocultural environments shaped their originating goals, the aspirations of the artisans involved, their perspectives on cultural property, and their benchmarks for success. For those scholars focusing on artisan enterprise development, attending to issues of capability development and enterprise evolution seems imperative for first understanding and then advocating for artisans to secure a place in the global fashion market. At the same time, acknowledging the constraints and opportunities within specific cultural contexts is vital to ensure that artisans retain control in shaping their cultural property as they enter the market.

NOTES

1. The following works provide insight on a broad variety of issues related to artisan enterprise development and the global economy: Basu 1995; Cockram 2005; Frater 2010; Grimes and Milgram 2000; Littrell and Dickson 2010; Milgram 2010; Morris 1996; Nash 1993; Norris 2010; Paige-Reeves 1998; Root 2005; Rosenbaum and Goldin 1997; Stephen 1991; Tice 1995; Turner 2007; Zorn 2004.
2. Data for the MarketPlace discussion were collected through field research across a two-year period from 2001 to 2003, funded by the Earthwatch Institute. As is common in such research, we drew on multiple sources of data including participant observation, photo documentation, and in-depth interviews with 161 artisans. Details of the interview and photo-documentation methodology, qualitative and statistical analysis, and extended findings can be found in the "Appendix: Methods" section of Littrell and Dickson 2010.
3. Across her twenty years as a development practitioner with Kala Raksha, Judy Frater has documented the Kala Raksha story through in-depth interviews with artisans to record their artistic and cultural heritage and to evaluate outcomes of various Kala Raksha initiatives, including the first six years of Kala Raksha Vidhyalaya (KRV), an institution of design education for traditional artisans of Kutch. These analyses are available through a series of DVDs available at http://www.kala-raksha.org. DVDs include *The Kala Raksha Story: Nurturing the Art of Craft; Needlecraft: A Way of Life; The Masters' Voices; The Stitches Speak*; and *Artisans Design: The Launch of Kala Raksha Vidhylaya.* In addition, current Kala Raksha activities can be accessed through the *KRV Newsletter*, also available at the Kala Raksha website.

BIBLIOGRAPHY

Basu, Kunal. 1995. "Marketing Developing Society Crafts: A Framework for Analysis and Change." In Janeen A. Costa and Gary J. Bamossy (eds.), *Marketing in a Multi-cultural World,* 257–98. Thousand Oaks, CA: Sage.

Boo, Katherine. 2012. *Beyond the Beautiful Forevers.* New York: Random House.

Chambers, Robert. 1997. *Whose Reality Counts? Putting the First Last.* London: Intermediate Technology.

Chatterjee, Ashoke. 2007. "Craft Crisis in India." *Hand/Eye: The Aid to Artisans Magazine,* Fall, p. 12.

Cockram, Mary. 2005. *Lessons Learned in Twenty Years: Honduras, Ghana, Hungary, Russia, Armenia, Central Asia, and Peru.* Hartford, CT: Aid to Artisans.

Frater, Judy. 1995. *Threads of Identity: Embroidery and Adornment of the Nomadic Rabaris.* Ahmedabad, India: Mapin.

Frater, Judy. 2003. "'This Is Ours,' Rabari Tradition and Identity in a Changing World." *Nomadic Peoples* 6 (2): 156–69.

Frater, Judy. 2010. "In the Artisan's Mind: Concepts of Design in Traditional Rabari Embroidery." In Kapila Vatsayan (ed.), *Sui Dhaga,* 84–93. New Delhi: Wisdom Tree with Indian International Centre.

Grimes, Kimberly M., and B. Lynne Milgram (eds.). 2000. *Artisans and Cooperatives: Developing Alternative Trade for the Global Economy.* Tucson: University of Arizona Press.

Handy, Femidy, Meenaz Kassam, Suzanne Feeney, and Bhagyashree Ranade. 2006. *Grass-Roots NGOs by Women for Women: The Driving Force of Development in India.* Thousand Oaks, CA: Sage.

Korten, David C. 1987. "Third Generation NGO Strategies: A Key to People-Centered Development." *World Development* 15 (Suppl.): 145–59.

Liebl, Maureen. 2005. "Jodhpur: The Most Creative of Communities." Paper presented at the Conference on Asia-Pacific Creative Communities: A Strategy for the 21st Century Senior Expert Symposium, Jodhpur, India, February 22–26.

Liebl, Maureen, and Tirthankar Roy. 2004. "Handmade in India: Traditional Craft Skills in a Changing World." In J. Michael Finger and Philip Schuler (eds.), *Poor People's Knowledge: Intellectual Property in Developing Countries,* 53–73. Washington, DC: World Bank and Oxford University Press.

Littrell, Mary A., and Marsha A. Dickson. 1999. *Social Responsibility in the Global Market: Fair Trade of Cultural Products.* Thousand Oaks, CA: Sage.

Littrell, Mary A., and Marsha A. Dickson. 2010. *Artisans and Fair Trade: Crafting Development.* Sterling, VA: Kumarian.

Milgram, B. Lynne. 2010. "From Trash to Totes: Recycled Production and Cooperative Economy Practice in the Philippines." *Human Organization* 69 (1): 75–85.

Morris, Walter F., Jr. 1996. *Handmade Money: Latin American Artisans in the Marketplace.* Washington, DC: Organization of American States.

Nash, June (ed.). 1993. *Crafts in the World Market.* New York: State University of New York Press.

Norris, Lucy. 2010. *Recycling Indian Clothing: Global Contexts of Reuse and Value.* Bloomington: Indiana University Press.

Nussbaum, Martha. 2000. *Women and Human Development: The Capabilities Approach.* Cambridge: Cambridge University Press.

Paige-Reeves, Janet. 1998. "Alpaca Sweater Design and Marketing: Problems and Prospects for Cooperative Knitting Organizations in Bolivia." *Human Organization* 57 (1): 83–93.

Robeyns, Ingrid. 2005. "The Capability Approach: A Theoretical Survey." *Journal of Human Development* 6 (1): 93–114.

Root, Regina A. (ed.). 2005. *The Latin American Fashion Reader.* Oxford: Berg.

Rosenbaum, Brenda, and Liliana Goldin. 1997. "New Exchange Processes in the International Market: The Re-making of Maya Artisan Production in Guatemala." *Museum Anthropology* 21 (2): 72–82.

Sen, Amartya. 1980. "Equality of What?" In Sterling McMurrin (ed.), *The Tanner Lectures on Human Values: I,* 195–220. Cambridge: Cambridge University Press.

Sen, Amartya. 1993. “Capability and Well-Being.” In Martha Nussbaum and Amartya Sen (eds.), *The Quality of Life*, 30–52. Oxford: Clarendon.

Stephen, Lynn. 1991. “Culture as a Resource: Four Cases of Self-Managed Indigenous Craft Production in Latin America.” *Economic Development and Cultural Change* 40 (1): 101–30.

Tice, Karen. 1995. *Kuna Crafts, Gender, and the Global Economy.* Austin: University of Texas Press.

Turner, Sarah. 2007. “Trading Old Textiles: The Selective Diversification of Highland Livelihoods in Northern Vietnam.” *Human Organization* 66 (4): 389–402.

Zorn, Elayne. 2004. *Weaving Future: Tourism, Cloth and Culture on an Andean Island.* Iowa City: University of Iowa Press.

18

Mapping Latin American Fashion

REGINA A. ROOT

During the bicentennial year of independence from Spanish colonialism for seven Latin American nations, fashion weeks throughout the region reassessed the symbols of cultural heritage with excitement and new seriousness. In Argentina, the press heralded retrospectives of national styles, pinpointing their evolution artificially to 1810; for the fashion show "Pasado de moda, 1810–2010" (a play on words with "past styles" and "out of fashion"), the city government of Buenos Aires explained that the objective was to "take back" fashion as "historical testimony" and demonstrate its critical influence on the formation of Argentine identity.[1] At the transnational fashion congress Ixel Moda one year earlier in Cartagena, Colombia, one collection by up-and-coming designers affiliated with Arturo Tejada Cano's design school advocated a "Sustainable Bicentennial" with upcycled materials: hats in the shape of Phrygian liberty caps, fashioned with gauze; military-style jackets with broken chains and top hats with poison warning signs, perhaps a reference to tyrannies past and new foreign invasions; and sheath dresses featuring colorful screenprints of Simón Bolívar, the nineteenth-century leader whose dreams of a unified revolutionary effort led to South American liberation from Spanish colonial oppression. At first glance, the collections seemed like proposals comprised of dissonant fragments, European in their tailoring and homegrown in outlook. Other garments evoked love, passion, peace, and empowerment, powerful tools with which to emerge from Colombia's drug-fed war. On many levels, these rescued clothes reimagined independence in light of contemporary human rights abuses and injustices, economic disparity, the loss of cultural identity, and the ecological crisis at hand. Piecing together fragments of old tires from military vehicles and retired uniforms, the designers had fashioned garments past into something completely different and new (see Figures 18.1 and 18.2).

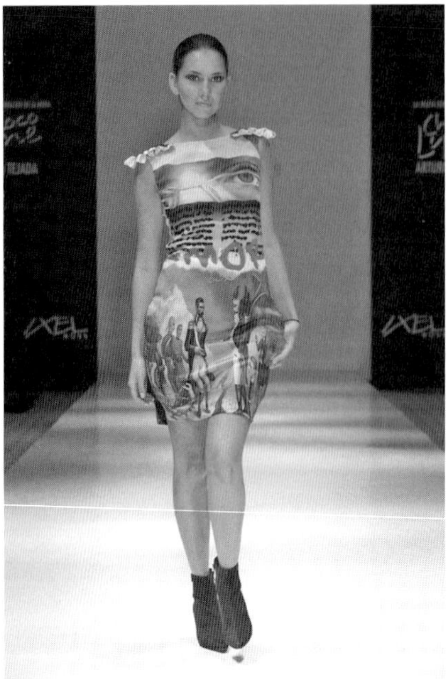

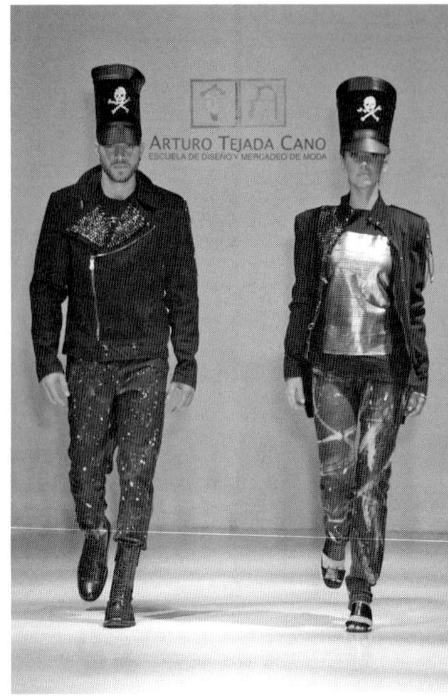

FIGURES 18.1 AND 18.2 The 2009 "Sustainable Bicentennial" collection included sheath dresses with images from independence and upcycled military uniforms. Figure 18.1: Dress designed by Darío Cárdenas. Figure 18.2: Denim garments and top hats by María Fernanda Alvarado.
Credit: Photographs by Sebastián Franco. Courtesy of Ixel Moda.

As several other countries look ahead to their independence bicentennials, a reassessment of national fashion histories throughout the region has predominated. At Ixel Moda's closing panel that same year, Laura Novik of Raíz Diseño (the nongovernmental organization at the forefront of Latin American sustainable design) referenced the need for more pan-American discussions on the origins of Latin American fashion. In light of current national fashion branding initiatives, she proclaimed, "We cannot brand ourselves if we don't know our own fashion history." And as the young designers of Ixel Moda had already revealed with symbols like the poison warning signs atop European-inspired top hats, fashion history has long replicated as much as it unmasked the legacies of colonialism and foreign intervention. As these countries move toward a third century of independence, several recent proposals call into question the historical erasure that has made mapping Latin American fashion such a challenge. Unlike a monument that commemorates with imposing permanence, twenty-first-century design proposals have modeled how independence itself constitutes a creative process in progress, both in terms of one's active role within its making and as a collective goal. Beyond any fibers or upcycled materials used, the "Sustainable Bicentennial" collection thus also opened an important entry point through which Colombian *and* Latin American fashion can and must be understood.

In spite of its vibrant history and significance to mass-market ranges around the globe, Latin American fashion design and history has long been overlooked. This chapter begins by briefly highlighting issues that have shaped dress and fashion in the region, noting key strands within and across which scholarship currently builds. Given the Latin American fashion industry's desire to capture its own history, analyzing the underpinnings of contemporary collections seems in high order. Here I focus on the power of colonial dress and the styles of independence, all of which informed the initial articulation and creation of uniquely national styles. Because newly found archival evidence has stimulated new insights into the role of fashion as a tool of agency and creative expression, I conclude with an illustrative example from the River Plate region following the retreat of Spanish colonialism. As scholars map Latin American fashion, the documentation of influences and in-depth analyses that bring together the fragments of a field represent an important step in the recovery and preservation of both Latin American and global fashion history.

WHAT IS LATIN AMERICAN FASHION?

This question was first addressed in the pages of *The Latin American Fashion Reader*, which brought together an international group of scholars whose research integrates the study of dress into the workings of culture, identity formation, and social change (Root 2005). Referring to the dress, body, and culture of a heterogeneous world culture region might seem all too impractical for the scholar wishing to compare and contrast the fashions of Mexico, Central America, the Caribbean, and South America. The "deliberate error" that the concept of Latin America itself represents provides an important paradox for scholars to unpack: invented in nineteenth-century France, the idea of "Latin America" took into account "French presence on the continent (Haiti, Guyana), [and] was favoured by South American exiles living in Paris who were keen to give their newly independent territories a supra-national continental identity" and differentiate this identity from that of Anglo-Americans (Davies 2002: 2). Recognizing the constructed nature of this world culture region's very naming, and still in search of an answer to the question often posed by design practitioners and scholars alike, What *is* Latin American fashion?, the volume focused on overlapping sociohistorical influences that have shaped the pursuit of elegance and transformed cultural dynamics to elucidate some general characteristics for the region. As a cultural process, fashion is a profoundly social experience that invites individual and collective bodies to assume certain identities and, at times, to transgress limits and create new ones. Grounded in aspects of human agency or self-fashioning, this volume initiated an interdisciplinary discussion on potential paths for research and revealed that the very object of study ultimately reveals whole worlds of culture.

Five central strands organized initial Latin American fashion studies research. Relying heavily on archival sources, the first strand unravels Latin American fashion history through the examination of the region's multicultural heritage and colonial and postcolonial legacies (Baptista 2010; Cahill 2007; Cruz de Amenábar 1996; Earle 2007; Meléndez 2005; Phipps 1996; Randall 2005; Root 2000, 2010; Rowe 2011; Schevill 2010; Sommer 2007; Tinajero 2005; Walker 2010). The second strand rethinks altered traditions through the points of contact between local knowledge and the global context (Demaray, Keim-Shenk, and Littrell 2005; Femenías 2005; Garcia 2010; Hendrickson 1995; López 2010; Scheinman 2005; Schevill 2010; Zorn 2004). At first glance, the resonances of fashion might seem limitless, as if the local were constantly remade for a world market. Despite the aggressive interactions of world trade, scholars have found that clear boundaries exist for individual—and particularly indigenous—communities to preserve the sacred attributes of their traditional rites and dress. The third strand analyzes the cultural imaginary, situating the articulations of dress within and beyond the parameters of urban, national, and transnational spaces (Castilho and García 2001; Goldgel 2013; Hershfield 2008; López-Gydosh and Dickson 2005; Majluf 2006; Montalva 2004; Rodríguez Lehmann 2008, 2013; Root 2010; Schevill 2010; Stephenson 1999). From the seminomadic Andean poncho confectioned for Parisian collections to the Brazilian bikini shown on the Cable News Network, the cultural imaginary links individual styles and collective fantasies to shifting understandings of myth and national identity (Aragón 2010; Arredondo 2010; Corcuera 2000; Earle 2003; Schevill 2010; Villaça 2005). The fourth strand highlights the mediation and consumption of culture, sometimes through the study of luxury goods or fashion icons (Andrade 2005; André 2005; Castilho and Villaça 2006; Hallstead 2009; Hallstead and Root 2014; Krischke Leitão, Nogueira de Oliveira Lima, and Pinheiro Machado 2006; Milian Arias 2005; Miller 2005; Moraña 2008; Orlove 1997). The fifth strand approaches the complexities of contemporary Latin American fashion, engaging the contested territories that make over the realm of the quotidian (Blanch, Novik, and Root 2008; Castilho and Galvão 2002; Forastelli 2005; Lescano 2004; Saulquin 2010; Schevill 2010). Scholars in the field likely engage more than one or perhaps all of these strands, as the recovery project implied by an inclusive fashion studies represents a comprehensive undertaking upon which to build and grow. The interpretations of the "Sustainable Bicentennial" presented by the Colombian designers at Ixel Moda, for example, would likely be considered incomplete without the engagement of all such strands.

UNRAVELING HISTORY

Museums of dress throughout Latin America often begin their fashion history with independence. In some regions, few samples of cloth and garments are generally available, leading to assertions that a full register of historical styles will never be possible (Anawalt 2010: 6; Saulquin 1990: 35). Furthermore, the founding fictions of Latin American independence projected what Antonio Cornejo Polar defined as the "socialized image of the national community," or the presentation of a national identity without always acknowledging the heterogeneous basis of the new nation (2003: 99). Postcolonial school textbooks throughout the region, for example, projected "the new world that Columbus gave us" and thereby integrated the colonial past into a narrative of heroic deeds that promoted the values of a "strong" national identity based on the domination of others (who were often scantily clothed in comparison to the steel-shell armor of the conquerors). Scholars of colonial and postcolonial fashion history therefore cover complex terrain when engaging the multivalent nature of dress in the region.

THE POWER OF COLONIAL DRESS

The first images and accounts of American natives that circulated throughout Europe reveal much about a sense of awe experienced by the first colonial invaders. They viewed the natives' "nakedness" with bewilderment and marveled at the presence of material goods such as cotton, woven cloth, and intricate feather work. In their descriptions, "everything in the European dream of possession rests on witnessing, a witnessing understood as a form of significant and representative seeing" (Greenblatt 1991: 122). The "New World" provided Europe with material goods as varied as silver, gold, sugar, chocolate, textiles, and dye. As colonial governments were established, native populations suffered the effects of brutal conquest, illness from pathogens, and tortures aimed to force conversion to Christianity. The term *black legend* coined by Friar Bartolomé de las Casas encompasses the most exploitative practices of settlers and the violent human rights abuses of those who had turned to slavery and systematic violence to establish ranches, mines, and textile industries.

During the colonial period, dress served as an important visual register in the construction of cultural, racial, and ethnic differences. In the early part of the sixteenth century, depictions of nakedness served to justify notions of European superiority (Meléndez 2005). Such images privileged the powerful, "civilized" colonizers and marked indigenous people as "barbarians" in need of governance. Because many native men and women had worn homespun and woven clothing for centuries before the conquest, Catholic missionaries often targeted the clothing of peoples from more tropical regions. Spanish priests insisted that women cover themselves, especially in more tropical regions, or "sew up their *anacus* for the sake of 'decency' so that they did not expose their legs as they walked" in the Andes (Phipps 1996: 153). Pre-Hispanic artifacts like the Mixtec codices depict recurring hair fashions, including symbolically dyed and "intricately designed" styles for women (Parker 2010: 53); in New Spain, hairstyles continued to vary tremendously, as one section of the Florentine Codex indicates, with women now assuming the Spanish wimple. Colonial powers dictated that men wear a Castilian shirt and white cotton trousers of Flemish origin (an immensely popular fashion in Spain) and crop their long hair (Bauer 2001: 71–73); ponchos, locally produced hats, and sandals were still used. While European-style dress was certainly promoted by colonial authorities, any "policy of co-optation" or excessive borrowing of styles was strongly discouraged. While some caciques, or noble Indians, distinguished themselves from common Indians by wearing shoes instead of sandals, dressing in silk or armor, and carrying arms, local authorities stripped those who tried to imitate the Spanish too closely (Bauer [2001] cites the Archivo General de Indias, Quito, leg. 211, fol. 73). In response to indigenous revolts, prohibitions against native garments in the Andean region were "often appended to the mandate for learning the Spanish language," meaning that dress and language "coupled as elements of cultural transformation" (Phipps 1996: 154).

Prior to colonization, dress and textiles served as indicators of social and religious identity and as mediums of exchange. Colonization also changed the terms of textile production with the introduction of steel shears and European methods involving spinning and rotary wheels, eventually replacing obsidian instruments, the drop spindle, and the backdrop loom (Anawalt 2010: 7; Bauer 2001: 105–8). Indigenous chronicler Guaman Poma de Ayala's *Nueva corónica y buen gobierno* (1615) represents the physical abuse of Incan women forced to produce woven clothing (see Figure 18.3). Some

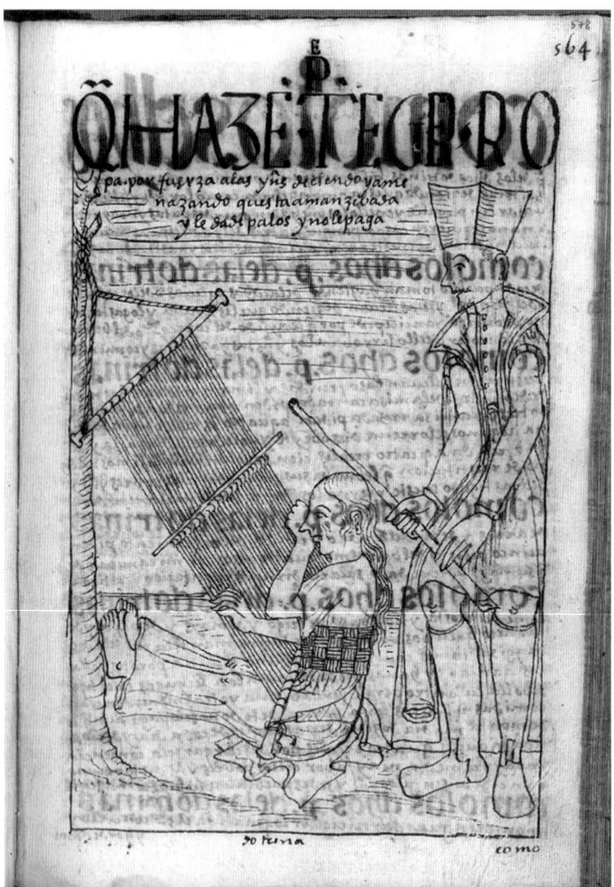

FIGURE 18.3 Forced to weave clothing, an Incan woman is abused by a parish priest. From Guaman Poma de Ayala's *Nueva corónica y buen gobierno* (1615).
Credit: Courtesy of the Royal Library.

religious orders, private investors, and even indigenous communities established textile workshops, or *obrajes,* in Mexico and the highlands of Ecuador and Peru for the production of wool, cotton, silk, and hemp fibers (Bauer 2001: 105–8; Miño Grijalva 1989; Villanueva 1985). Workers in these colonial textile factories toiled long hours in inhumane conditions. Local dependencies on cloth only grew, with each decade of colonialism creating more demand for "commercial, non-luxury fabrics in everyday use" produced in obrajes (Greenleaf 1967: 227). When Portugal's Queen Mary prohibited the manufacture of most textiles in Brazil in 1775, those same laws excluded only coarse cotton textiles used for African slave garments and the packing of dry goods (Andrade and Root 2010). With the emergence of alternate markets for cotton and the influx of goods from Asia (brought by the Spanish Empire's Manila Galleon) and Europe, many textile workshops were on the verge of ruin by the eighteenth century. Interregional trade exclusive of Spain began with the Spanish Free Trade Policy of 1778.

A caste system maintained a sense of hierarchy to privilege Europeans and respond to racial mixing, or *mestizaje.* From the onset of colonization, natives and African slaves had been forced to wear Western styles of dress, a system that reinforced the authority of the Spanish and Portuguese and, over time, their Creole descendants. Decrees prohibited the use of certain textiles by those who the caste system deemed as inferiors, thus leading to the prohibition of velvet, taffeta, or silk for specially fashioned Incan *unkus,* or tunics, in the Andean region (Iriarte 1993) or the woven rebozo scarves commonly worn by women in Mexico (Logan et al. 1994). A few colonial notarial inventories list that some of castes possessed a wide array of garments and items of jewelry. Archaeologists are still in the process of compiling records of colonial material culture, also through the lens of agency and policy; when it comes to the realm of fashion, surviving documents point to great movement between ethnic lines. The 1690 will of African descendant Sebastiana de Isla, while perhaps not completely representative, lists indigenous garments such as the *topo,* a kind of shawl pin, and the *lliglla,* or traditional shawl, in addition to eight cotton shirts, four petticoats, two wool skirts, and various adornments including Castilian garnets and a coral rosary (Jamieson 2004: 438–39).

Because the caste system could not be enforced completely, prominently displayed visual registers of racial mixing known as *casta* paintings utilized conventions in dress as worn by couples and their offspring and depicted the durable and nondurable goods available to them (Katzew 2004). Light-skinned *mestizos,* a term used to identify people of mixed European and indigenous descent, sometimes imitated the consumption patterns and styles of more socially preferable castes in order to be mistaken for one of them. Since hybridity had become a fact of daily life, some mestizos cut their hair or turned away from the hues of local dyes to distinguish themselves from Indians and thereby identify with higher castes with greater privileges (Bauer 2001: 111). Visible social groups of the seventeenth and eighteenth centuries, one could argue, manipulated dress codes to challenge a caste system that seemed to expand with increasingly hostile labels such as "coyote" and "lobo [wolf]" (Carrera 2003). Once racial miscegenation challenged the very categories of the caste system, however, any concept of colonial power began to disintegrate. Responding to a perceived threat, the Spanish crown issued a series of statements to emphasize the delineations of dress according to caste hierarchies, denouncing the ostentatious dress on the part of mestiza women but not the luxurious presence of clergymen. Sumptuary laws, like the Real Pragmática of 1716, further entrenched distinctions, limiting laborers to clothes made of wool, linen, or cotton (Konetzke 1962: 3:130). Dress figured prominently in punishments meted out for subversion of the caste system, with some members of the populace even taking enforcement into their own hands. According to *El lazarillo de ciegos caminantes,* a 1775–1776 travel guide for Buenos Aires to Lima, an elegantly dressed Creole woman invited an extravagantly dressed mulatta to her home, had her maids forcibly remove the mulatta's clothes, whipped her, and burned the discarded clothing (referred to as *las galas,* or formal dress), and finally re-dressed her in clothes deemed corresponding to her "birth" or status. The mulatta had apparently neglected to heed an earlier warning about dressing above her status (Concolorcorvo [1773] 1942: 72). Disruptive performances of dress may have served as early indicators of a cultural crisis that would bring about the subsequent fragmentation of the Spanish Empire.

FASHIONING INDEPENDENCE

By the early nineteenth century, the region experienced several calls for independence that deeply affected the way people consumed fashion. For Cuba and Puerto Rico, this struggle for independence would not materialize until the end of the nineteenth century, although the description of fashion and dance in several literary works began to plot the demise of Spanish rule and construct alternate political identities (Holland 1992). Under the colonial caste system, Creole descendants of Europeans had been designated as having inferior social status, although some boldly dared to appropriate subtle details in order to imitate their Spanish superiors, such as the usage of gold and silver threads or special fabrics in the construction of outfits (Bauer 2001: 112). As rivalries increased between factions and civil wars ensued, Creoles moved to Parisian styles that symbolized the legacy of "Liberty, Equality, and Fraternity" espoused by the French Revolution and advocated a society based on merit rather than inherited privilege (Root 2010). Portraits of Simón Bolívar of Venezuela, the independence leader referenced in the "Sustainable Bicentennial" collection, and José de San Martín of Argentina depicted new uniforms of their own design. By the late nineteenth century, one could find the garments of founding fathers represented in illustrated magazines without any hint of their wearer, as if the aura of the garments now on display for the national community represented some higher truth (see, for example, the renditions published by the *Papel Periódico Ilustrado* from late nineteenth-century Colombia).

Benedict Anderson (1991) argues that print capitalism played a pivotal role in the creation of a "new consciousness" in Latin America that aspired to independent thought without maintaining or imitating European ways. Of great interest here is the kind of discourse that emerged following the independence movement in response to the desire to configure civil and political identities for a national subject. The rhetoric of fashion helped form a model political body, or a symbolic form of liberation from Spanish domination. In real life, fashions began to mirror those of France and North America, although there may have been less change initially among the working classes. *Figurines,* or engraved fashion plates that were available for purchase and circulated in urban areas, responded to the increasing appetite for European—but not Spanish—styles. Women's fashions in Colombia, for example, appear to have been divided along class lines: wealthy Creole members appropriated French designs to distinguish themselves from Spanish women, while those with less buying power continued to integrate Spanish textiles and designs into their wardrobes. Believing their readership dispossessed of its colonial past, Argentine magazines (*La Moda, El Iniciador*) argued that the status of future nations rested on the respectability and decorum of their subjects. Fashion, whether in print or in practice, served as an important metaphor for political change and renovation.

NEW FASHION EMPIRES

The postcolonial relationship between center and periphery, or civilization and barbarism as Domingo Faustino Sarmiento ([1845] 2003) described it in his political treatise, became essential to debates about nation building in the nineteenth century. These debates often placed fashion at the heart of national constitution, as dress served to unite American patriots. While some garments still recalled Spanish tailoring, homegrown manifestations—such as the crimson civilian uniform of the Argentine Confederation under Juan Manuel de Rosas (1826–1852)—offered popular alternatives. According to Sarmiento, a civilized minority wore French-style clothing and risked persecution by the new regime. In response to Rosas's authoritarian practices and hoping to persuade others to adopt more fashion-forward politics, Miguel Cané recognized in 1839, "Fashion is the most flexible side of society, and because of this, it is perfected daily. . . . What will it take for us to *not* be what we are?" For Cané and other intellectuals of his generation, a change in fashion constituted revolutionary change, a historic moment to seize, to change, and "to march with the times, with fashion" (Cané 1838: 54).

Along with independence came shifts in consumption practices. Representations of other empires as superior to the Spanish regime further challenged the status quo. The British invasions of 1806 and 1807, while unsuccessful, marked a shift in the way inhabitants perceived themselves and their possessions. Mariquita Sánchez de Thompson, an elite member of society, equated the aesthetic of British soldiers with a kind of cultural supremacy: red-laced boots, foot-high black feathered hats, plaid sashes, and bright red jackets. By the 1820s, the colonial economy had collapsed, and foreign imports saturated the marketplace. English businessmen displayed a sartorial process much like diplomatic courting, thus making British etiquette and customs the model for the Buenos Aires elite. British ship captain Emeric Essex Vidal noted that the more privileged "adopted a style of dress between the English and French" and retained the Spanish *mantilla,* a shawl often made of silk (1820: 49). The poncho, a handwoven garment that recalled seminomadic indigenous origins and frontier culture, provides an interesting case within this context. British entrepreneurs not only appropriated the traditional designs but also supplanted Argentine-made ponchos with prefabricated garments churned out in the Manchester and Birmingham mills (Corcuera 2005). By 1838 Sir Woodbine Parish, a traveling diplomat and scientist, recalled that the gauchos (rural pampa dwellers) dressed almost exclusively in English-made ponchos (1852: 362). As the Creole manufactures were dismantled, use of the poncho—long a prominent part of the rural wardrobe—also waned. Similarly, if the gaucho's wife had a gown, then "ten to one it is from Manchester," Parish claimed (362), noting that those east of the Andes had long received their European goods from the River Plate region (Parish [1838] 1852: 349–50). At the same time, British reports touted Buenos Aires fashions as superior to those made at home. "If... any of the 'first chop' London milliners would condescend to visit Buenos Ayres, they would find many things that might be an addition to their fashionable vocabulary," wrote one reporter in the *British Packet* (April 20, 1833, pp. 2–3). From black English hats of superior quality to "black and buff Kid Gloves," advertisements in the 1830s and 1840s indicate a growing demand for all things British but also capture the emergence of a distinct Argentine aesthetic that challenged British fashion's inexpensive and "tasteless variations" (March 10, 1832, p. 3). As the report implied, British visitors would surely feel shame when comparing their misguided sartorial registers to this powerful new idiom.

As male leaders arranged political hierarchies, they found public spaces obstructed by groups of women whose political subjectivity they had overlooked. The *British Packet* routinely reported African Argentine marches, as when over 400 women with red-and-white turbans with gold bands and feathers, white dresses, red sashes, and ribands "marched through the streets in procession" shouting incessant "*vivas*" as part of a long series of political functions (January 21, 1837, pp. 2–3). Numerous spectators "encroached so much" on the women "that it was found necessary for soldiers to interfere to keep them back. ... Run, ladies, run!—there's nothing like beginning it," the report read. At other functions a "ponderous yet not inelegant comb" gave women's heads "a great deal of importance," a style also described by the *British Packet* as "very handsome, very dignified, and very knowing" (October 9, 1830, p. 1). The *peinetón,* a one-yard-square tortoiseshell hair comb that outsized any Spanish comb, paired best with contemporary French hairstyles (see Figure 18.4). With leg-of-mutton sleeves, corseted hourglass figures, and crowns as expansive as the pampas, fashionable women of the River Plate region left the confines of their homes with a fashion "presence" that critiqued those male leaders who professed the ideals of independence but then refused women the status of citizenship (Root 2010: 61–94).

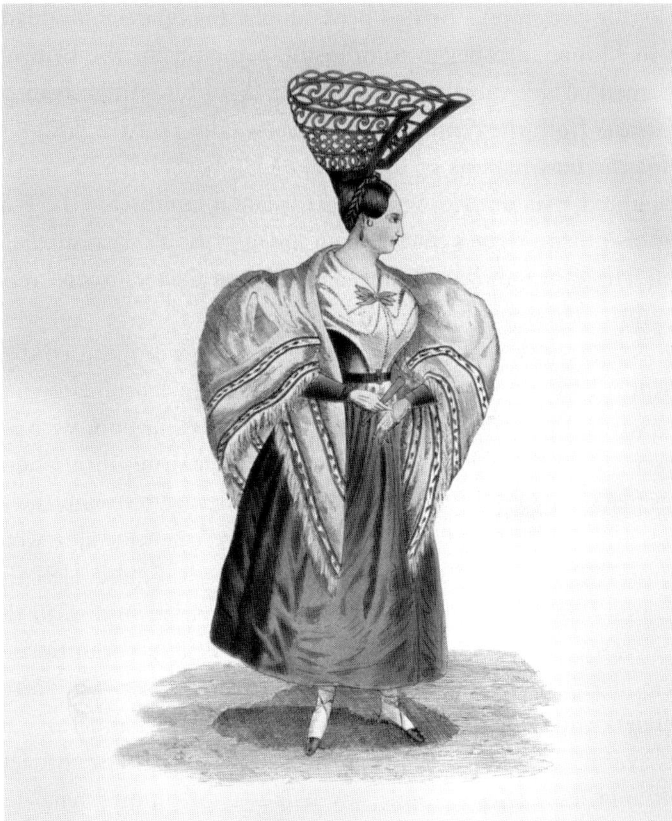

FIGURE 18.4 César Hipólito Bacle's *Trajes y costumbres de la provincia de Buenos Aires* depicted the peinetón-wearing woman of the 1830s. *Credit*: Courtesy of Argentina's Biblioteca Nacional.

As "Argentine" as such fashions may have appeared, a dose of irony resided in the fact that of the many tortoiseshell hair combs created in the 1820s and 1830s, the most noteworthy came from the workshop of a Spanish artisan. In 1825, two years after his arrival from Spain, Manuel Masculino opened up a shop that allowed female customers to consult with him on the designs of individual combs. To make the peinetón, African or Caribbean tortoiseshells were boiled, softened, shaped, overlapped, cut manually, dried, and then polished carefully to reveal original designs and motifs, including patriotic slogans. The peinetón combs made by Masculino quickly became costly status symbols, with women of the working classes seeking ones made of imitation tortoiseshell. Masculino's store thrived despite a depressed market in which most generally purchased the least expensive clothing and footwear possible, prohibitive tariffs, and vocal critics who disregarded the peinetón-wearing woman. Although some newspapers proclaimed, "Down with the Spanish!" as did one poem about a fictitious Spanish peinetón maker (Root 2010: 75), clients seemingly ignored the designer's peninsular heritage and sought his expertise when creating this female emblem associated with Argentine independence.

Just as the locally woven poncho had been supplanted by machine-made British versions, women in Montevideo began to drop the peinetón for the British bonnet. The *British Packet* lamented this substitution at length, describing English-inspired elegance as one that "detracts from the beauty of the wearers" and that the author believed "out of character" for the new nations of the region (October 31, 1835, p. 4). Another report further doubted that discarding the tortoiseshell combs for the English bonnet and French leg-of-mutton sleeves that were all the rage should last; surely, he wrote, Argentine women would not allow milliners and mantua makers to enslave them as they already had the British (September 19, 1835, p. 3).

For consumers, the idea that fashion symbolized the European continued well beyond the post-independence moment. As citizens of newly consolidated nations became readers well versed in the vocabulary of luxury and consumption, with a proliferation of fashion prescriptions from illustrated magazines circulating throughout the Americas, elite classes placed themselves at the center of modernity through the acquisition of European goods and markers of status. "In dress . . . the Argentine elite were determined to equal or outdo the wealthy of Europe," writes James R. Scobie (1974: 234). Newly arrived immigrants from Europe, on the other hand, tended to discard the rural styles with which they arrived, accessing a social mobility through adoptions like the coat and tie. With modernization, traditional styles were often discarded, writes James Higgins in a different context, "in favor of the styles of London and Paris . . . voluminous flounced skirts over hooped petticoats; high-necked dresses, blouses or jackets with lace sleeves; complicated hair styles . . . topped by hair-nets or plumed hats" (2005: 87). In 1898, once all of Spanish America had gained its independence, the popular Argentine version of the magazine *Caras y Caretas* projected visions of fashionable lifestyles for its readers. To commemorate the first independence bicentennial, its readers imagined a proliferation of publics through elegant illustrations associating empire not with colonialism but with new "tight skirts" unsuitable for dancing, advertisements on liberation from slavery referring to an antialcohol program, and "tintura l'Indienne" designed for fair-skinned complexions (using French to categorize autochthonous-inspired dyes or cosmetics; July 9, 1910, pp. 25, 114). The developing field of fashion marketing—ascribing new meaning to everything from skin whiteners to evening gowns—erased the heterogeneous reality of the now consolidated nation-state and further relegated indigenous peoples, African Argentines, and most rural inhabitants to the margins of European sophistication and distinction.

TOWARD AN INCLUSIVE FASHION STUDIES

Scholarly conversations on Latin American fashion inevitably draw on the contemporary practices of designers, producers, and consumers of fashion. An interdisciplinary approach to fashion studies allows, even forces, us to confront the complex nature of fashion history—a history very much still in the making. In finding meaning in dress and fashion, scholars will need to assess carefully and push forward definitive Latin American fashion histories in the future. Colonial authorities deemed their own traditions and styles to be superior, often ignoring or, worse, censoring those who practiced fashion in their own right. With independence, visible social sectors demanded political recognition through the use of dress and fashion accessories. These stories remain, for the most part, untold. Given the increasing number of books dedicated to contemporary global fashions, and the few that focus seriously on Latin America, we need to evaluate more carefully the blinders that have long caused us to overlook a most rich and compelling history. Refashioning the past and infusing fashion narratives with cultural memory, the young designers of Ixel Moda in search of a "Sustainable Bicentennial" actively deconstructed and reconstructed textiles, tendencies, and ideals. Had they chosen to write about this process instead of using fashion as a tool for reflection and change, their perspectives would likely have called into question discourses of power and privilege and the unfinished nature of the fashion canon. As scholars work to expand the concept of fashion and create a more inclusive fashion studies, recognizing all the potential interpretive chasms and including histories and communities ordinarily excluded from the field's purview will be vital work.

NOTE

1. "Pasado de moda 1810–2010," Campañas, Buenos Aires Ciudad, March 2010, http://www.buenosaires.edu.ar/areas/com_social/campanias/mas_info.php?campania=501 (accessed May 6, 2013).

BIBLIOGRAPHY

Anawalt, Patricia. 2010. "Regional Dress of Latin America in a European Context." In Margot Blum Schevill (ed.), *Berg Encyclopedia of World Dress and Fashion,* vol. 2, *Latin America and the Caribbean,* 5–11. Oxford: Berg.

Anderson, Benedict. 1991. *Imagined Communities.* London: Verso.

Andrade, Rita. 2005. "Mappin Stories: Adding an English Touch to the São Paulo Fashion Scene." In Regina A. Root (ed.), *Latin American Fashion Reader,* 176–87. Oxford: Berg.

Andrade, Rita, and Regina A. Root. 2010. "Dress, Body and Culture in Brazil." In Margot Blum Schevill (ed.), *Berg Encyclopedia of World Dress and Fashion,* vol. 2, *Latin America and the Caribbean,* 421–25. Oxford: Berg.

André, María Claudia. 2005. "Frida and Evita: Latin American Icons for Export." In Regina A. Root (ed.), *Latin American Fashion Reader,* 247–62. Oxford: Berg.

Aragón, Alba. 2010. "Film and Fashion." In Margot Blum Schevill (ed.), *Berg Encyclopedia of World Dress and Fashion,* vol. 2, *Latin America and the Caribbean,* 12–19. Oxford: Berg.

Arredondo, Isabel. 2010. "Dress in Mexican Cinema." In Margot Blum Schevill (ed.), *Berg Encyclopedia of World Dress and Fashion,* vol. 2, *Latin America and the Caribbean,* 142–46. Oxford: Berg.

Baptista, Asdrúbal (ed.). 2010. "Moda, subversión y ciudadanía." Special issue, *El Desafío de la Historia* 18 (3).

Bauer, Arnold. 2001. *Goods, Power, History: Latin America's Material Culture.* New York: Cambridge University Press.

Blanch, Alex, Laura Novik, and Regina A. Root. 2008. "La moda ética en América Latina." *Estudios* 16 (32): 305–14.

Cahill, David. 2007. "Refashioning the Inca: Costume, Political Power and Identity in Late Bourbon Peru." In Mina Roces and Louise Edwards (eds.), *The Politics of Dress in Asia and the Americas,* 182–99. Brighton, UK: Sussex Academic.

Cané, Miguel. 1838. "Modas." *El Iniciador,* May 15, 53–54.

Caras y Caretas. 1898–1939. Buenos Aires: Talleres de Caras y Caretas.

Carrera, Magalí M. 2003. *Imagining Identity in New Spain: Race, Lineage, and the Colonial Body in Portraiture and Casta Paintings.* Austin: University of Texas Press.

Castilho, Kathia, and Diana Galvão. 2002. *A moda do corpo o corpo da moda.* São Paulo, Brazil: Editora Esfera.

Castilho, Kathia, and Carol García. 2001. *Moda Brasil. Fragmentos de um Vestir Tropical.* São Paulo: Anhembi Morumbi.

Castilho, Kathia, and Nizia Villaça. 2006. *O Novo luxo.* São Paulo: Anhembi Morumbi.

Concolorcorvo [Alonso Carrió de la Vandera]. [1773] 1942. *El lazarillo de ciegos caminantes. De Buenos Aires hasta Lima.* Buenos Aires: Ediciones Argentinas Solar.

Corcuera, Ruth. 2000. *Ponchos de las tierras del Plata.* Buenos Aires: Fondo Nacional de las Artes and Vertraeten Editores.

Corcuera, Ruth. 2005. "Ponchos of the River Plate: Nostalgia for Eden." In Regina A. Root (ed.), *Latin American Fashion Reader,* 163–75. Oxford: Berg.

Cornejo Polar, Antonio. 2003. *Escribir en el aire. Ensayo sobre la heterogeneidad socio-cultural en las literaturas andinas.* Lima: Centro de Estudios Literarios "Antonio Cornejo Polar."

Cruz de Amenábar, Isabel. 1996. *El Traje. Transformaciones de una segunda piel.* Serie Arte y Sociedad en Chile, 1650–1820. Santiago: Ediciones Universidad Católica de Chile.

Davies, Catherine. 2002. "What Is Hispanic Studies?" In Catherine Davies (ed.), *The Companion to Hispanic Studies,* 1–12. London: Arnold.

Demaray, Elyse, Melody Keim-Shenk, and Mary Littrell. 2005. "Representations of Tradition in Latin American Boundary Textile Art." In Regina A. Root (ed.), *Latin American Fashion Reader,* 142–59. Oxford: Berg.

Earle, Rebecca. 2002. "Luxury, Clothing and Race in Colonial Spanish America." In Maxine Berg and Elizabeth Eger (eds.), *Luxury in the Eighteenth-Century: Debates, Desires, and Delectable Goods,* 219–27. Basingstoke, UK: Palgrave

Earle, Rebecca. 2007. "Nationalism and National Dress in Spanish America." In Mina Roces and Louise Edwards (eds.), *The Politics of Dress in Asia and the Americas,* 163–81. Brighton, UK: Sussex Academic.

Femenías, Blenda. 2005. *Gender and the Boundaries of Dress in Contemporary Peru.* Austin: University of Texas Press.

Forastelli, Fabricio. 2005. "Scattered Bodies, Unfashionable Flesh." In Regina A. Root (ed.), *Latin American Fashion Reader,* 283–89. Oxford: Berg.

Garcia, Carol. 2010. *Imagens Errantes. Ambiguidade, resistencia e cultura de moda.* São Paulo: Estaçao das Letras e Core.

Goldgel, Víctor. 2013. *Cuando lo nuevo conquistó América. Prensa, moda y literatura en el siglo XIX.* Buenos Aires: Siglo XIX.
Greenblatt, Stephen. 1991. *Marvelous Possessions: The Wonder of the New World.* Chicago: University of Chicago Press.
Greenleaf, Richard E. 1967. "The Obraje in the Late Mexican Colony." *The Americas* 23 (3): 227–50.
Hallstead, Susan. 2009. "Disease and Immorality: The Problem of Fashionable Dress in Buenos Aires (1862–1880)." *Latin American Literary Review* 37 (73): 90–117.
Hallstead, Susan, and Regina A. Root. 2014. *Pasado de moda: Expresiones culturales y consumo en la Argentina.* Buenos Aires: Edhasa.
Hendrickson, Carol. 1995. *Weaving Identities: Construction of Dress and Self in a Highland Guatemalan Town.* Austin: University of Texas Press.
Hershfield, Joanne. 2008. *Imagining la Chica Moderna: Women, Nation, and Visual Culture in Mexico, 1917–1936.* Durham and London: Duke University Press.
Higgins, James. 2005. *Lima: A Cultural History.* Oxford: Oxford University Press.
Holland, Norman. 1992. "Fashioning Cuba." In Andrew Parker, Mary Russo, Doris Sommer, and Patricia Yeager (eds.), *Nationalisms and Sexualities*, 147–56. London: Routledge.
Iriarte, Isabel. 1993. "Las túnicas incas en la pintura colonial." In Henrique Urbano (ed.), *Mito y simbolismo en los Andes,* 53–85. Cuzco, Peru: Centro "Bartolomé de las Casas."
Jamieson, Ross. 2004. "Bolts of Cloth and Shreds of Pottery: Impressions of Caste in Material Culture of the Seventeenth Century Audiencia of Quito." *Americas: A Quarterly Review of Inter-American Cultural History* 60 (3): 431–46.
Katzew, Ilona. 2004. *Casta Painting.* New Haven, CT: Yale University Press.
Konetzke, Richard. 1962. *Colección de documentos para la historia de la formación social de Hispanoamérica 1493–1810.* 5 vols. Madrid: Consejo Superior de Investigaciones.
Krischke Leitão, Débora, Diana Nogueira de Oliveira Lima, and Rosana Pinheiro Machado. 2006. *Antropología & Consumo. Diálogos entre Brazil e Argentina.* Porto Alegre, Brazil: Editora Age.
Lescano, Victoria. 2004. *Followers of Fashion: Falso Diccionario de la Moda.* Buenos Aires: Interzona.
Logan, Irene, Ruth Lechuga, Teresa Castelló Yturbide, Irmgard Weitlaner Johnson, and Chloë Sayer. 1994. *Rebozos de la Colección Robert Everts.* Colección Uso y Estilo. Mexico City: Museo Franz Meyer and Artes de México.
López, Rick. 2010. *Crafting Mexico: Intellectuals, Artisans and the State after Revolution.* Durham, NC: Duke University Press.
López-Gydosh, Dilia, and Marsha A. Dickson. 2005. "'Every Girl has a Fan which she Kept Always in Motion': Puerto Rican Women's Dress at a Time of Social and Cultural Transition." In Regina A. Root (ed.), *Latin American Fashion Reader,* 198–210. Oxford: Berg.
Majluf, Natalia (ed.). 2006. *Reproducing Nations: Types and Costumes in Asia and Latin America, ca. 1800–1860.* New York: Americas Society.
Meléndez, Mariselle. 2005. "Visualizing Difference: The Rhetoric of Clothing in Colonial Spanish America." In Regina A. Root (ed.), *Latin American Fashion Reader,* 17–30. Oxford: Berg.
Milian Arias, Claudia M. 2005. "Fashioning United States Salvadoranness: Unveiling the Faces of Christy Turlington and Rosa López." In Regina A. Root (ed.), *Latin American Fashion Reader,* 263–79. Oxford: Berg.

Miller, Marilyn. 2005. "*Guayaberismo* and the Essence of Cool." In Regina A. Root (ed.), *Latin American Fashion Reader,* 213–31. Oxford: Berg.

Miño Grijalva, Manuel. 1989. "El obraje colonial." *European Review of Latin American and Caribbean Studies* 47 (December): 3–19.

Montalva, Pía. 2004. *Morir un poco. Moda y sociedad en Chile, 1960–1976.* Biblioteca Todo es Historia. Editorial Sudamericana. Santiago, Chile: Random House Mondadori.

Moraña, Ana. 2008. "La propaganda, la moda y el consumo en la revista *Caras y Caretas* (Argentina, 1898–1910)." *Estudios* 16 (32): 249–73.

Orlove, Benjamin (ed.). 1997. *The Allure of the Foreign: Imported Goods in Postcolonial Latin America.* Ann Arbor: University of Michigan Press.

Parish, Sir Woodbine. [1838] 1852. *Buenos Ayres and the Provinces of the Rio de la Plata: From Their Discovery and Conquest by the Spaniards to the Establishment of Their Political Independence. With Some Account of Their Present State, Trade, Debt, etc.; an Appendix of Historical and Statistical Documents; and a Description of the Geology and Fossil Monsters of the Pampas. By Sir Woodbine Parish. . .* London: J. Murray.

Parker, Holly. 2010. "Mixtec Hairstyles." In Margot Blum Schevill (ed.), *Berg Encyclopedia of World Dress and Fashion,* vol. 2, *Latin America and the Caribbean,* 51–56. Oxford: Berg.

Phipps, Elena J. 1996. "Textiles as Cultural Memory: Andean Garments in the Colonial Period." In Diane Fane (ed.), *Converging Cultures: Art and Identity in Spanish America,* 144–56. New York: Brooklyn Museum/Harry N. Abrams.

Randall, Kimberly. 2005. "The Traveler's Eye: Chinas Poblanas and European-Inspired Costume in Postcolonial Mexico." In Regina A. Root (ed.), *Latin American Fashion Reader,* 44–65. Oxford: Berg.

Rodríguez Lehmann, Cecilia (ed.). 2008. "Retóricas banales. Moda, política y nación. Estudios." Special issue, *Revista de Investigaciones Literarias y Culturales* 16 (32).

Rodríguez Lehmann, Cecilia. 2013. *Con trazos de seda. Escrituras banales en el siglo XIX.* Caracas, Venezuela: Fundavag Ediciones.

Root, Regina A. 2000. "Tailoring the Nation: Fashion Writing in Nineteenth-Century Argentina." *Fashion Theory: The Journal of Dress, Body and Culture* 4 (1): 89–117.

Root, Regina A. (ed.). 2005. *The Latin American Fashion Reader.* Oxford: Berg.

Root, Regina A. 2010. *Couture and Consensus: Fashion and Politics in Postcolonial Argentina.* Minneapolis: University of Minnesota Press.

Rowe, Ann Pollard (ed.). 2011. *Costume and History in Highland Ecuador.* Austin: University of Texas Press.

Sarmiento, Domingo Faustino. [1845] 2003. *Facundo: Civilization and Barbarism.* Trans. Kathleen Ross. Berkeley: University of California Press.

Saulquin, Susana. 1990. *La moda en Argentina.* Buenos Aires: Emecé.

Saulquin, Susana. 2010. *La muerte de la moda, el día después.* Buenos Aires: Editorial Paidós.

Scheinman, Pamela. 2005. "Ixcacles: Maguey-Fiber Sandals in Modern Mexico." In Regina A. Root (ed.), *Latin American Fashion Reader,* 79–92. Oxford: Berg.

Schevill, Margot Blum (ed.). 2010. *Berg Encyclopedia of World Dress and Fashion.* Vol. 2, *Latin America and the Caribbean.* Oxford: Berg.

Scobie, James R. 1974. *Buenos Aires: Plaza to Suburb, 1870–1910.* New York: Oxford University Press.

Sommer, Barbara A. 2007. "Wigs, Weapons, Tattoos and Shoes: Getting Dressed in Colonial Amazonia and Brazil." In Mina Roces and Louise Edwards (eds.), *The Politics of Dress in Asia and the Americas,* 200–14. Brighton, UK: Sussex Academic.

Stephenson, Marcia. 1999. *Gender and Modernity in Andean Bolivia.* Austin: University of Texas Press.

Tinajero, Araceli. 2005. "Far Eastern Influences in Latin American Fashions." In Regina A. Root (ed.), *Latin American Fashion Reader,* 66–75. Oxford: Berg.

Vidal, Emeric Essex. 1820. *Picturesque Illustrations of Buenos Ayres and Monte Video Consisting of Twenty-Four Views: Accompanied with Descriptions of the Scenery and of the Costumes, Manners, &c. of the Inhabitants of Those Cities and Their Environs.* London: R. Ackermann.

Villaça, Nizia. 2005. "As She Walks to the Sea: A Semiology of Rio de Janeiro." In Regina A. Root (ed.), *Latin American Fashion Reader,* 188–97. Oxford: Berg.

Villanueva, Margaret A. 1985. "From Calpixqui to Corregidor: Appropriation of Women's Cotton Textile Production in Early Colonial Mexico." *Latin American Perspectives* 12 (1): 17–40.

Walker, Tamara J. 2010. "'He Outfitted His Family in Notable Decency': Slavery, Honour and Dress in Eighteenth-Century Lima, Peru." *Slavery & Abolition* 30 (3): 383–402.

Zorn, Elayne. 2004. *Weaving a Future: Tourism, Cloth and Culture on an Andean Island.* Iowa City: University of Iowa Press.

19

Secondhand Clothing and Africa: Global Fashion Influences, Local Dress Agency, and Policy Issues

KAREN TRANBERG HANSEN

Secondhand dress is a rich research topic for fashion scholars. When the focus turns, as in this chapter, to dress practices involving imported secondhand clothing in the developing world, a research setting with unparalleled scope opens up. As an emerging global fashion phenomenon, secondhand clothing offers important insights into questions about individual and group identity, agency, and power. What is more, research on secondhand dress fashion allows scholars to examine the place of the secondhand clothing industry within the global marketplace as well as in specific regional contexts.

This chapter approaches the secondhand clothing phenomenon both as a production system comprising processes from collection through distribution to sale and as a consumption system involving purchase, use, dress practice, and performance. The chapter explores what happens to the West's discarded garments once they are appropriated into everyday life in Africa, specifically in Zambia, the country in which the author has conducted long-term anthropological research on the urban economic landscape and consumption (Hansen 2000). Following an introduction that identifies some theoretical and methodological challenges to the study of secondhand clothing as a central, rather than marginal, aspect of fashion research, the chapter turns to secondhand clothing both as an industry and as a dress practice. This discussion briefly delineates the growth in secondhand clothing exports from the West to Africa since the liberalization of markets in many countries during the early 1990s. Next follow some examples from different parts of Africa. The focus then shifts to Zambia, highlighting how nationalism, market regulation, and dress conventions have been influenced by and in turn help shape economic and cultural politics in the postcolonial era. Showcasing markets and dress practices, the chapter then explores the changing relation of imported secondhand clothing from the West and garments and apparel from China to domestic garment production and their policy implications. The chapter also identifies specific markets and niches that satisfy the needs and desires of different population segments for everyday wear and fashionable design by local tailors and style entrepreneurs. The conclusion highlights the creative place of secondhand clothing consumption as a dress option in a local clothing market with global reach.

SECONDHAND CLOTHING AS FASHION: FRAMING CHALLENGES

In much of the contemporary West, secondhand clothing makes up fringe, or niche, markets. Today income distribution, purchasing power, and affordable mass-produced garments and apparel have reduced the need for large segments of the population to purchase used clothing. Yet in recent years, secondhand clothing has attracted the attention of fashion-conscious consumers who are on the lookout for specific period dress, distinct garments to complement existing outfits, or clothing that make them stand out against the uniformity of brand-name apparel. The charitable organizations that dominated the secondhand clothing retail scene in the 1960s and 1970s were joined during the 1980s by a variety of for-profit secondhand clothing stores, rarely featuring words like *used, secondhand,* or *thrift* in their names, targeting consumers keen on retro, vintage, and designer fashions. In effect, thrift shopping has become a popular pastime to which the news media, and scholars of cultural studies and popular culture, have begun paying attention (McRobbie 1989). So have scholars from a variety of disciplines, who, taken together, we may characterize as fashion scholars (Palmer and Clark 2005).

From receiving passing attention, secondhand clothing now has acquired a "new look," inspired by recent developments in dress and fashion scholarship as well as by global changes in the organization of garment production. The chief moves behind this shift are readily identifiable. Today we tend to view culture processually as created through agency, practice, and performance rather than as a specific society, bounded by customs and traditions. The most important medium through which these processes have been examined is consumption, conceived not only as markets and economic actors but also as identity-constructing processes. Some scholars view dress as a set of competing discourses, linked to the operation of power, that construct the body and its presentation. While many works on clothing focus on consumption, some scholars have gone further to link production and consumption when examining the significance of dress. Above all, globalization in the era of hypercommunication is helping to break down conventional fashion boundaries. In the process, our notion of fashion has changed its focus from an upscale property of the West's rapidly shifting style innovations to everyday preoccupations with multidirectional style shifts across the globe. In short, the worldwide circulation of garments and apparel, including secondhand clothing, has altered the availability of clothing both on high streets in the West and in open-air markets in the developing world. This widened accessibility inspires individualism at the same time as it propels the diversification of tastes in many directions.

Imported secondhand clothing is a common commodity in clothing markets across Africa, where it finds widespread use in everyday life by consumers who seek to satisfy both their clothing needs and desires. But Western observers have long tended to view Africa's secondhand clothing markets as dumping grounds for charitable clothing donations and the dress practices they gave rise to as faded imitations of Western fashion.

Influenced by reigning theoretical paradigms, scholars on their part were slow to recognize the significance of the trade and consumption of these garments. For specialist scholarship on textiles and dress in Africa described and cataloged details of form and fabric or focused on aesthetic appreciation and symbolic analysis (Picton 1995; Picton and Mack 1979). Other works analyzed clothing as an ethnic marker, an aspect of status and class and of political affiliation (Perani and Wolff 1999). In recent years, along with the cultural turn in dress and fashion scholarship in general, these trends have given way to a much more expansive approach that sees fashion as volatile, hybrid, and boundary crossing, highlighting the constantly changing ways in which personal, regional, and transnational interdependencies are influencing dress practices in Africa (Allman 2004; Gott and Loughran 2010: 2, 5; Rovine 2009).

To be sure, the incorporation of secondhand clothing into local dress repertoires offers a special exposure on the interaction between the local and the West. The cultural and political struggles that are played out on the body surface point to a continuing tension in the meeting between local practices and ideas and Western forms. This tension contributes importantly to the vitality and dynamism of the "new" cultural forms whose combination of elements is always in process. For clothes are not worn passively but require people's active collaboration. Aside from fulfilling basic clothing needs, secondhand clothing consumption is also about liking, wanting, and desiring, in this way constituting practices through which identities are both constructed and contested.

Because much of their work on dress falls outside the West's conventional fashion canon, anthropologists have played an important role in demonstrating that fashion is not an exclusive property of the West. In their research, anthropologists pay attention to what people wear, and when and where they wear it; what meanings wearers and viewers attribute to dress; and how such meanings should be interpreted. In my research I used several methods to examine both the supply and demand sides of the secondhand clothing market and to explore how wearers and viewers attributed meanings to dress in Zambia. I spent days and weeks in markets, observing clothing transactions, and my assistant and I went door-to-door in different residential areas, interviewing people about their clothing consumption practices. I also traveled across the country, following the journeys of secondhand clothing from the importers' warehouses in the capital to upcountry locations. What is more, participant observation in tailors' workshops enabled me to study how tailors and customers reached decisions about design and style, to discuss how tailors created and developed style, and to ask customers about their decision to go to the tailor rather than formal shops or the secondhand clothing market. Some tailors display photo albums of their styles, pattern books, and European and South African fashion magazines, while others use simple drawings. Many customers bring garments or photos of a dress they want copied, or they describe what they want the tailor to sew. In effect, going to the tailor offered rich insights into one phase of the meaning making of clothing.

Widespread repair and material alteration of secondhand clothing in tailors' workshops remake anonymous clothes into one-of-a-kind garments to fit their new wearers. But the cultural ideas that help refashion secondhand clothing into local ensembles achieve the effect of "the latest" through ongoing interaction. This is evident in everyday life on the street and in social gatherings, in what people wear and how, and in their commentaries about ensembles and the scrutiny with which they examine fabric quality, design features, and styling details.

THE INTERNATIONAL SECONDHAND CLOTHING TRADE

Vintage style on the fashion runway is merely one twist, though a glamorous one, on a rapidly expanding global trade that on the one hand grosses exporters of secondhand clothing millions of dollars and on the other fulfills clothing needs and desires in many developing countries. In the West today, the secondhand clothing trade in both domestic and foreign markets is dominated by nonprofit charitable organizations and private textile recycling/grading firms, often family owned. Its financial side has largely eluded public scrutiny. Thriving on an ethic of giving, the major charitable organizations look like patrons in a worldwide clothing donation project. Growing environmental concerns in the West in recent years have enhanced both the profitability and respectability of this trade, giving its practitioners a new cachet as textile salvagers and waste recyclers (Figure 19.1).

The charitable organizations are the largest single source of the garments that fuel the international trade in secondhand clothing from routine sales of a large proportion of their donated clothing. Textile recyclers/graders purchase used clothing in bulk from the enormous yield gathered by the charitable organizations, and they also buy surplus clothing from resale stores. The textile recycling business is lucrative because every piece of used clothing has many potential future lives. Clothes are transformed, for instance, into filler in roofing felts, loudspeaker cones, car dashboards, and panel lining; some end up as flock for mattresses, car seating or insulation, or wiper rags for industrial use.

The bulk of the clothing that has been sourced in this way is destined for new lives in the secondhand clothing export market, which yields more profit than the rag and fiber trade. At their warehouses and sorting plants, the clothing recyclers sort clothing by garment types, fabric, and quality before compressing them into bales. The standard weight is fifty kilograms (about 110 pounds), yet some firms compress bales of much higher

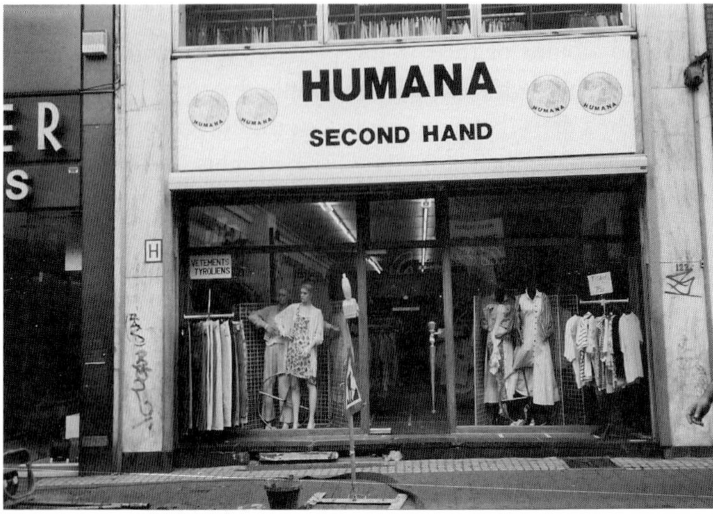

FIGURE 19.1 Secondhand resale store, Brussels, Belgium, 1997.
Credit: Photograph by Karen Tranberg Hansen.

weight, usually unsorted. The bottom quality goes to Africa, and medium quality to Latin America, while Japan receives a large portion of top-quality items, among which brand-name denim jeans and sneakers are in popular demand.

Although the secondhand clothing trade has a long history, its economic power and global scope were never as vast as they have been since the early 1990s in the wake of the liberalization of many Third World economies and the rise in demand from former Eastern Bloc countries. Worldwide the trade has grown more than tenfold since the early 1990s (United Nations 1996: 60, 2008: 121). The United States is the world's largest exporter in terms of volume and value, followed in 2006 by the United Kingdom, Germany, Belgium-Luxembourg, and the Netherlands (United Nations 2008: 121).

The countries of sub-Saharan Africa are the world's largest secondhand clothing destination, receiving close to 30 percent of total world exports in 2006. Several countries in Asia are also large net importers, among them Malaysia, Singapore, Pakistan, and Hong Kong, which all manufacture and export garments and apparel to the West. The export of secondhand clothing does not target developing countries exclusively. Sizable exports are shipped to Japan, Belgium-Luxembourg, and the Netherlands, which all import and reexport this commodity.

International secondhand clothing exports have grown in spurts, particularly during postwar periods when surplus army clothing flooded the market. The substantive increase in exports of secondhand clothing to Africa occurred after World War II. General economic growth, increased welfare in both Europe and the United States, and mass-produced affordable garments and apparel created a vast surplus of still wearable clothing. At the same time, rapid socioeconomic changes across much of the African continent made more and more people enter the clothing market as eager consumers.

AFRICAN CLOTHING MARKETS

At the turn of the millennium, there were three main types of garments in clothing markets in most African countries: imported secondhand, locally manufactured, and imported apparel from China. One source suggests that secondhand clothing makes up more than half of the clothing market by volume in many countries in sub-Saharan Africa (Baden and Barber 2005: 1). Many clothing industries declined in the wake of the economic liberalization policies of the 1980s and 1990s due to outmoded technology and declining local purchasing power. The same period saw a rapid growth in secondhand clothing imports. The popular media have sensationalized how this import has undermined domestic manufacture (Hansen 2004). Yet the interrelationship between the two is more complex. Secondhand clothing does not so much displace locally produced garments as it appeals to specific consumer segments. In fact, today in many countries secondhand clothing competes with Chinese apparel rather than with locally manufactured garments.

Secondhand clothing consumption practices in Africa are shaped by the policies that regulate the import and by distinct regional conventions and cultural norms concerning bodies and dress. Some African countries have at one time or another prohibited the import of secondhand clothing, for instance, Nigeria, Côte d'Ivoire, Kenya, and Malawi. Some countries have restrictive policies; for example, South Africa allows import of secondhand clothing only for charitable purposes and not for resale. And although secondhand clothing imports are banned in some countries, there is a brisk transborder trade in this commodity.

There is considerable regional variation in Africa's clothing markets. In Muslim-dominated North Africa, for example, secondhand clothing constitutes a much smaller portion of total garment imports than in sub-Saharan Africa. Dress conventions differ not only in terms of religious norms, for instance, whether people are Muslim or Christian, but also by gender, age, class, and region/ethnicity. Taken together, these factors inform the cultural norms of dress practice, influencing what types of garments which people will wear and when.

Briefly, in several countries in West Africa, distinct regional dress styles that are the products of long-standing textile crafts in weaving, dyeing, and printing today coexist with dress styles introduced during the colonial period and after. In Nigeria and Senegal, secondhand clothing has entered a specific niche. Although people from different socioeconomic groups, and not only the very poor, now purchase imported secondhand clothing and use it widely for everyday wear, Senegalese and Nigerians commonly follow long-standing regional style conventions, dressing with pride for purposes of displaying locally produced cloth in "African" styles. This is much in contrast to Zambia, where such textile crafts hardly existed in the precolonial period and where today people from across the socioeconomic spectrum except the top are dressing in the West's used clothing. In effect, people in Zambia have been wearing Western-styled clothing for so long that they have made it their own.

Last but not least, there are also invented dress traditions. In Zaire during the presidency of Mobuto Sese Seko, an authenticity code from the early 1970s prevented men from wearing Western coats and ties and women from wearing jeans. Instead, the *abacost* (*a bas la costume,* meaning "down [or out] with the suit"), a thigh-length jacket, was introduced. Since Mobuto's fall in 1997, the Western-style suit has returned, and men wear it now, as elsewhere, as one of several dress options. In South Africa after political independence from white minority rule in 1994, some of the new men in power began experimenting with fashion. President Nelson Mandela's Indonesian-inspired brightly patterned shirts worn without a tie and jacket were quickly appropriated into local fashion wear as "Mandela shirts" and became popular in the neighboring countries, too. Everywhere across Africa and in the diaspora today, the creative garments made by style entrepreneurs and designers are becoming more visible, drawing on a mix of references, style elements, fabrics, and accessories (Klopper 2000). Providing changing stylistic components that are incorporated into new tailor-made designs, imported secondhand clothing plays an active role in this process (Grabski 2010: 34).

THE SECONDHAND CLOTHING MARKET IN ZAMBIA

Zambia's secondhand clothing trade dates back to the colonial period, when imported used clothing reached Northern Rhodesia, as Zambia was called then, from across the border with the Belgian Congo, now the Democratic Republic of Congo (formerly Zaire). Direct importation of this commodity was prohibited in Zambia during the first decades after independence in 1964. When restrictive import and foreign exchange regulations were relaxed in the mid- to late 1980s, the secondhand clothing trade grew rapidly.

Across southern Africa today, people from Zambia are known as good dressers. Zambian women are noted for dressing more smartly and fashionably than women elsewhere in the region, and Zambian elite men for loving suits from Savile Row. Small-scale tailors in Lusaka produce highly styled outfits from *chitenge* fabric (colorful prints) for resale by suitcase traders in South Africa, where such outfits are called "Zambia." Women's chitenge outfits and men's suits are part of a dress universe that has diversified dramatically since the opening up of the economy when compared to the restricted clothing access during both the colonial period and the one-party state (1972–1991). When import restrictions were relaxed in the late 1980s, secondhand clothing from the United States and Europe quickly became a popular trade and consumption item. After a period of rapid growth during the first half of the 1990s, the import and local trade in secondhand clothes appears to have become an established part of the clothing market and in the 2000s rarely caused any public debate. In fact, with the growth of imported new garments from China in recent years, secondhand clothing's share of total clothing imports has actually declined.

Since the mid-1980s, imported secondhand clothing has been referred to as *salaula,* which in the Bemba language means approximately "selecting from a pile by rummaging" or, for short, "to pick." The term describes vividly the process that takes place once a bale of imported secondhand clothing has been opened in the market and consumers select garments to satisfy both their clothing needs and desires. The shopwindow of Zambia's secondhand clothing trade, the big public markets create an atmosphere much like shopping malls in the West, where consumers pursue almost unlimited desires with an abandon not possible in the formal stores, where Zambian consumers are often dealt with offhandedly or are pressured to purchase.

Consumers in Zambia go to secondhand clothing markets for many reasons. White-collar workers of both sexes in Lusaka's city center often spend their lunch hour going through the secondhand clothing stalls, sometimes making purchases at whim. Others go to find just that right item to match a particular garment. Some women who tailor in their homes search the markets for interesting buttons, belts, and trim to accent garments. And some go to purchase garments with the intention to resell. But the vast majority shop from salaula for clothing for themselves and their families.

On first sight, the salaula markets meet the nonlocal observer's eye as a chaotic mass of secondhand clothing hung up on flimsy wood contraptions, displayed on tables, or dumped in piles on the ground. That view is deceptive. A variety of informal rules organize vending spaces and structure sales practices. Both vendors and customers know these practices. A prospective customer looking for a specific garment will go to a particular part of the market. The vendors of men's suits, for example, one of the most expensive items, tend to be located in a part of the outdoor market that is near to major thoroughfares such as a main road passable by automobiles. So are vendors of other high-demand garments, such as women's skirts and blouses, and the best-selling item of all, at least in Zambia, baby clothes. There are spatial clusters of vendors selling shoes and, during the winter in the southern hemisphere, cold-weather clothing.

The display on most secondhand clothing stands is carefully designed. High-quality items are hung on clothes hangers on makeshift walls. A clothing line or a wood stand may display a row of cotton dresses. Everything that meets the eye has been carefully selected with a view to both presentation and sales strategy. Lively discussions and price negotiations accompany sales. The piles on the ground include damaged items and garments that have been around for a while.

Near the high end of the secondhand clothing display, and near the major roads of the market, cluster the "boutiques." Boutiques in these markets sell preselected items, coordinated to form matched outfits that are stylish. They tend to be operated by young vendors who "pick," in the language of the market. Once traders open secondhand clothing bales, the pickers descend on them, selecting garments on the spot. Then they make up, for instance, women's two-piece ensembles, men's suits, and leisure wear.

Secondhand clothing does not serve only poorer consumers. Yet only the very tiny high-income group in Zambia has an effective choice in the clothing market. This group, called *apamwamba,* a term in the Nyanja language that means approximately "those on the top," purchases clothing everywhere, including from upscale stores and boutiques in Lusaka's new shopping malls as well as from secondhand clothing markets. And people from these better-off households spend more money on tailor-made clothing than do members of poor households.

EXPERIMENTS WITH FASHION, STYLE, AND LOOKS

Clothing consumption is hard work. A vital dimension of the demand side involves cultural taste and style issues that come together in the creation of a "total look." Concerns with fabric quality, texture, and construction precede that creation, which in turn revolves around the anticipated dress needs of the specific situation. The chief attraction of garments from "outside" is style and variety, not price, which is why everyone, regardless of class, shops from salaula. Salaula fashions bring consumers into a bigger world: the world of awareness, of now. It is the search for the look, rather than brand names, that guides how people shop, although of course neither style issues nor clothing markets are ever static but develop in complex ways, one of which might be a preoccupation with brand names in the secondhand clothing markets in the future.

When shopping from secondhand clothing markets, consumers' preoccupation with creating particular appearances is inspired by trends from across the world. Consumers draw on these influences in ways that are informed by local norms about bodies and dress. The desired clothing silhouette for both adult women and men is neat and tidy. It is a product of immaculate garment care and of wearing clothes in ways that are not considered to be too revealing. Even then, women's and men's garments are understood differently. The cultural norms about how to dress weigh on women more heavily than on men. In effect, women feel restrained in their freedom to dress, so as not to provoke men. Women should not expose their shoulders. Above all, they must cover their "private parts," which in this region of Africa includes their thighs. This means that dress length, tightness, and fabric transparency become issues when women interact with men and elders both at home and in public.

The desire for uniqueness, to stand out, while dressing the body on Zambian terms entails considerable skill in the selection of items from the abundance of salaula, making discriminating decisions concerning quality, style, and value for money; in garment coordination to fit specific occasions and contexts; and in the overall presentation and comportment of the dressed body to produce a total look. Many consumers are extraordinarily savvy when purchasing clothing aimed to produce particular effects. In order to highlight that shopping from salaula does not mean that anything goes, I have called the skill that is critical to the successful work of consumption *clothing competence.* The underlying sensibility is a visual aesthetics that on first sight cultivates endless variation of dress yet on closer analysis also is in the service of continuity.

YOUNG MEN'S DRESS DILEMMAS

Unlike young women, who carefully monitor the way they dress in public, young men like to draw attention to themselves, in different ways to be sure, depending on their socioeconomic circumstances and regional location in Zambia's developing economy. They actively seek to present a smart appearance that is both fashionable and neat. Young men's self-conscious preoccupations with suits and jeans illustrate different constructions of these attributes of dress.

Suits are worn widely across the civil service ranks and for other white-collar jobs in Zambia. Formal suits index young urban men's desire to become adults, hold jobs, and become heads of households. Suits are associated with the patriarchal social power that is widespread throughout Zambia. Cutting a fine figure in a smart suit conveys something important about personal background, respectability, and responsibility. Most of the young men in their late teens or early twenties in a secondary school in Lusaka who in 1995 told me where they bought their clothes and how they liked to dress aspired to this dress practice and the ideal it conveys. "Suits are the clothes I like most," explained Simon, "because they make me look decent and soon I will be joining the society of workers." Morgan, his classmate, described a pair of trousers and a jacket he recently had received: "I was full of joy. . . . I like these clothes because a lot of people say that I look like a general manager and not only that, they also say that I look like a rich man." And Moses's delight in a double-breasted jacket his father had given him is evident: "I like jackets because they suit me like a second skin."

Other classmates liked jeans, particularly because they are durable but also because "they are in style now." But wearing jeans had a flip side that too readily called forth the image of scruffy youths and street vendors, who in the popular view are associated with illegal activities. According to Moses, "I hate wearing jeans because people may fail to distinguish between cigarette sellers and myself."

If suits and jeans frame young urban men's desires for a better life, young men in rural areas have similar desires but are more circumscribed by the conditions in which they live. Secondary school students in Mansa, a provincial town in Luapula Province, explained this clearly. Joshua explained, "Of all the clothes, I like strong ones which can serve me longer such as jeans. I like them because it is not easy for me to buy soap, and most of the time I do manual work in order to earn my living." The suit figures in the desires of these young rural men mostly by its absence. Describing why the suit combination did not fit his situation, Nicholas explained, "Such clothes can easily be torn and I think they are for office working people, so they don't suit me." Yet he added as an afterthought, "If I had a choice, I would really like to wear suits."

Jeans are a must in the evolving street vendor style. Lusaka's downtown streets are full of young male traders in all kinds of goods, many of whom put much effort into being seen and dress in a striking manner. In addition to the style explanations I describe below, the preference of street vendors for denim has a very practical reason. Jeans, one of them explained, "are durable; they are nice and easy to keep especially for bachelors like me who have no one to look after our clothes." What the young vendors my assistant interviewed in 1997 did for their own pleasure was to dress up in public in variations on the baggy-jeans look. The layered look was in vogue that year, as were knitted caps referred to as head socks and shoes with thick rubber soles, often worn without stockings.

The secondary school students and the young street vendors purchased their clothes from a variety of sources. Some bought imported clothing from suitcase traders who bring in garments from abroad, some went to the tailor for specific wear, and all of them scoured the salaula market for just the right items. As one of the street vendors explained, "In salaula you will find things you can't believe how good they are." When shopping for clothes, the young vendors look for garments that will contribute to the overall creation of a particular style, which in the late 1990s was "the big look," rather than for brand-name items. "I wear the big look because it is fashion," one of them said, while another explained how he liked to "move with time." I don't like "common clothes and imitations," said yet another.

Making associations between specific articles of clothing and behavior, young people construct an understanding of their world and how they inhabit it. Young male secondary students with high economic aspirations for themselves do not want to be mistaken for the school dropouts turned street vendors. They desire suits. The vendors for their part wear clothes they equate with the power and success achieved by popular performers both in Africa and beyond. Putting themselves together with clothing the major part of which is from salaula, both groups of young people are dressing to explore who they are and who they would like to become.

CULTURAL NORMS AND WOMEN'S DRESS OPTIONS

If suits are the garments to wear for young men who wish to be upwardly mobile, decent dress that does not reveal too much is the clothing style for young women, including young women of better means who have real options in the clothing market because of their economic background.

Interacting with young people of both sexes of mid- to upper-income backgrounds in 2002 and 2003, an assistant and I sought to learn where they hung out in their free time, with whom, and how they dressed on such occasions. Here I focus on the women we interviewed. Such women constitute a very small segment of Lusaka's huge youth population. Pursuing further education at a variety of colleges, training institutions, and universities, including some in Australia and the United States, most of these young women have the means, usually because of well-placed parents, to hang out with friends at Lusaka's new shopping malls, other shopping venues, popular pool halls, bars, and parks. There is a nightclub scene on which some of them also move. In their daytime interaction, aside from exchanging news about friends and talking about relationships, sex, the entertainment scene, and their futures, these young women spend considerable time discussing "looks," sharing information about the availability of particularly desired garments and about who has been seen wearing what and where. Most of them love clothes. The friends they move about with value their interest in dress in positive terms, and they all spend considerable time and effort discussing the latest fashion. "It is the combination of clothing," said a 22-year-old psychology student, "that demonstrates your sense of style."

"Clothes," said a 24-year-old marketing student, "place me in my class." Like many others, she did not like baggy jeans, "no boring loose slacks," as one expressed it, "because they are tomboyish, and gangsta," a comparison we also heard some young men make. During the daytime interactions when we interviewed the young women, they dressed decently but casually, meaning—controlling for body size—in tight jeans or knee-length jeans skirts resting on the hips with waistlines accentuated by cropped short tops. Young women who were heavyset wore long, fitted skirts with slits. A 22-year-old university student explained that her outfit, combining jeans, a matching top, and smart shoes, "make[s] me look mature and outline[s] my model body." Altogether, by Zambian norms, there was nothing too revealing in the way these young women dressed their bodies when moving about in public space. Their hair was either richly braided or cut short, the most popular women's hairstyles at the time. They accessorized their "total look" with cell phones, handbags, shoes, and jewelry.

These young women sourced most of their clothing from stores and boutiques, including from abroad. They also, as I indicated earlier, shop from salaula, but as a pastime, not a need. Some had never been to a tailor. They were not keen to wear chitenge dresses, and they did not all own one. Young women's attitude to wearing chitenge outfits revolves around body size and age. Looking best on "traditionally built women," these elaborately styled dresses evoke a level of maturity that some young women consider to be old, and they associate chitenge with their mothers' and grandmothers' attire. With such an outlook, it is no wonder that "casual" is the thing to wear.

"Everything I wear," said a 21-year-old woman, "should make people look and say 'wow, she is nice.'" In their concern to create their own fashion statements and demonstrate an individual sense of style, these young women make sure that they show off their apamwamba status. The reasons may have to do with Zambia's status as one of the world's least developed countries. In their self-styling through dress, apamwamba women seek to avoid "sliding down" in local socioeconomic terms. While they wear global fashions, the strategic presentation of their dressed bodies becomes meaningful on Zambian terms, that is, in the local context of economic decline, urban poverty, and other processes set in motion by Zambia's unequal place in the global economy.

CLOTHING MARKETS, NICHES, AND DRESS CHOICES

When I began exploring Zambia's clothing scene in the early 1990s, some observers feared that imported secondhand clothing might adversely affect the domestic textile and garment industry and even "kill" the small-scale tailoring craft. In fact, this has not happened. Rather, many tailors changed their physical location, moving, for example, from townships to city markets, and they reoriented their production. One tailor I knew from a periurban township had set himself up at Lusaka's oldest market, Kamwala, after closing shop in the local market. When I spoke to him in 1995, he told me, "I sat down for two hours to think of how to beat salaula." His solution, like that of many other tailors who continued working, was specialty production, in his case church uniforms, a regular part of many women's wardrobes in Zambia.

Many tailors in Lusaka's city center had followed a similar strategy, targeting niche production of garments and sizes rarely available in salaula (Figure 19.2). Such garments included women's slips, girls' frilly dresses, and a changing range of "office wear," meaning women's two-piece suits with varying details and trim. But perhaps above all, as one tailor noted, "There is no chitenge in salaula." Indeed, the production of chitenge wear has grown in recent years. Chitenge outfits have moved from serving largely as attire for special occasions to work dress for teachers and as free/casual wear on Fridays for office workers and bank clerks. Some of these tailors produced job lots, for example, of men's trousers, for formal boutiques as well as for up-country clients for resale in the villages, while others made chitenge dresses for suitcase traders to resell in Zimbabwe and South Africa. And recent years have witnessed the emergence of style entrepreneurs launching

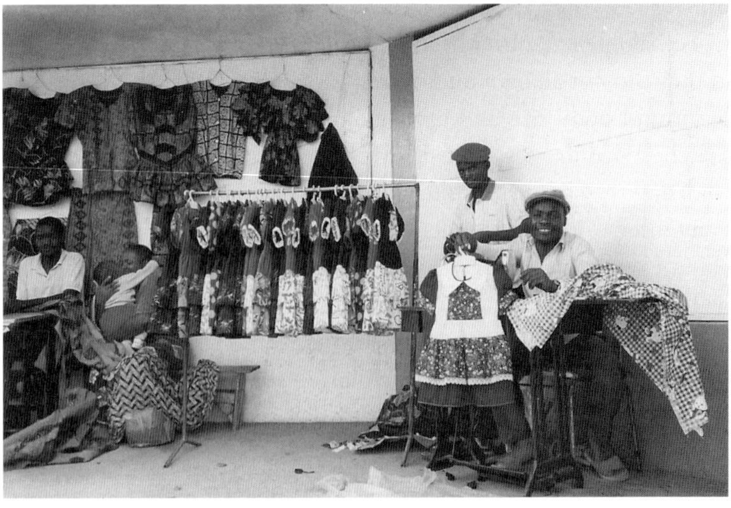

FIGURE 19.2 Niche production of girls' dresses in Lusaka, Zambia, 1995.
Credit: Photograph by Karen Tranberg Hansen.

themselves as local clothing designers, who are beginning to make a mark with "African designs" in chitenge fabrics that may add new value to the local fashion scene.

Since the turn of the millennium, the import of clothing and apparel from China has increased in Zambia. In many urban markets, traders from China rent a large number of stalls where Zambian workers sell clothing, shoes, and all kinds of accessories. In the nearby streets, formal stores sell a diversity of Chinese goods, especially clothing, apparel, and chitenge fabrics that appeal to consumers with limited means. Yet many consumers view Chinese clothes as cheap, and they complain about the quality. They compare them to salaula, which they consider to be far superior. "One day," a young female Zambian friend told me in 2005, "I wore a pair of new Chinese shoes to lunch. By the time I returned to the office, one of the heels had broken off." The Zambia Bureau of Standards does not apply any agreed-upon standard to regulate apparel imports from China (Springford 2010). Because they know consumers' concern with quality, suitcase traders from Zambia in fact travel to South Africa to purchase better-quality Chinese apparel for resale in Zambia.

Consumers not only consider Chinese clothing of poor quality but also view it as common (Springford 2010). In this view, Chinese clothes compare adversely to salaula. For salaula allows consumers to select specific garments they consider unique. Dressing in salaula enables a person to stand out, to present a special look that engages viewers' attention and is a cherished part of the experience of feeling good in clothes.

THE DEVELOPMENT OF A FORMAL FASHION SCENE

When women of means in Zambia today say, "I have a tailor," they have several things in mind. First, they may be clients of a particular male tailor, perhaps from the Democratic Republic of Congo, who supervises a workshop of male and female workers. Second, they may be clients of a particular female tailor, perhaps from the Democratic Republic of Congo, Nigeria, or Ghana, who runs a workshop with several workers of both sexes. Third, they may be clients of a woman entrepreneur who calls herself a designer, has her own clothing label, and either supervises a workshop of male and female tailors or subcontracts her designs to tailors whom she knows well. And, fourth, in fact the woman who says that she has a tailor is likely to draw on some or all of these sources at different times, depending on the occasion.

The design scene is the most recent twist on the ever-changing development of the organization of the tailor's craft in Zambia. In the mid-1990s, downtown Lusaka had several successful production units with boutique-style outlets, operated by well-educated women, often married to wealthy men. Such women were able to travel abroad, where some had taken design and fashion courses. They concentrated on producing "high quality fashion garments for high-income clients who prefer imported clothing from London, Paris, and New York" to what they perceive as cheap local wear (Kasengele 1998: 96–98). When I began to study the emerging fashion and design scene in 2007, these preferences had been challenged. Seasonally changing and creatively styled chitenge wear now takes center stage alongside other dress inspirations in fashionable women's wardrobes. Chitenge styles are displayed proudly by women who have the body to wear them. And young women who used to argue that chitenge outfits made them look "old" (Hansen 2000: 204) are getting attracted to the creatively styled chitenge fashions, made by a cohort of new designers who are deliberately modernizing the chitenge for young people to wear. "Chitenge," said Angela Mulenga in 2009 when I interviewed this 21-year-old designer with an educational background in business administration, "will stand the test of time." Angela's production of the Queen's Wear design label takes place in a tiny workshop in one of downtown Lusaka's old shopping venues, the Central Arcade, with four industrial sewing machines and one embroidery machine. Queen's Wear was started by Angela's mother, for whom the oldest of the four male tailors began working several years ago (Figure 19.3).

Between 1997 and 2009, more than five upscale shopping malls opened in Lusaka, and some are still under construction. New consumption spaces, clothing stores, and

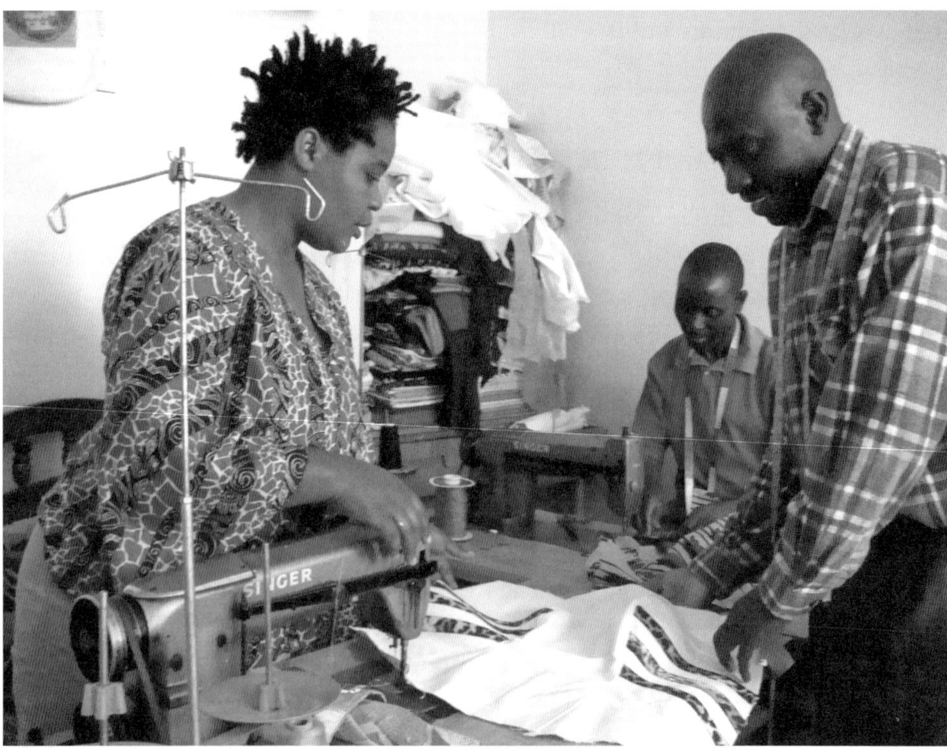

FIGURE 19.3 Designer in her atelier, instructing tailors, Lusaka, Zambia, 2009.
Credit: Photograph by Karen Tranberg Hansen.

boutiques appeal to urban residents with money to spend. Against this backdrop, two processes have helped fuel the growth of a more vibrant fashion design scene. For one, the production potential of these new designers has been greatly facilitated by the improved availability in recent years of imported sewing machines, dress fabric, and sewing notions. Second, and above all, their exposure to a global world of fashion and styles has expanded, and along with it so has the scope for local dress entrepreneurship. There now is a formal fashion circuit, complete with organizers, promoters, models, photographers, and a fashion magazine that was published from 2004 to 2010, *Beauty Zambia.* There are dress entrepreneurs who view themselves as designers and label their clothing lines, among them, Ubuntu Designs, Seyeni, Aglam Couture, Fay Design, and Dodo Wear Designs. The first organized Zambia Fashion Week unfolded in Lusaka in October 2005 and took place subsequently every year through 2009. Over these same years, other fashion shows and competitions have appeared. Some of the designers have joined in a group they call Ministry of Fashion to promote their lines.

Most of these self-proclaimed designers are women, although they include a few men. Among them are people of diverse national and cultural background; that is, not all of them are black Zambians. What they all share is a keen sense of style acquired from diverse experiences and exposures that do not always include formal training. Most of these designers do not sew themselves but hire tailors, mostly men, to carry out the basic tasks. A few put out their work for completion by tailors. Many operate from their own or their parents' homes or rented premises. They use several sewing machines, mostly their own but at times also rented, including, in addition to chain-stitch sewing machines, lockstitch machines and machines for embroidery and knitting. Some had several industrial sewing machines as well as old-fashioned treadle and hand-operated machines.

Who are the chief clients? My Choice, an upscale boutique in Lusaka's Manda Hill's shopping center, sells some garments produced by the new designers. This new crop of style entrepreneurs designs clothes, for example, for beauty pageant and Face of Africa contestants. In 2009 a group of them designed part of the wardrobe for the Zambian participant in the Miss Universe contest in Brazil. Designs produced for such events have ripple effects in the form of referrals. Women of means call on these designers to get special dresses made, particularly for kitchen parties (bridal showers) and weddings. Many designers have a special clientele that includes women in high-level jobs and public positions who are well known throughout Zambian society, some of whom are regarded as trendsetters when it comes to fashion. But more than anything else, it is the production of bridal wear and dresses for bridesmaids that ensures a flow of income for many of the new designers. And some would not be able to keep operating if they did not have the support of husbands in well-paid positions. Some of them pursue additional income-generating avenues to keep their creative design going, for example, producing uniforms for restaurants and sports teams and designing graphics for special-occasion stationery and invitation cards.

CONCLUSION

The interrelationship between imported secondhand clothing, imported apparel from China, and locally produced garments, including tailor- and designer-made outfits, is never stable but shifts over time, influenced by market regulations and the changing cultural politics of the day. As this chapter has demonstrated, the three parts of the clothing market serve distinct niches rather than competing with one another. What they share is fashion, that is, an aspect of dress practice that plays out on the body surface and gives both wearers and viewers a sense of good looks. What looks good in Zambia is a creative result of normative cultural dress conventions and local preoccupations with "the latest" that weigh on women's and men's bodies differently. Depending on their location in class and regional terms and on gender and age, people in Zambia attribute meanings about freedom from wants and normative constraints to secondhand clothing consumption, and in so doing they comment on their own position in a global world. In the process of selecting garments from a variety of sources, consumers are active in putting together an attractive and unique look reflecting an approach I saw expressed in a caption to a news story about fashion: "where others imitate, we originate" (*Post* 2005). In short, given their diverse clothing options, consumers in Zambia are arbiters of stylistic innovations that are contributing to the breakdown of fashion's Western hegemony.

BIBLIOGRAPHY

Allman, Jean (ed.). 2004. *Fashioning Africa: Power and the Politics of Dress.* Bloomington: Indiana University Press.

Baden, Sally, and Catherine Barber. 2005. *The Impact of the Second-Hand Clothing Trade on Developing Countries.* Oxford: Oxfam.

Gott, Suzanne, and Kristyne Loughran (eds.). 2010. *Contemporary African Fashion.* Bloomington: Indiana University Press.

Grabski, Jonna. 2010. "The Visual City: Tailors, Creativity, and Urban Life in Dakar, Senegal." In Suzanne Gott and Kristyne Loughran (eds.), *Contemporary African Fashion,* 29–37. Bloomington: Indiana University Press.

Hansen, Karen Tranberg. 2000. *Salaula: The World of Secondhand Clothing and Zambia.* Chicago: University of Chicago Press.

Hansen, Karen Tranberg. 2004. "Helping or Hindering? Controversies around the International Second-Hand Clothing Trade." *Anthropology Today* 20 (4): 3–9.

Kasengele, Mwango. 1998. "'Differentiation among Small-Scale Enterprises: The Zambian Clothing Industry in Lusaka." In Anita Spring and Barbara E. McDade (eds.), *African Entrepreneurship: Theory and Reality,* 93–106. Gainesville: University Press of Florida.

Klopper, Sandra. 2000. "Re-dressing the Past: The Africanisation of Sartorial Style in Contemporary South Africa." In Avtar Brah and Annie E. Coombes (eds.), *Hybridity and Its Discontents: Politics, Science, Culture,* 216–31. London: Routledge.

McRobbie, Angela. 1989. "Second-Hand Dress and the Role of the Ragmarket." In Angela McRobbie (ed.), *Zoot Suits and Second-Hand Dresses: An Anthology of Fashion and Music,* 23–49. Boston: Unwin Hyman.

Palmer, Alexandra, and Hazel Clark (eds.). 2005. *Old Clothes, New Looks: Second Hand Fashion.* Oxford: Berg.

Perani, Judith, and Norma H. Wolff. 1999. *Cloth, Dress, and Art Patronage in Africa.* Oxford: Berg.

Picton, John. 1995. *The Art of African Textiles: Technology, Tradition, and Lurex.* With Rayda Becker, Pauline Duponchel, Jackie Guille, Elizabeth Harney, David Heathcote, Julia Hilger, Atta Kwami, Pat Oyelola, and Simon Peers. London: Barbican Art Gallery; Lund Humphries.

Picton, John, and John Mack (eds.). 1979. *African Textiles.* London: British Museum.

The Post. 2005. "Trendsetters." December 2.

Rovine, Victoria L. 2009. "Viewing Africa through Fashion." *Fashion Theory: The Journal of Dress, Body, and Culture* 13 (2): 133–40.

Springford, James B. 2010. "Generating Values: Chinese Clothes in Lusaka." Master's thesis, Graduate School of Social Sciences, University of Amsterdam.

United Nations. 1996. *1995 International Trade Statistics Yearbook.* Vol. 2, *Trade by Commodity.* New York: United Nations.

United Nations. 2008. *2006 International Trade Statistics Yearbook.* Vol. 2, *Trade by Commodity.* New York: United Nations.

SECTION VI

Science, Technology, and New Fashion

Introduction

SANDY BLACK

Fashion has an affinity for the extreme, embracing novelty and the need to shock, surprise, and break boundaries, traditionally through the development of new silhouettes, designs, materials, fabrication processes, and contexts. Avant-garde concepts—either presented on the seasonal fashion catwalks or, increasingly, created in design collaborations and research groups—inspire others and gradually become normalized, to be continually replaced by new ideas, in the familiar cycles of the fashion system. In the twenty-first century, as digital technologies evolve and mature, the potential has been created for unprecedented convergence of disciplines to create intelligent and responsive textiles and fashion. Fashion is harnessing emerging science and technology to enhance both the functional and emotional experience of clothing, creating new scenarios that were previously only imagined. Integrating technologies such as digital and mobile communications within the fabrication and structure of fashion inevitably alters one's experience of and behavior toward clothing. The relationship of the individual to his or her clothing, in both public and personal spheres, will radically shift.

Both mobile and pervasive computing have already changed the technological landscape, providing the potential for seamless integration of computing power and functionality into objects (the "Internet of things") and environments. This is a world, at one time only the realm of science fiction, in which everything is connected and potentially responsive and in which context-relevant data can be continually retrieved. The spread of the QR (quick-response) code in advertising is testament to this development, allowing owners of smartphones to quickly connect to product information. Decades of research in scientific laboratories, especially for military and medical contexts, are emerging into the public and commercial spheres. New interdisciplinary research seeks to link information technology with micro-, nano-, and biotechnologies and even cognitive processes (Black 2007).

It is the proximity of textiles to the body through clothing, and their universal use, that gives the prospect of multifunctional and responsive textiles their powerful attraction for business. Pioneering research and development has been carried out by several companies including France Telecom and the Netherlands-based electronics giant Philips. Philips catalyzed new thinking by engaging textile and fashion designers with industrial designers and engineers in the 1990s, setting up a design lab within their UK research base with a specific remit to create clothing prototypes with embedded electronic functionality. Their many experimental ideas culminated in the launch of the ICD+ Levi's denim jacket, as documented in their influential publication *New Nomads* (Philips Electronics 2000). This early clothing with embedded electronic functionality (although not ultimately commercially viable) set a new benchmark, created the aspiration, and stimulated demand for such technologically enabled clothing and fashion, a goal that is becoming nearer with each new technical advance.

This section of the *Handbook* highlights several applications of scientific research and technological developments in materials, systems, and processes to fashion and identifies the shifts that have taken place over recent decades to create functionalized "smart" fashions. The impacts, opportunities, benefits, and risks associated with this growing phenomenon are discussed, and the potential for sustainability benefits is assessed. The four chapters examine the intersections between fashion, textiles, design, technology, and science through multidisciplinary, design-led research in smart and advanced materials and processes; the development and impact of wearable technologies; innovation through collaborations in science and fashion; and the contribution to future fashion made by scenarios envisaged in film and literature.

Since the end of the twentieth century, a new receptiveness to materials technology has led to increased interest from fashion designers in so-called technical fabrics, that is, those with specific functionalities, designed for specific purposes such as ballistic protection or abrasion resistance. A growing number of handbooks have emerged that gather together examples of innovations in the field. For example, Sarah Braddock Clarke and Marie O'Mahony produced the textile reference works *Techno Textiles, Sports-Tech,* and *Techno Textiles 2* (Braddock and O'Mahony 1998, 2002; Braddock Clarke and O'Mahony 2005), and O'Mahony authored *Advanced Textiles for Health and Wellbeing* (2011), in which the focus is the technology and technologists who are developing radical textiles linked to design outcomes that embrace the possibilities opened up. Similarly, fashion curator Andrew Bolton and writer Bradley Quinn have documented the interface of technical textiles and technology with avant-garde fashion designers and experimental artists in *The Supermodern Wardrobe* (Bolton 2002), *Techno Fashion* (Quinn 2002), and *The Fashion of Architecture* (Quinn 2003). Subsequent publications by fashion practitioners, such as Suzanne Lee's *Fashioning the Future* (2005), Sabine Seymour's *Fashionable Technology* (2008) and *Functional Aesthetics* (2010), and Sarah Braddock

Clarke and Jane Harris's *Digital Visions for Fashion and Textiles* (2012), have continued to chart the growth in the integration of digital technologies, electronics, and other scientific disciplines such as biotechnology and nanotechnology into fashion through a wide range of projects.

Perceptions of textiles have continued to evolve as the importance of both craft knowledge and advanced technology working in tandem is increasingly recognized. A major exhibition, Extreme Textiles, mounted in 2005 by the Cooper-Hewitt Museum at the Smithsonian Institute, helped to reposition textile technology, and its myriad applications, from the nineteenth-century mills to the forefront of twenty-first-century research and development (see McQuaid 2005). The exhibition's focus on designing for performance—stronger, faster, lighter, safer, smarter—proved inspirational to many. One such was Bradley Quinn, who describes this exhibition as igniting a "burning all-consuming interest" for the subject of textiles and its emerging applications (2010: 1). Quinn has continued to produce comprehensive surveys of emerging developments, including editing *Ultra Materials* (Beylerian and Dent 2007) and authoring *Textile Futures* (2010), *Design Futures* (2011) and *Fashion Futures* (2012).

In his chapter for this section, Quinn comments on the convergence of new fibers, fabric, and fashion with technology, creating a new "body technology": "technologized garments are changing how the body interacts with its surroundings and how designers and architects are fashioning the environments we live in." Quinn reminds us that textiles would not exist in the modern world without technology. He focuses on key examples of design practice over the last decade that merge electronics with designer fashion, where the emphasis is equally on the aesthetic experience and the functionality. For example, in the traditionally male-oriented world of wearable technology, New York–based fashion researcher Angel Chang created several collections of feminine technology-enabled clothing, in stark contrast to the typical outdoor male sportswear normally associated with the field. In the early twenty-first century, the entertainment world provides a global platform for the expression of extreme identities and extravagant staging. Here, the integration of LED lighting technology into clothing has become the new fashion currency for music artists and celebrities, moving beyond the spectacular theater of the radical fashion catwalks that evolved in the 1980s and 1990s (for example, from designers such as Issey Miyake, Alexander McQueen, Hussein Chalayan, Martin Margiela, Viktor & Rolf, and Rei Kawakubo). The London-based duo CuteCircuit, whose design-led practice merges fashion with interaction design[1] and custom-built electronic modules, are pioneering practitioners in illuminated fashions, as Quinn discusses. Their mission to "make technology beautiful, fun, and comfortable to wear" is found in projects such as the well-known Hug Shirt and designs commissioned for international celebrities and performers. Quinn concludes with the rather more sinister implications for surveillance that might follow from the embedded technology that surrounds us.

Following this overview of textiles, fashion, and technology, researcher Joanna Berzowska, director of XS Labs at Concordia University, Montreal, discusses in detail the development of her own experimental practice in wearable technology over more than a decade of interdisciplinary research projects that probe not just the enhanced functionality of electronic textiles and clothing but the sociocultural implications of on-body technology. Berzowska is a graduate of the Massachusetts Institute of Technology's Media Lab in Boston, an original cofounder with Maggie Orth of International Fashion Machines, and a pioneer of practice research in embedded electronics. The key to XS (Extra Soft) Lab research has been the development of "soft computation," using conductive threads and materials to integrate electronics into fashion clothing. Berzowska believes that the unique nature of wearable technology is that "it can be customized to be truly individual, it is ultimately portable, it can be used (and misused) in private, and it ultimately will allow us do the things we like to do in certain places and with certain people, while being remotely located." She goes on to discuss not just the benefits but the potential problematic qualities of wearable technologies, in projects that push the boundaries of technical possibilities while at the same time asking critical questions about their implementation. By challenging assumptions about utility and productivity, and developing and using "transitive materials," Berzowska hopes to show "the full potential of human expression," concluding that the future of wearable technology will be both social and cultural, where the inbuilt "programmatic behavior" of new materials is fully integrated with aesthetics.

Since the early twentieth century fashion designers have sought to shock with futuristic or outrageous-looking outfits, often inspired by a science fiction genre made popular in films and fiction. Fashion has inspired technology throughout history (as the late sixteenth-century development of the stocking-knitting frame attests), and conversely technology has inspired fashion, always an early adopter of new ideas and technologies. The concept of integrating greater functionality into clothing developed strongly in the post–World War II period, when investment was made in the technology of space exploration. This period is discussed in chapter 22 by Marie O'Mahony, author of several books exploring developments in textile technology and applications in fashion, sports, architecture, and health. O'Mahony has curated a number of exhibitions, including The Soft Machine: Design in the Cyborg Age (Amsterdam 1998–1999; see also O'Mahony 2002), which questioned whether the next phase of human evolution will be through artificial intelligence, robots, clones, and genetic engineering to create new cyborgs (man-machines). Her chapter identifies some of the many recent advances in textile technologies and discusses their role in future scenarios as represented in twentieth-century literature and film. She argues the depiction of textiles in literature and film is an indicator of how our lives might be transformed in the future. For example, the descriptions of textile technologies in the writing of authors such as Peter Carey and William Gibson, and films such as *Barbarella* and *The Matrix,* show "the expectations, excitement, and fears that such scientific advances elicit, touching on the social, cultural, political, and economic issues that impact on scientific research, development, and dissemination." Dresses and cars that change shape, carpets that track people's movement, and transparent buildings are all real-world developments but are also found in visions of the future from film and literature. Fiction and fashion and textiles can therefore be seen to be mutually supportive in inspiring each other.

The collaboration of art with science has a long history, art having provided the scientist with key methods of visual expression. For example, in the eighteenth century the major work of Carl Linnaeus in the classification of the living world would not have been possible without the ability of artists to capture for study the essential nature of and differences between animals and plants. Although this type of collaboration remains of value, new technologies have reduced its role. However, interest in the power of cross-disciplinary collaboration remains high. There is a wealth of commentary available that describes the output of specific collaborations, but perhaps little analysis of the context or methods utilized in these collaborations, especially from the perspective of science researchers working with the branch of art and design that is fashion. The fashion and textile sectors represent an aspect of design that has often been viewed as superficial and separated from the rest of the "serious" design sector, such as architecture and automotive and product design. Design research, itself emerging only in the mid-twentieth century, has until recent years provided minimal context and support in treating fashion and textiles design in a research context.

In the final chapter in this section, the interdisciplinary nature of several current UK-based fashion and science collaborative research projects is unpacked by myself and Philip Sams, a former industrial scientist with the fast-moving consumer goods conglomerate Unilever. Trained in chemistry, Sams worked in research and development for the laundry division and has, since 2000, actively engaged with fashion academics whose research projects span boundaries between art, design, science, and fashion. Through tracking several contemporary examples of long-term research projects and comparing these with the historical case of botany, Sams posits a simple taxonomy for such collaborations between science and "fashion-art," as he terms it: "artist seeking technology," "scientist seeking communication," or "fashion and science co-creation." Through this discussion, as well as proposing that fashion makes science and technology accessible, Sams and I argue for the strong advantages in combining art and design research with the mainstream STEM subjects (science, technology, engineering, and mathematics), acknowledging the key contribution that "fashion thinking" can make to future research. Taking the projects developed by artist/designer Helen Storey (London College of Fashion) and polymer scientist Tony Ryan (University of Sheffield) as a "gold standard" exemplar, we believe that cross-disciplinary research teams can co-create to achieve radical new solutions by collaboratively tackling major issues within the environmental sustainability agenda—the "grand challenges" put forward by the United Kingdom's Engineering and Physical Sciences Research Council and an agenda that is universally recognized. Such co-creative relationships can build on the great strength of fashion as social commentator and extend the impact of fashion to fields well beyond what is normally considered its territory.

While the major fashion companies are driven by the requirement for commercial returns, the industry as a whole looks for radical innovation to individuals and small design teams, often as they emerge from their respective academic institutions. In the volatile and fast-moving world of techno fashion, as in mainstream fashion, it is usual for experimental design projects to emerge, inspire, delight, and then disappear within a short time frame, like a firefly. As Berzowska points out, the research effort being carried out in academia needs to be supported and translated beyond the prototype into industry and the wider community. This, however, requires vision and, not least, financial investment. It remains to be seen, as research progresses, how soon it will be feasible to realize the vision Philips Design expressed in *New Nomads*:

> To create a seamless integration between people, textiles and electronics that will enable us to reach out to the world to stretch our capabilities and possibilities, while at the same time conserving our own and, as our research continues, the planet's energy. (Josephine Green, quoted in Philips Electronics 2000: 13)

As experimental fashion designer Iris van Herpen, who collaboratively develops innovative 3D-printed showpiece dresses, states, "I hope designers will be able to manipulate materials more efficiently than we can today...I hope there will be a new generation of 'super materials' that do not exist today." Perhaps her vision of a "non material" future for fashion in which people could be dressed in "smoke, drops of water, coloured vapour or radio waves" (Quinn 2012: 50) might sustain the planet.

NOTE

1. *Interaction design* is defined by CuteCircuit as "the design of the relationship between people and technology, and the way people use technology" (Black 2010: 107).

BIBLIOGRAPHY

Beylerian, George M., and Andrew Dent. 2007. *Ultra Materials: How Materials Innovation Is Changing the World.* Ed. Bradley Quinn. London: Thames and Hudson.

Black, Sandy. 2007. "Trends in Smart Medical Textiles." In Lieva van Langenhove (ed.), *Smart Textiles for Medicine and Healthcare,* 3–26. Cambridge, UK: Woodhead.

Black, Sandy. 2010. "Reconciling Electronics and Fashion: CuteCircuit in Conversation with Sandy Black." *Fashion Practice: The Journal of Design, Creative Process and the Fashion Industry* 2 (1): 105–20.

Bolton, Andrew. 2002. *The Supermodern Wardrobe.* London: V&A Publications.

Braddock, Sarah E., and Marie O'Mahony. 1998. *Techno Textiles.* London: Thames and Hudson.

Braddock, Sarah E., and Marie O'Mahony. 2002. *SportsTech.* London: Thames and Hudson.

Braddock Clarke, Sarah E., and Jane Harris. 2012. *Digital Visions for Fashion and Textiles.* London: Thames and Hudson.

Braddock Clarke, Sarah E., and Marie O'Mahony. 2005. *Techno Textiles 2.* London: Thames and Hudson.

Lee, Suzanne. 2005. *Fashioning the Future: Tomorrow's Wardrobe.* London: Thames and Hudson.
McQuaid, Matilda (ed.). 2005. *Extreme Textiles: Designing for High Performance.* London: Thames and Hudson; New York: Princeton Architectural Press.
O'Mahony, Marie. 2002. *Cyborg: The Man-Machine.* London: Thames and Hudson.
O'Mahony, Marie. 2011. *Advanced Textiles for Health and Wellbeing.* London: Thames and Hudson.
Philips Electronics. 2000. *New Nomads: An Exploration of Wearable Electronics by Philips.* Rotterdam: 010 Publishers.
Quinn, Bradley. 2002. *Techno Fashion.* Oxford: Berg.
Quinn, Bradley. 2003. *The Fashion of Architecture.* Oxford: Berg.
Quinn, Bradley. 2010. *Textile Futures: Fashion, Design and Technology.* Oxford: Berg.
Quinn, Bradley. 2011. *Design Futures.* London: Merrell.
Quinn, Bradley. 2012. *Fashion Futures.* London: Merrell.
Seymour, Sabine. 2008. *Fashionable Technology: The Intersection of Design, Fashion, Science and Technology.* Vienna: Springer.
Seymour, Sabine. 2010. *Functional Aesthetics: Visions in Fashionable Technology.* Vienna: Springer.

20

Technology and Future Fashion: Body Technology for the Twenty-First Century

BRADLEY QUINN

INTRODUCTION

Fashion and technology are a perfect fit. Wearable technology can transform garments into information hubs that gather data from the environment around them and even exchange data with other technological systems. Embellished with sensors and electroluminescent wires, garments can detect ambient sound and light around them. By interconnecting wearable optic sensors, microcontrollers, and LED (light-emitting diode) lighting, garments are able to respond to light and noise around them and display their reactions on the surface of the fabric.

The fast-paced progress of technology complements fashion's ever-evolving aesthetic, and the portable nature of garments makes wireless technology even more mobile. Each gives the other a wider frame of reference and more scope for new horizons to dawn. Technologized garments are changing how the body interacts with its surroundings and how designers and architects are fashioning the environments we live in. And as fashion and technology come together now more dramatically than ever before, they reveal their capacity to transform the human experience more than technology alone ever could.

FUTURE FIBERS

Fibers form the basis for most of the garments worn today. Fiber technology is fundamental to textile production and is one of the most advanced areas of materials science. Some of the high-tech fibers and superstrong filaments created today are refined enough to craft the couture garments of Parisian fashion yet strong enough to hoist a satellite into space. Twenty-first-century fibers are strong enough to create rigid, architectural components yet still soft enough to cradle a baby's skin (McQuaid 2005). And while some of them look more like space-age materials than conventional fabrics, many recreate the look and performance of traditional textiles.

Without sophisticated fibers, integrating garments and technology would be nearly impossible. Fabrics are usually perceived as flammable, vulnerable to water, impermanent, and weak, while technology is equated with resilience, electricity, and hardware parts. Although heavy-duty hardware and delicate fibers may seem irreconcilably diverse, technological advances are making each of them lighter in weight and sleeker in appearance. Ultimately, this makes the experience of wearing technology more comfortable and more practical.

Because many of our earliest haptic experiences are fiber based, a single textile can evoke a lifetime of memories and sensations.[1] Identifying a fiber with the fingertips provides unique physical and sensorial information about surfaces and textures. Touch is one of the earliest senses to develop, and its relationship to the development of other senses, especially vision, is generating new areas of research. As haptic technologies evolve, textile researchers are gaining a deeper understanding of why fibers hold eternal appeal (Grunwald 2008; Robles-de-la-Torre 2006).

It is interesting to note that initiatives to promote local ecosystems, such as the slow food movement in Italy,[2] have generated greater awareness of how fibers are grown and how textiles feel against the skin. Textiles can make the wearer feel good and, like certain foods, can be emotionally uplifting and even boost mood (Andrews 2008). Advanced textiles promise to do just that, by becoming somatic interfaces that can alter the wearer's emotional set point in a number of ways. "Smarter" textiles promise to monitor mood and heighten awareness, administer medication, broadcast our feelings or dampen them, and transmit information about our well-being to the environments around us. Classifying textiles in terms of their emotional, sensory, and empathic capabilities shows how far forward they have moved in a relatively short time frame. As the examples in this chapter reveal, textiles are moving beyond notions of embedded and electronic; consequently, terms such as *techno fashion, e-textiles,* and *i-wear* already seem out of date.

Despite the high-tech allure of futuristic fabrics, the appeal of natural fibers continues to endure. Many contemporary textiles may surpass them in performance, but the natural fibers that have dressed the human race for several millennia have a feel-good factor that is likely to persist. Natural fibers are almost as ancient as the earth itself and are inextricably linked to humanity's long history. Fibers are nourished by the earth and nurtured by the sun, and their growth reflects the processes that sustain human life. Water, nutrients, sunshine, and oxygen transform dry seeds into rich fields and sustain whole forests of fibers. Natural textiles bring nature's bounty to the artificial environments of humans, where they provide reminders of our connections to the earth.

Reverence for the "natural" has formed the basis for modern movements to slow down and rediscover low-tech, Luddite approaches.[3] Advocates of such movements sometimes wear natural fibers and hemp-heavy fabrics to symbolize an alternative approach, or perhaps antidote, to modern technology. At a time when the textile is virtually indistinguishable from technology, making it a cipher for analog forms is paradoxical. Technology pervades every aspect of the fibers' growth, harvest, production, and manufacture, and the drive for efficiency continues to govern the wearer's experience also.

TECHNO FASHION

Wearable technologies promise to transform the fashioned body forever. As technologized textiles redefine garments as mobile, networked environments, they anchor the cerebral world of intelligence to the intimate environments of the modern human. The exchanges between them are facilitated by fabrics woven from fibers capable of conducting electrical impulses and transferring information. Known as electronic textiles (e-textiles), the new generation of fabrics are fibrous substrates into which microelectronic components and connectors have been seamlessly integrated. As technical hardware and tactile textures become one, the fabrics that result are free from the bulky external components that made earlier generations awkward to wear.

Like computing devices, electronic textiles can relay information via conductors, switches, and sensors and can exchange signals with remote systems via transistors and woven antennae. Threads coated with metals such as silver and nickel make excellent conductors, and ductile fibers made from materials such as carbon, polymers, and finely drawn copper sit snugly on the body. Advances in wire-bonding technology have resulted in electrically isolated wires encapsulated in polyurethane to eliminate bodily contact or friction with other fibers. Minute silicon chips and sensors can be downscaled to fiber size and interwoven with plastic-threaded chip carriers and tiny flexible circuit boards (Van Langenhove 2007). Like most types of programmable hardware, the networks created by these parts can sustain a range of software applications and easily adapt to changes in the computational and sensing requirements of an application.

Although high-street fashions and high-tech devices may seem irreconcilably diverse, electronic textiles were developed in order to integrate garments and technology in medical and technical sectors. They have the drape, flexibility, and resilience of most fashion fabrics, and like conventional textiles, they can be engineered for the desired resistance, thickness, density, weightlessness, porosity, surface texture, and flame resistance. Whether sewn and stitched, bonded together, or simply draped around the body, electronic textiles can be worn for everyday use. As fashion designers and technologists create garments from electronic textiles, they reconceive clothing as a system of active materials that have the ability to change color, form, and texture over time. At the same time, collaborations like these forge a uniquely neutral space as the traditionally feminine-gendered practices of garment making meet the previously male-dominated worlds of technology and materials science.

The process of integrating textiles and technology is not just surface deep; it actually begins at a molecular level. Fresh developments in molecular templating processes led to a stronger bond between the conductive polymers and the electronic circuitry integrated into the fabric. A patented technique developed collaboratively by scientists at Australia's Commonwealth Scientific and Industrial Research Organisation and the University of Wollongong dramatically heightens the textiles' electroconductive properties by binding the indissoluble inherently conductive polymers to the fabric's fibers (Wu et al. 2009). This makes electronic conduction more stable, so that the garment becomes more durable as a result, even capable of withstanding the hostile environment of the domestic washing machine. Novel research conducted at the University of Manchester (Dias et al. 2008) and Nottingham Trent University in the United Kingdom embeds microelectronic components such as LEDs into the yarn-spinning stage, using it to knit or weave electronically enabled fabrics (Hunter 2013).

The earliest garments made with electronic textiles were "Smart Shirts" designed by researchers at the University of Virginia's Department of Electrical and Computer Engineering and at Georgia Institute of Technology. The shirt, developed by Sundaresan Jayaraman and patented by the Georgia Institute of Technology, was funded by the Defense Advanced Research Projects Agency, the primary research and development arm of the U.S. Department of Defense (Park and Jayaraman 2001). Jayaraman engineered a supple textile substrate from a mixture of natural fibers, gossamer wires, and optical fibers. The garment revealed that virtually any type of fabric fiber could be bonded with a conductive fiber to create a sensor system. The system woven into the Smart Shirt was designed specifically to calibrate heart rate, respiration, and body temperature and relay the data to a remote system in real time for analysis.

Similarly, a range of smart garments developed by Thomas Martin, an associate professor at the University of Virginia, bonded electrical wires, sensors, and actuators to fibers and wove them into an electronic textile. Crafted into apparel similar to sportswear, Martin's garments were able to sense their own shapes and monitor the movements of the wearer (Martin et al. 2004).

The clothing developed by Jayaraman and Martin highlights the importance of configuring the sensor networks so that the garment can monitor itself at the same time that it monitors the wearer. For example, if the wearer decided to roll up the sleeves while sensors in the cuffs are monitoring the pulse, the sensors should inform the network to temporarily suspend their function. Where the network senses areas of damage, strain, or power shortages, it should reroute the surveillance to other parts of the garment so that monitoring can proceed without being short-circuited. Such capabilities are essential for electronic textiles worn in battle, medical diagnostics, and chemical biosensing.

If smart garments were able to sense stimuli in the ambient environment, they would be able to "see" and "smell" on behalf of the wearer. A shirt for the blind, for example, could be woven with indicators that provide warnings about approaching objects. Workers in the chemical industry could wear overalls that "smell" leaching toxins and detect them before they cause harm to the wearers.

All electronic textiles rely heavily on fiber strength to create structures with specific architectures and properties. Classes of fibers are usually categorized according to filament length and the type of material they are made from. Glass, carbon, and polymer fibers are widely used, and each has a distinct advantage. Glass is regarded as inexpensive and versatile, while carbon fibers are said to have the highest strength and durability. Polymer fibers tend to be chosen for technical fabrics with specific properties or for the production of fibers for high-tech applications. Long fibers of any type provide more tensile strength, creating fabrics that are highly flexible, impact-resistant, and less likely to fracture. Shorter fibers provide reinforcement and absorb impact, providing an easy and inexpensive way to improve strength and stiffness.

The, type, length, and surface compatibility of fibers can be engineered to maximize a textile's performance, enabling it to achieve strength-to-weight values unparalleled elsewhere in the world of materials. Superstrong fabrics aren't created through fiber technology alone; their strength is augmented by the construction techniques used to craft them. Bundling fibers together has a "strength in numbers" effect that makes them more resilient, while braided fibers are even stronger (Beylerian and Dent 2007).

The buildup of individual flexible filaments into a warp and a weft enables any abrasion or impact to be distributed among a large number of filaments, making it less likely to fracture a single fiber. This is the main reason that woven construction is the best choice for electronic textiles. Although it is possible to get the same fit, texture, tactility, and washability from nonwoven textiles, they rarely have the comfort that woven or knit fabric has. Weaving is an ancient technique that creates a simple and effective system today, one that continues to be at the forefront of materials innovation.

Biopolymer and polymer science are forging exchanges between biopolymer molecular structure, fiber behavior, and the coloration of polymers. Technologists from both fields are working to develop organic, plant-based polymers that can be utilized to replace oil-based nonwoven fabrics. Polymer fibers are generally lighter, smaller, softer, less expensive, safer, and more colorful than other types of fibers, and clear polymers can create fibers with translucent properties. Polymer foams have a density, hardness, moldability, and printability that make them perfect for fashion applications, and technologists are currently developing ways to adapt them for electronic textiles.

Although advances in polymer development have led to superstrong plastic filaments such as Spectra (by Honeywell) or Dyneema (by DSM), carbon fibers still have the highest tensile strength; experiments have shown that a filament just one millimeter (0.039 inches) in diameter is strong enough to hoist a four-door car above the ground (Beylerian and Dent 2007: 27). Although carbon fibers are strong, they lack tenacity and impact absorption. Whereas a carbon fiber is likely to shatter when impacted, a polymer fiber yields easily and absorbs the impact. Polymer fibers such as polyethylene are stronger, and aramid fibers such as Kevlar (by DuPont) and Twaron (by Teijin) are uniquely impact-resistant. Developments in embedding carbon nanotubes into films prove substantially more robust than the indium tin oxide films commonly used to make computer screens and mobile phone displays, which makes them ideal for the touch screens and flexible displays developed for electronic textiles.

Such innovations are made possible by technical fibers, such as AmberStrand by Syscom, which is electrically conductive, lightweight, flexible, and strong. AmberStrand's base is the high-modulus Zylon fiber, a filament technically known as polyphenylene bisoxazole, which is a polymer/metal hybrid. Zylon is coated with metal through a proprietary process that produces strong, flexible strands that are bundled together to form yarn. The yarn contains conductive metals such as silver, copper, and nickel and is said to be less toxic to manufacture than copper beryllium alloy wire, another popular conductive material. AmberStrand is mostly used in aerospace applications and in computing devices, but it is gaining ground in electronic textiles, too.[4]

Microfibers are responsible for making synthetic fibers chic again. They can create textiles that are lighter, softer, more elastic, and more durable than those made from natural fibers. Microfibers (that is, fibers with a diameter measured in microns—a micrometer is one-millionth or $1/10^6$ of a meter) are a popular choice for fabrics ranging from faux suedes and furs to high-performance textiles made for sportswear. By working at molecular and atomic scale, nanoscale engineering (at dimensions between 1 and 100 nanometers—a nanometer is one-billionth or $1/10^9$ of a meter) has succeeded in making it possible for individual fibers to repel liquids, and as a result, stain resistance took a quantum leap. Previously, stain resistance resulted from coating the fabric's surface with materials such as Teflon, which disintegrated with wear. Nanotechnology alters individual fibers on a molecular level, making their ability to repel liquid an inherent part of a fiber's composition, and subsequently it can be maintained throughout the life span of the fiber. Nanotextiles, as such fabrics are called, result from the production and manipulation of nanoscale fibers, including those created through the processes of electrospinning, and the synthesis of carbon nanotubes, polymer nanofiber processing, and the extrusion of nanocomposite fibers.

Advances in fiber and manufacturing technology have made three-dimensional textiles possible. Typically produced on Raschel double-bar warp-knitting machines, three-dimensional fabrics (sometimes known as spacer fabrics) transform textiles from two-dimensional surfaces into materials that have volume and depth. Developed for use in cushioning, these textiles are rapidly replacing foam, especially in the sneaker and sportswear markets. They eliminate the need for an additional decorative textile layered onto the surface of the foam, precluding the use of adhesive to bond the two together. Synthetics such as polyesters and nylons can be used as well as cottons and other natural fibers, and the density and cushioning properties can be varied throughout the textile. Because the thickness is customizable and variable from area to area, it makes it possible to cushion sensitive electronic components or reinforce critical subfabric interfaces.

Not all electronic textiles are based on fiber construction. The composite materials known as quantum tunneling composites consist of metals and nonconducting elastomeric binders that function as pressure sensors and become conductive when they come into contact.[5] The material's name refers to the quantum tunneling process that results when the composite materials are compressed. Without pressure, the conductive elements are not close enough to conduct electricity. Applying pressure moves them into contact with each other, enabling the electrons to "tunnel" through the material.

ILLUMINATING FABRIC

For most of their long history, fabric surfaces were made to communicate, and given their capacity to transfer information, it's no surprise that today's textiles continue to relay data in the digital age. As a wearable communication platform, an electronic textile designates a dynamic surface around the body that interconnects people and places. Electronic fabrics are capable of absorbing mobile phone technology, and as they do so, they provide the perfect interfaces for Bluetooth technology and iPhone and similar smartphone systems. Speakers and microphones are weaving their way into collars and cuffs, and flexible, battery-powered optical fiber screens are being woven into sleeves and jacket linings. Made from flexible plastic fiber-optic threads and illuminated by tiny LEDs fixed along the edge of the display screen, they are controlled by microchip interfaces. The optical fibers will be configured into pixels as they designate sections that remain dark and areas that illuminate when the LEDs are activated. One of the early prototype screens developed by France Telecom displayed crude, but readable, symbols. As the prototypes evolved, research organizations such as International Fashion Machines (see below) developed more sophisticated versions that displayed text characters, advertising logos, and a range of geometric ciphers (Lee 2005; McQuaid 2005).

Textiles woven from optical fibers harness their luminous quality to create illuminating textiles.[6] The Italian-made, nonreflective Luminex fabric, which is produced from fiber optics and colored LEDs, can be cut and handled like any other tailoring material. Luminex uses energy-efficient LEDs to transmit light at low voltages and can be powered by rechargeable batteries. Luminex can also incorporate microchips into the fabric to create a variety of radiant effects. Microchips could also transform Luminex into an interface capable of processing signals and responding to environmental stimuli. A different technology features in the Lumalive fabric developed by Philips, which has the potential to display as many as 16 million colors in a detachable, flexible panel sandwiched between layers of fabric. Lumalive textiles are comprised of colored LEDs that have been fully integrated into the fabric without compromising the softness of the cloth. Their surfaces can broadcast texts, graphics, or multicolored motifs, as shown in the work of experimental fashion designer Anke Loh (Figures 20.1 and 20.2).[7]

Made from plastic, optical fibers can be woven into a fabric's structure during the fabric-production process using a three-dimensional technique. The technique employs

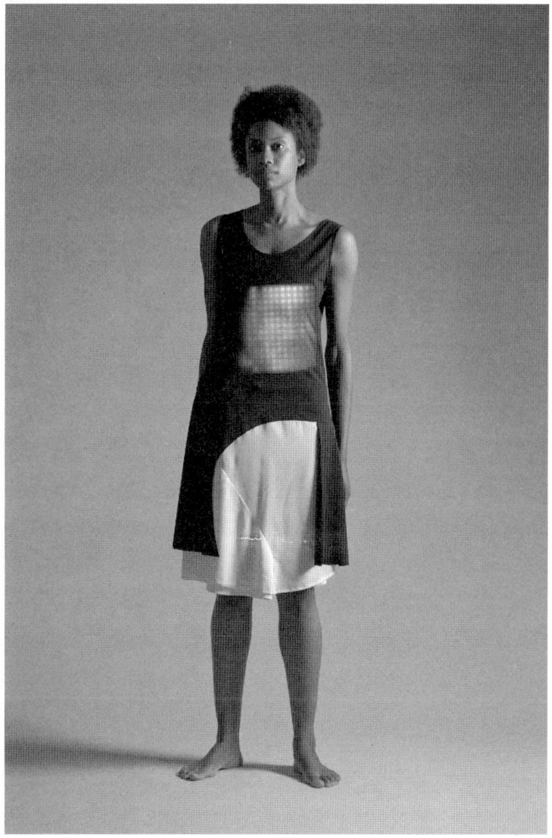

FIGURE 20.1 Anke Loh, Dressing Light collection, 2006. Experimental designer Anke Loh created dresses and skirts incorporating Philips Lumalive soft embedded LED panels programmed with a video display of faces.
Credit: Photograph by James Prinz. Courtesy of Anke Loh.

spiraling movements that prevent any discontinuities at the armholes, hems, or seams using a novel modification in the weaving process. This process eclipses the need for traditional "cut-and-sew" operations that produce fabric two-dimensionally. This process was a significant breakthrough in textile engineering as it enabled a fully finished fashion garment to be completed on a weaving machine.

Electroluminescent wires appear similar to optical fibers in their luminescence and have the same flexibility and versatility. Their durability and weatherproof characteristics make them ideal for outerwear applications. Like optical fibers, they do not generate heat and can easily be woven into a variety of textile forms. Electroluminescent wires have a very low current draw that makes it possible to power a thirty-meter (thirty-nine-yard) length with just a single one-amp fuse. However, a driver (similar to a transformer) is necessary. The type of driver is chosen according to the volume of wire, the voltage, and the degree of brightness desired. The color tones are determined by the optic

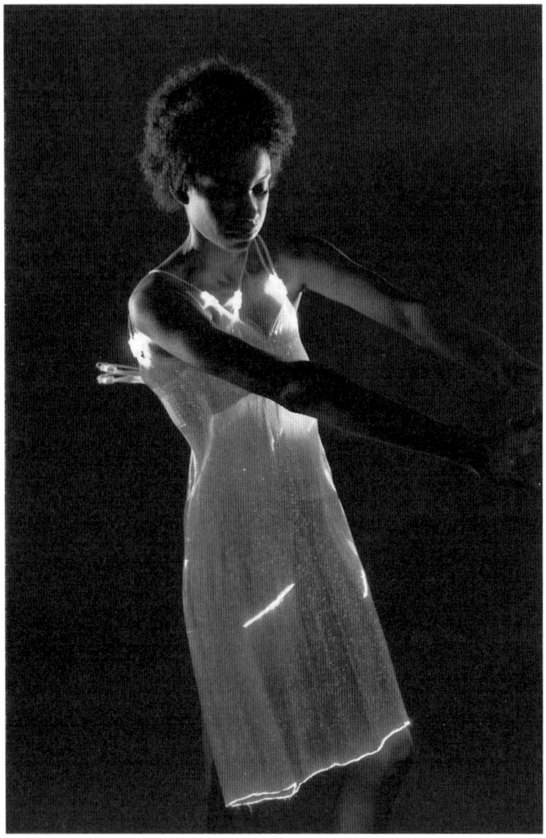

FIGURE 20.2 Anke Loh, Dressing Light collection, 2006. Anke Loh created vibrant light-emitting dresses using Luminex fabric. The dress glows a rich blue color in the dark.
Credit: Photograph by Saverio Trugli. Courtesy of Anke Loh.

wavelengths rather than color particles. Lower frequencies give the fabrics softer shades of primary colors or pastel hues, while higher frequencies make the colors appear deeper and more solid (Debevec 2005).

Fabrics made from optical fibers and electroluminescent wires show that, in addition to data, both light and power can be transmitted through a textile substrate. The batteries that power electronic textiles are now smaller and lighter and are seldom cumbersome for the wearer. Although equipping textiles with an integral energy source is a breakthrough for textile technology, concerns about the health risks associated with wearing batteries and other power sources in close proximity to the human body raise questions regarding the viability of these fabrics.

Marin Soljačić, a technologist based at the Massachusetts Institute of Technology, foresees a future when electronic textiles will not need an integral power source at all. Soljačić's vision for nonradiative energy transfer draws on an experiment conducted in 1831 by the physicist Michael Faraday, who discovered that an electric current flowing through one wire invariably induces a secondary current in a neighboring wire.

Faraday was unable to confine the electrical current to the two wires; the power was transmitted in all directions, meaning that the energy dissipated with distance.

Soljačić's experiments with nonradiative energy transfer have shown how near-field magnetic resonance between two strongly coupled induction coils can transfer sixty watts of electrical power with 40 percent efficiency across a distance of two meters (about 2.2 yards) (Handley 2007; Kurs et al. 2007). Because the external fields of this transmission process are magnetic rather than radioactive, the health risks are believed to be less than for power transmission in systems that emit electrical fields. Soljačić's experiments were able to recharge an object the size of a laptop within a few yards of the power source. Soljačić and colleagues intend to extend the range of nonradiative wireless power and create a system that could provide coverage throughout the office or home, meaning that electronic textiles and other devices could be recharged ambiently when positioned within range of a power source.[8] At present, electronic textiles are not equipped with hardware and software systems to route the power efficiently throughout the garment. A single electronic textile or smart garment may include a wide array of sensors—including accelerometers, gyroscopes, and detectors that pinpoint location, as well as microphones, ultrasonic emitters, and piezoelectric films that change voltage in response to shape changes.

Low-tech experiments with conductive fibers have revealed that solar power can be harnessed by fabric and interspersed throughout the fabric's structure. Designer Andrew Schneider created a prototype solar-powered bikini made by overlaying narrow strips of photovoltaic film onto a swimsuit and sewing them on with conductive thread. The swimsuit produced a five-volt output that, via the attached USB connector, could slowly recharge electronic gadgets like an iPod.[9]

WEARABLE TECHNOLOGY

Equipped with cameras, microphones, speakers, and sensors, "embedded" textiles once held the promise of the future. To describe an object as *embedded* implies that it can be removed or detached, resulting in a portal that other devices can be linked into. An electronic textile, for example, could also be embedded with portals to facilitate information exchanges with systems not yet capable of transferring data wirelessly. Embedded portals could also accept power transfers, audiovisual exchanges, and debugging diagnostics.

The first "wearable computer" prototypes of the early 1990s were actually body-mounted devices attached to jackets, waistcoats, and vests. Their cables and connectors were anchored in place by fasteners and stitching or crudely fed through seams, and wireless antennae were attached to collars and cuffs. Gadgets such as the MP3 player were among the first to be embedded in textiles and garments; fitted to denim jackets and water-repellent metallic-coated nylon parkas, their wiring and hardware were encased between layers of fabric (Philips Electronics 2000). Although such garments were often described as interactive, the wearer triggered various interfaces manually rather than activating them in a truly integrated system that interacted with the wearer and the textile itself.

The embedded interfaces of such "intelligent" garments proved to be awkward for the wearer and frustrating for the designers, and subsequently sparked the demand for a new generation of fully integrated electronic textiles. Although the success of electronic fabrics will soon make embedded textiles a thing of the past, embedded technology continues to play an important role in the development of technically enhanced clothing.

Hussein Chalayan was one of the first fashion designers to engage with technological systems, and many of his collections have pioneered garments that feature wireless technology, electrical circuitry, and embedded connectors. Some of Chalayan's most groundbreaking uses of materials and processes were presented in his spring/summer 2007 collection, titled One Hundred and Eleven, when he designed dresses powered by machine-driven levers that opened and closed to reconfigure the garment's shape and silhouette. The technology embedded in the garments enabled hemlines to rise autonomously, a bustier to open of its own accord, and a jacket to unfasten itself and pull away from the model's torso. These designs were made possible through collaboration with the team behind the special effects for the *Harry Potter* films such as *The Prisoner of Azkaban,* who incorporated microchips into fabric panels so that they would move according to the sequences Chalayan programmed them to (Violette 2011).

The mechanical dresses were ingeniously fitted with electronic components and engineered pulley systems. The garments' surfaces were painstakingly embroidered with thousands of Swarovski crystals (Swarovski having sponsored the collection), giving them the dual appeal of opulent elegance and high-tech savviness. Although the technology was streamlined and embedded into corsets and pads worn beneath the garments, it was still cumbersome to the models wearing the garments. Further research is needed to reconfigure the shape-changing features of the embedded system into an electronic textile that can assume different shapes and morph back to its starting point again.

Chalayan's 2007 collections marked a radical departure from a world where distinctions between body and technology, body and dress, natural and artificial, once seemed clear. This illustrates how, as Michel Foucault (1977) described, social and cultural discourses construct our bodies in a way that makes us as analogous to a machine as possible. The design of the dress is imbued with technologies that make interaction efficient, productive, and empowered, akin to the machine-like principles of controlled automation. The presence of high-tech systems in fashion fuses its body-conscious ideals with a belief in automation, speed, and accuracy as the means to achieve it.

U.S.-based International Fashion Machines (founded by Maggie Orth and Joanna Berzowska) was one of the first companies to pioneer a new generation of fashion based on interactive technology, electronic textiles, and embedded computer interfaces. In 1998 they designed the Firefly dress, a garment constructed from two layers of conductive metallic silk organza separated by a layer of tulle embedded with LEDs and conductive Velcro brushes. When the wearer moved, the Velcro conductors came into contact with the LEDs, completing the circuit and causing the LEDs to light up. International Fashion Machines also created a jacket with an integrated synthesizer and embroidered keypad that functions as a musical instrument. The jacket is embedded with sensing electronics, speakers, a customized MIDI synthesizer, and batteries. By touching sensors embedded in the jacket and pressing keys embroidered in conductive thread, the wearer can create music. The keypad uses a capacitive sensing method to discern pressure and emits a small electrical charge when the individual keys are touched (McQuaid 2005).

New York fashion designer Angel Chang was one of the first designers to bring wearable technology to the catwalks of New York Fashion Week, creating garments that explored the potentials of smart fabrics. Chang uses technology to amplify the concepts underpinning her designs, imbuing many of her garments with multifunctionality and the ability to transform their surfaces. Her designs defy the boundaries between streetwear, daywear, formal wear, and casual wear. Organic fabrics are gently stitched to produce gossamer surfaces, while nylons and industrial plastics are used to give her clothing unexpected details. Chang's streamlined silhouettes and precise tailoring suggest a utilitarian or futuristic identity. Functional and original, Chang's clothing is designed with a high degree of comfort in mind.

Chang collaborates with engineers and interactive designers to develop ways of moving fashion forward and also to create garments that would solve some of the problems facing urban women. "My generation of women is so different from previous ones," she says. "We are multi-tasking more, traveling around the world, and managing all aspects of our lives through hand-held organisers, mobile phones and the Internet."[10] Noting that women's lifestyles have changed drastically in recent years, Chang was perplexed to realize that wardrobes have not. Chang advocates the integration of clothing and technology to make wireless communication easier and Internet access more available, which she believes can be achieved without compromising comfort or aesthetics. "Technology can easily be concealed within the garment's design," Chang says, "as it is in my metallic-finished knit hoodie with iPod controls. And my Edwardian-inspired jacket, also made from conductive textiles, which functions as an MP3 player. I love embroidery, so it was a natural choice for me to hand embroider buttons on the sleeve that cue the MP3 player to play, stop, fast forward and rewind, and control volume" (Figure 20.3).

Chang designed a jacket hand-embroidered with LEDs and conductive "X-static" silver fibers sourced from Noble Biomaterials, who also supply the fiber to the U.S. military.[11] "The X-static fiber is coated in a layer of pure silver permanently bonded to its surface," Chang explains. "The fiber remains soft after the coating process, retaining its traditional tactile characteristics. It can be made into a filament or spun yarn and used in knits, wovens and non-wovens." It was used to create a battery-powered self-heating jacket that was temperature regulated for the person wearing it.

While Chang has a strong vision for incorporating wireless technology into fabric, her work also explores dye techniques and surface coatings. "My interest in technological innovation is strong, and so is my desire to adapt fabric to provide the technological solutions that women need," Chang said. "I'm aligning with technology little by little, also exploring thermochromic inks and UV-activated motifs. They're affordable and fun, and a springboard to bigger ideas."

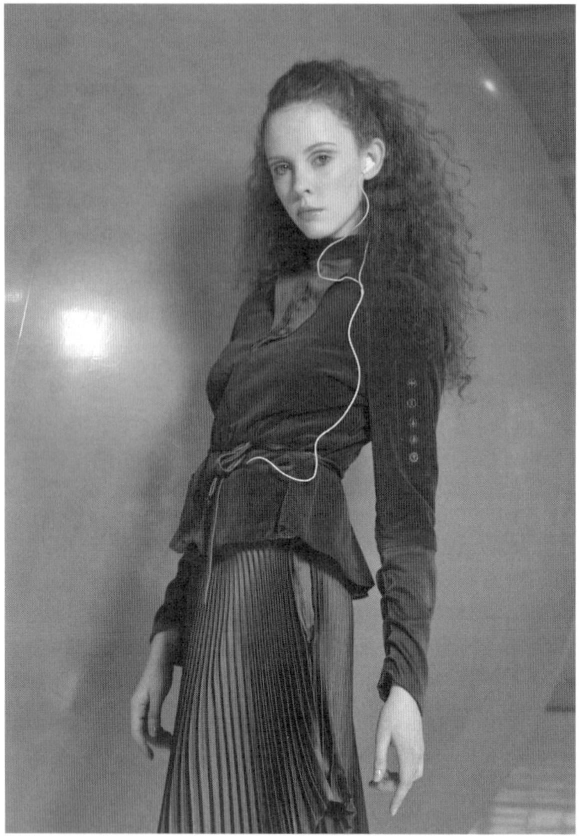

FIGURE 20.3 Angel Chang, Edwardian-inspired velvet jacket with MP3 player control buttons embroidered on sleeve using conductive thread, 2007. This feminine jacket incorporates Eleksen pressure-sensing technology (now part of Peratech, United Kingdom), in contrast to the masculine sports outerwear normally seen with such technology.
Credit: Photograph by Lee Clower. Courtesy of Angel Chang.

Embedded technology can also effect color changes in fabric or configure new techniques. CuteCircuit is a London-based wearable technology company with a mandate to make technology beautiful, fun, and comfortable to wear: hard shells, trailing wires, and pockets full of batteries are banished from their design methodology. In the twelve years that CuteCircuit has been active, founding directors Francesca Rosella, an Italian fashion designer, and Ryan Genz, an American design engineer, have made technologized garments that are beautiful to look at and comfortable to wear.

Each of CuteCircuit's designs begins at the fiber and fabric level, where Rosella and Genz embed conductive threads and integrate microelectronic systems and telecommunication technology. By incorporating miniature LEDs, they create fashion fabrics capable of changing color and motif. When these are combined with integrated sensors that detect movement or body heat, the clothing that results seems to come alive as it is worn. Garments such as the Kinetic dress, which is activated by the wearer's movements, respond to specific movements to cue a blue color to emerge on the surface via electroluminescent embroidery thread. Although the dress is made with a surprising number of independent microelectronic systems and integrated sensors, none of them are visible in the fabric itself. Whereas other examples of wearable technology are often characterized by hard plastic pieces, trailing wires, and pockets full of batteries, CuteCircuit's designs have the look and feel of ordinary garments. Their recent Twitter dress is a sophisticated evening gown designed to light up in response to tweets (Figure 20.4).

CuteCircuit designed the pioneering Hug Shirt to recreate the experience of being hugged by a loved one. The shirt was conceived as a wearable haptic device that interfaces with mobile phones as a Bluetooth accessory: "We made the garments by integrating Bluetooth technology into the shirts," Rosella explains, "which enabled it to receive data from mobile phones as simply as receiving a text message."[12] The shirts are

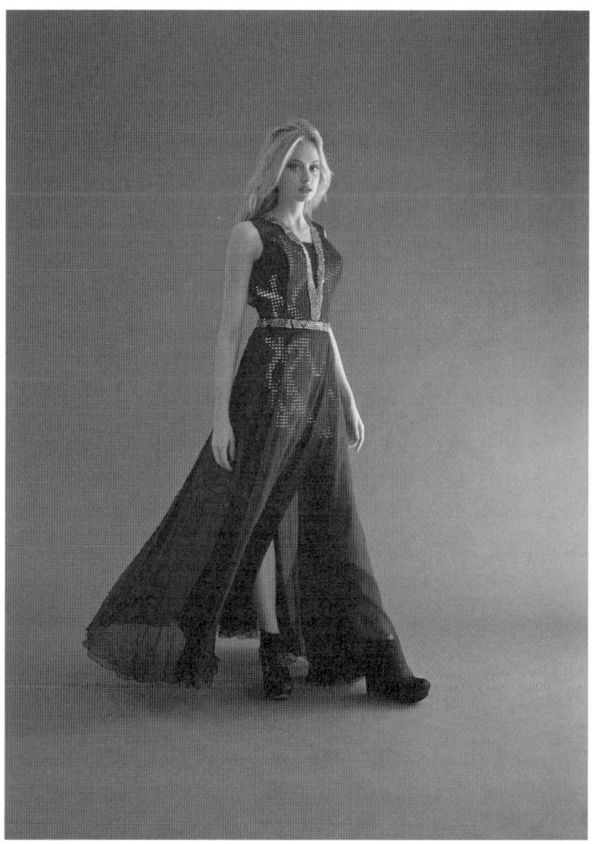

FIGURE 20.4 Twitter dress designed by CuteCircuit as worn by singer Nicole Scherzinger, November 2012. The Twitter dress is an elegant "digital couture" black chiffon evening gown adorned with hematite Swarovski crystals. The dress incorporates high-density LEDs that light up with animations that move around the body and show direct real-time responses to tweets for @twitterdress.
Credit: Photograph by CuteCircuit.

embedded with sensors that can receive and transmit information to any smartphone. The wearers touch sensorized areas on their own shirt to send simulated caresses to each other by using them as wearable mouse pads to activate the pressure-sensitive areas. Embedded sensors monitor the pressure and duration of the hug, detect the sender's heart rate and skin temperature, and relay it to the other wearer's shirt via the mobile phone network. The system even enables those without a Hug Shirt to transmit virtual hugs to Hug Shirt wearers. A software application known as HugMe transmits hugs via Bluetooth, effectively transmitting a touch message from person to person.

To create the Hug system, CuteCircuit experimented with several different types of fabrics and materials, including balloons and sponges. "We mapped out the positioning of arms and hands as people hugged each other, and recorded the positions on the textile," Rosella says. "Areas such as the upper arms, upper back, neck, shoulders and around the waist, were fitted with detachable pads containing the hugging output actuators, which compress the fabric to create the sensation of a hug."

In 2009 the Museum of Science and Industry in Chicago commissioned CuteCircuit to design the groundbreaking Galaxy dress for its permanent collection (Figure 20.5). Embroidered with 24,000 full-color LEDs and 4,000 Swarovski crystals, the dress was the largest wearable digital display in the world. The dress was made from four layers of silk chiffon, onto which tiny LEDs were embroidered using conductive threads to interconnect them with extrathin, flexible circuits. "Although the surface of the dress contained an extensive layer of technological parts, the embroidery techniques we used enabled the fabric to drape smoothly across the body and move with lightness and fluidity," says Rosella. "Because the LEDs' energy consumption is low, the dress is powered by normal iPod batteries without any risk of overheating."

CuteCircuit has also designed the Embedded Theatre, a wearable device that analyzes the wearer's location and delivers audio narrative and navigational information via a headset. The headset exchanges information with a garment embedded with sensors and wireless network capabilities. The technology embedded in the garment contains a mobile device (like a personal digital assistant or cell phone) and headphones fitted with digital sensors. The system uses Wi-Fi triangulation to gauge the wearer's location, and its sensors identify the direction the wearer is facing. These two data sources make it possible to recreate the physical landscape in an ephemeral guise that corresponds precisely to real-world objects and locations. For example, the technology pinpoints where the wearer is standing, and the sensors detect that he or she is looking at a particular building. At that point, the sensors trigger audio files to begin describing its architectural history. When the technology senses that the wearer is about to head in a certain direction, it uses audio files to advise them about any unseen hindrances further ahead.

Austrian-born designer Sabine Seymour established Moondial in 1998, a fashion technology lab with studios in Austria and New York. Seymour utilizes conductive fibers, explores the potential that nanotechnology has for smart textiles, and designs electronic fabrics. Seymour's dynamic View jacket features an embedded Lumalive display

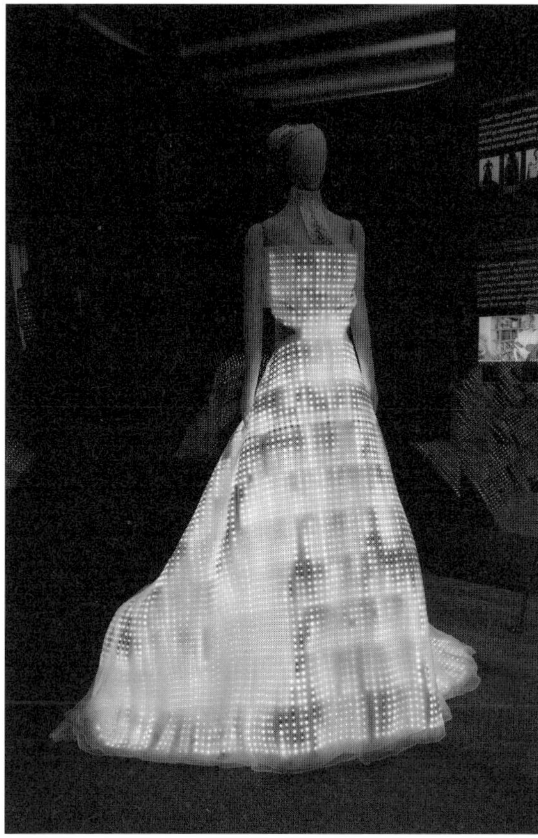

FIGURE 20.5 CuteCircuit, Galaxy dress, 2009. Commissioned by the Chicago Museum of Science and Industry for their permanent display, this dramatic dress comprised the largest visual array to date, containing 24,000 LED lights, powered by just one small battery. Colors change and move across the surface continually.
Credit: Photograph by J. B. Spector, Museum of Science and Industry, Chicago, United States. Courtesy of CuteCircuit.

made by Philips Design. The display can project pictures, moving images, scrolling texts, and morphing patterns, transforming the jacket into an animated surface. "The design of the jacket is contextualized for specific events," Seymour explains.[13] "The dynamic movement on the surface draws attention. It could be programmed to broadcast brand logos or advertising slogans, which would make it a great tool for guerrilla marketing. Programmed with patterns, images or animations that the wearer likes, it can become a fashion statement." Seymour plans to create future versions of the jacket made with a fully integrated digital display and technological components. "The goal is to enhance the fibers so that the display potential is built into them as they are manufactured, rather than adding electronics to them after they have been woven into fabric."

Other designs transfer a basic garment into a dynamic design, such as Seymour's light-reactive Sun T-shirt, which uses simple UV light to morph the graphics printed on the front into shapes. "The shirt functions as a canvas to tell a story," Seymour says, "and the sun provides the switch that turns on the graphics and enables them to reveal new images." Another T-shirt, the Sun N°01 Zebra, was made in a limited edition and launched at the Ars Electronica Festival in 2009; it is now considered to be a collector's item.

As Seymour develops novel techniques and creates supply chains that streamline the production of wearable technology, she is faced with issues that affect the industry as a whole. "Because wearable technology is still a new area, designers are faced with issues that need to resolved before techno textiles and wearables can move forward," Seymour explains. "IP-related issues, venture capital investment and specialist manufacturing can restrict designers." Seymour's contact with consumers has enabled her to identify how they could contribute to the process. "Some consumers would like to self-assemble wearable garments and techno textiles," she says. "Customized 3D printing or on-the-fly knitting could be made a part of the retail experience. I think the pairing of a gallery-like store with an Apple-style genius bar would enable consumers to customize wearable technology, making it simpler to buy and easier to use." Seymour's pioneering research is setting new standards for smart garments and taking the industry forward as a result. In 2008 Seymour published *Fashionable Technology,* one of the first surveys of the field, identifying experimental projects in fashion and technology, followed in 2010 by a second volume, *Functional Aesthetics.*

SURVEILLANCE?

Technology also has a sinister side, and when intelligence is embedded into textiles, it reveals that the startling reach of surveillance even pervades the fabrics we wear. Like the body-rig devices worn by undercover police, the cameras and recording devices embedded into fabric could easily slip past detection or be used in areas where audiovisual technology has been banned. Not only can embedded electronics store information on computer circuits, but they can also transmit and receive data when activated by an external signal.

Textiles that can monitor vital signs, such as those used by the military and by physicians, reveal that surveillance can play an important role in health and safety. Made into a diagnostic garment, the textiles can relay information about the wearer's health to a physician to ensure real-time assessment of the patient's health. This technology is also being investigated by the U.S. military, as part of research into more interactive uniforms for soldiers on the ground.

When, in 2003, it was reported that Benetton's clothing brand Sisley planned to embed a radio frequency identification (RFID) chip into the label of every new garment, consumer watchdog organizations protested. An RFID chip emits an electronic product code (ePC) that provides a unique ID for a garment. The ePC is intended to replace the UPC bar code used to tag garments. Because the ePC actually assigns a unique number to each individual item, it goes beyond identifying product categories. Once the ePC has been assigned, it is transmitted by an RFID tag embedded in the product. The chips can vary in size but are generally smaller than most fibers, comparable to the size of a grain of sand or a speck of dust. Electronic scanners or reader devices are used to detect the signal transmitted by the RFID chip. Retailers claim that RFID chips could revolutionize quality control by enabling them to retrace a garment's production cycle and identify where defects could have originated.

The claim that chips are necessary to keep track of a garment's journey through production stages, shipping, and retail is contested by organizations such as CASPIAN (Consumers against Supermarket Privacy Invasion and Numbering). CASPIAN reveals that devices embedded in clothing would enable retailers to track individuals by linking the customers' names and credit card information with the serial number assigned to the garment. According to Katherine Albrecht and Liz McIntyre, CASPIAN's directors, "selling a pair of shoes that doubles as a tracking device without telling consumers about the RFID device it contains is essentially a form of fraud. When a shopper buys a pair of shoes, she has a reasonable expectation that she is getting shoes—not something else. Once mandatory labelling is in place, if people chose to buy shoes that can track them, that should be their free choice. But consumers must be informed of what that choice means."[14] CASPIAN, and many other consumer organizations, envisions a global network of millions of scanners and reading devices along the entire garment supply chain. The devices would be found not only in factories, seaports, transport hubs, distribution centers, warehouses, and retail outlets but even in the home.

Embedded chips also raise issues of ownership. The chips embedded in bankcards remain the property of the bank at all times, irrespective of being held by the consumer. Applied to fashion companies, who could assert ownership of the embedded chip because of its integral relationship to their data system, it could mean that the garment was merely licensed to the consumer for the duration of its life span.

Although the RFID system described here remains current, today's retailers are more likely to tag garments with ultra-high-frequency (UHF) chips. UHF tags are a new generation of RFID technology that facilitates faster data transfer speeds and longer read ranges. UHF chips were first used in retail sectors where a larger distance between the reader devices and the chip was necessary.

CONCLUSION

As fashion forges connections with science and technology, clothing takes a radical departure from a world where distinctions between body and technology, body and dress, natural and artificial, once seemed clear. Wearable technology can invite social and cultural discourses about how we choose to fashion our bodies and even enable us to construct new identities. While the familiar folds of fashion create second skins for the human form, the technology embedded within them could transform the wearer into a hybrid of machine and human being.

NOTES

1. *Haptic technology* refers to systems operated by touch. This emerging technology has wide-reaching applications in many different fields.
2. The Slow Food movement, which has developed in Italy from the late 1980s, has stimulated other movements, including Slow Fashion and Slow Textiles (Fletcher 2007).
3. The Luddites were an early nineteenth-century social movement of British textile artisans who demonstrated, sometimes violently, against the changes brought about by the Industrial Revolution. Mechanized looms led to less work, and artisans often mobilized and destroyed them.
4. See http://www.amberstrand.com for more information.
5. Peratech is a leading developer of quantum tunneling composite technology. See http://www.peratech.com for further information.
6. Optical fibers are made from glass or plastic and transport light along their entire length. They are widely used in fiber-optic communication because their bandwidth permits data transmission over longer distances and at higher data rates than many other forms of communications.
7. For Luminex, see http://www.luminex.it/. For Lumalive, see http://www.research.philips.com/newscenter/.
8. See Jennifer Chu, "TR10—Wireless Power," *MIT Technology Review* - 10 Breakthrough technologies, March/April 2008, http://www2.technologyreview.com/article/409599/tr10-wireless-power (accessed February 25, 2013).
9. Paul Ridden, "Solar Bikini Goes into Very Limited Production," *Gizmag* online magazine, June 15, 2011, http://www.gizmag.com/solar-bikini-goes-into-limited-production/18920/; see also "Solar Bikini" on Andrew Schneider's website, http://andrewjs.com/solarbikini.html (accessed February 25, 2013).
10. Angel Chang, interview by the author, New York, April 10, 2006.
11. The X-static fiber is coated in a layer of 99.9 percent pure silver, which is permanently bonded to the surface. It was developed as an industrial and medical product, made for high-tech healthcare applications and smart military garments. In addition to being conductive, X-static is antimicrobial and antistatic. See http://www.x-staticfiber.com for further information.
12. Francesca Rosella, interview by the author, London, February 1, 2008.
13. Sabine Seymour, interview by the author, London, March 1, 2011.
14. CASPIAN, "Where Does CASPIAN Stand on Legislation?" http://www.spychips.com/about_us.html (accessed January 30, 2013).

BIBLIOGRAPHY

Andrews, Geoff. 2008. *The Slow Food Story.* Montreal, Canada: McGill-Queen's University Press.

Beylerian, George, and Andrew Dent. 2007. *Ultra Materials: How Materials Innovation Is Changing the World.* Ed. Bradley Quinn. London: Thames and Hudson.

Debevec, Paul. 2005. *High Dynamic Range Imaging: Acquisition, Display, and Image-Based Lighting.* Burlington, MA: Morgan Kaufmann.

Dias, Tilak, William Hurley, Ravindra Monaragala, and R. Wijeyesiriwardana. 2008. "Development of Electrically-Active Textiles." *Advances in Science and Technology* 60: 74–84. http://www.scientific.net/AST.60.74 (accessed February 28, 2013).

Fletcher, Kate. 2007. "Slow Fashion." *The Ecologist,* June 1. http://www.theecologist.org/green_green_living/clothing/269245/slow_fashion.html (accessed January 30, 2013).

Foucault, Michel. 1977. *Discipline and Punish.* London: Penguin.

Grunwald, Martin (ed.). 2008. *Human Haptic Perception: Basics and Applications.* Basel: Birkhäuser.

Handley, Frank. 2007. "Goodbye Wires." WiTricity press release, MIT Institute for Soldier Nanotechnologies, June 7. http://www.mit.edu/~soljacic/MIT_WiTricity_Press_Release.pdf (accessed February 28, 2013).

Hunter, Billy. 2013. "Researchers Develop Washable Wearable Computing." Innovation in Textiles, January 30. http://www.innovationintextiles.com/researchers-develop-washable-wearable-computing/ (accessed January 30, 2013).

Kurs, André, Aristeidis Karalis, Robert Moffatt, J. D. Joannopoulos, Peter Fisher, and Marin Soljačić. 2007. "Wireless Power Transfer via Strongly Coupled Magnetic Resonances." *Science* 317 (5834): 83–86.

Lee, Suzanne. 2005. *Fashioning the Future: Tomorrow's Wardrobe.* London: Thames and Hudson.

Martin, Thomas, Mark Jones, Joshua Edmison, Tanwir Sheikh, and Zahir Nakad. 2004. "Modeling and Simulating Electronic Textile Applications." In Proceedings of ACM SIGPLAN/SIGBED conference on Languages, Compilers and Tools for Embedded Systems, June 11–13, 10–19. New York: Association for Computing Machinery (ACM).

McQuaid, Matilda (ed.). 2005. *Extreme Textiles.* London: Thames and Hudson; New York: Princeton Architectural Press.

Park, Sungmee, and Sundaresan Jayaraman. 2001. "Adaptive and Responsive Textile Structures." In Xiaoming Tao (ed.), *Smart Fibres, Fabrics and Clothing*, 226–45. Cambridge, UK: Woodhead; Boston: CRC.

Philips Electronics. 2000. *New Nomads: An Exploration of Wearable Electronics by Philips.* Rotterdam: 010 Publishers.

Robles-de-la-Torre, Gabriel. 2006. "The Importance of the Sense of Touch in Virtual and Real Environments." *IEEE Multimedia* 13 (3): 24–30.

Seymour, Sabine. 2008. *Fashionable Technology: The Intersection of Design, Fashion, Science and Technology.* Vienna: Springer.

Seymour, Sabine. 2010. *Functional Aesthetics: Visions in Fashionable Technology.* Vienna: Springer.

Van Langenhove, Lieva (ed.). 2007. *Smart Textiles for Medicine and Healthcare.* Cambridge, UK: Woodhead.

Violette, Robert (ed.). 2011. *Hussein Chalayan.* New York: Rizzoli.

Wu, J., D. Zhou, M. G. Looney, P. J. Waters, G. G. Wallace, and C. O. Too. 2009. "A Molecular Template Approach to Integration of Polyaniline into Textiles." *Synthetic Metals* 159 (12): 1135–40. http://www.sciencedirect.com/science/article/pii/S0379677909000757 (accessed February 28, 2013).

21

XS Labs: Electronic Textiles and Reactive Garments as Sociocultural Interventions

JOANNA BERZOWSKA

WEARABLE TECHNOLOGIES

Wearable technologies, in the form of electronically enabled garments and accessories, have entered mainstream consumer markets. They have emerged from decades of research and development that was mostly rooted in military, medical, and sports performance (often involving biometric monitoring and tracking applications) and include current areas of interest such as wellness, quality of life, serious play, and fitness. Numetrex is one company that produces a collection of athletic apparel with integrated textile-based electronic heart rate monitoring technology developed by Textronics in 2005.[1] These shirts and tops, used with a watch-based display, provide a more seamless and natural way to track one's heart rate when exercising, since they move with the body like a traditional sports shirt, rather than a cumbersome chest strap. Another notable product in the category of fitness and wellness monitoring is the Fitbit, a wearable device that tracks one's daily physical activity (walking, climbing steps, sleeping) and, in tandem with various mobile and online applications, allows users to track, analyze, and compare personal data, so as to change daily habits, become more active, or lose weight.[2] The applications allow users to monitor their behavior, find patterns in their data, and, by sharing their stats, to leverage the appeal of social networking. These types of activities form the basis of the recently popular "quantified self" movement, which involves collecting and tracking one's own data through hardware and software in order to improve one's quality of life and become a "better self" (*Economist* 2012). In addition, there has been demonstrable interest in wearable technologies from consumer electronics companies such as Philips, as evidenced by their patenting history, and from experimental fashion designers such as Hussein Chalayan, as seen in his runway shows, but the true and full potential of wearable technologies as sociocultural artifacts is yet to be truly unleashed, outside of the context of research labs. The field of wearable technology is still, in my opinion, too firmly anchored in the tradition of consumer electronics, with narrow definitions of functionality, which does not include more esoteric and poetic expressive forms, more easily explored in a research context.

XS LABS

XS Labs has been active since 2002 as a design research studio with a focus on innovation in electronic textiles and reactive garments. The lab is located within the Faculty of Fine Arts at Concordia University, where I am a professor and chair of the design and computation arts program. I work with students, both graduate and undergraduate, from a variety of disciplines that include fibers, design, computation arts, computer science, and studio arts. We experiment with various design and research methods: some that approximate art practice or industrial design, some that are inspired by research models from engineering and materials science. Our research is supported by a wide range of funding agencies, including the Canada Council for the Arts, the National Sciences and Engineering Research Council of Canada, the Hexagram Institute for Research/Creation in Media Arts and Technologies, the Canada Foundation for Innovation, the Social Sciences and Humanities Research Council of Canada, and Canadian Heritage Fonds québécois de recherche sur la société et la culture.

The range of XS Labs projects described in this chapter include several research directions and specifically address social and cultural concerns that emerge from the integration of computational and electronic forms on the human body. It is important to note that many practitioners in this field have arrived either from a traditional textile or fashion background or from a traditional consumer electronics background. What shaped XS Labs, however, was not a history or practice in weaving, fashion design, or even fiber arts. It emerged from a concern with the lack of "softness" in human–computer interaction (HCI) and the desire to explore and exploit a wider range of material properties in the development of physical interfaces. HCI is a field of research and practice in computer science that focuses on the interfaces between people (referred to as users) and computers. It is often regarded as the intersection of computer science, cognitive science, and human factors engineering (Carroll 2009). "The original and abiding technical focus of HCI was and is the concept of usability. . . . However, inside HCI the concept of usability has been re-articulated and reconstructed almost continually, and has become increasingly rich and intriguingly problematic. Usability now often subsumes qualities like fun, well being, collective efficacy, aesthetic tension, enhanced creativity, flow, support for human development, and others" (Carroll 2009).

My own interest in electronic textiles grew out of a desire to raise concerns with aesthetics, personal expression, and critique, as opposed to the prevalent utilitarian focus of wearable technology design on universal connectivity and productivity applications.

BEYOND-THE-WRIST INTERACTION

In the 1990s, we foresaw the exciting potential of electronic textiles for their ability to conform to the human body and bring softness to physical interfaces. Most work conducted in HCI at that time focused on tangible interaction and involved the manipulation of physical objects with the human hand. We anticipated that electronic textiles would be one of the building blocks that would allow us to expand the realm of physical interaction into a wearable, everyday context and to explore the boundaries of what XS Labs calls "beyond-the-wrist" interaction. Indeed, the boundaries of the tangible evolved over time to include embedded as well as embodied interaction.

As researchers and designers in this new field, we find satisfaction in the fact that Mark Weiser's (1991) prophetic vision of ubiquitous computing has largely become reality, and computing technology is truly receding into the background of our awareness. At the same time, we need to realize that much work remains to be done and that, especially, the relationship between computational technologies and design practices needs to evolve. The research directions that shape the field of HCI are still too often predicated on traditional definitions of computers and their intended uses. They do not consider the broad range of computational expression, technologies, and materials available to designers today.

In recent history, accelerating progress in all branches of scientific research has been redefining our fundamental design materials (Addington and Schodek 2005). Materials such as conductive fibers, reactive inks, photoelectrics, and shape-memory alloys are already shaping new physical forms and new experiences that are redefining our relationship with materiality and with technology (Coelho et al. 2007). Our design philosophy at XS Labs focuses on the use of these new materials and technologies as fundamental design elements.

The projects at XS Labs often demonstrate a preoccupation with—and a resistance to—task-based, utilitarian definitions of functionality in HCI. Our definition of *function* simultaneously looks at the materiality and the magic of computing technologies; it incorporates the concepts of beauty and pleasure. We are particularly concerned with the exploration of interactive forms that emphasize the natural expressive qualities of "transitive materials," a new class of responsive materials that bridge, physically and computationally, the distinctions designers traditionally make between form and function, or structures and membranes, and that "blur the gap between computation and structure, . . . and between disciplines that have traditionally stood apart" (Coelho et al. 2007: 1). We focus on the aesthetics of interaction, which compels us to interrogate and recontextualize the materials themselves. The interaction narratives function as entry points to question some of the fundamental assumptions we make about the technologies and the materials that drive our designs.

A core component of our research at XS Labs involves the development of enabling technologies, methods, and materials—in the form of soft electronic circuits and composite fibers—as well as the exploration of the expressive potential of soft reactive structures. Many of our electronic textile innovations are informed by the technical and the cultural history of how textiles have been made for generations—weaving, stitching, embroidering, knitting, beading, or quilting—but use a range of materials with different electromechanical properties. We consider the soft, playful, and magical aspects of these materials, so as to better adapt them to the contours of the human body and the complexities of human needs and desires. Our approach often engages subtle elements of the absurd, the perverse, and the transgressive. We construct narratives that involve dark humor and romanticism as a way to drive design innovation. These integrative approaches allow us to construct composite textiles with complex functionality and sophisticated behaviors.

Research labs and experimental design collectives have been exploring the social and cultural dimensions of wearable technologies, delving into areas such as memory representation, tactile communication, remote intimacy, and social critique. What makes wearable technology unique is that it can be customized to be truly individual, it is ultimately portable, it can be used (and misused) in private, and it ultimately will allow us do the things we like to do in certain places and with certain people, while being remotely located. Because this work is inherently multidisciplinary, the multiplicity of research methods, which include empirical as well as design-led explorations, has given rise to a rich landscape of wearable technology projects. This landscape includes the more traditional concerns with productivity and task-based applications but, more important, also allows artists and designers to highlight the more subtle, complex, and potentially problematic qualities of these materials and technologies. Projects such as Memory Rich Clothing from XS Labs both push the boundaries of technical possibilities while at the same time asking crucial critical questions about the implementations of these technologies. Our overarching research themes include (a) transitive materials and soft electronics, (b) textiles as dynamic displays (color and shape changes, sensing fabric substrates), (c) conceptual explorations (history and memory, pattern and repetition), (d) parasitic power (human-generated power), (e) fiber-scale functionality, and (f) programming materiality. This chapter focuses on a subset of our work, dealing more specifically with memory, communication, power, and discomfort.

MEMORY REPRESENTATION AND SURVEILLANCE

One of the important research concerns at XS Labs focuses on the ever-evolving concept of memory. We love to collect and store not only physical possessions but also disembodied memories in the form of experiences, in order to create mementos, diaries, and personal as well as shared histories. With the remarkable contemporary advances in potential memory-storage capacity, we need to ask ourselves some serious questions about our design approaches and the creative capacities of the "memory-rich" devices and materials that we create. What models of memory and mind are used in designing and creating technologies that remember? And, most important, how do we include the need, capacity, and desire to forget?

One approach is to step away from the disembodied model of memory implicit in memory-storage devices such as memory sticks and the representation of memories through digital artifacts such as digital photos cross-referenced in Facebook and to look at embodied models of memory: how physical memories are represented in the world. Physical artifacts such as garments become stained, worn, torn, or scratched over time. They accumulate traces of use and carry the evidence of our identity and our history (Berzowska 2005b).

The idea that a trace acquired in past experience somehow represents that experience, or carries information about it, is at the heart of representative realism in the philosophy of memory. This has been the dominant view of memory in modern philosophy of mind, and it is assumed in much work on memory in cognitive science (Sutton 2004). How can we scratch the surface of the digital spaces that we now inhabit, so as to leave personal histories and stories? How do the technologies that we use allow us to remember, and what do they allow us to remember? How do our own devices decide what is worth remembering? Contextual factors are important, but how do we define context?

MEMORY RICH CLOTHING

The Memory Rich Clothing (MRC) series of projects from 2002 to 2006 focused on the development of reactive garments that display their physical memory or "history of use." The term *physical memory* is used to describe spatial and tactile memory inherent in experiencing things through the body. Garments build up physical memory insofar as they retain some traces of the presence of the user, through the accumulation of sweat, hair, stains, or tears. They sense and record personal histories that can be communicated visually or through other senses. Our primary objective was to produce garments that show personal data, such as where and when they have last been touched, including subtle evidence of intimate contact (Berzowska 2005b).

The MRC dresses explored touch, embodied intimacy, and the technical implementation and construction of visually reactive substrates for manipulating use data on a textile. The conceptual framework consisted of the gathering and displaying of intimate touch events but also explored social choreographies that emerge when bodies actively inhabit identical reactive costumes. Wearable artifacts, by virtue of the fact that they are worn on the body, are a very intimate technology. Social and cultural changes are implicit in any new technology. The project explored the idea of wearable technologies that encourage physical touch and contribute to creating embodied as opposed to virtual proximity between people. Examples such as the Hug Shirt by CuteCircuit and the Love Jackets by Despina Papadopoulos both promote physical (haptic and visual) displays of intimacy (Quinn 2010: 29; see chapter 20 in this volume). The Hug Shirt, developed by Francesca Rosella and Ryan Genz, allows the sensation of a hug to be communicated and recreated over a distance. "Embedded in the shirt there are sensors that feel the strength of the touch, the skin warmth and the heartbeat rate of the sender and actuators that recreate the sensation of touch, warmth and emotion of the hug to the shirt of the distant loved one."[3] The Love Jackets by Despina Papadopoulos similarly allow for physical displays of affection but also set the stage for imagining new patterns of communication and social interaction. Each jacket emits a particular infrared signal (a technology used for remote control devices). The partner jacket can recognize the specific frequency when its paired garment is in sight and in range (no more than ten feet [three meters] apart, facing each other). The jackets then emit a sound and a pattern of lights (Quinn 2010: 29). Embrace-Me, another project by the Papadopoulos-owned Studio 5050, features a hoodie overprinted with a conductive silver logo, which acts as a switch and connection between two garments. "When two people wearing the hoodies embrace they actually power each other up through that pattern. The symbolic energy transfer becomes fully actualized and the embrace is instantly translated into an explosion of light and sound."[4]

SPOTTY, FEATHERY, AND INTIMATE

Several pieces within the MRC series specifically address physical memory and the physical display of intimate communications, but from a critical point of view rather than a utilitarian one: the Spotty Dresses, Feathery Dresses, and the Intimate Memory Shirt & Skirt. The first are light cotton dresses overprinted with an irregular pattern of thermochromic spots, based on animal camouflage patterns. Thermochromic ink changes color at various temperatures, and the inks used for these particular dresses become transparent when heated to thirty-two degrees Celsius, the average temperature of a human hand at a comfortable ambient temperature. The dresses remember traces of presence, in the form of physical touch, and show when and where a garment—and the body that wears it—has been touched. Body contact—whether touching, rubbing, or pressing the fabric against the wearers' bodies or the bodies of another—makes the inks change color and effectively disappear, so that direct physical contact erases the pattern. Metaphorically, this refers to an erasure of social camouflage, which is enabled by digital technologies that promote intimacy but disappears when that intimacy is enacted. The end result is that physical touch strips us of our camouflage, and, to continue the metaphor, our naked selves are revealed.

The Feathery Dresses are embellished with three touch sensors (soft, conductive textile switches) that record touch events. These events act as input into the simple program running on the microcontroller integrated in the garment and affect the pattern of illuminated feathers embroidered on the dress. Each sensitive area on the dress is directly mapped to illuminate a different area of feathers. The microcontroller allows us to use much less conductive material in the body of the dresses and reduces failure rates due to broken connections. It also allows us to experiment with different representations, behaviors, and timing to explore different interaction models relating touch and illumination. Both the Spotty and Feathery Dresses were completed during a 2004 residency with Sara Diamond, thematically related to her CodeZebra project, built to facilitate debates between artists and scientists and based on a visual aesthetic that draws from zoomorphic imagery. "The CodeZebra Project was inspired by shape shifting, a form of ritual where humans perform animal identities in ritual contexts to challenge social roles" (Diamond 2009: 216). These animal identities, referencing camouflage (hiding and revealing) as well as emotions that include fear, desire, and anticipation, allowed us to explore critical aspects of the physical representation of intimate events rather than presenting the projects as product prototypes. The performative and playful environment allowed us to build a more complex narrative fostered by the critical and exploratory approaches to the notions of digital communication and physical intimacy.

The Intimate Memory Shirt & Skirt was our first experiment in MRC. The outfit consists of a shirt and a skirt that employ two different input and output methodologies to record acts of physical intimacy and indicate the time elapsed since those intimacy events occurred. The shirt deploys a microphone in the collar and a series of light-emitting diodes (LEDs) stitched in a curved line across the front. When someone whispers something into the wearer's ear, or blows on the wearer's neck, the shirt lights up, showing that an intimacy event has occurred. The number of lights represents the intensity of the intimacy event, similar to the volume indicator on a stereo. Over time, the lights turn off, one by one, to show the time elapsed since the event took place. The skirt incorporates soft switches, sewn out of conductive metallic silk organza and connected with conductive threads to a stitched analog circuit. When the wearer is touched, regardless of the context of the touch, LEDs illuminate in the embroidery to register the intimacy event. In a similar fashion to how our skin registers touch, the illumination fades over time to indicate the time elapsed since the event. The light registers not only intensity but also the way in which the event unfolds over time. This project allowed us to develop a multitude of scenarios, from the most "positive," which positioned the garment as a disco product, to the most "negative," which involved inappropriate and violent touch. Because of the overtly sexual nature of touching someone's thighs, this garment highlights the fact that many memory technologies are invasive:

> Most people remark that they would not want their partners to see that they had been groped by someone else. They claim that this information, and this physical memory, is a private one, it is a memory that they might not want to share with others. This piece reveals ways in which our actions and our personal histories can be recorded, stored, and displayed. It highlights aspects of surveillance that we are often happy to forget when dealing with more conventional wearable technologies. Many people do not question issues of surveillance and loss of privacy implicit in the deployment of wearable technologies, whatever they may be. (Berzowska 2005b: 34)

BIOMETRICS AND MEMORY

In an information-saturated world, increased memory storage and pervasive distributed computational architectures promise instantaneous access to shared stored information. The sensing infrastructure necessary to implement this vision presents many challenges to computer science; the sheer amount of data challenges the human mind. From a neurological standpoint, the semantic and episodic memory systems are each considered to be "essentially unlimited in their capacity" (Emilien 2004: 27). From a personal position, each of us recognizes the extreme stress of living in a perpetual data avalanche. Our mental structures require digital augmentation, yet our essence requires tactility, effervescence, and the spontaneous.

In psychology and philosophy, the term *memory* is used to refer to the diverse set of cognitive capacities by which we retain information and reconstruct past experiences. Some memories are encoded through language, others through images, sounds, or smells. In many ways, memory—our ability to invoke past episodes of our lives—is both familiar and puzzling. It differs from perception or imagination, because we remember experiences and events that actually happened but are not happening at the present moment (Sutton 2004).

Humans, as research into false memories has undeniably shown, also remember things that did not necessarily happen (Schacter 2001). Humans construct memories. All major cultural initiatives since prehistory can be interpreted in the light of the human instinct to preserve events from extinction. Wearable technologies are the contemporary representatives on that continuum. There are two main ways that memory is constructed in the mobile and social media industry: those devices that help capture, store, and retrieve data and those that help to manage these ingredients into a subsequent story. We all share a universal need to create and collect experiences, since these very experiences form the core of our social glue: they enable us to connect and to engage one another.

To allow more flexibility in our investigations of physical memory, integrating biometric data, we developed the Octopus modules: compact, body-worn displays that support a range of possible interactions. Several devices, approximately five to fifteen, are affixed to a single person, using magnetic snaps that can be attached and rearranged on a reconfigurable garment substrate. Three types of events can be sensed using the Octopus modules: body movement (an accelerometer detects shaking and tilting; thus simple changes in posture or gait can be detected), contact (a capacitive sensor and an infrared reflectance sensor detect the contact of hands or objects with the front surface), and communications (the devices can interact over the line of sight using an infrared remote control protocol).

Finally, we created the BUG module: a brooch that attaches to the body and travels through the world, recording events such as touch, the movement of the body during the course of the day, and changing levels of illumination in the environment. The BUG is constructed of two very different kinds of materials. Its shell and enclosure are crafted by a metalsmith out of silver. Its "brain" is engineered out of electronic components on a printed circuit board. The electronics integrate a light sensor, a touch sensor, and a movement sensor, as well as a microcontroller. The BUG can record its history of use (or history of interaction), and when attached to a conductive textile substrate, it will beam/communicate this data to a central microcontroller, which will then represent the data. The textile is embroidered with highly conductive tracks, which allow the BUG to attach with its legs and draw electricity as well as communicate the sensor data. Each BUG senses and remembers

- how the body moves and shakes during the day (accelerometer);
- how much light a person is exposed to during the day (photo sensor); and
- whether it has been touched (capacitive sensor).

These biometric data can potentially help us address the questions within the current wave of mobile devices (no longer the "calm technology" of Mark Weiser, the wave is being described as "continuous computing") about defining the ways that memories are captured, stored, cataloged, parsed, represented, and retrieved. The challenges will not be technical but will involve the social and cultural aspects of memory creation, because the term *memory* should not be defined solely as a collection of biometric data. There are many ways to think of memory, including genetic memory, cultural memory, personal histories, or the rewriting of history.

POWER AND DISCOMFORT

The 2005 Constellation Dresses and the Leeches raise specific questions regarding our increasing need for power—electric energy—to feed the electronic devices we wear on our bodies and will soon be integrating into our electronic garments. These projects address ecological concerns through the design of garments that directly tackle issues of power consumption and sustainability through the exploration of different parasitic metaphors, where electronic modules suck power from our bodies and electronic garments suck power from each other. Central to this exploration are the questions: where does power come from in a wearable context, and how do we connect to various power sources?

The Constellation Dresses are covered with twelve magnetic snaps arranged over the torso and thighs and connected in pairs through a single line of conductive thread. LEDs are integrated into the dresses in a design that resembles a constellation, with a cluster of stars connected to each other through short and straight lines. One set of snaps acts as a switch for the LED circuit; when connected to the snaps from another dress, the circuit on the garment is closed and the LEDs light up. The magnetic snaps act as a mechanical and electrical connection between bodies, and their irregular placement induces wearers to create playful and compelling choreographies to connect their circuits.

Rather than being complete and functional electronic pieces in themselves, the Constellation Dresses work as meshes on a circuit network and depend on the physical contact of the magnetic snaps to function. By bringing people together mechanically and electronically, the garments explore metaphors for building electronic or social networks. In addition, the dresses compel people to draw power from each other, hinting at a parasitic model for powering our mobile technologies.[5]

The Leeches dress, constructed with stitched conductive organza stripes, functions as a soft, wearable, and reconfigurable power-distribution substrate for attaching individual silicone-coated electronic modules that illuminate the dress. The Leeches can be attached in a variety of positions and configurations. They are held in place by magnetic snaps, which act as both mechanical and electrical connections. A single power module can be attached at the shoulder. This module can power up to ten Leeches scattered around the body. The red LEDs inside the Leeches resemble power-hungry creatures that, once attached, suck or draw power (the metaphoric "blood") from the body and reference the potential dangers of electromagnetic fields emanating from electronic garments (Figure 21.1).[6]

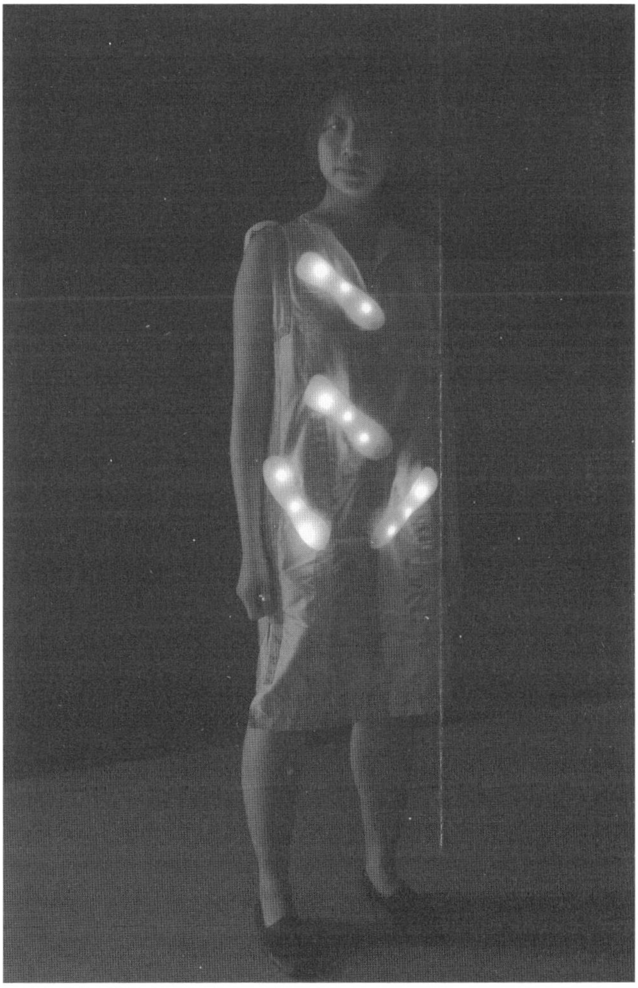

FIGURE 21.1 Leeches dress by Joanna Berzowska, 2004. The electronic modules are attached to the Leeches garment, which feeds them power so they can illuminate red. Photograph by Hugues Bruyère. *Credit*: Courtesy of Joanna Berzowska.

Captain Electric is XS Labs' most complex project exploring this research direction. Completed in 2010, it is a collection of three garments that passively harness energy from the body but also allow active power generation by the user. They convert kinetic energy from the human body into electric energy. Continuing fashion's historic relationship between discomfort and style, the electronic dresses restrict the body and, through mechanical constraints, produce sufficient energy to actuate light and sound events. Rather than attempting to conceal the generators and their operation, they overtly integrate them into the concept and design. The group Itchy, Sticky, and Stiff comprises three garments that conceptually reference safety apparel and personal protection as well as our fears of natural disasters and other states of emergency, personal phobias, anxieties, and paranoia (Berzowska et al. 2010a, 2010b; Figure 21.2).

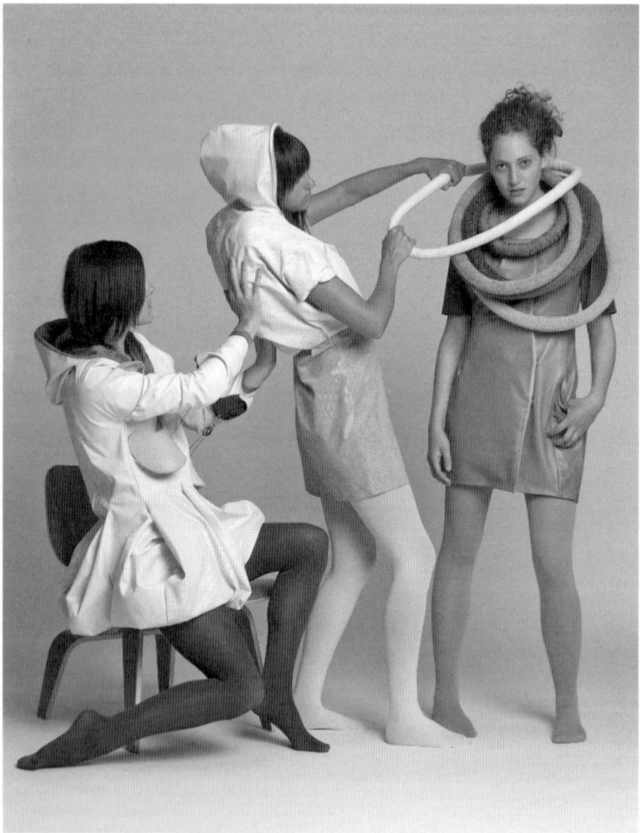

FIGURE 21.2 Sticky, Stiff, and Itchy. From Captain Electric by Joanna Berzowska with Marc Beaulieu, Anne-Marie Laflamme, Gaïa Orain, and Vincent Leclerc, 2009.
Credit: Photograph by Guillaume Pelletier. Courtesy of Joanna Berzowska.

Sticky is a hooded leather dress that impedes natural body movement by restricting the arms, keeping them close to the body. This restriction forces the body to move in more pronounced motions, actively generating energy to fuel the dress, to feed a series of LEDs integrated in silicone forms sewn into the pocket, concealed from view (Figure 21.3). When the futility of the effort compels stillness, a gentle phosphorescent glow remains. The tailored leather silhouette of the Itchy dress is decorated with large reconfigurable wool necklaces that disturb the body because they are, literally, itchy. One of the necklaces is attached to a power generator, while a smaller one is augmented with a series of LEDs, illuminating the wearer's face. The pattern of the lights that rotate around the neckline of the dress is reminiscent of safety buoys, lighthouses, and emergency sirens. The individual's discomfort and nervous energy perversely direct attention to her face. Reminiscent of the posture caused by muscular stiffness, the silhouette of Stiff draws emphasis to the individual's back and shoulders. As she attempts to straighten her back, the energy that is generated activates a speaker integrated into the hood, which plays soothing and comforting (though often conflicting) messages, in an effort to reduce social and personal anxiety.[7]

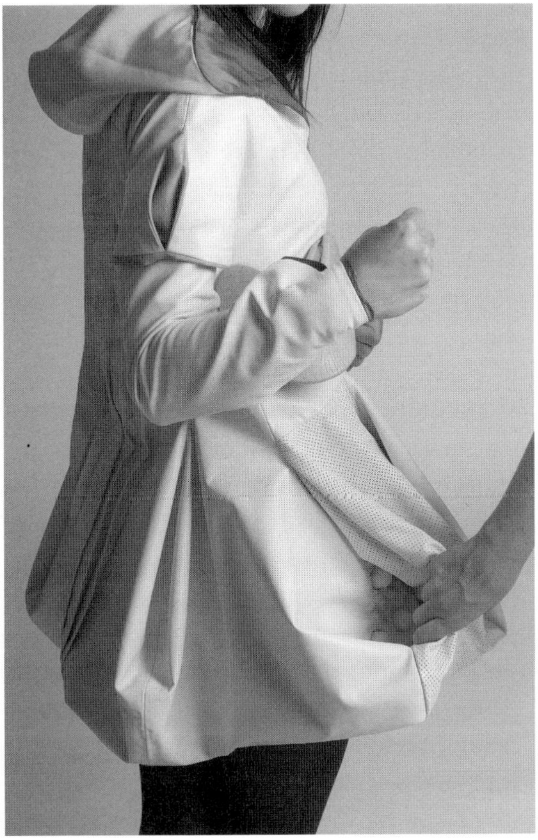

FIGURE 21.3 Detail of the leather Sticky dress showing hidden silicone forms containing LEDs that glow with blue light, 2009.
Credit: Photograph by Guillaume Pelletier. Courtesy of Joanna Berzowska.

AUGMENTING THE BODY AND COMMUNICATION

Social networking technologies (which have traditionally been situated on the body in the form of uniforms, fashion, and decorations) have become disembodied in recent years. Social networking companies such as Facebook, YouTube, Flickr, and Blogger have deployed new environments for constructing our identities, personal and collective, on networked devices. Through several XS Labs projects, we have been exploring how these social networks can, once again, move back onto the body through electronic textiles and responsive garments.

The SMOKS, for instance, are a pair of electronically enhanced suits, an experimental platform for constructing individual and collective memories, for creating and nurturing social networks, and for engaging in personal communication and intimacy. They capture physical memories, represent traces of human touch, record and play sounds, and provide hiding places for physical mementos. In my opinion, the whole point of making a technology wearable is to render it individual and personal, comfortable, and efficient. The only reason to make a technology soft and worn on the body is to allow us to do something more efficiently, in more comfort, and alone. The future of wearable technologies is deeply centered in the social and cultural sphere. The future of "smart textiles" is to do what "dumb textiles" have been doing (with incredible success) for generations but to do it remotely and perhaps in seclusion. "Dumb textiles" have been very successful throughout history and across different cultures in communicating many (both subtle and overt) aspects of our personal and cultural identities. "We have learned to use garments effectively to hide, reveal, and distort the self that we present to the world. We use fashion to express social, cultural, economic, religious, sexual, and professional aspects of our identity, among others" (Berzowska 2005b: 35). Garments "also collect and reflect some of our most intimate moments and are marked by our sweat, food stains, and tears" (Berzowska 2005a: 61).

Garments will soon become the new playground for digital social networking technologies, as software slowly seeps off mobile phones and into (for example) illuminated zippers that display when you have been "poked" on Facebook, flowers that open and close to reveal the status of your social relationships, or furry spots that appear when a new post has been uploaded. The future is social. We want to know when our friends are thinking about us, and we want to show this information to those around us. We want to show off our social networks in the same way we like to show off brand names and labels. We want to integrate some of our networked personas back into our physical reality.

The much sought-after "killer application" will not involve reading e-mail on my sleeve, increasing my productivity by receiving vibrating reminders of my appointments in my jacket, or keeping track of my calorie intake through my necklace. Those are specialized applications that are not social nor personal in a meaningful way. One of the important futures for electronic textiles and wearable technologies is to perpetuate the "function" of fashion: to have fun, to connect with friends, and to bring social networking information back onto the body, exploring the emotional resonance of personal space. XS Labs projects experiment in that space, by presenting garments that can change shape, make sounds, or display messages in ways that are reminiscent of social technologies but truly embodied and material.

The 2004 XS Labs Inflatable Distract Dress contains a network of interconnected bulges. Influenced by animals such as the puffer fish, which inflate by pumping water into special sacs when in their natural environment, and air when out of water, the dress can be mouth-inflated to intimidate and confuse the "enemy" (e.g., unwanted attention). The Inflatable Reclaim Dress deploys two large silicone inflatable balloons placed at the hips, which can be inflated with a portable bottle of compressed air to increase needed personal space. In a crowded situation, or in a situation where more personal privacy is required, the dress can be inflated to create a (personal) physical buffer between the wearer and public space.[8]

The Accouphène tuxedo, a 2006 XS Labs project, is decorated with thirteen soft textile speakers, created by embroidering decorative coils of highly conductive yarn on the front of the jacket. The coils are connected to a central circuit, which sends pulses of energy through the coils. Sounds are generated when the sleeve of Accouphène, which contains a magnet, is moved over the coils. The speaker coils, when powered, generate a weak magnetic field that reacts to a strong magnet. The magnet's strength and its distance from the embroidered coil determine the amplitude of the sounds. By electronically pulsing the embroidered coils at different frequencies, Accouphène can play different notes. As such, Accouphène creates a three-dimensional sonic environment around the human body that can be activated and modulated through hand movement.[9]

The 2003 project Blazer, developed by Vincent Leclerc, is a light-emitting bracelet integrated in the cuff of a very long striped sleeve. Text can be displayed in space by moving the arm or the whole body. This simple emissive display takes advantage of retinal persistence to create visual images (in this case, typography) as the viewer makes sense of an apparently random pattern of flashing lights. When the body is still, we see noise. When the body is in motion, the noise becomes a message: text is displayed.[10]

The SoundSleeves is a 2003 XS Labs project consisting of a set of disembodied sleeves, joined at the back and covered with conductive strips of silver metallic organza. The sleeves react to movement and physical contact. When users flex or cross their arms, a sound is synthesized within the sleeves and output through miniature flat speakers. The strips, when considered as a whole, are in fact a body-scale flex sensor that controls the sounds. This simple design illustrates the possible emergent behaviors of many soft switches, which, when dispersed on the body, can be deployed to create a larger wearable sensate surface. SoundSleeves augment our natural body language with sound. They become an extension of the body: when our body language is tense and protective (crossing our arms, for instance), the pitch of the sounds becomes higher, as if signaling danger. When our body language is more relaxed, the pitch shifts down, becoming more comfortable, like the purring of a cat.[11]

EXPRESSIVE COMPUTATIONAL FORMS

Other projects that seek to engage the whole body through physical transformation include XS Labs' work with shape-memory alloys, most notably Nitinol. Kukkia and Vilkas, from 2005, were XS Labs' first kinetic electronic garments (Berzowska and Coelho 2005c). The Kukkia flowers around the face slowly open and close, like a caress. It is an expressive and behavioral kinetic sculpture that develops a visceral relationship with the wearer. Vilkas is a dress with a kinetic hemline that rises to reveal the knee and lower thigh. The hemline is programmed to rise autonomously, not in response to any external or internal input. This initiates a physical conversation between the wearer and the garment, as they fight over control of the body's real estate. Developed a year later, Skorpions is a set of more complex kinetic electronic garments with anthropomorphic qualities, referencing parasites that inhabit the skin of the host. These dresses are not "interactive" artifacts in the usual sense of the word but instead reference the history of garments as objects of discomfort and desire. Their programming does not respond to sensor data but exploits emotional and affective characteristics such as control, anticipation, and unpredictability (Berzowska and Mainstone 2008; Figure 21.4).

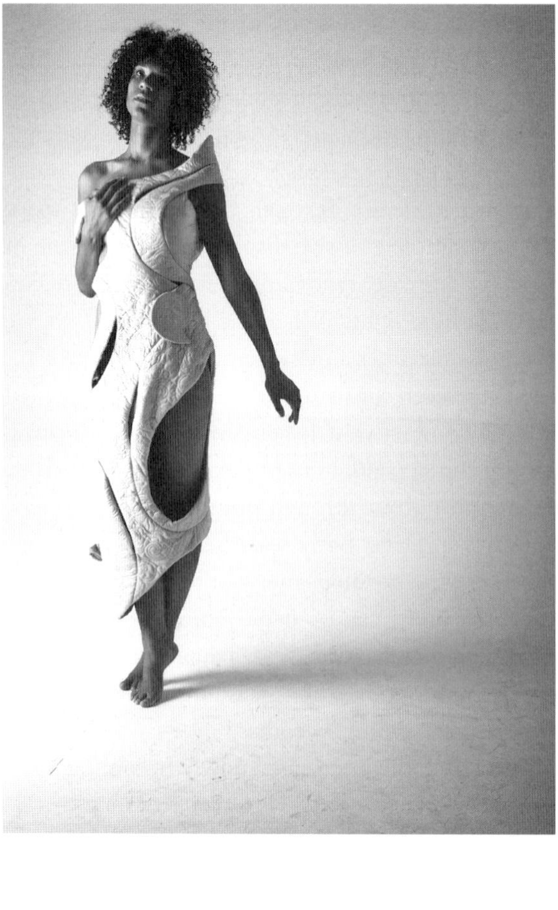

FIGURE 21.4 Luttergill from Skorpions by Joanna Berzowska with Di Mainstone, 2007. The Skorpions dresses "breathe" and pulse, controlled by their own internal programming. They are not "interactive" artifacts; they are living, behavioral kinetic sculptures that exploit characteristics such as control, anticipation, and unpredictability. *Credit*: Photograph by Nico Stinghe. Courtesy of Joanna Berzowska.

The future of computational forms will be enabled by the development of new textiles, through the development of new fibers and composite materials with more complex functionality. These may include fibers that collect energy from the body and from the environment and that are able to store this energy (like a battery or a capacitor) but also to use kinetic or electric energy to transform themselves: to move, change color, or change shape. Indeed, since 2009, we have been working with Professor Maksim Skorobogatiy from the Polytechnique de Montreal to develop this new generation of composite fibers and textiles. We are using complex manufacturing techniques to create fibers made up of multiple layers of polymers, which, when stretched and drawn out to a small diameter, begin to interact at the nanoscale, known as photonic band gap fibers. Such fibers exploit changes in energy to change their own visual properties. The goal of this project, entitled Karma Chameleon, is to develop a prototype for an all-fiber-based textile that can harness, sense, and display energy. One of the first prototypes is the PLEET dress, in which the woven photonic elements create different patterns and textures when illuminated (Berzowska 2011). We developed the Sparkl panels that change in response to the angle and intensity of light, both transmitted and reflected, in their design, creating illusions of depth. Different layers of imagery and color are revealed. The panels are woven on a computer-controlled electronic Jacquard loom with cotton, linen, and photonic band gap fibers that reflect one color when side-illuminated with ambient light and emit a different color when transmitting white light. We can dynamically change the color of an individual fiber by controlling the relative intensity of guided and ambient light (Figure 21.5).

The core technical innovation in this work involves shifting this functionality entirely within the fiber itself, which, conceptually, constitutes a radical deviation from the dominant model of a textile substrate with attached mechano-electronics to that of a seamless composite material (Berzowska and Skorobogatiy 2010). The concept of "programming materiality" refers to the use of these new materials, where seemingly simple decisions such as cutting two-fifths of an inch (one centimeter) to the left or to the right of the seam will alter the very behavior of that material. Imagine a textile that changes color when we cut it, where the shape of a pattern piece will control the speed at which it curls up, or where a stitch can be used to connect two circuit components together to make a larger sensor array. This new materiality, which includes the computational, is what we talk about when we attempt to define "transitive materials" (Coelho et al. 2007). The future must be integrated, as discussed at a recent conference on tangible and embedded interaction:

> Designers need to consider the programmatic behavior of each material when making aesthetic decisions. The two can never again exist independently from one another. One of our great opportunities... is to define a new language for talking about materiality, interactivity, and physical interaction design. This new language should integrate performative concepts so as to provide roadmaps for the training of future designers who will unquestionably be working with materials that not only drive behavior through their physical properties but also through their computational nature. (Berzowska 2012: 24)

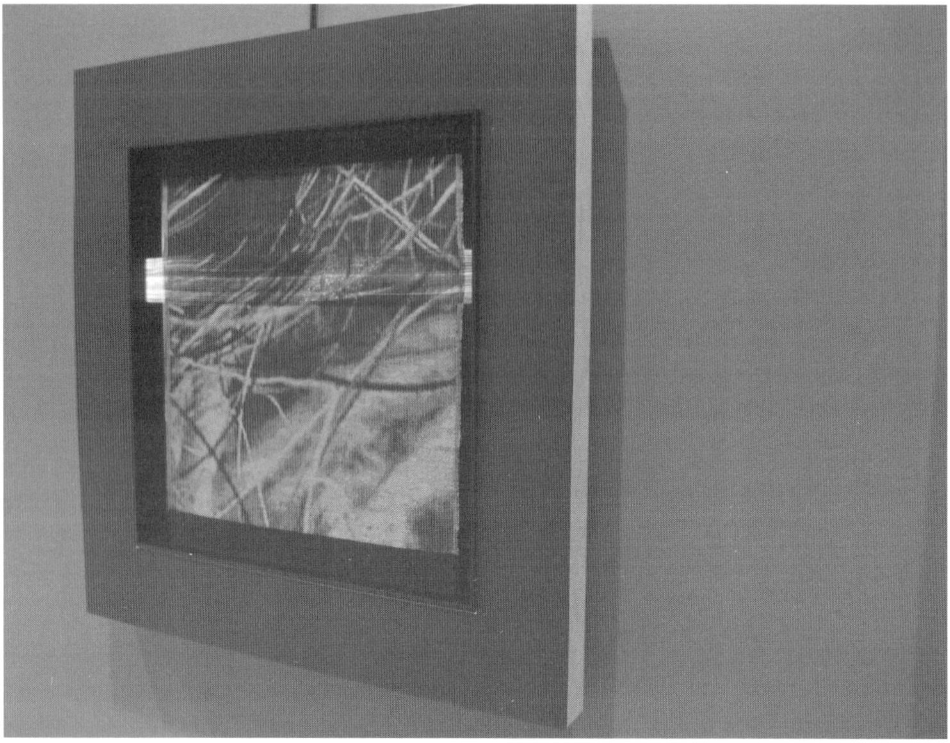

FIGURE 21.5 Sparkl panel by Joanna Berzowska in collaboration with Maksim Skorobogatiy, 2011. Sparkl panels change in response to the angle and intensity of light, both transmitted and reflected, in their design, creating illusions of depth. The tangled imagery contrasts the orthogonal weave structures and suggests a seaside landscape where the reflected and transmitted light collapses sea and grass, creating dynamic ripples.
Credit: Courtesy of Joanna Berzowska.

FROM RESEARCH TO CONSUMERS

The research lab allows us to develop work that is poetic and exploratory and that functions as both technology research and sociocultural intervention. It is challenging to move beyond the academic context and transition into a space where we develop consumer products that embody some of these questions and respond to some larger research themes, including augmenting the body, communication, biometrics, memory, power, and discomfort. Since the beginning of 2012, I have been consulting for the company OM Signal, developing wearable technology products that focus on wellness and well-being. OM Signal aims to be the first-ever bio-lifestyle company. This approach is influenced by the fact that over 20 million Americans practice yoga, a fivefold increase in a mere decade, and countless others seek greater health and well-being through other activities. Responding to the growing need in our society to find balance in our lives, through the concepts of wellness and well-being, the first product will be a designer shirt that is continually connected with the iPhone. The shirt tracks various biosignatures from the body and provides feedback. It tracks events through textile-based sensors and provides a few insightful indicators of health and well-being, including (a) the relative state of well-being or arousal (indirect measure of autonomic system), (b) heart rhythms (including full electrocardiogram signature), (c) breathing rhythms (including full respiration), and (d) activity level (from accelerometer). Through the iPhone, OM Signal offers a variety of engaging biofeedback to help (a) improve your well-being, (b) increase self-knowledge, (c) achieve greater self-mastery, and (d) reduce stress. The development team includes experts from the fields of software engineering, medicine and physiology, biosignal processing, machine learning, fashion, and design. Inspired by the "quantified self" movement, we aim to deploy the full promise of wearable technologies as sociocultural artifacts by challenging HCI assumptions about utility and productivity, while trying to focus on a more complex and nuanced definition of functionality. This is the future of wearable technologies, a future where the definition of usability is no longer dictated by traditional HCI priorities and where the full potential of human expression can be achieved.

NOTES

1. Numetrex, http://www.numetrex.com/ (accessed November 16, 2012).
2. Fitbit, http://www.fitbit.com/ (accessed November 16, 2012).
3. "Hug Shirt," CuteCircuit website, http://www.cutecircuit.com/hug-shirt/ (accessed November 16, 2012).
4. "Embrace-Me," Studio5050 website, http://www.5050ltd.com/embrace_me.php (accessed November 16, 2012).
5. XS Labs, http://www.xslabs.net/constellation/constellations.html (accessed November 24, 2012).
6. XS Labs, http://www.xslabs.net/constellation/leeches.html (accessed November 16, 2012).
7. Captain Electric, http://captain-electric.net/ (accessed November 16, 2012).
8. XS Labs, http://www.xslabs.net/work-pages/distract.html; http://www.xslabs.net/work-pages/reclaim.html.
9. XS Labs, http://www.xslabs.net/acouphene.
10. Blazer, http://www.uttermatter.com/blazer/012 (accessed November 16, 2012).
11. XS Labs, http://www.uttermatter.com/sleeev/.

BIBLIOGRAPHY

Addington, Michelle, and Daniel L. Schodek. 2005. *Smart Materials and Technologies for the Architecture and Design Professions.* Oxford: Architectural Press.

Berzowska, Joanna. 2005a. "Electronic Textiles: Wearable Computers, Reactive Fashion, and Soft Computation." *Textile: The Journal of Cloth and Culture* 3 (1): 58–75.

Berzowska, Joanna. 2005b. "Memory Rich Clothing: Second Skins That Communicate Physical Memory." In Linda Candy (ed.), *Proceedings of the 5th Conference on Creativity and Cognition,* 32–40. New York: Association for Computing Machinery (ACM).

Berzowska, Joanna. 2011. "PLEET: Light-Emitting Electronic Garment." *Fashion Practice: The Journal of Design, Creative Process and the Fashion Industry* 3 (1): 11–28.

Berzowska, Joanna. 2012. "Programming Materiality." In Stephen N. Spencer (ed.), *Proceedings of the Sixth International Conference on Tangible, Embedded and Embodied Interaction (TEI '12),* 23–24. New York: Association for Computing Machinery (ACM).

Berzowska, Joanna, and Marcelo Coelho. 2005. "Kukkia and Vilkas: Kinetic Electronic Garments." In Eiji Shimizu and Masatsugu Kidode (eds.), *Proceedings of the Ninth IEEE International Symposium on Wearable Computers (ISWC '05),* 82–85. Washington, DC: IEEE Computer Society.

Berzowska, Joanna, and Di Mainstone. 2008. "Skorpions: Kinetic Electronic Garments." In Lina Yamaguchi (ed.), *ACM SIGGRAPH 2008 Art Gallery (SIGGRAPH '08),* 92. New York: Association for Computing Machinery (ACM).

Berzowska, Joanna, and Maksim Skorobogatiy. 2010. "Karma Chameleon: Bragg Fiber Jacquard-Woven Photonic Textiles." In Hiroshi Ishii, Robert J.K. Jacob, Pattie Maes, Marcelo Coelho, Jamie Zigelbaum, Thomas Pederson, Orit Shaer, and Ron Wakkary (eds.), *Proceedings of the Fourth International Conference on Tangible, Embedded, and Embodied interaction (TEI '10),* 297–98. New York: Association for Computing Machinery (ACM).

Berzowska, Joanna, Marc Beaulieu, Vincent Leclerc, Gaia Orain, Catharine Marchand, Catou Cornoyer, Emily Paris, Lois Frankel, and Miliana Sesartic. 2010a. "Captain Electric and Battery Boy: Prototypes for Wearable Power-Generating Artifacts." In Marcelo Coelho, Jamie Zigelbaum, Hiroshi Ishii, Robert J.K. Jacob, Pattie Maes, Thomas Pederson, Orit Shaer, and Ron Wakkary (eds.), *Proceedings of the Fourth International Conference on Tangible, Embedded, and Embodied interaction (TEI '10),* 129–36. New York: Association for Computing Machinery (ACM).

Berzowska, Joanna, Marc Beaulieu, Gaia Orain, and Anne-Marie Laflamme. 2010b. "Captain Electric: Human Powered Electronic Garments." In Keiichi Sato, Pieter Desmet, Paul Hekkert, Geke Ludden, and A. Mathew (eds.), *Proceedings of the 7th International Conference on Design and Emotion, Craft of Design and Emotions, Chicago (IL, USA), October 4–7, 2010.* Chicago: Design and Emotion Society and Institute of Design, Illinois Institute of Technology. http://www.designandemotion.org/library/page/viewDoc/126 (accessed November 16, 2012).

Carroll, John M. 2009. "Human Computer Interaction (HCI)." In Mads Soegaard and Rikke Friis Dam (eds.), *Encyclopedia of Human-Computer Interaction.* Aarhus, Denmark: The Interaction Design Foundation. http://www.interaction-design.org/encyclopedia/human_computer_interaction_hci.html (accessed September 24, 2012).

Coelho, Marcelo, Sajid Sadi, Pattie Maes, Joanna Berzowska, and Neri Oxman. 2007. "Transitive Materials: Towards an Integrated Approach to Material Technology." Presented at the 9th International Conference on Ubiquitous Computing (Ubicomp '07), Innsbruck, Austria.

Diamond, Sara. 2009. "A Tool for Collaborative Online Dialogue: CodeZebraOS." PhD diss., University of East London, London.

The Economist. 2012. "Counting Every Moment." March 3.

Emilien, Gerard, Cecile Durlach, Elena Antoniadis, Martial Van Der Linden, and Jean-Marie Maloteaux. 2004. *Memory: Neuropsychological, Imaging and Psychopharmacological Perspectives.* Hove, UK and New York: Psychology Press.

Quinn, Bradley. 2010. *Textile Futures: Fashion, Design and Technology.* Oxford: Berg.

Schacter, Daniel L. 2001. *The Seven Sins of Memory: How the Mind Forgets and Remembers.* Boston: Houghton Mifflin.

Sutton, John. 2004. "Memory." In Edward N. Zalta (ed.), *Stanford Encyclopedia of Philosophy.* Stanford: Center for Study of Language and Information, Stanford University. http://plato.stanford.edu/archives/sum2004/entries/memory/ (accessed September 24, 2012).

Weiser, Mark. 1991. "The Computer for the Twenty-First Century." *Scientific American* 265 (3): 94–104.

22

Advanced Textiles for Fashion in Science, Literature, and Film

MARIE O'MAHONY

INTRODUCTION

What is now proved was once only imagined.

—William Blake (1757–1827)

Blake's words were written at the time of the Industrial Revolution in England, a time when scientific discovery and technological development were making real their promises of manufacturing capability, not least in the textile industry (Basalla 1989; Mokyr 2011).

This chapter examines the role of science fiction in the development of new concepts and assesses its importance in bridging the gap between science and advanced textiles for fashion. It examines the scientific concepts and contemporary culture behind futuristic textiles in laboratories and on the catwalk, and discusses the depiction of textiles in literature and film as an indicator of how our lives might be transformed. The descriptions of actual textile technologies are compared to the depictions of textiles in the writing of authors such as Peter Carey and William Gibson and in films such as *Barbarella* (Roger Vadim, 1968). In the history of technological materials we see both fiction (or fantasy) and fashion contributing to the development of identity. The blurring of distinctions between fact and fiction shows the expectations, excitement, and fears that scientific advances elicit, touching on the social, cultural, political, and economic issues that impact on scientific research, development, and dissemination.

Simulation is used in fiction, particularly in film, to engage the viewer by the use of relatively low-technology materials to suggest more futuristic ones. In Jacques Fonteray and Paco Rabanne's costumes for *Barbarella*, we see an example of this. The film was set in 40,000 C.E. but filmed in 1968, and costumes used plastic and metals in part because they look futuristic but also because they have a visual malleability that allows for many identities to be projected onto them by the viewer. When treated as textile materials for fashion, both plastic and metals have since this time become highly technical materials, while the first man-made fiber, rayon, has found its own identity as a fabric rather than a mere mimic of silk. The question posed here is this: how important has fiction (in the form of literature and film) been to this evolution? Does the medium of film, as Adrienne Munich (2011) attests, provide the perfect vehicle for fashion to look to the past in order to design for the future, affording it a "Janus-like" quality?

The role that fiction has played in the development of material identity is exemplified by the American, European, and Soviet space programs and the earlier fictional work of German filmmaker Fritz Lang (*The Girl in the Moon,* 1929). A dialogue between space technology and fashion continues today in the spin-off programs of the U.S. National

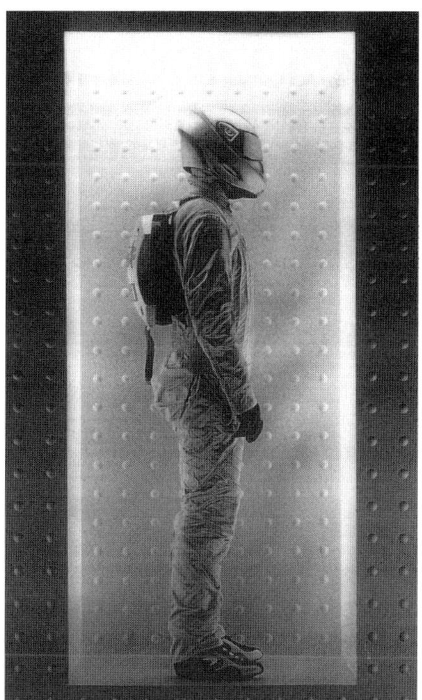

FIGURE 22.1 This cooling suit was designed by Grado Zero Espace with European Space Agency technologies for use by the McLaren Formula One team (2002). Collaboration between diverse industries is leading to new and unexpected fashion in terms of both functionality and aesthetics. *Credit*: Photograph by Grado Zero Espace.

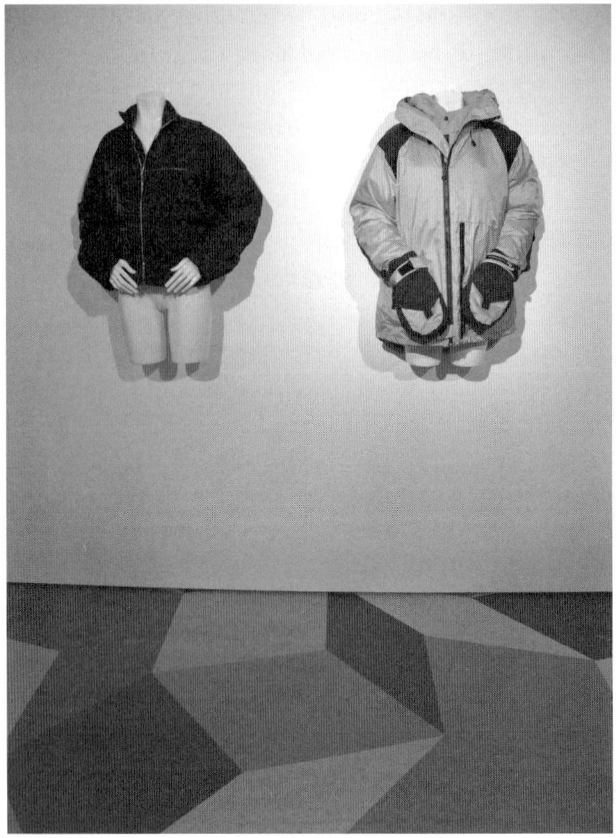

FIGURE 22.2 In cooperation with the European Space Agency, Grado Zero Espace applies space technologies such as the highly insulating Aerogel to sportswear and other terrestrial applications. *Credit*: Photograph by Marie O'Mahony at the TechnoThreads exhibition at Science Gallery, Trinity College, Dublin, 2008.

Aeronautics and Space Administration (NASA) and the European Space Agency. The latter agency's collaboration includes work with the Italian manufacturer and research laboratory Grado Zero Espace in the search for commercial applications for such technologies as Aerogel (the lightest high-insulation man-made material) and shape-memory materials. By applying design considerations, the Italian company brings a fashion aesthetic to technologies that were primarily developed for their high performance (Figures 22.1, 22.2, and 22.3).

The dynamic between technology and fashion can be seen in the work of designer Hussein Chalayan as he collaborates with technologists, sculptors, engineers, filmmakers, and so on in the realization of his work, for example, his well-known video dress and motion dresses from his 2007 collections One Hundred and Eleven and Airborne (Black 2009;

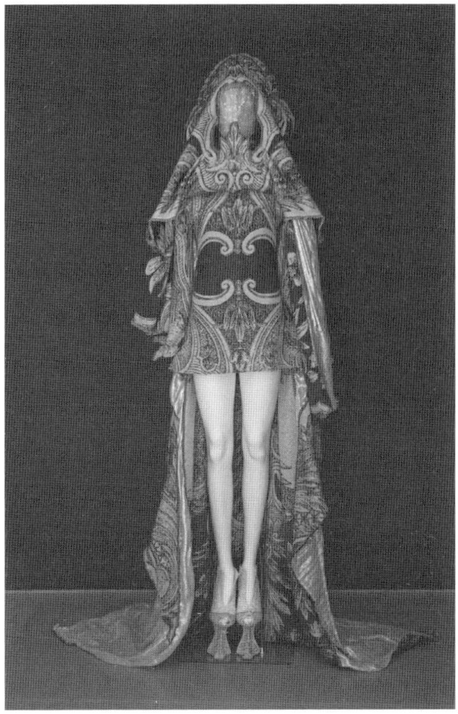

FIGURE 22.3. A reflective print is used by JANTAMINIAU in the Irradiance collection to lend a space or otherworldly aesthetic quality to the work (2011).
Credit: Photograph by Joep Vogels. Courtesy of Textielmuseum Tilburg, the Netherlands.

Violette 2011). Fiction has the ability to act as a catalyst for fashion, providing a narrative for the technology. In doing this, fashion is not simply a "technological portal" (Quinn 2012).

THE FORMATION OF NEW FIBER AND FABRIC IDENTITY

Humans' use of natural fibers, both animal and plant, has a long history dating from the Stone Age. The emergence of synthetic fibers in the early part of the twentieth century offered a myriad of new possibilities for a new type of fiber born in the materials laboratory and produced in a factory. In the 1930s, rayon was developed as a manufactured-fiber alternative to silk (Kauffman 1988), whereas DuPont's Kevlar from the late 1960s was entirely new.[1] With no provenance to draw on, the early synthetics could literally be molded to take on different forms and identities—it was up to the materials scientist or manufacturer to imbue the material with its final properties. However, despite limitless possibilities, scientists often resorted to the familiar. The new synthetic materials—for example, nylon and plastic—were used as alternatives to existing materials, and their own potential was not immediately realized. Plastic was first introduced and marketed as a cheap substitute for more expensive materials such as ivory and wood (Sparke 1994) and suffered for decades from a poor image and lack of a strong identity of its own. Designers were reluctant to use plastic for high-priced work, which meant that good design using plastic material was slow to emerge, delaying plastic's acceptance by the discerning consumer. In contrast, this nonspecific, open identity of plastic had great appeal in the cinema, where ambiguity is positively sought, heightening the viewers' suspension of reality and engaging their own imagination in the process. Thus the identity of plastic became at once everything and nothing, a core problem that Sparke identifies, stating "there is no one truth but rather a plurality of 'possibilities'" (Sparke 1994: 8). Examples of the materials suggested by plastics in several science fiction films have now been realized. The transparent cocoon-like bed seen in *Barbarella* (1968) visually resembles inflatable cushions and membranes made of ethylene tetrafluoroethylene that are now used in architecture, enabling transparency and curved forms (O'Mahony 2011: 110). In *Tron: Legacy* (Joseph Kosinski, 2010) electroluminescent flat lights are used to provide illumination in a more technically advanced version of the original illuminated costume designs for the 1982 Steven Lisberger cult film *Tron* (McCarthy 2010). The flexibility of the television screen envisioned in David Cronenberg's *Videodrome* (1983) is now emerging in flexible organic light-emitting diode technologies, with the Apple corporation recently filing a patent for their use in a flexible bracelet watch (Rothkopf, Wright, and Myers 2013).

THE AESTHETICS OF SPACE

The space age of the mid-twentieth century promised to reveal the secrets of the unexplored universe. The costs of the ambitious space programs had to be supported by state funding, for which public support was essential. At the same time, the cinema as a medium was also relatively young and captured the public imagination with fantastic scenarios. The two fields, space exploration and film, became natural allies: space gave film subject matter, while the cinema engaged the public with space long before the first man set foot on the moon. This link with cinema was vital in the development of technology and the aesthetics of textiles and clothing for survival in outer space and other extreme environments.

The Soviet space program in the early twentieth century offered a technical utopianism that was co-opted by the mystic occultism of cosmism (Siddiqi 2008). Russian cosmism flourished between the late nineteenth and mid-twentieth century and was sufficiently well regarded to influence government science policy. Cosmism sought to link humanity with the cosmos and attracted a range of theologians, poets, philosophers, painters, and spaceflight theorists such as Konstantin Tsiolkovsky (Lytkin, Finney, and Alepko 1995). It combined both Eastern and Western philosophical traditions along with Russian Orthodox religion, theosophy, and pan-Slavism. This blurring of fact and fiction is reflected in the writing and career of Alexi Tolstoy, son of Leo Tolstoy and one of the first Russian science fiction writers (Tolstoy 1983). Tolstoy was also a member of the USSR Academy of Sciences with a planet, 3771 Alexejtolstoj, named in his honor. Tolstoy's science fiction novel *Aelita; or, The Decline of Mars* ([1922] 1985) was the inspiration for Yakov Protazanov's 1924 film *Aelita—Queen of Mars.* The interplanetary love story provides a Russian cosmic view of the human place in the cosmos. The set design for the film was undertaken by a number of designers, including Sergei Kozlovsky and Aleksandra Ekster, the latter also working on the costumes, including costumes that appear to be made of plastic tubes and robot-like outfits. The film is heavily inspired by the Russian futurist and Russian constructivist movements of the period, echoing these artistic movements' homage to the machine, speed, and the future (Neumann 1999). The film and the spectacle that accompanied its showing were hugely popular at the time, but its real importance is its influence on the development of subsequent science fiction films and the development of a futuristic aesthetic in fashion.

A futuristic fashion aesthetic can challenge today's notions of beauty. Science fiction author William Gibson and novelist Peter Carey have explored this concept, and both speculate on a future reaction to the aesthetic of beauty, developing a technological or machine aesthetic or even an aesthetic of ugliness. In the opening chapter of *Neuromancer* Gibson writes, "The bartender's smile widened. His ugliness was the stuff of legend. In an age of affordable beauty, there was something heraldic about his lack of it" (Gibson 1984: 3). In *The Fat Man in History* (1993), Carey depicts a counterrevolutionary future where obesity and disfigurement are "utopian" for certain sectors of society—those who have everything. Gibson's writing is echoed in the visual and physical development of wearable technology, which had in its initial stages a very utilitarian aesthetic. Carey's dystopian vision can be compared to the use of the asymmetrical bustle in the avant-garde collections of designers Vivienne Westwood and Rei Kawakubo (especially in the mid-1990s), as both challenge notions of beauty while ultimately reimagining it.

At the premiere of Fritz Lang's last silent film, *The Girl in the Moon* (1929),[2] in Berlin's UFA Palace cinema, the public was astonished to find that a real rocket was launched. Many of the details of the film, such as weightlessness, were quite accurate, although other aspects appeared more unlikely; for example, the clothing worn by the astronauts included a cable-knit cardigan, shirt, and tie. The rocket was devised by Professor Herman Oberth, who had already written *The Rocket into Interplanetary Space* (1923). Oberth agreed to help Lang in return for the filmmaker's assistance in raising money for the development of a real rocket program. The film inspired the establishment of the Rocketport Group,[3] rocket specialists that included Oberth's assistant Wernher von Braun, who it is believed also worked on the film (Frayling 2009). The Gestapo were sufficiently convinced by the accuracy of the rockets in the film to seize the models as state secrets when they rose to power. Von Braun worked on the German V-2 rocket and after World War II on the American rocket missile and space program. To engage public interest (and obtain government funding), von Braun also made a television series, *Tomorrowland,* with Walt Disney. While the film rocket influenced the appearance of the real rocket program, the early spacesuit design and aesthetic were guided by existing extreme-weather clothing. This early connection between science and science fiction has continued to inspire both, particularly in terms of clothing for the space environment.

THE SPACE SUIT

The American spacesuit design evolved from the Wiley Post pressure suit that in turn was inspired by early designs for a pressurized deep-sea diving suit (Braddock Clarke and O'Mahony 2005). Moving and working outside the spaceship necessitate the use of an extra-vehicular mobility unit that regulates pressure and temperature, supplies oxygen, allows communication, and protects against debris and other physical hazards while allowing ease of movement. The Apollo spacesuits are made up of twenty to twenty-four layers of advanced textiles such as Dacron, Mylar, Teflon-coated fiberglass textiles, and polyvinyl chloride (PVC; Chullen et al. 2011). Many of these textiles were originally developed for the space industry, and the brand names used were designed to evoke futuristic high technology and imply a high technical performance. The use of such names also created some distance from the early marketing of synthetics as low-cost and low-quality alternatives to natural fibers.

The success and excitement generated by the moon landing in 1969 inspired an enthusiasm for all things futuristic, including the aesthetics of fashion and the performance of textiles. Cristóbal Balenciaga's 1967 silk gazar one-seam gown with matching hat evokes the seamless aesthetic suggested by images of the astronauts encased in their sealed portable environments. Seamlessness often suggests a futuristic aesthetic, derived from its one-piece production process—intriguing and deceptively simple in appearance. In his 1957 review of the Citroen Deesse car, Roland Barthes evoked the mood of the time in his appreciation of the aerodynamic, apparently seamless design of the car: "Smoothness is always an attribute of perfection because its opposite reveals a technical and typically human operation of assembling: Christ's robe was seamless, just as the airships of science-fiction are made of unbroken metal" (reprinted in Barthes 1992: 88). Several contemporary designers have exaggerated seamless attributes, resulting in an overall aesthetic with a futuristic "otherworldly" quality. In 1966 Paco Rabanne launched his fashion career with dresses embellished with rhodoid sequins and plaques in a collection entitled 12 Unwearable Dresses in Contemporary Materials. His architectural training brought an unconventional vision to bear on his treatment of three-dimensional form in fashion, particularly in his disregard for conventional seams. More recently, the shoe designer Marloes ten Bhömer designed an unusual molded resin shoe without a separated heel (Figure 22.4).

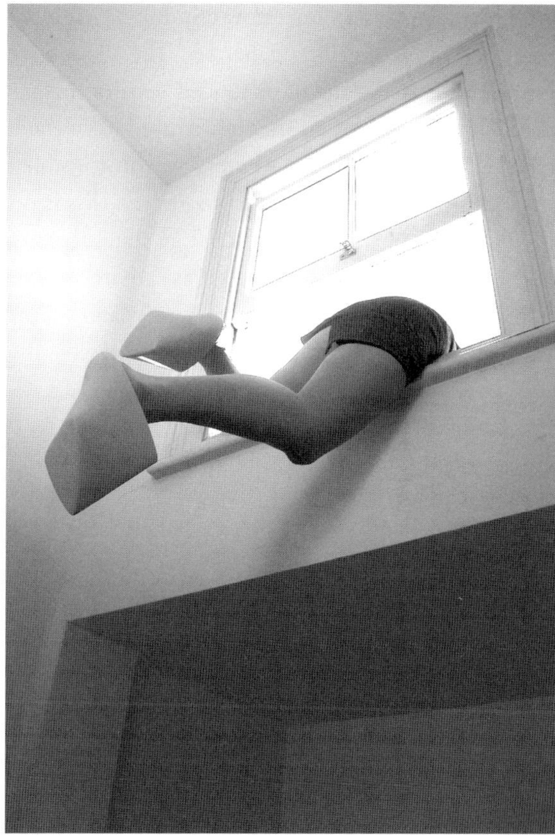

FIGURE 22.4 The Noheelshoe by Marloes ten Bhömer Shoes cast in polyurethane resin in a two-piece mould re-invent existing footwear typologies. The design effectively erases the heel to create an entirely different foot form and aesthetic (2003).
Credit: Photograph by Marloes ten Bhömer.

THE SPACESUIT OF THE FUTURE

In the twenty-first century, the future design of the spacesuit has looked to science fiction, sportswear, and nature for inspiration in an effort to improve comfort and fit. In 2011 the Virgin Galactic company turned to film for inspiration for their space tourist clothes for use by passengers on the SpaceShipTwo spacecraft.[4] In this instance the film was *Moonraker* (John Glenn, 1997) from the James Bond series, featuring personalized flight suits, soft helmets equipped with microphones and headphones, and soft-soled shoes. Jacques Fonteray, the costume designer on *Moonraker,* also designed the costumes for *Barbarella.* Barbarella, played by Jane Fonda, wears a wardrobe that evokes past, present, and futuristic spacesuits in the design of the garments and in the choice of shiny silver-colored or transparent fabrics, although high-performance fabrics are implied rather than actually used.

In contrast, recent textile developments now combine a futuristic aesthetic with contemporary technology to confer specific properties. The innovative Swiss manufacturer Schoeller Technology produces a range of advanced textiles for particular end uses. For example, SchoellerPCM is a neoprene rubber fabric used for wetsuits that incorporates a phase-change material (PCM) to keep the wearer at a comfortable temperature whether actively surfing or standing waiting for the surf to arrive. This is one of over 500 phase-change materials identified by NASA that can change state depending on external stimuli (O'Mahony 2011). Such materials are classed as "smart" or "responsive"—they can sense and respond appropriately to fluctuations in the wearer's temperature via encapsulated chemicals that change between solid and liquid states by absorbing and releasing heat. Further examples of smart materials include Schoeller's Coldblack and Energear fabric developments. The Coldblack technology is a finishing treatment applied to the textile and is designed to overcome the problem of black cloth attracting and storing heat at high temperatures, ensuring the fabric remains at a temperature comparable to white material even in extreme heat. Schoeller's Energear technology ensures that radiated heat from the body is recovered via the use of a mineral matrix embedded in the fabric. It is designed to help prevent premature fatigue and to promote faster warm-up and muscular regeneration, and works by reflecting the body's far-infrared rays back to the wearer without compromising fabric breathability, weather protection, or stretch.

THE HYBRID IDENTITY AND THE CYBORG

Ovid (43 B.C.E.–17 C.E.) in his epic poem *Metamorphoses* presents the philosophical idea that the soul does not die with the body but rather moves from one form to another, taking on other shapes while maintaining its spiritual identity. The notion of the hybrid form represents a partial transformation that, unlike a full metamorphosis, retains a high proportion of the original form.

Today's material hybrids bring together two or more different substances, combining the qualities of each to produce a new material with enhanced characteristics that the original materials do not possess individually. Materials that are part ceramic and part textile, or part metal and part textile, are now commercially available, driven by both performance requirements and aesthetic values. The work of Iris van Herpen, for example, explores this hybridity in materials (Thys and Conellan 2012). Using leather as a base material she transforms it with the addition of ceramic and lacquer to create a surreal "other" quality. The original nature of the materials is transformed both by the surface treatment and by the designer's manipulation of the leather into body-conforming garments and extreme footwear. Van Herpen's use of materials relates to an architectural treatment of space or the work of sculptors such as Barbara Hepworth (1903–1975) or László Moholy-Nagy (1895–1946). To achieve her visionary sculptural pieces created using digital design and three-dimensional printing, van Herpen collaborates with contemporary architects including Daniel Widrig (Figures 22.5 and 22.6; Braddock Clarke and Harris 2012).

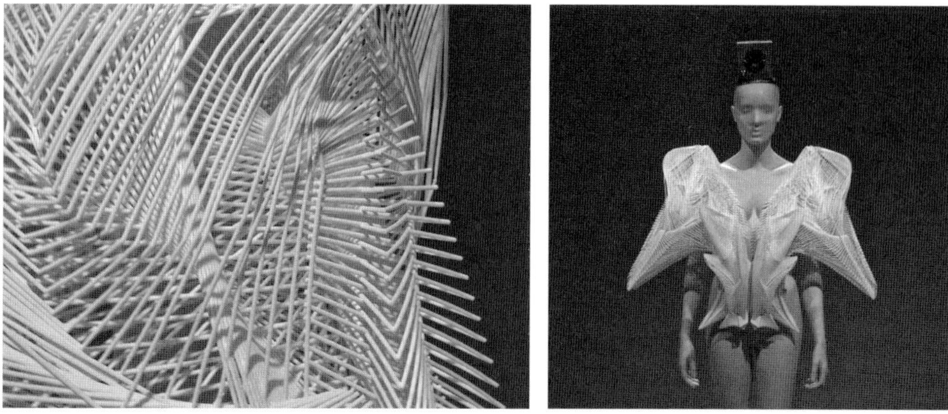

FIGURE 22.5 Iris van Herpen, Escapism, January 2011 (plus detail). In this collection the designer considers how we use addictive digital entertainment to escape from reality. In the collection a wide range of materials and processes are used, such as metal satin, burned copper gauze, smocked leather, and polyamide (seen here) digitally printed using a three-dimensional additive manufacturing process. The highly tactile nature of the materials is in sharp contrast to the absence of material experience in digital entertainment.
Credit: Photographs by Marie O'Mahony, at the exhibition Iris van Herpen, Groninger Museum, the Netherlands, 2012.

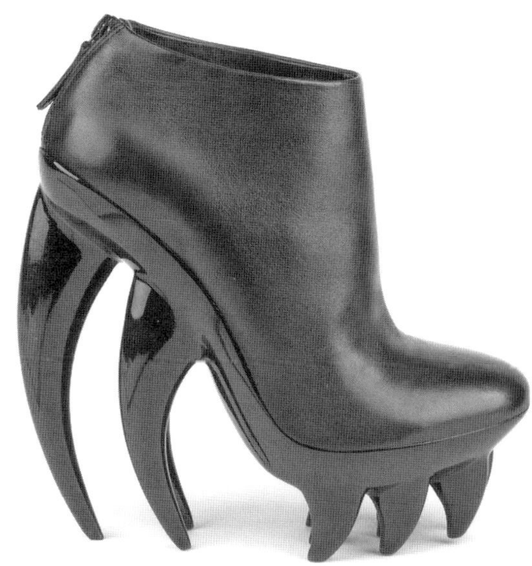

FIGURE 22.6 Fang shoes, United Nude/Iris van Herpen, 2012. In Iris van Herpen's fifth collaboration with the innovative footwear company United Nude, she designed shoes in which ten "fangs" are supported by high-technology carbon and glass fiber composites that combine strength with lightness.
Credit: Courtesy of United Nude.

The concept of a hybrid human has a long history, with some of the earliest examples found in mythology. Sarah Bakewell (1998) suggests that the origin of mermaids can be found in the dugong, a mammal native to warm coastal waters and sometimes found to breathe by "standing" on its tail with its head showing above water. In Fortuny Liceti's *De Monstris* (O'Mahony 2002), we see a selection of monsters that includes a scaly hybrid, part human with an elephant foot in place of her right hand, bird-of-prey claws for feet, and a donkey's head.[5]

At the turn of the new millennium, these fantastical beings have served as inspiration to avant-garde contemporary fashion designers from Walter van Beirendonck to Gareth Pugh, as humans move toward what Manfred Clynes and Nathan Kline referred to as a new "cyborg state." They coined the term *cyborg* (from *cybernetic organism*) in 1960, referring to a human-machine hybrid that had the capability of surviving in extraterrestrial conditions (Clynes and Kline 1960).[6] Their neologism derived from the Greek word for "steersman" and refers to the study of control systems and comparison between artificial and biological systems, the second syllable emphasizing the importance of the human to the cyborg (O'Mahony 2002). Clynes and Kline argue that the cyborg state is essential not only to exist in an extraterrestrial environment but to be more human. They also propose that the cyborg state offers the potential to become heightened or "hyper" humans.

Umberto Eco in *Travels in Hyper-reality* (1990) argues that in our hyperreal world, the real is no longer enough, and we must instead look to create the ultimate fake by blurring or even eliminating boundaries between game and illusion. The fact that the cyborg theme appears in fiction with such regularity and in such a range of forms (Gibson 1984; Ishinomori 2003) serves to diffuse the distinction between reality and fiction. Fashion designers exploit this duality conceptually and aesthetically. In Belgian designer Walter van Beirendonck's Sexclown (spring/summer 2008) series, the designer considers the nature of future fetishism. Avatars, digital life forms, and African Sogobo rituals combine to create an aesthetic that celebrates body diversity and masculinity. Van Beirendonck's designs give the appearance of the models having just stepped out of a digital world.[7] In the collection he portrays a hyperreality where shoulders, hips, and waistlines are accentuated (Figure 22.7).

Donna Haraway in her *Manifesto for Cyborgs* (1985) argues that the cyborg must be seen as far more than a man/machine hybrid, as a creature of both social reality and fiction. An illustration of this can be seen in the work of multimedia artist Suzi Webster, where she considers the impact of technology on humans. In her interactive dress titled Electric Skin she has created a space that is neither internal nor external; instead, it evokes a third space between. The white garment has the appearance of a dress/coat with a hood that reaches over the wearer's head and face. It is bioresponsive, sensing and responding to the inhalation and exhalation of the wearer's breath, utilizing electroluminescent wires to create pulses of light with each breath. The work has an ethereal quality as it changes from static pure white to emitting a pale then more intense glow around the hood. The wearer experiences a technically altered state of perception and enhanced awareness of self through breath, as she is immersed in pale blue aquatic light.

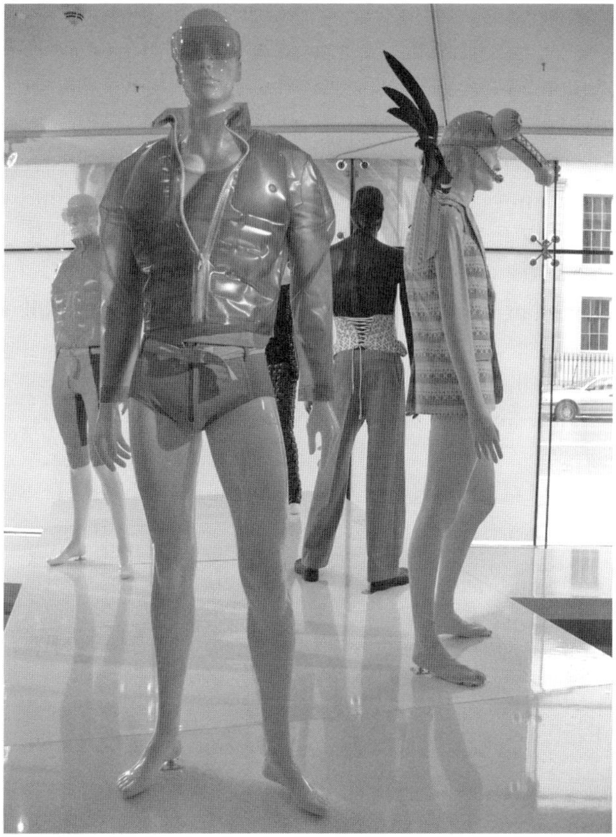

FIGURE 22.7 The vinyl Killer jacket (spring/summer 1999) for Walter van Beirendonck's W&LT (Wild and Lethal Trash) line was designed to reshape the body. In place of vigorous workouts it encouraged the wearers to just blow up their "muscles" using nozzles like those on a pool toy. The work blurs the line between science and science fiction in the way it deals with subjects such as cloning and the idea of artificially extending the life of the body. *Credit*: Photograph by Marie O'Mahony at the TechnoThreads exhibition at Science Gallery, Trinity College, Dublin, 2008.

As technology becomes increasingly embedded in everyday objects and closer to the body (see, for example, the work of computer scientist Steve Mann[8] or the performance artist Stelarc[9]) it can be speculated that the era of the cyborg could soon be within reach, especially in a medical context.

NEW NAMES FOR NEW MATERIALS

In the mid-twentieth century new synthetic textiles gained predominance over the natural fibers they emulated, but by the end of the century the pendulum had swung back and natural fibers were presented as an alternative to synthetics. In the early twenty-first century the balance is changing again as new fiber and fabrication methods are making it possible to create hybrids of both. New natural fibers (such as milk- and soy-based fibers) and enhancements to existing materials have been developed to exhibit advanced technological properties. The materials scientist, designer, and manufacturer have to communicate both the natural and enhanced aspects simultaneously, using word combinations such as TechnoNaturals (Braddock Clarke and O'Mahony 2005) and new names like milk protein fiber, technically known as casein, which is useful for its antibacterial properties. Although the production process is more closely aligned to synthetic-fiber methods than that of a natural fiber, the reference to milk was found to be appealing to consumers, who liked the idea of wearing milk, perhaps with echoes of Cleopatra bathing in milk (Braddock Clarke and O'Mahony 2005).

NANOTECHNOLOGY AND BIOMIMETICS

Nanotechnology is the term used to refer to the manufacturing, processing, and rearrangement of atoms to fabricate custom products (Forrest 1995). The ability to design products at a molecular level was first proposed by Richard P. Feynman, who included the suggestion that "it would be interesting in surgery if you could swallow the surgeon. You put the mechanical surgeon inside the blood vessel and it goes into the heart and 'looks' around" (1959: 64). This became the basis for the 1966 science fiction film *Fantastic Voyage* (Richard Fleischer, 1966), in which a medical team and submarine were reduced in size and injected into the bloodstream of the patient. In the Irish satirist and columnist Flann O'Brien's book *The Third Policeman* we see a man, or to be precise a policeman, and a bicycle morph together "as a result of the interchanging of the atoms of each of them and you would be surprised at the number of people in these parts who are nearly half people and half bicycles" (reprinted 2006: 296).[10] This he attributes to the inordinate length of time that people in 1950s rural Ireland spent on their bicycles. Some years later, Speedo launched their Fastskin fabric, which really did integrate with humans to enhance their performance.[11]

The design of Speedo's Fastskin is based on the microscopic surface topology of the skin of the shark. Launched at the 2000 Olympics in Sydney, it immediately created controversy as swimmers wearing the suit broke thirteen of the fifteen world records, winning 83 percent of the swimming medals at the games. Like a shark's skin, the polyurethane fabric appears smooth but on closer analysis is seen to have tiny ridges that serve to reduce viscous drag and skin friction. Scanning electron microscopes have allowed materials scientists to design at this extremely small scale. The importance of imaging was understood by Feynman, who complained that 1950s imaging technology was holding back scientific development and understanding, stating, "Make the microscope one hundred times more powerful, and many of the problems of biology would be made very much easier" (1959: 62).

The field of biomimetics is based on the extraction of good design from nature (van Hinte 1998), a rich source of inspiration in the development of nanotechnologies for

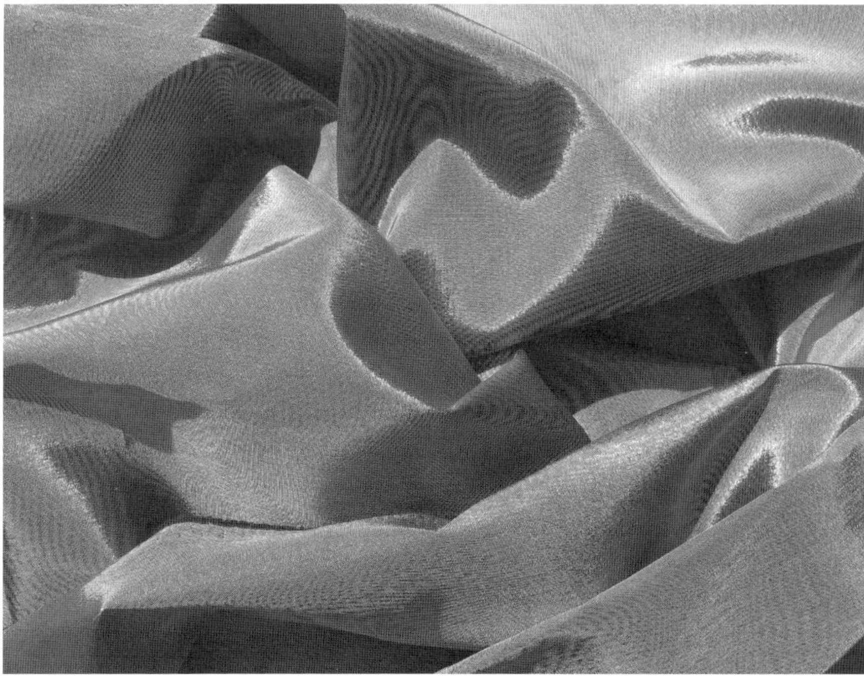

FIGURE 22.8 Teijin Fibers Ltd. has developed the Morphotex fabric based on the wing of the *Morpho* butterfly (2009). Inspired by nature, the function of the fabric's structure changes in the textile, where it is valued for its optical rather than camouflage qualities.
Credit: Photograph by Marie O'Mahony.

textiles. Schoeller Textiles has developed NanoSphere, a stain- and water-resistant coating for textiles. This is based on the nanoscale surface structure of the lotus leaf, which, like shark skin, looks smooth but has small bumps over its surface, making it difficult for water and dirt to adhere to the leaf's surface. While the majority of nanotechnology applications in textiles are used in coating and finishing treatments for fabrics, research is being undertaken whereby the fibers themselves are coated. In the Textiles Nanotechnology Laboratory at Cornell University, researchers are developing fiber coatings with polyelectrolytes, inorganic and metallic nanolayers for use in high-performance and smart materials. Cotton with nanoparticles of silver and gold produces an antibacterial fiber that uses a minimum of the precious metal, keeping the cost lower than would be possible in a conventional coating technique (O'Mahony 2011: 32–33). A research group based in Turkey and Austria is developing a process that allows them to enclose fiber optics with a dye-sensitive photovoltaic nanocoating. The intention is to then weave the fibers into a fabric and maximize the conversion of solar to electrical energy for use in wearable technology applications (Bedeloglu et al. 2009).

Speculating on the future of nanotechnology in textiles in 1995, David R. Forrest envisaged materials changing at a molecular level such that a solid might become fluid so that "distinctions between fabrics and other types of materials would blur" (1995: 14). Current research into hybrid and treated materials appears to confirm this potential.

The Russian author Vladimir Nabokov (1899–1977) combined artistic and scientific vision in his passion for butterflies. In the United States he worked at Harvard as a research fellow and curator in lepidoptera at the Museum of Comparative Zoology. He displayed an expert eye for anatomical distinctions and was especially interested in mimicry. The passion and frustration of the amateur lepidopterist is revealed in his novel *The Gift* (1937) and a short story, *The Aurelian* (1941).[12] Nabokov's literature goes beyond repeating the scientific view of the world and instead sets about combining the known with the unknown. He suggests instead that "physical reality fully exists only when it is actively, creatively perceived" (Blackwell 2003: 259). In *The Aurelian,* we see the protagonist lament that he (like Nabokov) has not been able to see his butterflies in their natural habitat: "He had more difficulty in imagining the tropics, but experienced still keener pangs when he did, for never would he catch the loftily flapping Brazilian Morphos, so ample and radiant that they cast an azure reflection upon one's hand" (Nabokov 1941: 1). In flight, the butterfly seems to appear, then disappear, camouflaged against the blue of the sky.

The Japanese textile company Teijin Fibers Ltd. took inspiration for their Morphotex fiber (now discontinued) from the wings of the *Morpho* butterfly, whose vivid blue iridescent color is the result of microscopic scales on the backs of the wings (Kambe, Zhu, and Kinoshita 2011). This type of color, known as "structural colour," is derived from periodic natural phase changes or biophotonic materials (Ding, Xu, and Wang 2009). Teijin created a filament yarn using multiple layers of ultrathin nanoscale film to structure the surface to reflect the blue wavelength of light (Figure 22.8). The fiber is therefore engineered to produce color without the need for dyes, more sustainably than using conventional dye processes.

CONCLUSION

Advances in fashion and textiles have many connections with science, literature, and film, as seen in the examples above. The emergence of novel technologies for use in textiles is a source of excitement as well as consternation. Historically there was provenance to draw on: Jacquard weaving could look back to the tradition of handweaving, digital printing to silk screen printing, and so on. New technologies do not necessarily have these points of reference. For example, today's three-dimensional printers are so far removed from conventional notions of printing that the term is potentially a barrier to its perceived capabilities. Fiction and imagination will continue to play a role in the development of enhanced performance, aesthetics, products, and clothing that new processes might deliver. Roland Barthes maintains that "any material can arbitrarily be endowed with meaning" (1992: 110), which is a reminder of the power of narrative in defining physical objects. Context and use are also important: for example, each time a particular sports clothing technology is worn by an Olympic gold medalist, meaning is imparted to reinforce the idea that it is a winning fabric.

A tyranny of association has been seen in the development of plastics (Sparke 1994), but the converse can also be true in terms of a lack of association. Philosopher

Jean Baudrillard (cited in Sparke 1994: 112) describes synthetics as having freedom from a natural symbolism that enables them to gravitate "towards a superior level of abstraction which enables a game of the universal association of materials to take place" (1994: 112). A new material can draw on provenance, if not directly its own, and pursue its identity in a fluid way. The ability to morph and change is essential for textiles and their associated technologies to develop and, most important, to innovate.

Looking ahead, new possibilities are opening up to continue the relationship between fashion and textiles, science and fiction. Rapid changes continue in the digital media world of e-books, games, and other forms of user experience where recent developments aim to create greater physical engagement and immersive interaction with the senses. A parallel trajectory can be seen with textiles, where the emerging field of e-textiles carries the potential to bring both physical and digital together—literally. The fabric of the future may be experienced as a truly cyclical process where the real and the imagined constantly overlap: inspired by fiction, engineered by the textile technologist, and mediated by the user.

NOTES

1. "Kevlar Brand: Better, Stronger and Safer with Kevlar® Fiber," DuPont website, http://www2.dupont.com/personal-protection/en-us/dpt/kevlar.html (accessed February 22, 2013).
2. Translated from the German original *Frau im Mond.* It is also known as *Woman in the Moon.*
3. Translated from the German *Raketenflugplatz.*
4. "Virgin Galactic Ponders Spacesuit Design Options," Virgin Galactic website, October 26, 2011, http://news.softpedia.com/news/Virgin-Galactic-Ponders-Spacesuit-Design-Options-230110.shtml (accessed November 18, 2011).
5. Malcolm Letts (1949) describes Mandeville's use of extracts from Pliny, Solinius, Jerome, Isidore of Seville, the Alexander romances, and the early bestiaries.
6. The article is based on a paper delivered by the authors under the title Drugs, Space and Cybernetics, presented at the Psychophysiological Aspects of Space Flight Symposium in San Antonio, Texas, USA, May 1960.
7. Personal correspondence with Walter van Beirendonck during the author's research for the exhibition TechnoThreads, Science Gallery Trinity College, Dublin, Ireland, April 26–July 26, 2008, http://www.sciencegallery.com/whatsgone_exhibits.
8. Steve Mann, now at the University of Toronto, founded the Wearable Computing group at the Massachusetts Institute of Technology in the United States. He developed the "Digital Eye Glass" (wearable computer and augmented reality systems) from the early 1980s to the present. See also Mann and Niedzviecki (2001).
9. Australian artist Stelarc's projects with robotics have included Third Arm and Exoskeleton, investigating control and involuntary movement. See http://stelarc.org (accessed May 10, 2013).
10. Although *The Third Policeman* was not published until 1969, there is strong evidence to suggest that it was written in the late 1930s or early 1940s.
11. "Speedo History," Speedo, http://www.speedocanada.com/_controller/index.cfm?categoryID=4 (accessed January 20, 2012).

12. "Aurelian is an archaic word for lepidopterist, one who is interested in butterflies. The term is derived from aurelia, meaning chrysalis, and relates to the golden color it may attain just before the butterfly emerges; the Latin word for gold is aurum." Note from *The Atlantic* online. The magazine was the original publisher of the short story (see Nabokov 1941).

BIBLIOGRAPHY

Bakewell, Sarah. 1998. "Illustrations from the Wellcome Institute Library: Images of Bodily Transformation." *Medical History* 42 (4): 503–17.

Barthes, Roland. 1992. *Mythologies.* New York: Noonday Press.

Basalla, George. 1989. *The Evolution of Technology.* Cambridge: Cambridge University Press.

Bedeloglu, Ayse, Ali Demir, Yalcin Bozkurt, and Niyazi Serdar Sariciftci. 2009. "A Photovoltaic Fiber Design for Smart Textiles." *Textile Research Journal* 80 (11): 1065–74.

Black, Sandy. 2009. "Designer Hussein Chalayan in Conversation with Sandy Black." *Fashion Practice: The Journal of Design, Creative Process and the Fashion Industry* 1 (2): 239–50.

Blackwell, Stephen H. 2003. "The Poetics of Science in, and around, Nabokov's The Gift." *The Russian Review* 62 (2): 243–61.

Braddock Clarke, Sarah E., and Jane Harris. 2012. *Digital Visions for Fashion and Textiles.* London: Thames and Hudson.

Braddock Clarke, Sarah E., and Marie O'Mahony. 2005. *TechnoTextiles 2.* London: Thames and Hudson.

Carey, Peter. 1993. *The Fat Man in History.* London: Vintage.

Chullen, Cinda, Ken Thomas, Joe McMann, Kristi Dolan, Rose Bitterly, and Cathleen Lewis. 2011. "US Spacesuit Knowledge Capture." *Proceedings of the International Conference on Environmental Systems* 41 (July): 1–27. http://hdl.handle.net/2060/20110010282 (accessed July 20, 2012).

Clynes, Manfred E., and Nathan S. Kline. 1960. "Cyborgs and Space." *Astronautics Magazine,* September.

Ding, Y., S. Xu, and Z. L. Wang. 2009. "Structural Colours from *Morpho peleides* Butterfly Wing Scales." *Journal of Applied Physics* 106 (074702): 1–6.

Eco, Umberto. 1990. *Travels in Hyper-reality.* Boston: Mariner Books.

Feynman, Richard P. 1959. "There's Plenty of Room at the Bottom." Lecture presented at the Annual Meeting of the American Physical Society, California Institute of Technology, December 29. Published in 1960 in *Caltech Engineering and Science* 23 (5): 22–36. http://www.zyvex.com/nanotech/feynman.html (accessed May 14, 2013).

Fletcher R. Rothkopf, Derek W. Wright, and Scott A. Myers. Bi-stable Spring with Flexible Display. U.S. Patent Application 20130044215, filed August 17, 2011, and issued February 21, 2013.

Forrest, David R. 1995. "The Future Impact of Molecular Nanotechnology on Textile Technology and on the Textile Industry." Paper presented at Discover Expo '95, Industrial Fabric and Equipment Exposition, Charlotte, North Carolina, October 12.

Frayling, Christopher. 2009. "Rotwang and Sons: The Soul of the Designer in the Machine Age." In Jeremy Aynsley and H. Atkinson (eds.), *The Banham Lectures—Essays on Designing the Future,* 266–79. Oxford: Berg.

Gibson, William. 1984. *Neuromancer.* New York: Ace Hardcover.

Haraway, Donna. 1985. "Manifesto for Cyborgs: Science, Technology, and Socialist Feminism in the 1980s." *Socialist Review* 80: 65–108.

Ishinomori, Shotaro. 2003. *Cyborg 2009.* Vol. 1. Los Angeles: TokyoPop.

Kambe, Makoto, Dong, Zhu, and Shuichi, Kinoshita. 2011. "Origin of Retroreflection from a Wing of the *Morpho* Butterfly. "*Journal of the Physical Society of Japan* 80 (5): 1–10.

Kauffman, George B. 1988. "Rayon: The First Semi-synthetic Fiber Product." *Journal of Chemical Education* 70 (11): 887–93.

Letts, Malcolm. 1949. *Sir John Mandeville: The Man and His Book.* London: Blatchford.

Lytkin, Vladimir, Ben Finney, and Liudmila Alepko. 1995. "Tsiolkovsky—Russian Cosmism and Extraterrestrial Intelligence." *Quarterly Journal of the Royal Astronomical Society* 36 (4): 369–76.

Mann, Steve, and Hal Niedzviecki. 2001. *Cyborg: Digital Destiny and Human Possibility in the Age of the Wearable Computer.* New York: Random House.

McCarthy, Erin 2010. "Creating Tron: Legacy's Lightsuits." *Popular Mechanics,* December 9. http://www.popularmechanics.com/technology/digital/visual-effects/tron-legacy-lightsuit-costume-vfx (accessed February 24, 2013).

Mokyr, Joel. (ed.). 2011. *The Economics of the Industrial Revolution.* London: Routledge.

Munich, Adrienne. (ed.). 2011. *Fashion in Film.* Bloomington: Indiana University Press.

Nabokov, Vladimir. 1941. "The Aurelian." *The Atlantic Magazine,* November. http://www.theatlantic.com/magazine/archive/1941/11/the-aurelian/306224/ (accessed November 18, 2012).

Neumann, Dietrich. 1999. *Film Architecture: Set Designs from Metropolis to Blade Runner.* Munich: Prestel.

O'Brien, Flann. 2006. *The Complete Novels of Flann O'Brien.* New York: Everyman's Library.

O'Mahony, Marie. 2002. *Cyborg: The Man-Machine.* London: Thames and Hudson.

O'Mahony, Marie. 2011. *Advanced Textiles for Health and Wellbeing.* London: Thames and Hudson.

Ovid. 2008. *Metamorphoses.* Oxford: Oxford Paperbacks.

Quinn, Bradley. 2012. *Fashion Futures.* London: Merrell.

Siddiqi, Asif A. 2008. "Imagining the Cosmos: Utopians, Mystics, and the Popular Culture of Spaceflight in Revolutionary Russia." *Osiris* 23 (1): 260–88.

Sparke, Penny (ed.). 1994. *Plastics Age.* New York: Overlook.

Thys, Marianne, and Lise Conellan (eds.). 2012. *Iris van Herpen.* Schotten, Belgium: BAi Publishing.

Tolstoy, Aleksey Nikolayevich. [1922] 1985. *Aelita; or, The Decline of Mars.* Ann Arbor, MI: Ardis.

Tolstoy, Nikolai 1983. *The Tolstoys: Twenty-Four Generations of Russian History.* London: Hamish Hamilton.

Van Hinte, Ed (ed.). 1998. *Smart Design.* Workshop report. Amsterdam: The Netherlands Design Institute.

Violette, Robert (ed.). 2011. *Hussein Chalayan.* New York: Rizzoli.

23

Fashion and Science Intersections: Collaborations across Disciplines

PHILIP SAMS AND SANDY BLACK

This chapter discusses an interdisciplinary culture of science and the arts that (re)-emerged from the mid-1990s in the United Kingdom. During this period, a number of innovative research projects were nurtured by public funding bodies and within educational institutions. For example, the Royal College of Art in London pioneered art and design practice-led research projects in the framework of doctoral research, and the Wellcome Trust (a UK national institute for biomedical research) launched its groundbreaking SciArt initiative in 1997.[1] In 1998 the National Endowment for Science, Technology and the Arts (NESTA) was established by the UK government to foster original ideas and support economic growth. Elsewhere, innovative research institutions such as the Massachusetts Institute of Technology (MIT) Media Lab in the United States (established in the 1980s) and the Interaction Design Institute Ivrea in Italy (operating from 2001 to 2005) nurtured a radical interdisciplinary approach to the emerging digital world, in which interaction design became significant, providing a new human-centered approach to the development of products, technology, and services.

A distinctive common factor within the collaborative projects discussed in this chapter is their origins within the disciplines of fashion and textiles. This industry sector is often dismissed as purely commercial due to its enormous economic significance worldwide, initiated by the Industrial Revolution. The fashion industry in particular, due to its inherent business and cultural imperatives (crudely summarized as speed, cost, and novelty), has been notable for a lack of investment in or a culture of academic research and development. Of course, the lifeblood of the fashion system is its focus on novelty and innovation, at first disseminated by the slow "trickle-down" process, a theory proposed by Thorstein Veblen in 1899 in *The Theory of the Leisure Class* and applied to fashion by Georg Simmel in 1904. Now fashion (as proposed by the seasonal catwalk presentations) is disseminated through many digital media channels almost instantaneously. The cultural significance of fashion and textiles has long been recognized within a historical context; however, the embodied practice of fashion via design, aesthetics, and materiality harnessed to individuals' emotional and symbolic needs has only recently been embraced within fashion cultural studies and material culture (Entwistle 2000; see also chapter 1 by Lou Taylor).

This chapter highlights the concept of interdisciplinary practice as research (Frayling 1993) using the lens of innovative fashion-related projects. It examines the collaborative co-creation process across disciplines that span science, technology, art, and design through the experience of a participant observer, Philip Sams. Through observations made by Sams, as a scientist working for one of the major global corporations within the fast-moving consumer goods industry, evidence is presented of an "outsider's" understanding of fashion's collaboration with science and technology, across what C. P. Snow famously referred to as *The Two Cultures* ([1959] 2001), discussing the humanities and sciences. From observation and interviews with practitioners working at these interfaces in the context of fashion and textiles, a simple taxonomy is proposed to describe and categorize the relationships that have emerged and through which new research territory has developed.

Such cross-disciplinary collaborations are not new, but have served different purposes throughout history and have regained considerable momentum in the late twentieth and early twenty-first centuries. Historically, in the early Renaissance period the academy drew distinctions only between natural philosophy, medicine, and mathematics. The work of Leonardo da Vinci (1452–1519) is testament to the integrated practices of art and engineering, of visualization and experimentation, that he and his contemporaries embodied. As the scientific revolution evolved into the eighteenth century, with the work of key figures including Isaac Newton (1642–1727) and Gottfried Wilhelm Leibniz (1646–1716), the disciplines of science became increasingly delineated, continuing into the nineteenth century. Taking here the historical development of botany and the communication of its knowledge as an example of collaboration between the arts and science, parallels and differences can be traced with regard to contemporary collaborations within academia, and across academia and industry.

THE CONTEMPORARY COLLABORATIVE CONTEXT ACROSS FASHION AND SCIENCE

In the late 1990s, industrial research scientist Philip Sams (a physical chemist, expert in soap and bubbles) was establishing a clothes care research program in Unilever's Laundry Research Department, based at Port Sunlight in the United Kingdom. It became clear to Sams that as the company was a partner in one-fifth of the world's washing days (based on its roughly 20 percent share of the global washing powder market) he should build an in-depth understanding of clothes that went well beyond how to clean them. His journey into clothing started, perhaps predictably, with the technology and properties of new textiles, but in 2000 a chance encounter with a fashion academic (Sandy Black) at a textile and clothing conference that was presenting work outside the more usual science parameters introduced fashion and a wider "fashion thinking" into his research landscape.[2] Already pursuing an interdisciplinary agenda, Black persuaded Sams to work with her embryonic master's in fashion studies program at London College of Fashion, acting in effect as a scientist in residence. This led to several seed-corn projects with fashion students (Black and Sams 2005), and an annual student award Fashion Meets Unilever, which ran for eight years. However, this collaboration with fashion (at first sight an unlikely branch of academia for the Unilever organization) had to be justified to the science team and the key question "why fashion and science?" satisfactorily answered.

Fashion is an inherently multidisciplinary subject, ranging from hard business economics (the fifth-largest global employment sector) to sociocultural theory, via design, technology, production, management, marketing communication, and consumption. It is about manufactured artifacts, and, as such, fashion has a history intertwined with and inseparable from science and technology. At Unilever Research and Development the community, predominantly of chemists, was fully aware that the successful push for synthetic dyes to satisfy a growing appetite for fashion in the nineteenth century had led to the creation of the global chemical industry. This is well documented, but a pertinent comment can be found in the monograph *Chemistry Triumphant,* written between the two World Wars by the then director of organic chemistry at the U.S. giant Dow Chemical Company. Here, the enthusiasm and ability of German chemists is recognized, and lamented: "no instance of such extreme stupidity has ever been recorded in the history of the world as when France and England gave up the dye industry to Germany" (Hale 1932: 47). The paradigm shift from technology for fashion to technology for a new military-industrial society was then, and continues to be, revolutionary.

A second example of links between science and fashion can be seen in the rise of polymer chemistry, which has been aided by the development and important economic value of synthetic fibers. In *Nylon: The Man-Made Fashion Revolution* (1999) Susannah Handley charts the invention of synthetic fibers. Particularly compelling is Handley's analysis of the way the chemicals company DuPont, owner of the nylon patents and brand name, courted high fashion as a means to publicize the technology and engage the public.

The power of fashion to use and drive science is thus the first reason for the scientist to be interested in working with fashion practitioners. There is, however, far more to it than that. Fashion is at the heart of human personality. A well-known quote from Virginia Woolf in *Orlando* resonates: "Vain trifles as they seem, clothes have, they say, more important offices than merely to keep us warm. They change our view of the world and the world's view of us" (1928: 170). The author articulates very effectively the intense, ubiquitous power of clothing as a form of human communication. This is absolutely the territory of fashion; fashion is about people's dreams and aspirations, about our sense of self. In Sam's view we are all, to some extent, slaves to fashion.

In many respects it is the second, cultural role of fashion that is most compelling to a research scientist. It is particularly relevant to the brand-driven world of fast-moving consumer goods but goes well beyond the realms of fashion simply as a metaphor for less glamorous products. As a totality, fashion makes science and technology acceptable and accessible to people. Fashion and science need each other, and this provides good reason for industrial and academic scientists to take fashion very seriously indeed, and for fashion practitioners to seek out science collaborations.

Interest in the power and opportunity of such cross-disciplinary collaboration with fashion is high. Thus a wealth of commentary has become available in textile handbooks describing the output of specific partnerships (Braddock and O'Mahony 1998, 2002; Braddock Clarke and O'Mahony 2005; O'Mahony 2011). Others have documented the interface of technical textiles and technology with avant-garde fashion designers and experimental artists (Bolton 2002; Lee 2005; Quinn 2002; Seymour 2008).

Taking a more conceptual approach, in *Fashioning the Future* (2005) Suzanne Lee, herself a fashion designer/researcher, provided inspirational visions celebrating a series of new fashion narratives that emerge when designers work with science and technology, including some of the case studies in this chapter. A key narrative in Lee's book is "The Programmable Jacket"—describing the development of wearable electronics seeded in the Media Lab at MIT, an incubator of "new thinking" with a pivotal role in the late twentieth century. Lee's current practice, developed from her research for *Fashioning the Future,* "grows" experimental bacterial cellulose-based materials in collaboration with scientist David Hepworth of the biotech company Cellucomp, for their Biocouture project, to create prototype biodegradable garments, a long-term project with exciting prospects.[3]

To return to the original question: why should science and technology engage with the world of fashion, and how do successful collaborations work? These questions are explored by examining a scientist's journey into this multidisciplinary world, together with observations on the experiences of a range of practitioners. Coming from a background that is clearly outside fashion, fashion thinking has always been more relevant to Sams than fashion output. Accordingly, the intention is to explore the context of, and the methods utilized in, collaborations between science and that branch of art and design that can be labeled fashion. The focus here is on people rather than product—an analysis of personality and style of working rather than a description of project aims and output, documented elsewhere (see above). It is a fuzzy landscape, and the terms *art, design, science,* and *technology* are of necessity used imprecisely. Although the case studies are UK based, they can simply be considered as experimental data—the insights and implications arising are, it is proposed, general.

WHEN SCIENCE SEEKS OUT ART: LEARNING FROM HISTORY

In the past, the science and art disciplines might have been considered inseparable—partners in a single cultural drive. Well-known examples in European culture include Leonardo da Vinci and Michelangelo (1475–1564). Should da Vinci be classified as artist or engineer? Such a split of definition is unhelpful for such a polymath, as a single label diminishes rather than defines his achievements and vision.

Before exploring the nature of modern fashion-science collaboration, it is instructive to examine a more general science/art partnership with a long and honorable history. Sams was introduced to the work of Robert Hooke (1635–1703) by his one-time chemistry master, Eric Clayton, also a polymath. Although Hooke is best known for his law on the extension of elastic materials, Clayton pointed to the quality of the drawings in Hooke's *Micrographia* (1665), a volume of observations through a microscope that showed a significant artistic ability far beyond simple illustration and that were important in the development of physical science. A further example of a historical need for science and art to work together can be found in the science of botany. Richard Mabey in his book *Weeds* (2010) makes the point that plant drawings were of little help or use to natural philosophers making early attempts to classify plants until the mid-sixteenth century, when the vision of the artist Albrecht Dürer (1471–1528) radically changed the paradigm. Dürer's etching *Large Piece of Turf* (*Dass grosse Rasenstueck*) is described by Mabey as "the first truly naturalistic flower-painting... herald of a new humanistic attitude toward painting" (2010: 58). Art thus brought a new way of looking at plants, out of which, ultimately, came the great work of Carl Linnaeus (1707–1778) on the plant kingdom, part of his classification of the living world (Linnaeus 1735). Linnaeus's classification would not have been possible without the ability of art and artists to capture for study the essence of and differences between plants. This work changed the focus of what had become botanical art and illustration toward flowers. Taxonomy—the ordered process of naming and grouping showing links and relationships—is one of the greatest scientific methods. It builds on a very human desire to classify things, to put them in categories. This approach has been applied below in the proposed model.

The botanist requires an accurate portrayal of plants, artistry has been a secondary consideration as in the following description: "The main goal of botanical illustration is not art but scientific accuracy. It must portray a plant with precision and level of detail for it to be recognized and distinguished from another species."[4] An abundance of literature exists on botanical art and illustration (e.g., Blunt and Raphael 1979; DeBray 2001), and new ways of developing botanical art and communication continue to emerge. Between 2001 and 2004 ceramic artist Rob Kesseler worked with botanists at Kew Gardens in London (the world-renowned scientific research center and repository) to find inspirational new ways to visualize the microscopic detail of seeds and similar small plant structures.[5] Funded by a NESTA fellowship, Kesseler's digital artworks based on electron microscopy tackle the inherent problems of "seeing" and understanding the invisible, providing both scientific and aesthetic benefits.

Botanical art communicates very clearly to the outside world what the scientist is talking about, but the relationship between art and botany goes much further. Botany is a fine historical example of science seeking art, where art has provided the scientist with key skills and methods. Building on this honorable collaborative history, botany is also a relevant place to start when considering fashion, as it likewise concerns the definition of external appearance and the communication of a form of "self," for example, in the way flowers—the sexual components of plants—have developed to attract and work synergistically with pollinators. As attraction is recognized as a key part of the communication role for clothes, botany is a suitable springboard from which to return to significant contemporary fashion-led collaborations with science.

WHEN ART SEEKS SCIENCE: PIONEERING FASHION AND ARTS-BASED PHD RESEARCH AT THE ROYAL COLLEGE OF ART

In the mid-1990s, inspirational cross-disciplinary research blossomed under the guidance of Professor John Miles in the Fashion and Textiles School at the Royal College of Art (RCA), London. This was a significant contribution to a role taken on by the RCA at the time as pioneers of the art- and design-based PhD, then a new and experimental journey for academic research. In 1993 Christopher Frayling, then rector of the RCA, discussed this new type of practice-led research, building on Herbert Read's concept of "teaching through art" to define it as "research *through* art and design" (as distinguished from research *into* or *for* art and design; Frayling 1993). Four of the key PhD candidates from that time have here shared their insights into collaborative arts/science research. Three (Torres, Tillotson, and Harris) are grouped under the concept of "artist/designer seeking technology" and the fourth (Geesin) as "artist communicating science."

The Artist/Designer Seeking Technology: Manel Torres, Jenny Tillotson, and Jane Harris

Fashion designer Manel Torres had a deceptively simple idea for a medium through which to produce radical fashion items—fabric in a can. This became the subject of his PhD research (Torres 2001) and has since taken him deep into the chemical engineering laboratories at Imperial College in London for over ten years of research and development. He describes how the Fabrican idea was born, when at a wedding in the early 1990s he saw the bride sprayed with Silly String as the couple left the church:

> I was an aspiring fashion designer and thought, "what a great idea it would be if you could literally dress someone from an aerosol can". I set about looking to buy such a product, but found that fabric from an aerosol can didn't exist. So I decided to embark on the project of creating spray-on fabric myself.[6]

Torres is very aware of the significant opportunity of place that working at the RCA provided, facilitating his science and technology collaboration at the neighboring Imperial College. He comments on the co-location of major London arts and science institutions:

> When I walk around the famous colleges and museums of South Kensington in London, I really sense the optimism and ambition of the Victorian era and strongly identify with it. The Royal College of Art, Imperial College, the Royal College of Music, were all set up in close proximity to one another by the Victorians. The area of London

> that was once called Albertopolis was a concentration of the highest learning in the arts and sciences. A hundred years later, crossing the disciplines of science and fashion, I am the modern beneficiary of this nineteenth-century vision. Ironically, the first materials I produced with the new technology were not unlike the crinolines so beloved by Victorian high fashion.

From the start of his PhD, Torres was a designer seeking technology. His concept was well developed, and he had started working with fibers and sprays. Then he was fortunate to meet Dr. Paul Luckham, an expert on polymer technology and professor in the Department of Chemical Engineering, Imperial College. Torres was given both mental and physical space to experiment, surrounded by an excellent science environment with an enthusiastic science community ready to help him. Under the experienced technology mentoring of Luckham, by the end of the PhD in 2003 Torres had patents sufficient for himself and Luckham to set up Fabrican Ltd. as a venture company at Imperial (Figure 23.1).

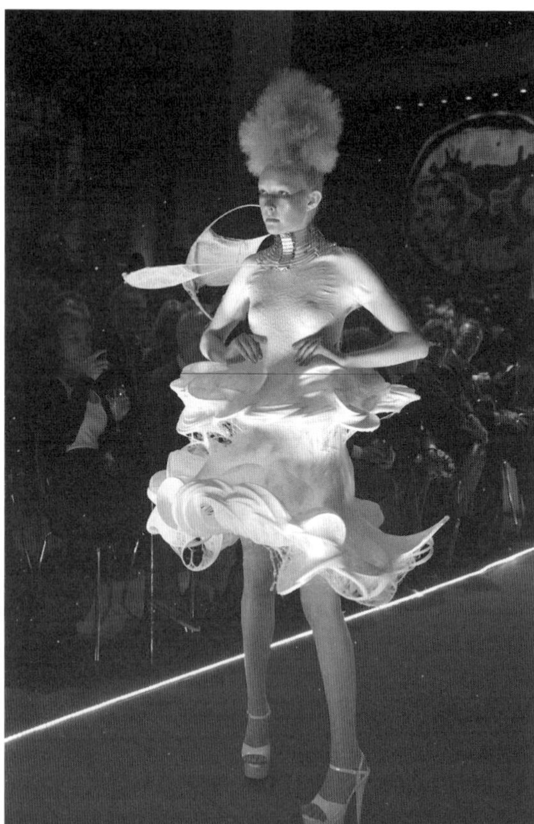

FIGURE 23.1 Fabrican spray-on dress by Manel Torres, First Fabrican Fashion Show, September 2010.
Credit: Photograph by Ian Cole.

Around the same time that the concept of spray-on fabric was crystallizing in Torres's mind, Jenny Tillotson left the world of fashion marketing and media to enroll at the RCA to study for a PhD in printed textiles (Tillotson 1997). Her concept "wellness through sensory design" reflected her personal experience, for example, as a volunteer caring for people living with HIV and AIDS. However, she attributes as her key influence her fashion designer husband. From his perspective designing for the radical French label Thierry Mugler from 1979 to 1994 he encouraged Tillotson to fuse fashion with well-being. A Mugler comment on the future of fashion became a driver for her passion and motivation: "Fashion will change dramatically in the years to come. It will be more human, closer to the needs of the people in terms of their wellbeing, not wellshowing" (Khornak 1982: 7).

Tillotson was able to use her PhD research to define a long-term vision to "re-cable fashion" to provide the required "wellness," initially through volatile chemicals embedded in and delivered from clothing and accessories. It might also be argued that the PhD process "used" Tillotson, capturing her for a life in research following the quest to deliver this vision. When she was a new research fellow at Central Saint Martins, University of the Arts London, an early visit to MIT's Media Lab introduced her to the emerging world of wearable computers, after which she started exploring the potential application and impact of nanotechnology on health care, finally resulting in realizable designs for scent-delivery systems embedded in fashion.

Tillotson's PhD entailed a long concept research phase, with much dialogue with scientists, until she reached the stage so clearly defined in the case of Torres: a designer looking for technology. The scene was set for her first really important collaboration with a science partner. Tillotson heard about microfluidics and "lab on a chip" technologies (Manz, Graber, and Widmer 1990) that turned out to be just the technology that would mimic a human heart, its arteries and veins, to facilitate the sought-after scent delivery for well-being benefits. Like for Torres, being in the right place played its part, and Tillotson contacted Professor Andreas Manz at, once again, Imperial College London, next to her previous base at the RCA and not far from Central Saint Martins. She describes how he understood her vision, and as a result they have worked together periodically since 2000. Several projects progressed, ultimately resulting in the formation of a venture company, eScent (Figure 23.2; Tillotson 2009).

This perfumery-on-a-chip concept stimulates the sense of smell to trigger emotion, an olfactory keyboard in a similar vein to the "scent organ" in Aldous Huxley's *Brave New World* (1932). By this time the collaboration was moving into a new stage: "His [Manz's] team developed a wireless technology and I transformed this into a story called 'Scent By A Wireless Web' based on the defence mechanisms in insects, the superhero 'spiderman,' and scent communication."[7] Tillotson has since begun a second in-depth science partnership with Professor Chris Lowe at the Institute of Biotechnology at the University of Cambridge. This moves away from liquids to computer-controlled delivery of "solid scent" from a small disposable cartridge to give selective delivery of multiple scents in a range of contexts.

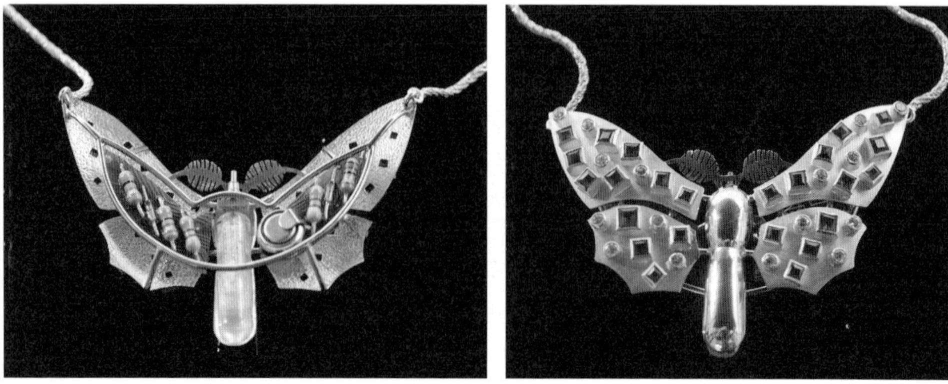

FIGURE 23.2 Butterfly Perfume eScent by Jenny Tillotson. Back and front views of a gold ruby-encrusted pendant by Don Baxendale with microelectromechanical systems (MEMS) scent-dispensing system developed with the Institute of Analytical Sciences.
Credit: Courtesy of Jenny Tillotson.

Jane Harris, the third of the RCA fashion-based PhDs, was determined to show that virtual textiles and fashion can have their own craft and beauty (Harris 2000). Her journey into digital three-dimensional textiles that move and perform as real clothes are worn was inspired early by radical thinking:

> In 1990, a visionary mentor with a textile background, from the 1960s generation, suggested that I look at Virtual Reality. I could barely type, and had no computer—they were still beasts at the time and hugely expensive with visual results pretty crude. But he had this view that the nature of my material practice would find synergies with computing and particularly the visualisation of "things" in general, imagineering how computers and their "add-ons" may become used.[8]

From then on, like Torres and Tillotson, Harris knew what she needed from technology and set out to find it. She sought out information and communications technology partners in the 1990s, such as Vicon Optical Motion Capture, who contributed expertise in three-dimensional modeling and have remained with her ever since. She comments that her role in the collaboration is, in many ways, similar to that of a film director who draws together many different components, connecting the complexities of language and meaning that cross over from one world to the other (Figure 23.3).

Harris was subsequently supported with a three-year NESTA Fellowship, from 2006 to 2009, to develop her practice. These fellowships were awarded to a selected group of emerging UK talent in the arts, science, or industry (see also the above discussion of Kesseler's work) to help expand their potential as key contributors to culture and enterprise in the United Kingdom. Harris started the fellowship with a strong

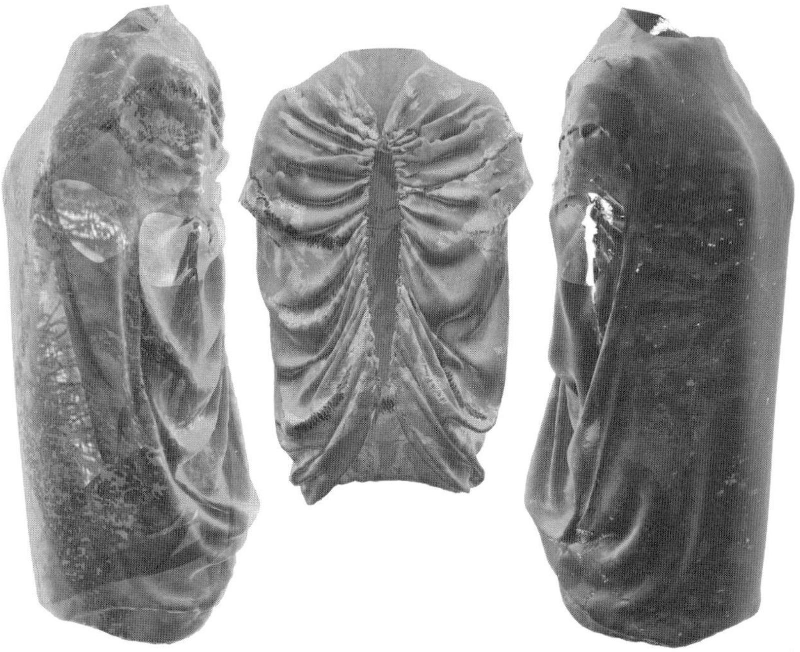

FIGURE 23.3 Balloon Top by Jane Harris with Shelley Fox and Mike Dawson, 2003–2004. Digital simulation of a garment from Shelley Fox's Collection 7 (autumn/winter 1999/2000). Using three-dimensional computer graphic animation, the bodiless garment is simulated, morphing from a flat circle to a drawstring-backed top, a fully three-dimensional garment.
Credit: Courtesy of Jane Harris.

vision, using her virtual art focused on the moving body to build a brave new world of "enhanced reality" performance with cloth at the core; in 2004 she collaborated with the Museum of London to "animate" an eighteenth-century dress, moving through space, achieved by digitally constructing the three-dimensional form in wire frame from motion capture, then applying digital textile surfaces. The opportunity to travel widely created new connections that impacted positively on Harris's academic research. Her influence in taking the voice of art and design to the technology sector increased significantly, and she became reader in digital imaging design at University of the Arts London.

In responding to the question, "why might cross-disciplinary relationships work (or not)?" Harris notes that while language can be a problem in the multidisciplinary context, success often depends on personality and time. Tillotson also commented on style and personality in collaborations:

> From experience, the only way for cross-disciplinary relationships to work is if the scientist is considerate about the design aspect from the beginning of the journey. . . . It has to be a two-way process for it to work. What tends to happen is the science dominates

> the relationship and the design suffers.... However, I consider Manz and Lowe to be my two science fashion partners.

Comparing these accounts of Manel Torres, Jenny Tillotson, and Jane Harris there is perhaps a corollary to Tillotson's comment above. The three artist-designers have immersed themselves in science, in part becoming scientists themselves, and have been highly considerate of the scientists who are, in Tillotson's description, their "science fashion" partners. On the one hand, they have taught these scientists the power of their fashion thinking to create real yet unusual applications of science and technology that could touch people's lives; on the other hand, the scientists have taught them the power of "slow," the long, never-ending dance that is science research and development.

After more than a decade of research and development these three pioneers have moved forward with their projects and careers. Harris has continued her virtual textile/art practice as professor of design at Kingston University, London. Tillotson has worked on a fellowship project entitled Smell the Colour of the Rainbow with the consumer products company Philips, which is interested in the power of scent to reduce stress and improve sleep. Fabrican is developing applications in the automotive, health care, and household product sectors and seeking partners in the fashion arena. The company has emerged onto the public stage: it was awarded a gold medal for the Science in Style, Spray-On Fabric Fashion Show from the Council for the Advancement and Support of Education, and was featured in films and fashion events in London and Moscow and on the cover of *Time* magazine as one of the 50 Best Inventions of 2010, together, incidentally with Suzanne Lee's BioCouture project.

Artistic Invention and Science Communication: Frances Geesin

As the earliest of the RCA arts-based PhDs (Geesin 1995), Frances Geesin started in a similar manner to the cases above but progressed differently. Already a well-established textile artist when she enrolled for her PhD in 1990, Geesin's unusual research journey led from textiles to her invention of the technology that would fulfill a quest to produce textile art that could make sounds. At the beginning, Geesin, like Tillotson, was influenced by the creative opportunities to "question possibilities" that working with her "creative composer lateral-thinking partner" Ron Geesin presented.

Geesin's initial aim was to stiffen fabric to capture its drape and fluidity, in the same manner that freezing creates a type of permanence. Like Torres, she started researching available technology and experimenting with materials and processes herself in other departments at the RCA, including metalwork and jewelry:

> With the support of the technician John Bartholomew I began electroplating fabrics by making them conductive with a silver-based ink, imparting rigidity and true permanence—this I understand was a first. I then went into industry and used electrolysis

> plating, the same technique used for car components and bathroom fittings. With Dr Russell House we metallised a net fabric used for fruit and vegetables with gold . . . and were overjoyed at creating something precious out of the ordinary. I attended numerous trade shows and came across a fibre manufactured by BASF that was designed for anti-static applications. Because I knew the fibre was conductive, I knitted and wove these yarns into small sample fabrics and wired them for electroplating. To my delight they changed to copper and opened the door for me to explore the potential of conductive fibres and fabrics.[9]

Geesin had by then personally developed a technology good enough to work with electronics design engineer Spencer Childs at the RCA. She knitted a piano keyboard, Spencer assembled the electronics, and "yes it worked it could be played." Prototype sound- and light-emitting fabrics, *Tri-ora,* were exhibited in the Science Museum London in 1996.

The next stages of Geesin's journey took a new direction, bringing an applied context for science and technology into the picture. The (autonomous) group Philips Design approached Geesin to work with them on their emerging, and at the time radical, "wearable electronics" ideas. From the familiar design environment at Philips Design, Geesin was pulled deeper into the Philips technology community in their UK research laboratory at Redhill, Surrey. Some years later, one of the top engineers at Redhill referred to this presence as an unusual case of the artist influencing the scientists, functioning as a catalyst in their multidisciplinary environment. Throughout this time, Geesin maintained her independence as a freelance artist, working with, but not for, the corporation. With the "intellectual generosity" of the artist (a phrase coined by Helen Storey to describe a different group of multidisciplinary collaborators) she also shared her thinking with other academic design researchers for them to make of it what they would, and Geesin's influence on work at other academic incubators such as Brunel University and Central Saint Martins, University of the Arts London, should be noted. For example, Geesin's pioneering work with conductive yarns and wearable computing was embraced by other designers as stimulus for the development of new generations of wearable technology via woven textiles.[10]

The Philips experience is a reminder of the historical case studies discussed earlier, for it describes the scientists reaching out to and working with the artist to provide new methods and approaches. This leads toward a more recent focus for Geesin's work that arose from a serendipitous encounter with the then chief executive officer of the Institute of Nanotechnology, Ottilia Saxl. Saxl recruited Geesin to her nanotechnology cause, seeding new collaborations with scientists in the field. The strange, complex, metal-plated nonwoven textiles that are Geesin's artistic medium of choice have proved ideal to help with the difficult task of communicating advances in nanotechnology, interpreted from research into the science (Figure 23.4). This demonstrates another driver that can be observed in forming many arts/science partnerships, the power of personality interlaced with opportunistic collisions and serendipitous networking.

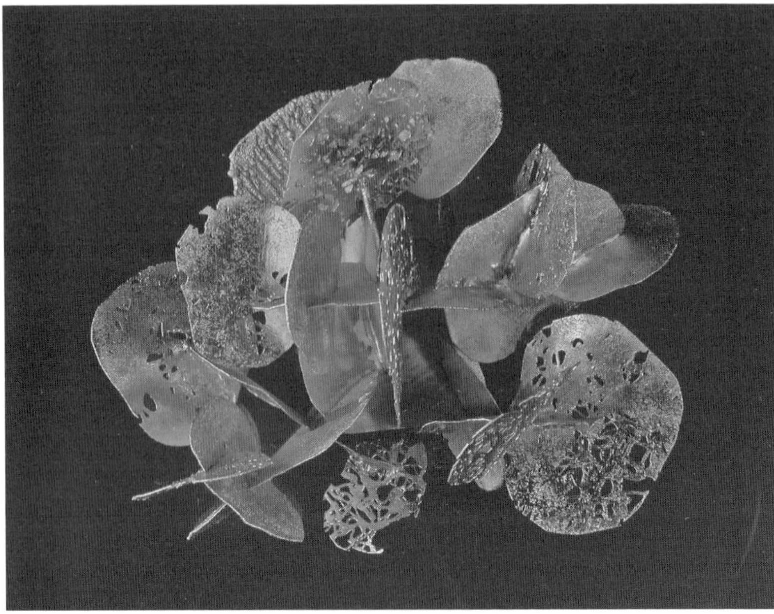

FIGURE 23.4 Cell Group Zinc by Frances Geesin, 2007. This work is informed by images describing nanostructures that can exhibit complex electronic properties. The interleaved structures are assembled from two contrasting industrial materials, a nonwoven and a conductive shielding fabric. It describes an internal energy and creates shadows by the light falling on and through it, revealing both absence and presence.
Credit: Photograph by Ron Geesin.

FROM COMMUNICATION TO CO-CREATION: HELEN STOREY, KATE STOREY, AND TONY RYAN

When Ottilia Saxl asked Frances Geesin to engage with nanotechnology, Geesin began the now familiar approach of the SciArt genre pioneered in 1997 by the Wellcome Trust[11] where "scientist seeks artist for communication." This is perhaps the natural successor to the "scientist seeks methodology" scenario described in the discussion on botany. Science is quite capable of developing its own methodologies, but new science bases are often extremely complex. As a result, science is often hard to understand—even by its practitioners—and the key role for art and artists has shifted from method to communication, as the next example demonstrates.

Fashion designer Helen Storey stepped away from the catwalk in the mid-1990s, planning to apply her fashion art to new challenges with social value. Her first project was part of the earliest tranche of Wellcome Trust SciArt collaborations, funded in 1997 with her sister, developmental biologist Kate Storey. The innovative Primitive Streak project elucidated key early stages in the development of the human fetus.[12] This fashion-art collection demonstrates the strength of a genre (fashion) in which sometimes difficult, challenging pieces of art are grounded by the ultimate relationship with humanity that flows from their intimate position on the human form; however experimental, fashion-art is always grounded. With regard to earlier comments on "why fashion," Primitive Streak is the stuff of dreams. It has successfully traveled the world since 1997, seen by over 11 million people, and in 2011 was relaunched in partnership with the Wellcome Trust Arts Award.

Primitive Streak is well articulated by Helen and Kate Storey on the project website and has undoubtedly been a shared journey. However, at its core, it is a fine example of what can happen when the scientist seeks communication (to engage with a broad public, in this case). But does such a project influence the science, and what is the perception of the scientist? In conversation with Helen Storey she revealed that whenever her sister has been asked if the work has changed her science, the answer is always no.

Since the success of Primitive Streak, Helen Storey has continued her research journey into science. In 2005 Storey heard leading materials scientist Professor Tony Ryan of Sheffield University talking on the radio. Ryan (one-time professor of public understanding of science) is a superb communicator, explaining what polymers are and advocating what they can do for us. Storey was intrigued and decided to find out more. She simply telephoned with some questions and was invited up to Sheffield to "muck around" in the polymer laboratory. From this has grown an extraordinary research partnership, one that can be viewed as a "gold standard" of science/fashion-art collaboration.

The first project from the partnership, Wonderland, directly tackles the challenge of degradation of the environment through excess waste, in particular plastics.[13] The art output is succinctly described on the leading fashion website SHOWstudio: "Wonderland used fashion as a 'Trojan Horse' to progress a radical, two-year exploration into biodegradable materials. This project showcases the life—and death—of Helen Storey's collection of incredible dissolving dresses" (Figure 23.5).[14] However, the project also generated a first-rate science and technology output of patentable product possibilities for a better, more sustainable world, such as water-purification devices for use in sub-Saharan Africa.

The question arises, what are Tony Ryan and Helen Storey doing when they collaborate? They co-create new research agendas on major social issues—and then find ways to take them forward. They influence each other on a shared journey into the unknown, through dialogue and experimentation. In his BBC Reith lectures of 2005, engineer Alec Broers stated bluntly, "Technology will determine the future of the human race."[15] Around the same time fashion journalist Annalisa Barbieri (2005) commented that "fashion is actually a wonder force, an invention more useful than radio." These quotations suggest a tension between fashion, science, and technology, an intangible but valuable force that Helen Storey and Tony Ryan are able to harness to great effect.

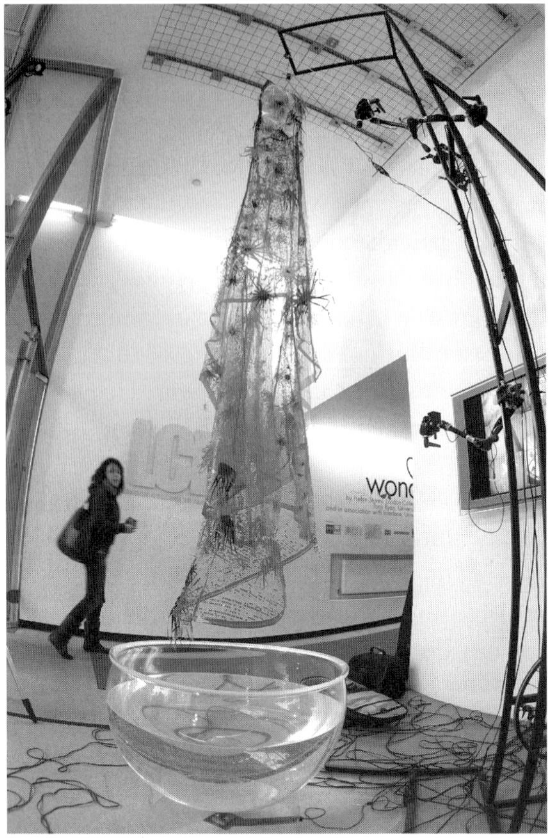

FIGURE 23.5 Wonderland "disappearing dress" installation, London College of Fashion, 2008. This plastic dress slowly dissolved into the water over twenty-eight days, highlighting an alternative future for plastics.
Credit: Photograph by Alex Maguire. Courtesy of Helen Storey.

A SIMPLE TAXONOMY FOR COLLABORATIVE ART/DESIGN/SCIENCE PROJECTS

A further champion of design and technology working together is Raymond Oliver, a chemical engineer with a track record of industrial research and development leadership who embraces design to the extent that he holds a professorial research post in the Faculty of Art, Design and Social Science at Northumbria University. He has seen first-hand the way scientists/technologists frequently fail to deliver the potential value of their work, and so he advocates "D-STEM" projects, that is, design working with science, technology, engineering, and mathematics, as a key methodology to create genuine, inspiring innovation. Adding art into that, AD-STEM is a suitable acronym for the family of projects that have sprung from the collaborations between art/design and science/technology discussed so far.

TABLE 23.1 AD-STEM COLLABORATIONS

ARTIST/DESIGNER SEEKING TECHNOLOGY	SCIENTIST SEEKING (E.G., COMMUNICATION, METHODS)	SCIENTISTS + ARTISTS CO-CREATING
Fabrican (Torres from Luckham)	Plant taxonomy (Linnaeus)	Wonderland and Catalytic Clothing (Ryan and Storey)
	Plant Structure (Kew Gardens from Kesseler)	
Wellness (Tillotson from Manz)	Philips wearables (Philips from Geesin)	
Interactive textile (Geesin from, e.g., BASF)	Nanotechnology sector (Saxl from Geesin)	
Digital textile (Harris from, e.g., Vicon)	Primitive Streak (Storey and Storey)	

To return to the aim of this chapter, and building on the observation that botany is a good metaphor for fashion, the very simple classification of AD-STEM projects in Table 23.1 is proposed. This self-explanatory structure comes from identification by the boundary questions—who is seeking, who is providing? The model is what taxonomists would call "high level," and although it would be possible to sketch out more detailed lower orders, the effort expended may not justify this. Care should be taken that co-creation is not confused with development. Most high-performing partnerships will reach a stage of developing ideas together; for example, technology is developed as the design requirements move on to new ideas. However, co-creation is a phase when the seeking/providing question cannot be answered, where the partnership takes on challenges external to what might normally be expected from them to create an inspirational experiment together.

Although simple, there are a number of reasons why this structure has value and is worth considering by practitioners. First, analysis of the projects in this way reflects on the nature of the partnerships making them happen; it is always good to be clear about what a partnership is offering—and to identify whether it is the sort of relationship that the practitioner wants to be part of. Second, it is good for communication—both within the partnership and to the outside world. Collaborative projects often appear to the observer as a complex web of activity, and it has been the experience of the coauthor, Philip Sams, that it is not always clear why the partnership has been formed. The simple definitions above can provide helpful guidance.

COLLABORATIVE METHODS OF WORKING

In 2009 researchers at London College of Fashion explored the clash of arts/science disciplines and the practice of collaboration in a series of public events, culminating in a discussion between scientists, artists, and designers all experienced in working at the intersection of science and the arts.[16] The questions focused on what has been described above as co-creation, asking, when does it happen, what is needed, how can it be encouraged? The key messages were simple. First, a consensus quickly emerged that co-creative collaborations are driven by personal chemistry and trust. Although it might be argued that these will always play a part in any partnership, they are essential in a situation that starts voluntarily, beyond a need for any particular skills, and where either party is free to walk away. This freedom and lack of structured dependency is also reflected in the way that co-creative partnerships frequently arise—the power of serendipity and random collisions were articulated as important factors. Finally, it was recognized that co-creation is potentially possible when the challenge is fuzzy and significantly bigger than the participating co-creators. The Ryan and Storey partnership described above, starting with the Wonderland project, fulfills all of these criteria—a chance connection through radio resulted in their taking on the major challenge of sustainable consumption, framed by the mutually supportive personalities of the protagonists. Ryan and Storey have developed further projects, including the notion of "catalytic clothing," a concept crystallized through discussions in a research workshop comprising a mix of science, design, and humanities academics. It is important to note that although synergies can be serendipitous when diverse people are brought into a room together, the workshop methodology requires structured discussion in order to achieve viable outcomes.

The Catalytic Clothing project tackles the significant global problem of air pollution in cities by the fusion of the technology of surface science and catalysis with the communal power of masses of people, motivated through fashion and clothing. At the time of writing, the Catalytic Clothing message has reached many millions of people worldwide through a viral film campaign, tracked and communicated through a new visual mapping mechanism.[17] While Wonderland provided output that was obviously directly relevant and useful to both Storey's fashion college and Ryan's department of science and technology, there are fewer academic recognition benefits for Ryan with Catalytic Clothing than with the Wonderland project. Storey comments that Ryan provides "intellectual generosity" by accessing technology for the project from outside his research group. In other words, this co-creating partnership exists beyond direct mutual self-interest.

INTO THE FUTURE

One interesting question arises—is it fashion-art or science individuals who usually initiate the partnerships? In the modern case studies above, the lead has, in the main, been taken by the artist/designer. Even in cases that turned into "scientist seeking..." observations suggest that the conversation has tended to be opened by the artist, with the scientist then realizing that this was indeed needed! Raymond Oliver moved from the chemical industry to design academia via the concept of D-STEM. He describes how in his experience of chemical synthesis and processing, potentially great materials were often, in his words, "left hanging in the ether. . . . [T]he challenge of creating materials-based products that matter to people, became quite compelling." His path took him first to the RCA, where designers were eager to try new materials, and "the upshot is that creative design meeting active and interactive materials opens a broad fusion of opportunities, starting from fashion as a driver of human innovation." In pursuit of this aim, in late 2012, funded by Northumbria University in the north of England, Oliver launched a new London center dubbed P^3i[18]—"the first D:STEM interaction studio in the UK," following the example of international institutions such as MIT's Media Lab, Ivrea, and XS Labs in Montreal, Canada (see chapter 21).[19]

As noted earlier in this chapter, historically, art and science were closely connected contributors to a single culture. C. P. Snow stated in his 1959 Rede Lecture *The Two Cultures*, "The intellectual life of the whole of Western society is increasingly being split into two polar groups" ([1959] 2001: 3). Snow was describing what he saw as an emerging rift between scientists and writers. A more recent essay on the subject of "two cultures" draws attention to the core message in Snow's work that scientists will save the world, whereas traditional intellectuals would hold this back (Dizikes 2009). Thus the "two cultures" concept has taken on a life of its own as a description of a schism between scientists (as the leaders into the future) and artists in general (as the followers), becoming a cliché easily used without study of the original text. This schism is still reflected in current discourse by use of the terms *scientists* and *creatives* as oppositional, implying that arts and the humanities have a monopoly on creativity.

What might drive scientists to downgrade the role that arts can have? While there is a desire by science to gain new insights through artistic engagement, this is not a clearly defined need for much contemporary work. The "sci-art" role is primarily that of communicating the science to a wider public—important but not leading the work. Two signposts toward a more balanced partnership emerge. First is the key role that design schools (rather than art schools) can have when they grasp the future through inspired leadership. Nicholas Negroponte founded and directed the Media Lab, in the school of architecture at MIT, to achieve his vision of designing for a digital, wired-up world, captured in his book *Being Digital* (1999). This inspirational fusion of design onto science and technology has defined current understandings of how creative multidisciplinary activity can work at its very best. While design schools can be groundbreaking and highly influential, as in the Bauhaus, for example, without necessarily falling directly in step with radical science, there will no doubt be new examples. Perhaps universities in the twenty-first-century powerhouses in Asia might create radical partnerships between design and science.

Second is the serendipitous partnership that leads to co-creation. We have seen how this flourishes when addressing major social issues, and there are many challenges that can usefully be taken on, for example, how to reduce the stress of migration that will potentially be required to deal with shifts in global food and water availability. Fashion-art is perhaps a particularly good partner for this because of its human-centered thinking.

In the United Kingdom, there is a new wave of enthusiasm and support for cross-disciplinary initiatives. For example, the UK Crafts Council, traditionally focused on handcrafts, in its 2012 conference Assemble embraced the potential for collaborations between craft practitioners and makers, and emerging science and technology. In this context, Suzanne Lee, director of the BioCouture project (mentioned earlier), suggests that "the future of craft and fashion lies in the relationship between scientists and makers."[20] The future for design, and particularly fashion/science partnerships, seems positive, a fruitful route into a new single-culture future.

NOTES

1. The Wellcome Trust (UK) instigated the "SciArt" series of competitions in 1997 to foster collaborative cross-disciplinary exploration and communication of scientific research in the biomedical science sector through visual arts projects. Over the course of a decade SciArt supported 118 projects with nearly £3 million of funding.
2. Design thinking is a term now widely used in business to indicate the approach and methods of ideation and problem solving used by designers (see, for example, Cross 2011). Fashion thinking is an emerging concept within design thinking (see also Nixon and Blakley 2012).
3. BioCouture, http://www.biocouture.com (accessed November 15, 2012).
4. BGCI (Botanic Gardens Conservation International), http://www.bgci.org/resources/botanical_illustration/ (accessed April 20, 2012).
5. Rob Kesseler, http://www.robkesseler.co.uk (accessed November 30, 2012).
6. Manel Torres, personal communication with Philip Sams, October 25, 2011. The following quote is also from this source.
7. Jenny Tillotson, personal communication with Philip Sams, October 25, 2011. Subsequent quotations from Tillotson are from this source.
8. Jane Harris, personal communication with Philip Sams, November 16, 2011.
9. Frances Geesin, personal communication with Philip Sams, October 31, 2011. The following quote is also from this source.
10. See, for example, Intelligent Textiles, http://www.intelligenttextiles.com.
11. See note 1.
12. Helen Storey and Kate Storey, Primitive Streak, http://www.primitive-streak.org (accessed April 24, 2012).
13. Helen Storey and Anthony Ryan, Wonderland, http://www.wonderland-sheffield.co.uk (accessed April 24, 2012).
14. "Wonderland," SHOWstudio, http://showstudio.com/project/wonderland (accessed April 24, 2012).
15. Alec Broers, "Technology Will Determine the Future of the Human Race," BBC Reith Lecture no. 1, April 6, 2005, http://www.bbc.co.uk/radio4/reith2005/lecturer.shtml (accessed April 20, 2012).
16. The panel comprised the scientists Tony Ryan of Sheffield University (polymer scientist), Matt Wyon of the University of Wolverhampton (dance and sports scientist), and Philip

Sams (industrial chemist) while the designer-artists were represented by Susan Benn (Performing Arts Lab), Alec Robertson (DeMontfort University and 4D Design), Helen Storey (artist/researcher LCF), and Sandy Black (designer/researcher LCF).

17. Catalytic Clothing, http://www.cataytic-clothing.com (accessed April 20, 2012).
18. P3i is an acronym for "printable, paintable, programmable (intelligent) materials."
19. Raymond Oliver, personal communication with Philip Sams, November 24, 2011.
20. Suzanne Lee speaking at Assemble, the UK Crafts Council conference in London, September 17, 2012.

BIBLIOGRAPHY

Barbieri, Annalisa. 2005. "First Impressions." *The Guardian,* April 12.

Black, Sandy, and Philip Sams. 2005. "Seeds for the Future—How Fashion and Science Can Help Each Other." In Textile Institute Proceedings of 84th Annual World Conference, USA, March 22–25. CD-ROM.

Blunt, Wilfrid, and Sandra Raphael. 1979. *The Illustrated Herbal.* London: Frances Lincoln.

Bolton, Andrew. 2002. *The Supermodern Wardrobe.* London: V&A Publications.

Braddock, Sarah E., and Marie O'Mahony. 1998. *Techno Textiles.* London: Thames and Hudson.

Braddock, Sarah E., and Marie O'Mahony. 2002. *SportsTech.* London: Thames and Hudson.

Braddock Clarke, Sarah E., and Marie O'Mahony. 2005. *Techno Textiles 2.* London: Thames and Hudson.

Cross, Nigel. 2011. *Design Thinking.* London: Berg.

DeBray, Lys. 2001. *The Art of Botanical Illustration.* London: Quantum.

Dizikes, Peter. 2009. "Our Two Cultures." *New York Times,* March 19.

Entwistle, Joanne. 2000. *The Fashioned Body.* Cambridge, UK: Polity.

Frayling, Christopher. 1993. "Research in Art and Design." RCA Research Papers 1 (1). London: Royal College of Art.

Geesin, Frances. 1995. "The Chemical and Structural Manipulation of Fabrics and Fibres." PhD diss., Royal College of Art, London.

Hale, William. 1932. *Chemistry Triumphant.* Baltimore: Williams & Wilkins.

Handley, Susannah. 1999. *Nylon: The Man-Made Fashion Revolution.* London: Bloomsbury.

Harris, Jane. 2000. "Surface Tension—the Aesthetic Fabrication of Digital Textiles." PhD diss., Royal College of Art, London.

Hooke, Robert. 1665. *Micrographia.* London: Martyn and Allestrey.

Huxley, Aldous. 1932. *Brave New World.* London: Chatto & Windus.

Khornak, L. 1982. *Fashion 2001.* London: Columbus Books.

Lee, Suzanne. 2005. *Fashioning the Future: Tomorrow's Wardrobe.* London: Thames and Hudson.

Linnaeus, Carolus. 1735. *Systema Naturae.* Leiden, the Netherlands: Apud Theodorum Haak.

Mabey, Richard. 2010. *Weeds.* London: Profile.

Manz, Andreas, N. Graber, and H. M. Widmer. 1990. "Miniaturized Total Chemical Analysis Systems: A Novel Concept for Chemical Sensing." *Sensors and Actuators* B1: 244–48.

Negroponte, Nicholas. 1999. *Being Digital.* New York: Alfred Knopf.

Nixon, Natalie, and Johanna Blakley. 2012. "Fashion Thinking: Towards an Actionable Methodology." *Fashion Practice: The Journal of Design, Creative Process and the Fashion Industry* 4 (2): 153–76.

O'Mahony, Marie. 2011. *Advanced Textiles for Health and Wellbeing.* London: Thames and Hudson.

Quinn, Bradley. 2002. *Techno Fashion.* Oxford: Berg.

Seymour, Sabine. 2008. *Fashionable Technology: The Intersection of Design, Fashion, Science and Technology.* Vienna: Springer.

Simmel, Georg. 1904. "Fashion." *International Quarterly* 10: 130–55.

Snow, C. P. [1959] 2001. *The Two Cultures.* Cambridge: Cambridge University Press.

Tillotson, Jenny. 1997. "Interactive Olfactory Surfaces: The Wellness Collection—a Science Fashion Story." PhD diss., Royal College of Art, London.

Tillotson, Jenny. 2009. "Scentsory Design: A Holistic Approach to Fashion as a Vehicle to Deliver Emotional Wellbeing." *Fashion Practice* 1 (1): 33–61.

Torres, Manel. 2001. "Fabric in a Can—the Future." PhD diss., Royal College of Art, London.

Veblen, Thorstein. 1899. *The Theory of the Leisure Class: An Economic Study in the Evolution of Institutions.* New York: Macmillan.

Woolf, Virginia. 1928. *Orlando.* London: Hogarth.

SECTION VII

Sustainable Fashion in a Globalized World

Introduction

SANDY BLACK AND REGINA A. ROOT

While the *Fashion Studies Handbook* approaches sustainability and globalization throughout fashion theory and history, especially as related to practice, this concluding section highlights the cultural and economic realignments that already inform and challenge everyday fashion practices around the globe. It considers the fast-changing practices within fashion production and consumption, precipitated by the global environmental and economic imperatives that have impacted fashion since the Industrial Revolution. Both practical and cultural shifts have resulted, and are still emerging, due to increased awareness of issues endemic to the complex fashion system of global manufacturing and the pressing need for enhanced sustainability. This section discusses issues pertaining to sustainable fashion from a range of perspectives and indicates future directions for the practice of fashion. Through radical shifts in business culture from actors across the industry spectrum—such as retail companies and brands, buyers, manufacturers, and designers—to new modes of operation, it is envisaged that the principles of sustainability can become increasingly embedded in fashion manufacturing processes and the retail offer. Nor are consumers of fashion absolved from responsibility for nurturing a more sustainable fashion system. Consumer choices are intimately connected to success and failure within the fashion system, but influencing consumer behavior toward more sustainable goals is a quest still in its infancy.

The fashion and apparel industry is intrinsically wasteful, as fashion cycles through style changes and encourages obsolescence in favor of the new season's merchandise. However, since the mid-1990s, significant shifts in trading have combined to accelerate the traditional twice-yearly fashion seasons, a commercial infrastructure familiar since the mid-twentieth century. With the abolition of the General Agreement on Tariffs and Trade in 1995 (a post–World War II measure) and the establishment of the World Trade

Organization, a relaxation of protectionist trading quotas and tariffs saw a rapid migration of garment production offshore from developed countries such as the United States and Britain to lower-wage areas for more competitive pricing. As competition in such saturated markets has grown, short-lived transseasonal collections—known as "fast fashion"—have become commonplace in the early twenty-first century, with eight to ten new collections a year the norm in mass-market fashion. As the rate of fashion production and consumption has increased, so has competitive pressure, resulting in a continuing reduction in retail prices that has in turn created iniquitous pressures on producers at the lower end of the supply chain (a practice known in industry parlance as the "race to the bottom"). In this distributed global industry, new markets for fashion are constantly being opened up in developing countries, exacerbating the problems with the fashion life cycle of high-turnover production, consumption, and waste.

Given the complexity of the major issues apparent throughout the fashion system, it is unsurprising that its endemic problems were largely sidestepped within the fashion and textile industries until a major reawakening at the turn of the new millennium. A confluence of natural disasters and economic and political crises forced a reexamination of business cultures, questioning their ethical dimensions, and created a demand for greater transparency in the age of instant digital communication. Through a combination of sustained media exposé and commentary, the 2007 Nobel Peace Prize laureate Al Gore challenged with *An Inconvenient Truth* (Guggenheim 2006), and Naomi Klein (2000) delved into the political challenges of addressing global climate change and corporate social responsibility (also see Achbar, Abbott, and Bakan 2003; Rivoli 2005; Stern 2006). A groundswell of public opinion mobilized toward greater awareness of sustainability, building further on the Brundtland Commission's report on *Our Common Future* (United Nations World Commission on Environment and Development 1987). Major initiatives followed at the government level in the United Kingdom (the Defra Sustainable Clothing Action Plan, 2007[1]) and retail (Marks & Spencer's Plan A, 2007) and in the United States (Gap, Nike). Later, new academic/industry partnerships to develop sustainable fashion were established in Scandinavia (the Nordic Initiative, Clean and Ethical, or NICE, 2008;[2] the Swedish Foundation for Strategic Environmental Research [MISTRA], 2010). In the United States in 2010, the largest third-party fair trade certifier, Fair Trade USA, began to certify linens and apparel. The 2010 California Transparency in Supply Chains Act requires high-level retailers and manufacturers to make transparent "efforts to eradicate slavery and human trafficking from [their] direct supply chain for tangible goods offered for sale."[3] Made in a Free World[4] created a mobile phone app, partially funded by the U.S. State Department Office to Monitor and Combat Trafficking in Persons, to help consumers determine their slavery footprint. In 2005 the luxury sportswear brand Patagonia, which makes transparent its environmental impact with its carbon "footprint chronicles," began the Common Threads Initiative with a pledge asking consumers to pledge to buy only what they need, "repair what breaks," reuse, and recycle.[5] In 2011 a group of global apparel industry players, including Patagonia, adidas, Levis, and many more brands, set up the Sustainable Apparel Coalition. All of these initiatives have drawn on academic research to inform the practices of the fashion industry and its supply chains.

Historically, the business of fashion has not been the province of fashion theory, which primarily addresses cultural practice and meaning associated with dressing the body. However, the issues underlying sustainability serve as a unifying agenda in which interdisciplinary research—interfacing academia and industry, theory and practice—now recognize and learn from each other's approaches and methods. "Eco" or "green" fashion sprouted alongside Rachel Carson's *Silent Spring* (1962) and this renowned biologist's unwavering argument against the use of pesticides to which industrial sectors had long attributed health benefits (e.g., the "DDT is good for me-e-e" Pennsalt campaign). The photograph of Earth from the 1968 Apollo space mission, which appeared on the Whole Earth catalog (Brand 1972) and in fashion spreads, significantly altered the way in which consumers saw themselves. The counterculture of the 1970s, despite the fact that hippie dress was often itself mass-manufactured, sported natural looks and trends (Welters 2008). In response to conspicuous consumption in the 1980s, the Esprit Ecollection designed by Lynda Grose introduced "environmentally conscious style"; Grose went on to initiate the Sustainable Cotton Project (Black 2008). This approach has matured in the twenty-first century and now (of necessity) represents a permanent shift toward sustainable practice across fashion, general apparel, and the textile industry, to parallel similar shifts in food, architecture, and the automotive industries, among others. The discourse of fashion has evolved to adopt the terminology of sustainability, encompassing the three pillars of sustainable thinking: ecology, economics, and humanity. This section integrates a fourth dimension—culture and aesthetics—that scholars and design professionals seek to integrate into the holistic thinking required for sustainability.

The fashion system in the early twenty-first century is a globalized system of design, marketing, materials, and manufacturing sourced in disparate locations worldwide, especially South Asia, and transported internationally for retail sale in high-value markets in developed and developing countries. A few scholars have expanded the purview of sustainable fashion history with analysis of pioneering work in various world culture regions, recognizing the integration of local forms of knowledge into the design process and the terms of consumption (Blanch, Novik, and Root 2008; Clark 2008; Hansen 2000). The major issues for fashion-related research include ethical business practices and social justice for garment workers in factories or manual workers and artisans in the home, extraction of materials (both agriculturally derived and synthetic), apparel-production methods and associated technical processes, global sourcing remote from markets and consequent transportation, the increasing demand for natural resources, short life cycles, disposal and waste, the role of design and designers, and the economic models and cultural contexts in which the fashion system operates. Although these issues are large and complex, both academic research and industry initiatives have gained new vitality to envision and generate a range of solutions addressing many of the issues while endeavoring to retain the economic, social, and symbolic benefits that fashion confers.

Following the early seminal literature on the sustainable imperative for ecology and design practice in architecture (Brand 1972; Carson 1962; Manzini 2003; Papanek 1972, 1995; Whitely 1992), a new wave of publications specific to product design (Chapman 2005; McDonough and Braungart 2002; Walker 2006), and then fashion and textile design (Black 2007, 2008, 2012; Brown 2010; Fletcher 2008; Fletcher and Grose 2012; Gwilt and Rissanen 2011; Hethorn and Ulasewicz 2008; Root 2008; Siegle 2011), appeared in the first decade of the twenty-first century examining theories, concepts, practices, and strategies for increasing sustainability through the fashion life cycle. At the same time economists have set out their critiques of contemporary business and posited the need for dynamic changes in strategic models (Hawken 1993, 1999; Jackson 2011).

As the ethos of sustainability in fashion becomes established, the four chapters in this section offer a range of perspectives mapping the contemporary industry landscape and culture. Marsha A. Dickson focuses on the progress toward and barriers to improvements in garment workers' conditions in the global apparel industry. Guiding readers through ways in which to approach human rights and corporate social responsibility initiatives, Dickson reminds scholars not to get "stuck" in the eruption of novelty but rather to engage critical approaches that push the field further through arguments grounded in sound fieldwork, archival research, and methodology. Margaret Maynard examines the fast fashion phenomenon in the context of labor issues and sustainability, analyzing carefully the terms implied with "sustainability of attire," cultural practices, and the impact of discarded clothing on recipient countries. She acknowledges a need for transnational dialogue within sustainable fashion studies in order to decenter the European perspectives that currently prevail in the field. Kate Fletcher discusses the role and influence of design for sustainability within the fashion and textiles industries, exploring design innovation at the level of product, service, and system and contextualizing a number of approaches for improving the environmental and social quality of the sector. Drawing on examples from large- and small-scale industry and a wide range of product types, Fletcher highlights both the opportunity and potential for change toward sustainability in fashion and textiles, with a focus on the potential of local, artisan-based textile and fashion production. Globalization is at once challenging and changing the field of fashion studies and the terms of its engagement. In a fruitful intellectual exchange, Simonetta Carbonaro and David Goldsmith discuss new, more holistic concepts for sustainable business models within the fashion sector that disrupt unsustainable "business as usual." Two exemplars, rooted in their professional practice, trace the differences and links between a large organization, Coop Italia, and a small Indian producer of textiles, Gudi Mudi, via their production chains. The integration of cultural and visual aesthetics within new business models aims to design and engender a new type of prosperity.

Theoretically speaking, sustainable fashion has forged a new path for fashion studies. In the context of globalization, this growing subfield reevaluates design history, analyzes carefully the impacts of innovations and design solutions, and at times represents scholarship in action. As institutions and industries reconsider the creative process and the supply chain in the pursuit of sustainable fashion, design professionals also recognize the significance of their role as facilitators to a larger production process that will require sustainable materials and sustained livelihoods for the people involved. Sustainable fashion demands a new way of thinking: it involves slowing down fashion cycles, understanding why and how a garment is made, treading lightly on the earth, and seeking workable solutions in an era of urgency and crisis. The directions highlighted in this section signal a new, more holistic approach to the notion of sustainable fashion, as both scholars and practitioners search for solutions to the question: can fashion ever be sustainable?

NOTES

1. "Sustainable Clothing Action Plan," UK Department for the Environment, Food and Rural Affairs, March 30, 2011, http://www.defra.gov.uk/publications/2011/03/30/pb13206-clothing-action-plan/ (accessed May 8, 2013).
2. Nordic Initiative, Clean and Ethical, http://www.nicefashion.org/en/ (accessed December 17, 2012).
3. California Transparency in Supply Chains Act of 2010, http://www.state.gov/documents/organization/164934.pdf (accessed December 17, 2012).
4. Made in a Free World, http://slaveryfootprint.org (accessed December 17, 2012).
5. Common Threads Initiative, Patagonia, http://www.patagonia.com/us/common-threads/ (accessed December 19, 2012).

BIBLIOGRAPHY

Achbar, Mark, Jennifer Abbott, and Joel Bakan (dirs.). 2003. *The Corporation. British Columbia,* Canada: Big Picture Media Corporation.

Black, Sandy. 2007. "Interrogating Fashion." In Tom Inns (ed.), *Insights and Questions: Designing for the 21st Century*, 299–314. Aldershot, UK: Gower.

Black, Sandy. 2008. *Eco Chic: The Fashion Paradox.* London: Black Dog.

Black, Sandy. 2012. *The Sustainable Fashion Handbook.* London: Thames and Hudson.

Blanch, Alex, Laura Novik, and Regina A. Root. 2008. "La moda ética en América Latina." *Estudios* 16 (32): 305–14.

Brand, Stewart (ed.). 1972. *The Last Whole Earth Catalog.* Menlo Park, CA: Portola Institute.

Brown, Sass. 2010. *Eco Fashion.* London: Laurence King.

Carson, Rachel. 1962. *Silent Spring.* Boston: Houghton Mifflin.

Chapman, Jonathan. 2005. *Emotionally Durable Design: Objects, Experience and Empathy.* London: Earthscan.

Clark, Hazel. 2008. "SLOW + FASHION—an Oxymoron—or a Promise for the Future...?" *Fashion Theory* 12 (4): 427–46.
Fletcher, Kate. 2008. *Sustainable Fashion and Textiles: Design Journeys.* London: Earthscan.
Fletcher, Kate, and Lynda Grose. 2012. *Fashion and Sustainability: Design for Change.* London: Laurence King.
Guggenheim, Davis. 2006. *An Inconvenient Truth.* Film. Los Angeles, CA: Paramount Classics and Participant Productions.
Gwilt, Alison, and Timo Rissanen. 2011. *Shaping Sustainable Fashion: Changing the Way We Make and Use Clothes.* London: Earthscan.
Hansen, Karen Tranberg. 2000. *Salaula: The World of Secondhand Clothing and Zambia.* Chicago: University of Chicago Press.
Hawken, Paul. 1993. *Ecology of Commerce: How Business Can Save the Planet.* London: Weidenfeld and Nicolson.
Hawken, Paul. 1999. *Natural Capitalism: The Next Industrial Revolution.* London: Earthscan.
Hethorn, Janet, and Connie Ulasewicz (eds.). 2008. *Sustainable Fashion: Why Now? A Conversation Exploring Issues, Practices, and Possibilities.* New York: Fairchild Books.
Jackson, Tim. 2011. *Prosperity without Growth: Economics for a Finite Planet.* London: Routledge.
Klein, Naomi. 2000. *No Logo.* New York: Flamingo.
Manzini, Ezio. 2003. *Sustainable Everyday: Scenarios of Urban Life.* Milan: Ambiente.
McDonough, William, and Michael Braungart. 2002. *Cradle to Cradle: Remaking the Way We Make Things.* New York: North Point.
Papanek, Victor. 1972. *Design for the Real World.* London: Thames and Hudson.
Papanek, Victor. 1995. *The Green Imperative: Ecology and Ethics in Design and Architecture.* London: Thames and Hudson.
Rivoli, Pietra. 2005. *The Travels of a T-Shirt in the Global Economy: An Economist Examines the Markets, Power and Politics of World Trade.* Hoboken, NJ: John Wiley.
Root, Regina A. (ed.). 2008. "Ecofashion." Special issue, *Fashion Theory* 12 (4).
Siegle, Lucy. 2011. *To Die For: Is Fashion Wearing Out the World?* London: Fourth Estate.
Stern, Nicholas. 2006. *Review on the Economics of Climate Change.* London: Her Majesty's Treasury.
United Nations World Commission on Environment and Development. 1987. *Our Common Future.* http://www.un-documents.net/our-common-future.pdf (accessed December 17, 2012).
Walker, Stuart. 2006. *Sustainable by Design: Explorations in Theory and Practice.* London: Earthscan.
Welters, Linda. 2008. "The Natural Look: American Style in the 1970s." *Fashion Theory* 12 (4): 489–510.
Whitely, Nigel. 1992. *Design for Society.* London: Reaktion Books.

24

Corporate Responsibility in the Global Apparel Industry: Toward an Integrated Human Rights–Based Approach

MARSHA A. DICKSON

In 1997 *Beautiful Flowers of the Maquiladora* was translated into English. Based on field research in Mexico in the 1970s, the book shared the life histories of ten Mexican women who had migrated to work in maquiladoras along the United States–Mexico border. Most of the women were very young; had little work experience and few alternatives for work, limited formal education, and no knowledge about their rights as workers; and hailed from poor families (Iglesias Prieto 1997). The research illuminated the conditions faced by women at the bottom of the vast global supply chains, which were rapidly developing to support the fashion industry. The abuses shared by the women included the following:

- Discriminatory hiring and promotion practices
- Little or no development of skills/intellect
- Repetitive, monotonous tasks that alienate workers and create health problems
- Poorly ventilated workplaces/unsafe conditions/poor lighting or toxin-filled air
- Limits to bathroom breaks
- Poor pay without increases to cover increased prices of basic needs
- Extreme disciplinary measures
- Psychological manipulation/abuse to compel faster work, longer hours, and fewer troublemakers

- Sexual harassment/abuse
- Intense/unrealistic production quotas not based on professional time and method studies that take physical toll on workers, who work to exhaustion
- Last-minute changes to schedules requiring mothers to be away from children overnight
- Union busting, including closing factories where workers strike, threats and harassment, and blacklisting
- No job security

An often-cited U.S.-centric definition of a sweatshop is "an employer that violates more than one federal or state labor law governing minimum wage and overtime, child labor, industrial homework, occupational safety and health, workers' compensation, or industry registration" (U.S. General Accounting Office 1994). But most would agree that the characteristics Iglesias Prieto described vividly illustrated sweatshop conditions. Likewise, the findings exemplified the fashion industry's negative impacts on social sustainability as Mexico's young workers were exploited and communities divided for others' gains. By the early 1990s the media had begun to link sweatshop conditions with the U.S. brand-name manufacturers and retailers contracting the work (Varley 1998). In the twenty years that followed, amid an onslaught of questions from media and activist campaigns, apparel companies shifted from denial of responsibility for their contractors' labor practices and began taking steps to reform the industry. However, many of the problems observed by Iglesias Prieto remain, as does the social responsibility work to resolve them (Dickson, Loker, and Eckman 2009).

Social responsibility includes the range of activities companies and other stakeholders carry out to assure workers making their products experience fair labor standards and safe and healthy working conditions. Social responsibility is embedded in the societal context and cuts across nodes of the global value chain involving brands and retailers, factories and suppliers, and a host of stakeholders—consumers, investors, nongovernmental organizations (NGOs), workers themselves, and others. Social responsibility involves the policies and practices carried out in support of the end goal of sustainability where human rights for all individuals in the value chain are achieved (Dickson, Loker, and Eckman 2009).

A comprehensive review of literature on social responsibility in the apparel industry would include content on contextual and historical events, including the student anti-sweatshop movement (e.g., Bender and Greenwald 2003), the role of trade policy (e.g., Rosen 2002), efforts of multistakeholder initiatives (e.g., Casey 2006; O'Rourke 2003, 2006), consumer behavior (e.g., Dickson 2013), industry structure (e.g., Hale and Wills 2007), and other topics. This chapter focuses exclusively on the evolving policies and practices of corporate social responsibility (CSR) in the apparel industry and reviews the literature studying various initiatives, measuring their effectiveness, and exploring new strategies for improving working conditions in global apparel supply chains. The review is not exhaustive; rather, papers reviewed include only those that present unique empirical research or extend progressive theories and conceptual frameworks.

LAWS AND RIGHTS FRAMING CSR

The United Nations' (UN) "Guiding Principles on Business and Human Rights" provide an understanding of CSR in the context of the business responsibility to respect human rights. The guiding principles require businesses to avoid impinging on the human rights of others and to address any negative impacts that result directly from their business activities or indirectly through their relationships with others, including suppliers producing their goods (Ruggie 2011). For example, if a retailer found that a supplier was using forced or child labor, the retailer would be expected to mitigate the human rights violation. Human rights frame sweatshop issues broadly and are fundamental to individuals living freely and with dignity. They apply to all individuals regardless of the country they reside in and the wealth of that country, and in every context of their lives, including at work. The responsibility to respect human rights applies to businesses of all sizes and ownership structures and means at minimum businesses must "do no harm" all the time and in all situations (Ruggie 2011).

In order for companies to be aware of, prevent, and address negative human rights impacts, they carry out due diligence encompassing four main areas: adopting human rights policies, integrating the policies throughout the company, identifying how current/potential activities impact human rights, and tracking and communicating performance. Additionally, anticipating that due diligence may not uncover all violations of human rights, companies put in place grievance systems that allow victims to report problems and have them addressed (Ruggie 2011). The characteristics of human rights due diligence are summarized in Table 24.1 and provide broad topics for organizing this literature review. The topics are presented in the chronological order in which CSR developed in the industry.

Few apparel companies seem to approach CSR with the goal of assuring garment workers' rights. Instead, most focus their programs on reducing legal and reputational risk. Papers in law journals from the early 1990s considered the role and adequacy of laws for addressing some of the key issues found in the global apparel industry (Lam 1992). One particular issue of concern was how to address exploitation of children in manufacturing industries with production outside U.S. jurisdiction. Nicole Krug (1998) and Christopher Kern (2000) extended examples of the efforts private corporations were making to address the issue.

In the early 1990s, the industry was rapidly globalizing, and while national governments had the responsibility to protect the rights of their citizens, they were not always doing so. This placed unique responsibilities on businesses, which have the potential to impact virtually all human rights (see Ruggie 2011). Using as a springboard the discovery of scores of Thai women who were psychologically and physically abused and

TABLE 24.1 ELEMENTS AND CHARACTERISTICS OF HUMAN RIGHTS DUE DILIGENCE

DUE DILIGENCE ELEMENT	CHARACTERISTICS
Adopt a human rights policy	• Reference the United Nations' Declaration of Human Rights, International Labour Organization's Fundamental Principles and Rights at Work • Provide detail necessary to make policies meaningful to the company's various functions • Have top management endorse the policy • Identify who is responsible
Integrate human rights policies throughout the company	• Align company policies and procedures with the human rights commitment • Communicate the human rights expectations internally and externally to employees, business partners, and other relevant stakeholders • Seek management ownership of the policies • Train employees so they have the capacity to respond to situations that arise
Identify how current and potential business activities impact human rights	• Identify what the specific human rights risks are in the countries the company is involved with, how company activities impact those risks, and whether through the relationships they have with others (for example, business partners and suppliers) the company might contribute to human rights abuses • Draw on human rights experts and other resources in identifying impacts, including meaningful engagement with relevant stakeholders • Engage directly with factory workers • Have contracts requiring all suppliers who will potentially affect human rights to respect those, and gather evidence that they are willing and able to do so, using leverage if necessary
Track and communicate performance	• Conduct monitoring to determine the company's human rights impacts • Address the human rights violations found • Track performance improvements with qualitative and quantitative metrics • Share information and best practices with other companies to improve their due diligence • Communicate publicly with stakeholders expressing concerns about responses to actual/potential human rights impacts • Report regularly to expand sense of accountability and increase transparency with stakeholders

enslaved in El Monte, California, to sew garments for less than minimum wage, Laura Ho, Catherine Powell, and Leti Volpp (1996) connected sweatshop conditions with international human rights law and internationally agreed-upon conventions meant to assure rights at work. The conventions, developed by governments, industry, and labor involved with the International Labour Organization (ILO), encouraged decent working conditions and promoted rights at work. While many countries had not ratified the ILO conventions and thus were not expected to enforce them (Ho, Powell, and Volpp 1996), in 1998 eight core conventions related to discrimination, child labor, forced labor, and freedom of association and collective bargaining were designated the *Fundamental Principles and Rights at Work,* and enforcement was required of every UN member country, regardless of whether the conventions had been ratified (Dickson, Loker, and Eckman 2009).

BRAND AND RETAILER CSR AND HUMAN RIGHTS INITIATIVES

By the mid-1990s there was widespread recognition of the labor issues associated with garment production and wide-ranging viewpoints on how they should be approached. *The Sweatshop Quandary: Corporate Responsibility on the Global Frontier* (Varley 1998) gave background information on the issues and unfolding approaches to social responsibility. The book was also significant because its contributors were deeply engaged practitioners with NGOs. Their field research captured diverse viewpoints and provided an understanding of challenges faced by garment workers and those attempting to ensure their rights in a range of countries.

Adopting Human Rights Policies

Adopting codes of conduct was one of the first steps taken by brands and retailers as they recognized their responsibilities to workers (Elliott and Freeman 2003; Ho, Powell, and Volpp 1996). A code of conduct sets out in writing the standards and working conditions expected of contractors in the production of apparel (Diller 1999; Esbenshade 2004b). Research using content analysis to compare codes of conduct was conducted by practitioners in the field and academic researchers (Diller 1999; Emmelhanz and Adams 1999; Kolk and Van Tulder 2002, 2004; Pearson and Seyfang 2001; Van Tulder and Kolk 2001; Varley 1998; Wolfe and Dickson 2002). The studies examined the major provisions addressed in the codes of conduct with special attention given to child labor, the details of the code, and the commitment and processes of companies to monitor and enforce the codes (Emmelhanz and Adams 1999; Kolk and Van Tulder 2002, 2004; Varley 1998; Van Tulder and Kolk 2001; Wolfe and Dickson 2002). Some studies compared codes from the apparel industry with those from other industries

(Diller 1999) or compared company codes of conduct with ones developed by campaign organizations or by multifirm and government-related initiatives (Kolk and Van Tulder 2002; Pearson and Seyfang 2001; Van Tulder and Kolk 2001; Varley 1998).

Pamela Varley (1998) noted confusion about which rights should be the focus of the codes (e.g., child labor or unions). Most early codes of conduct were written by companies and lacked detail; they more often referenced national laws than international conventions (Diller 1999; Emmelhanz and Adams 1999; Kolk and Van Tulder 2002, 2004; Varley 1998). For example, codes did not define the age of a "child," indicated a minimum age of fourteen, or defined child labor by reference to local laws, which often conflicted with ILO conventions (Diller 1999; Kolk and Van Tulder 2002; Wolfe and Dickson 2002).

Private companies adopted less strict codes of conduct than groups that had involved civil society in formulating and implementing the codes (Van Tulder and Kolk 2001). Likewise, the codes developed by business associations were less detailed than those developed by NGOs (Kolk and Van Tulder 2002). Kimberly Elliott and Richard Freeman (2003) suggested that companies preferred weaker codes that their suppliers could more feasibly meet, whereas activists preferred stronger (aspirational) ones that could be used to push companies to further action once they had adopted these codes. The most contentious code elements related to wages and freedom of association. Limited information was provided about how the codes of conduct were monitored and enforced, or the sanctions that would be used when companies were out of compliance (Emmelhanz and Adams 1999; Kolk and Van Tulder 2002; Wolfe and Dickson 2002). Without evidence of how the codes of conduct would be implemented, companies gave the appearance that they intended to "cut and run" rather than stick with their suppliers to resolve the issues (Varley 1998).

Tracking and Communicating Performance with Monitoring

Many apparel companies had adopted codes of conduct and implemented them by requiring contractors to sign a guarantee of their compliance. Others, however, began conducting monitoring investigations within their contractors' facilities to assess compliance (Elliott and Freeman 2003; Esbenshade 2004b). Monitoring quickly became the prevalent strategy for addressing workplace issues, essentially sparking a new industry that spanned the globe. Monitoring also became the center of contentious debates among NGOs, manufacturers, unions, academics, and others who were concerned whether it should substitute for government investigations and enforcement and under what circumstances monitors could be trusted (Esbenshade 2001, 2004a, 2004b; O'Rourke 2003; Varley 1998). Several studies involving field research in a range of garment-producing countries focused on private monitoring that was conducted by a manufacturer's own employees (internal monitoring) or a commercial firm hired by the manufacturer (external monitoring). The following problems were identified (Clean

Clothes Campaign 2005; Esbenshade 2001, 2004a, 2004b; Locke, Amengual, and Mangla 2009; O'Rourke 2003):

- Erratic monitoring practices involving short and superficial visits
- Lack of thoroughness/failure to identify gross violations of the code of conduct
- Lack of interviewer confidentiality
- Lack of monitoring on rights of freedom of association and collective bargaining
- Exclusion of workers from a process that is meant to "protect" them rather than empower them to protect themselves by monitoring their own working conditions on a day-to-day basis
- Minimal training and qualifications for monitoring
- Lack of oversight regarding the quality of monitoring and credentials of monitoring firms
- Conflicts of interest regarding who the monitors were working for and their relationships with the companies paying them
- Lack of transparency of suppliers in company supply chains with potential for undisclosed or hidden factories
- Fraudulent efforts taken by contractors to hide violations of the code
- Confidentiality of the monitoring findings where only the manufacturer knew the extent of a contractor's compliance
- Lack of follow-up and sanctions to correct problems

By the mid-2000s, the majority of the apparel industry remained reliant on monitoring. A few brands had recognized its shortcomings, though, and were moving on to more comprehensive approaches to solve labor problems (Clean Clothes Campaign 2005).

Establishing Internal Programs and Communicating Expectations Internally

Developing comprehensive programs for CSR required companies to establish who would be responsible for this work. Qualitative research conducted by Ivana Mamic (2005) and Sandra Waddock and Charles Bodwell (2003) described CSR programs in the apparel, footwear, retail, and other sectors. Common steps for managing CSR included creating a vision and obtaining the commitment of senior management, developing understanding among employees and suppliers, operationally integrating the vision through business strategies and practices, remediating violations of their codes, and working to continuously improve CSR programs based on assessment of effectiveness. Mamic (2005) found that the footwear industry had the most advanced CSR practices.

Communicating Best Practices

Case studies began to be conducted on how companies were addressing working conditions in their global operations (Hartman, Arnold, and Wokutch 2003). The case studies involved qualitative field research where programs were reviewed and interviews conducted with multiple stakeholders. These studies revealed the complexities of operating innovative programs. One study examined Nike's efforts in Vietnam to provide education and microenterprise loans to workers and to train management in cultural sensitivity (Hartman and Wokutch 2003). Another focused on how adidas implemented its code of conduct in Thailand and Brazil and analyzed its programs focused on health and safety and child labor in Vietnam (Hartman, Wokutch, and French 2003). Yet another case study described Levi Strauss & Co.'s implementation of its code of conduct in Mexico, El Salvador, and Guatemala (Radin 2003). Small businesses requiring suppliers to certify compliance with SA8000, a factory-certification program operated by Social Accountability International, were the focus of a more recent case study (Ciliberti et al. 2011). Forthcoming publications provide insight on contemporary best practices as the industry passes through a second decade of CSR work, with case study research on the human rights due diligence practiced by adidas during a labor dispute with an Indonesian factory (Dickson and Anderson 2012) and the managerial and operational activities necessary for an apparel company to be the first small business following industry giants like Nike and adidas to have its labor compliance program accredited by the Fair Labor Association (FLA), a multistakeholder initiative working to improve labor conditions in factories around the world (Milne, Dickson, and Keene forthcoming).

In addition to CSR efforts in factories, research expanded to consider aspects of programs that indirectly supported CSR implementation in factories, particularly engagement with civil society stakeholders. N. Craig Smith, Sean Ansett, and Lior Erez (2011) used qualitative research methods to describe the stakeholder engagement process carried out by Gap, Inc., and illustrated the benefits of that work in controversial cases where young children in India were found embroidering Gap clothing and Gap contractors were exposed for dumping toxic materials into landfills and a river, putting at risk the health of local communities. Another case study shared why Gildan, Inc., began participating with the FLA after facing backlash from campaign groups that criticized the company's initial certification of its factories by the industry-sponsored Worldwide Responsible Accredited Production (WRAP; Turcotte, de Bellefeuille, and den Hond 2007). WRAP had been criticized from its inception by labor activists and others who believed it was impossible for the industry to adequately police itself (Dickson, Loker, and Eckman 2009).

Tracking Performance Improvements

From consultation with nearly 400 workers and company/organization representatives, Helle Jorgensen and colleagues (2003) examined barriers to improving suppliers' social performance and considered options for overcoming them. While the content and form of many codes had converged by the time of their work, inconsistent interpretation and application of the codes created challenges for suppliers. The varied demands companies had for the height of a fire extinguisher was a frequently cited example of the confusion caused in applying codes of conduct. Comprehensive field research confirmed that only marginal improvements had been experienced by factory workers making products for companies associated with the United Kingdom's Ethical Trading Initiative, a learning forum involving multiple stakeholders focused on developing best practices for implementing CSR. Improvements were mixed and uneven for workers depending on whether they were permanent, full-time employees or on temporary contracts. The majority of workers were experiencing better health and safety provisions and reduced working hours. Wages had increased but not to the point of a living wage (Barrientos and Smith 2007).

Looking at factory compliance with Nike's code of conduct, Richard Locke, Fei Qin, and Alberto Brause (2007) analyzed the results of hundreds of monitoring visits, determining that compliance varied widely by the country of factory location, age and size of the factories, and the relationship factories had with Nike. Nearly half of the factories showed no improvements, and over one-third declined in compliance with Nike's code during the period of activity studied. Case study research examined the implementation of Reebok's code of conduct with a footwear supplier in China, whereby factory management had cooperated with less costly remediation to bring the factory into compliance on issues of forced overtime, child labor, and safety and health. The factory, however, had resisted making changes that would significantly increase labor costs. The supplier faced fines and sanctions for noncompliance at a time when prices paid to the factory for Reebok's shoes were reduced. As a result, the supplier could not afford to comply and resorted to maintaining double books to feign compliance. Efforts to increase productivity were successful, but reduced working hours increased worker stress, and wage ceilings set by management prevented the workers from earning more for the increased productivity (Yu 2008).

One comprehensive approach to improving labor conditions tied to trade incentives was the ILO's Better Work program in Cambodia. A collaboration between the ILO and the International Finance Corporation, Better Work aims to improve compliance with labor standards in global supply chains. Anna Shea, Mariko Nakayama, and Jody Heymann (2010) conducted field research in Cambodia, interviewing multiple stakeholders involved in the project; observing various project activities, including factory monitoring and training programs for government, factory management, and union leaders; and reviewing data from factory monitoring. Similarly, Gunseli Berik and Yana van der Meulen Rodgers (2008) examined compliance with codes of conduct in Bangladesh and Cambodia using primary data from surveys and focus groups and secondary data from the FLA's publicly reported tracking charts of factory violations. Both research teams found certain labor conditions had improved slightly in Cambodia; however, major violations continued, with forced overtime and excessive hours of work, discrimination, and violations related to freedom of association and collective bargaining. Low wages persisted as well (Berik and Meulen Rodgers

2008; Shea, Nakayama, and Heymann 2010). Researchers have noted problems with monitoring procedures, including advance notification of when the visit would take place and factory management's coaching of workers to report conditions that were better than they really were (Berik and Meulen Rodgers 2008; Shea, Nakayama, and Heymann 2010).

EMERGING RESEARCH AGENDAS FOR IMPROVING EFFECTIVENESS

Human rights due diligence is ongoing work with the goal of avoiding or lessening the impacts of company activities on human rights (Ruggie 2011). Recent research related to improving the effectiveness of CSR includes three key themes: increasing the very low wages of workers, expanding transparency and public reporting about CSR practices, and strengthening partnerships between buying companies and their suppliers. Researchers are encouraged to explore these topics or others where they can make a difference.

How to Address Low Wages

Companies need to prioritize their work with suppliers on human rights issues. The guiding principles recommend prioritizing based on severity of impact (Ruggie 2011). Field research involving interviews and surveys with workers, factory management, supply-chain agents, brand and retail staff, union and government officials, and others, aimed at refining and clarifying ongoing issues in the apparel and agricultural sectors, identified wage levels as a long-standing issue in the apparel industry. Wages paid to garment workers have been the basis for contentious engagements between companies, activists, and NGOs (Raworth 2004) and continue to be an urgent topic marked by worker strikes in Cambodia, Vietnam, Bangladesh, and elsewhere in protest of poor wages. The primary focus has been on workers earning a living wage that covers basic needs and provides some discretionary income for a number of family members in contrast to payment of minimum wages (Dickson, Loker, and Eckman 2009; Miller and Williams 2009; Pollin, Burns, and Heintz 2004).

Robert Pollin, Justine Burns, and James Heintz (2004) used publicly available secondary data on labor costs and garment pricing to calculate whether paying living wages to garment workers would have unintended consequences. The authors determined that workers would be unlikely to be laid off in countries with large-scale apparel industries, and those countries and regions would not lose advantage, if living wages were implemented gradually. Assuming a 100 percent increase in wages, the authors estimated increases in the final retail price of garments made in the United States and Mexico would rise 4.5 percent and 2.8 percent respectively. Also considering living wage, Doug Miller and Peter Williams (2009) explored various mechanisms that might be used to implement it, including government regulations and productivity increases. The authors determined that long-term and collaborative commitments involving sharing data on unit labor costs would be necessary between buyers and their suppliers. They advocated a negotiated rather than a formula approach to living wages whereby workers or their representatives would bargain with management to set appropriate remuneration.

An innovative strategy for addressing low wage levels was proposed by Daniel Vaughn-Whitehead (2010), who suggested too much emphasis was placed on a living wage. His comprehensive concept of fair wages included twelve dimensions. Actual payment of wages, wage discrimination, wage share, negotiation of wages, minimum wage levels, prevailing wage levels, living wage, and others were analyzed with an aim to improve wages. The findings of wage monitoring conducted in collaboration with the FLA was revealing in illustrating the urgency of addressing fair wages. Of thirty-one suppliers studied in five Asian countries (most in China), 77 percent were not providing legally required social benefits, 68 percent had difficulty paying for overtime, 58 percent falsified wage and hour records, and 58 percent were underpaying wages earned by their workers. Other startling findings included that one-quarter of the companies were not paying wages or paying them late, and 23 percent were not paying legally required minimum wages. Additional research is needed to explore how to address legal and human rights violations related to wages and assure workers are paid fairly.

How to Increase Transparency and Public Reporting about CSR

Reporting publicly to interested stakeholders about company policies and practices in support of human rights is an important component of tracking and communication, especially in industries where human rights risks are known to exist (Ruggie 2011). Until recently, public reporting by apparel brands and retailers was limited to a few large and well-known companies. In a website analysis of 119 high-grossing apparel brands and retailers, Marsha Dickson and Kevin Kovaleski (2007, as reported in Dickson, Loker, and Eckman 2009) found only 8 that provided information about code-of-conduct adoption and implementation. Lack of public reporting may be linked to the lawsuit filed against Nike by Marc Kasky, claiming that Nike had engaged in false advertising in the various letters, opinion editorials, press releases, reports, and other public information the company had disclosed. A case study detailed the series of events that resulted in the U.S. Supreme Court leaving issues about disclosure unresolved and raising fears among other U.S. companies considering public reporting about CSR initiatives (DeTienne and Lewis 2005).

Recognizing company concerns, Marsha Dickson and Molly Eckman (2008) analyzed the content of media stories related to public reporting activities conducted by the FLA during 2003 through 2005. On the basis of the content, the authors advised that worries about negative consequences from reporting were unfounded. Additional case studies suggested that as their CSR programs matured, companies were becoming more confident about public reporting and the collaborations and joint remediation it facilitated (Doorey 2011). Additionally, involvement with multistakeholder initiatives strengthened credibility and supported communications with NGOs (Valero and Dickson 2013). Although it is difficult to determine motivations from content analysis of text, some studies proposed that public reporting allowed companies to correct negative publicity and update stakeholders on the progress that was being made with their CSR programs (Gaskill-Fox 2010; Islam and Deegan 2010; Waller and Conaway 2011).

In 2012 the California Transparency in Supply Chains Act 2010 required manufacturers and retailers doing business in California to disclose their efforts to identify and mitigate the risks of human trafficking and modern-day slavery. The legislation provided a new opportunity to learn about apparel brands' and retailers' CSR programs. Content analysis of the disclosures of eighty-six high-volume apparel companies soon after the law went into effect on January 1, 2012, showed variability in the quality and amount of information provided; one-quarter had not made the required disclosure easily accessible (Dickson and Warren 2012). Tiffany Rogers (2012) more deeply analyzed the content of twelve apparel companies' CSR reporting, including their responses to the act, using the UN guiding principles as a framework for analysis. The research provided deep understanding of the components of strong human rights–focused CSR programs (e.g., adidas Group) and revealed the areas where companies can improve their programs and reporting for more thorough due diligence.

Human rights abuses are material risks to investors, and they impact the value of the firm (Ruggie 2011). An event study of changes in company value associated with negative and positive news about sweatshops found the value of affected firms declined with negative press about labor conditions, but in a single example where Reebok addressed sweatshop concerns, the value of the firm went up (Rock 2003). Jeffrey Katz and colleagues (2008) observed similar downturns in company value as a result of public reports issued by the FLA, but in subsequent reports in which the companies were mentioned there were no losses. Interest continued in using information about human rights due diligence as material evidence in firm valuation, as indicated by investor commitment to a collaboration between the FLA and Harvard Law School's Pension and Capital Stewardship project that was developing measures of company CSR practices (Investor Responsibility Research Center Institute 2012).

How to Strengthen Buyer and Supplier Partnerships

Suppliers have the same responsibility as brands and retailers to respect human rights (Ruggie 2011), and the relationship buyers have with them is influential on code compliance (Raworth 2004). Stephen Frenkel and Duncan Scott (2002) distinguished two ways that companies worked with suppliers. The compliance approach involved a top-down approach by the buying companies in developing the code, communicating its importance, and enforcing it with suppliers. In contrast, a collaborative approach involved a partnership with frequent communications between buying companies and suppliers in support of continuous improvement in working conditions. Through qualitative field research, the authors observed that the compliance approach encouraged adherence to adidas's code by setting rules and pressuring suppliers to conform to those. On the other hand, the collaborative approach engaged suppliers to work with the company to improve working conditions and pay as well as productivity and quality, reduce health and safety issues, improve worker turnover, and reduce monitoring costs.

Field research continued to demonstrate the differing effects of collaborative partnerships as contrasted with traditional compliance approaches for Ethical Trading Initiative member companies and their suppliers (Barrientos and Smith 2007), Nike's suppliers in Vietnam (Lim and Phillips 2008), and an anonymous buyer company's commitment to resolve labor issues with suppliers in Bangladesh, China, the Dominican Republic, Honduras, and India (Locke, Amengual, and Mangla 2009). A lack of incentives provided to suppliers for compliance with codes of conduct diminished their efforts in compliance as well (Chang 2010; Locke, Amengual, and Mangla 2009; Raworth 2004). A survey incorporating sourcing managers' perspectives about CSR partnerships found that companies emphasizing product development and differentiation and therefore control over their supply chains were more likely to be engaged in a CSR partnership with suppliers. In contrast, those companies emphasizing a low-price strategy had less engagement with supply-chain partners (Park and Dickson 2008).

The value of collaborative relationships with suppliers for improved compliance with codes of conduct was also supported from suppliers' perspectives through a survey in China's apparel industry. To improve relationships with suppliers, buying companies were encouraged to carry out respectful dialogue with them, setting mutually agreeable and achievable goals, working together on corrective action plans, and acknowledging improvements even if they did not result in full compliance (Jiang 2009). Theoretically, suppliers' commitment to deeper and broader social responsibility initiatives grows as they shift to more central positions in supply networks and take on more participative roles in supply-chain management (Vurro, Russo, and Perrini 2009).

APPROACHES TO FUTURE RESEARCH

This chapter has outlined the evolution of CSR in the apparel industry from a human rights perspective. Key topics covered, including adoption of codes of conduct, evaluation of monitoring, establishment of CSR programs, communication of best practices, and tracking of performance improvements, demonstrate how research has also evolved with the progression of industry practice. In support of human rights in the apparel industry, it is critical for researchers to understand how far the field has come and how to develop research programs that make a difference to factory workers around the world. Toward this goal, the chapter concludes with two recommendations.

Appreciate the Diversity of Research

Literature on CSR and human rights for workers in the apparel industry is conducted from a wide range of academic fields as well as by practitioners. The research reviewed for this chapter was drawn from fashion studies, anthropology, development studies, environmental science, business management, law, political science, sociology, women's studies, and others. It included the work of academics and practitioners, sometimes in collaborative teams. To fully understand the state of research in the field, it is important to examine peer-reviewed publications from all these fields and others but also reports generated by practitioners in the field. Strong practitioner reports often reflect leading-edge thinking on high-priority issues that are central to the evolution and improvement of CSR.

When reading widely, researchers will encounter different approaches used by disciplines to approach and report research. A scholar accustomed to defending in great detail every methodological decision made in a study may be frustrated by research reporting in some fields that includes only a sentence or two about the methods, essentially asking readers to trust the "arguments" the authors want to "prove" from their studies. It will be important not to dismiss immediately as biased research that has been conducted in ways different from one's own. Researchers engaging in critical thinking about the limitations and opportunities of different disciplinary perspectives and the contributions of diverse research may be better able to test results and position their own research in ways that move the field forward. Rather than moving timidly to explore the smallest next step from a previous study, it may be more valuable for researchers to take bold steps to test hypotheses and approaches that have the potential for immediate impact on human rights.

Go into the Field

In the process of reviewing literature for this chapter, publications from peer-reviewed journals were eliminated from inclusion because some did not provide new knowledge or innovative theories about CSR in the apparel industry. Publications relying on a few news stories and short lists of academic literature advanced arguments based on "conceptual thought," which in the absence of empirical data or deep experience in the field simply did not make strong contributions. The strongest publications collected empirical data with comprehensive studies that addressed current issues of concern among leading businesses. Researchers are encouraged to set aside theorizing from the comfort of their offices for empirical research that takes them into the field in contact with the workers, factory management, company representatives, NGOs, and others working on CSR and human rights. Preparing for field research can be challenging since researchers must work with their institutional review boards to avoid unintended consequences or harm to their informants. Additionally, the most relevant research will take a participatory action approach and include the needs of the study's subjects in formulating research questions and interpreting results (see Hale and Wills 2007). Collaboration with practitioners can also be challenging because of their agendas and time frames but rewarding because of the impacts that can result. Practitioners are interested in implementing innovative processes for CSR and are less interested in waiting for research that supports their ideas. Working with practitioners, academics can capture relevant data so that others learn from the experiments. In the end, an integrated human rights–based approach to CSR puts the workers and their needs before any other.

BIBLIOGRAPHY

Barrientos, Stephanie, and Sally Smith. 2007. "Do Workers Benefit from Ethical Trade? Assessing Codes of Labour Practice in Global Production Systems." *Third World Quarterly* 28: 713–29.

Bender, Daniel E., and Richard A. Greenwald. 2003. *Sweatshop USA: The American Sweatshop in Historical and Global Perspective.* New York: Routledge.

Berik, Gunseli, and Yana van der Meulen Rodgers. 2008. "Options for Enforcing Labour Standards: Lessons from Bangladesh and Cambodia." *Journal of International Development* 22: 55–85.

Casey, Roseann. 2006. "Meaningful Change: Raising the Bar in Supply Chain Workplace Standards." Corporate Social Responsibility Initiative, Working Paper no. 29. Cambridge, MA: John F. Kennedy School of Government. http://www.hks.harvard.edu/m-rcbg/CSRI/publications/workingpaper_29_casey.pdf (accessed July 1, 2012).

Chang, Rita K. 2010. "World Class Corporate Social Responsibility: Policies and Practices of Apparel Manufacturers." Senior honor's thesis, University of Delaware.

Ciliberti, Francesco, Job de Haan, Gerard de Groot, and Pierpaolo Pantrandolfo. 2011. "CSR Codes and the Principal-Agent Problem in Supply Chains: Four Case Studies." *Journal of Cleaner Production* 19: 885–94.

Clean Clothes Campaign. 2005. "Looking for a Quick Fix: How Weak Social Auditing Is Keeping Workers in Sweatshops." Clean Clothes Campaign, Amsterdam. http://www.cleanclothes.org/resources/publications/05-quick-fix.pdf/view (accessed July 1, 2012).

DeTienne, Kristen B., and Lee W. Lewis. 2005. "The Pragmatic and Ethical Barriers to Corporate Social Responsibility Disclosure: The Nike Case." *Journal of Business Ethics* 60: 359–76.

Dickson, Marsha A. 2013. "Identifying and Understanding Ethical Consumer Behavior: Reflections on 15 Years of Research." In Jennifer Bair, Marsha A. Dickson, and Doug Miller (eds.), *Workers' Rights and Labor Compliance in Global Supply Chains.* Abingdon, UK: Taylor and Francis.

Dickson, Marsha A., and William Anderson. 2012. "Implementing Human Rights Due Diligence in Global Apparel and Footwear Supply Chains: Case Study of adidas Group and PT Panarub." Unpublished manuscript.

Dickson, Marsha A., and Molly Eckman. 2008. "Media Portrayal of Voluntary Public Reporting about Corporate Social Responsibility Performance: Does Coverage Encourage or Discourage Ethical Management?" *Journal of Business Ethics* 83: 725–43.

Dickson, Marsha A., Suzanne Loker, and Molly Eckman. 2009. *Social Responsibility in the Global Apparel Industry.* New York: Fairchild Books.

Dickson, Marsha A., and Haley Warren. 2012. "Best Practices for Addressing Risks of Human Trafficking and Slavery in Global Apparel Supply Chains: Content Analysis of Disclosures under the California Transparency in Supply Chains Act 2010." Unpublished manuscript.

Diller, Janelle. 1999. "A Social Conscience in the Global Marketplace? Labour Dimensions of Codes of Conduct, Social Labelling, and Investor Initiatives." *International Labour Review* 138: 99–129.

Doorey, David J. 2011. "The Transparent Supply Chain: From Resistance to Implementation at Nike and Levi-Strauss." *Journal of Business Ethics* 103: 587–603.

Elliott, Kimberly A., and Richard B. Freeman. 2003. *Can Labor Standards Improve under Globalization?* Washington, DC: Institute for International Economics.

Emmelhanz, Margaret A., and Ronald J. Adams. 1999. "The Apparel Industry Response to 'Sweatshop' Concerns: A Review and Analysis of Codes of Conduct." *Journal of Supply Chain Management* 35 (3): 51–57.

Esbenshade, Jill. 2001. "The Social Accountability Contract: Private Monitoring from Los Angeles to the Global Apparel Industry." *Labor Studies Journal* 26 (1): 98–120.

Esbenshade, Jill. 2004a. "Codes of Conduct: Challenges and Opportunities for Workers' Rights." *Social Justice* 31 (3): 40–59.

Esbenshade, Jill. 2004b. *Monitoring Sweatshops: Workers, Consumers, and the Global Apparel Industry.* Philadelphia: Temple University Press.

Frenkel, Stephen J., and Duncan Scott. 2002. "Compliance, Collaboration, and Codes of Labor Practice: The adidas Connection." *California Management Review* 45: 29–49.

Gaskill-Fox, Jennifer N. 2010. "How Apparel Companies Communicate Corporate Social Responsibility on Their Websites: A Longitudinal Study." Master's thesis, Colorado State University.

Hale, Angela, and Jane Wills (eds.). 2007. *Threads of Labour: Garment Industry Supply Chains from the Workers' Perspective.* Malden, MA: Blackwell.

Hartman, Laura P., Denis G. Arnold, and Richard E. Wokutch (eds.). 2003. *Rising above Sweatshops: Innovative Approaches to Global Labor Challenges.* Westport, CT: Praeger.

Hartman, Laura P., and Richard E. Wokutch. 2003. "Nike, Inc.: Corporate Social Responsibility and Workplace Standard Initiatives in Vietnam." In Laura P. Hartman, Denis G. Arnold, and Richard E. Wokutch (eds.), *Rising above Sweatshops: Innovative Approaches to Global Labor Challenges,* 145–90. Westport, CT: Praeger.

Hartman, Laura P., Richard E. Wokutch, and J. Lawrence French. 2003. "Adidas-Salomon: Child Labor and Health and Safety Initiatives in Vietnam and Brazil." In Laura P. Hartman, Denis G. Arnold, and Richard E. Wokutch (eds.), *Rising above Sweatshops: Innovative Approaches to Global Labor Challenges,* 191–248. Westport, CT: Praeger.

Ho, Laura, Catherine Powell, and Leti Volpp. 1996. "(Dis)assembling Rights of Women Workers along the Global Assembly Line: Human Rights and the Garment Industry." *Harvard Civil Rights-Civil Liberties Law Review* 31: 383–414.

Iglesias Prieto, Norma. 1997. *Beautiful Flowers of the Maquiladora.* Austin: University of Texas Press.

Investor Responsibility Research Center Institute. 2012. "Key Performance Indicators for Investors to Assess Labor and Human Rights Risks Faced by Global Corporations in Supply Chains." http://www.irrcinstitute.org/projects.php?project=52 (accessed July 1, 2012).

Islam, Muhammad A., and Craig Deegan. 2010. "Media Pressures and Corporate Disclosure of Social Responsibility Performance Information: A Study of Two Global Clothing and Sports Retail Companies." *Accounting and Business Research* 40: 131–48.

Jiang, Bin. 2009. "Implementing Supplier Codes of Conduct in Global Supply Chains: Process Explanations from Theoretic and Empirical Perspectives." *Journal of Business Ethics* 85: 77–92.

Jorgensen, Helle B., Michael Pruzan-Jorgensen, Margaret Jungk, and Aron Cramer. 2003. "Strengthening Implementation of Corporate Social Responsibility in Global Supply Chains." The World Bank/International Finance Corporation, Washington, DC. http://siteresources.worldbank.org/INTPSD/Resources/CSR/Strengthening_Implementatio.pdf (accessed July 1, 2012).

Katz, Jeffrey P., Eric Higgins, Marsha A. Dickson, and Molly Eckman. 2008. "The Impact of External Monitoring and Public Reporting on Business Performance in a Global Manufacturing Industry." *Business & Society* 20 (10): 1–22.

Kern, Christopher M. 2000. "Child Labor: The International Law and Corporate Impact." *Syracuse Journal of International Law and Commerce* 27: 177–98.

Kolk, Aris, and Rob Van Tulder. 2002. "Child Labor and Multinational Conduct: A Comparison of International Business and Stakeholder Codes." *Journal of Business Ethics* 36: 291–301.

Kolk, Aris, and Rob Van Tulder. 2004. "Ethics in International Business: Multinational Approaches to Child Labor." *Journal of World Business* 39: 49–60.

Krug, Nicole J. 1998. "Exploiting Child Labor: Corporate Responsibility and the Role of Corporate Codes of Conduct." *New York Law School Journal of Human Rights* 14: 651–76.

Lam, Leo L. 1992. "Designer Duty: Extending Liability to Manufacturers for Violations of Labor Standards in Garment Industry Sweatshops." *University of Pennsylvania Law Review* 141: 623–67.

Lim, Suk-Jun, and Joe Phillips. 2008. "Embedding CSR Values: The Global Footwear Industry's Evolving Governance Structure." *Journal of Business Ethics* 81: 143–56.

Locke, Richard, Matthew Amengual, and Akshay Mangla. 2009. "Virtue out of Necessity? Compliance, Commitment, and the Improvement of Labor Conditions in Global Supply Chains." *Politics & Society* 37: 319–51.

Locke, Richard, Fei Qin, and Alberto Brause. 2007. "Does Monitoring Improve Labor Standards? Lessons from Nike." *Industrial & Labor Relations Review* 61: 3–31.

Mamic, Ivana. 2005. "Managing Global Supply Chain: The Sports Footwear, Apparel and Retail Sectors." *Journal of Business Ethics* 59: 81–100.

Miller, Doug, and Peter Williams. 2009. "What Price a Living Wage? Implementation Issues in the Quest for Decent Wages in the Global Apparel Sector." *Global Social Policy* 9: 99–125.

Milne, Allison T. C., Marsha A. Dickson, and Kelsey Keene. Forthcoming. "Small Business Implementation of CSR for Fair Labor Association Accreditation: The Case of Zephyr Graf-X." *Journal of Corporate Citizenship*.

O'Rourke, Dara. 2003. "Outsourcing Regulation: Analyzing Nongovernmental Systems of Labor Standards and Monitoring." *Policy Studies Journal* 31: 1–29.

O'Rourke, Dara. 2006. "Multi-stakeholder Regulation: Privatizing or Socializing Global Labor Standards?" *World Development* 24: 899–918.

Park, Haesun, and Marsha A. Dickson. 2008. "Engaging in Buyer-Seller Partnership for Fair Labor Management: The Role of a Buyer Firm's Strategic Emphasis." *Clothing and Textiles Research Journal* 26: 41–56.

Pearson, Ruth, and Gill Seyfang. 2001. "New Hope or False Dawn? Voluntary Codes of Conduct, Labour Regulation and Social Policy in a Globalizing World." *Global Social Policy* 1: 49–78.

Pollin, Robert, Justine Burns, and James Heintz. 2004. "Global Apparel Production and Sweatshop Labour: Can Raising Retail Prices Finance Living Wages?" *Cambridge Journal of Economics* 28: 153–71.

Radin, Tara J. 2003. "Levi Strauss & Co.: Implementation of Global Sourcing and Operating Guidelines in Latin America." In Laura P. Hartman, Denis G. Arnold, and Richard E. Wokutch (eds.), *Rising above Sweatshops: Innovative Approaches to Global Labor Challenges,* 249–92. Westport, CT: Praeger.

Raworth, Kate. 2004. "Trading Away Our Rights: Women Working in Global Supply Chains." Oxfam International, Oxford. http://www.maketradefair.com/en/assets/english/taor.pdf (accessed July 1, 2012).

Rock, Michael T. 2003. "Public Disclosure of the Sweatshop Practices of American Multinational Garment/Shoe Makers/Retailers: Impacts on Their Stock Prices." *Competition & Change* 7 (1): 23–38.

Rogers, Tiffany. 2012. "The Influence of the California Transparency in Supply Chains Act on Apparel Company Due Diligence for Corporate Social Responsibility." Master's thesis, University of Delaware.

Rosen, Ellen I. 2002. *Making Sweatshops.* Berkeley: University of California Press.

Ruggie, John. 2011. "Guiding Principles on Business and Human Rights: Implementing the United Nations 'Protect, Respect and Remedy' Framework." United Nations, New York. http://www.ohchr.org/documents/issues/business/A.HRC.17.31.pdf (accessed July 1, 2012).

Shea, Anna, Mariko Nakayama, and Jody Heymann. 2010. "Improving Labour Standards in Clothing Factories: Lessons from Stakeholder Views and Monitoring Results in Cambodia." *Global Social Policy* 10: 85–110.

Smith, N. Craig, Sean Ansett, and Lior Erez. 2011. "How Gap Inc. Engaged with Its Stakeholders." *MIT Sloan Management Review* 52: 69–76.

Turcotte, Marie-France B., Stephanie de Bellefeuille, and Frank den Hond. 2007. "Gildan, Inc.: Influencing Corporate Governance in the Textile Sector." *Journal of Corporate Citizenship* 27: 23–36.

U.S. General Accounting Office. 1994. *Garment Industry Efforts to Address the Prevalence and Conditions of Sweatshops.* Washington, DC: U.S. General Accounting Office.

Valero, Theadora, and Marsha A. Dickson. 2013. "Motivations and Concerns for Public Reporting about Corporate Social Responsibility and Compliance with Labor Standards: A Case Study of the Apparel Industry." In Jennifer Bair, Marsha A. Dickson, and Doug Miller (eds.), *Workers' Rights and Labor Compliance in Global Supply Chains.* Abingdon, UK: Taylor and Francis.

Van Tulder, Rob, and Aris Kolk. 2001. "Multinationality and Corporate Ethics: Codes of Conduct in the Sporting Goods Industry." *Journal of International Business Studies* 32: 267–83.

Varley, Pamela (ed.). 1998. *The Sweatshop Quandary: Corporate Responsibility on the Global Frontier.* Washington, DC: Investor Responsibility Research Center.

Vaughn-Whitehead, Daniel. 2010. *Fair Wages: Strengthening Corporate Social Responsibility.* Cheltenham, UK: Edward Elgar.

Vurro, Clodia, Angeloantonio Russo, and Francesco Perrini. 2009. "Shaping Sustainable Value Chains: Network Determinants of Supply Chain Governance Models." *Journal of Business Ethics* 90: 607–21.

Waddock, Sandra, and Charles Bodwell. 2003. "Philosophy Applied II: Total Responsibility Management." In Laura P. Hartman, Denis G. Arnold, and Richard E. Wokutch (eds.), *Rising above Sweatshops: Innovative Approaches to Global Labor Challenges,* 119–41. Westport, CT: Praeger.

Waller, Randall L., and Roger N. Conaway. 2011. "Framing and Counterframing the Issue of Corporate Social Responsibility: The Communication Strategies of Nikebiz.com." *Journal of Business Communication* 48: 83–106.

Wolfe, Jennifer H., and Marsha A. Dickson. 2002. "Apparel Manufacturer and Retailer Efforts to Reduce Child Labor: An Ethics of Virtue Perspective on Codes of Conduct." *Clothing and Textiles Research Journal* 20: 183–95.

Yu, Xiaomin. 2008. "Impacts of Corporate Code of Conduct on Labor Standards: A Case Study of Reebok's Athletic Footwear Supplier Factory in China." *Journal of Business Ethics* 81: 513–29.

25

Fast Fashion and Sustainability

MARGARET MAYNARD

A basic tenet of capitalism is the generation of profit from consumption of new things. Can "fast" fashion, a particular phenomenon that emerged globally toward the end of the 1990s, characterized by rapid changes of stylish attire, ever be socially and environmentally sustainable? Fashion is big business, a crucial indicator of economic growth and employment. As one of the drivers of success, constant gratification of fashion consumers is a key way in which capitalist investment measures its progress. Profit margins for conglomerates and their shareholders remain their most significant priority. But can this pressure for the new be channeled into desires for longer-lasting garments? The advent of rapid production of fashions relatively cheaply, no longer seasonal but based on trend spotting, makes it important to analyze how it affects eco-viability. In order to explore this issue we need first to consider what is meant by *sustainability,* for it is a slippery term. In the case of fashion it refers primarily to the ability to maintain economic growth (constant production of new types of attire) without depletion of resources or damage to the environment.

In relation to clothing production generally, the goal of sustainability brings with it problematic ramifications. For example, the manufacture of constantly changing small runs of fashion is an important creator of employment, as indeed is its relative, mass-produced generic clothing. This is especially so in the underdeveloped parts of the world and has occurred increasingly in countries that provide cheap exploitable labor. Transnational companies, for example, source cheap garments anywhere that trade barriers do not apply, be it Central America, the Caribbean, Mexico, eastern Europe, sub-Saharan Africa, China, Bangladesh, Samoa, or Southeast Asia, including Vietnam (Maynard 2010: 254). While exploitation is a serious problem in itself,[1] such manufacturing is a vital, perhaps only, source of income for workers in impoverished countries. It has particular benefits. Could any economy remain viable into the future, in terms of supply and demand, and still dispense with the entire business of volume fashion as we know it? How, for instance, could the capacity for employment be replaced in the underdeveloped, newly developing, or even to some extent developed world if eco-sustainability gained serious purchase?

There is a further aspect to sustainability. Ironically, overproduction, signaling sound employment figures, is an important sign of a corporation's economic success. Increasingly inexpensive fashion of diminishing quality, such as fast fashion, leads in turn to greater volumes of discarded clothing becoming available for export and reuse. It becomes a crucial source of secondhand clothing for those living beyond the developed world. In this aspect, it provides a second and even third tier of profit and is an important resource for the world's poorest people. Take away these products, and you take away the ability of multitudes of less fortunate peoples to clothe themselves and thus maintain their livelihoods within cultures that are modernizing economically. Finally, sustainability of attire in the widest application of the term can also refer to certain indigenous cultures, in parts of Asia and the South Pacific, for instance, where there are powerful desires to maintain, even revive, cultural practices, including forms of customary dress, outside mainstream global styles.

Central to this discussion, though, is whether so-called fast fashion, a highly resource-hungry aspect of the middle range of the industry, can be compatible with long-term care for the environment? Since the later twentieth century, public commentary and vigorous political polemic surrounding all aspects of environmental degradation have grown more strident. The practices and materials of the fashion and textile industries (now truly global enterprises) have until recently been somewhat less subject to criticism than other products. Yet in 1998 environmental scientist Michael S. Bahorsky estimated up to 50 percent of world textile pollutant chemicals had processes linked to garments (1998: 691). Over a decade later Bradley Quinn, in his book *Textile Futures,* still suggests textiles mean toxins, with fashion manufacturers using a range of procedures "that place clothing fabrication on a par with petro-chemical production" (2010: 109). Fast fashion, by its use of excessive but finite resources, its production methods, and its encouragement of rapidly changing stylish consumption, thus lies at the heart of debates about environmental protection. Although all manner of less damaging, stable forms of dress and organic textiles are being marketed, there are few signs that the seemingly insatiable consumer taste for never-ending novel types of attire will seriously diminish.

During the first decade of the twenty-first century, activist organizations have been sources of pressure on major clothing corporations to become more environmentally responsible, but company chains of supply are so complicated that lack of transparency has been a problematic factor (Kunz and Garner 2011: 103–5). Naomi Klein's best seller *No Logo* (2000) had an instant effect on both the public and activists. Not a text about dress per se, it is a piece of sustained investigative journalism exposing highly dubious activities (promotional and production methods) of huge U.S. clothing brands especially equated with the 1990s—Nike and Gap, for instance. It fearlessly highlights the unethical practices of these clothing corporations and cynical attempts to divert attention from their real aims. It is also a brilliant insight into the activities of radical ecologists and anti-corporate activists, such as the RTS (Reclaim the Streets) movement, Adbusters, and culture jamming, which intend to subvert the activities of corporate power.

Can alternative forms of demand-led dressing (characteristic of fast fashion) emerge that will both be ethical and also satisfy consumers captivated by fresh, inventive styles and novel color combinations, the hallmark of this form of clothing? Sandy Black argues that ecofashion is moving beyond niche products toward the mainstream (2010: 259). Undoubtedly, many so-called slow or alternative fashions are highly creative and socially aware forms of fashion, favoring reuse and opposing global standardization (Clark 2008: 428–29). Hazel Clark suggests these are posing a potential challenge to the global fashion system. One wonders, though, if this is a realistic assessment, for many appear to be small-scale solutions, with only an ecological veneer. And some fashion companies like Ecouterre seem at face value only to exploit "green" terminology, conveniently blurring boundaries between different categories of products. The question is, how much of this is genuine concern for the environment, and how much mere lip service, niche marketing, or sheer experimentation? Despite annual events like Source Expo (in the United Kingdom), an industry event concerned with stylish dress and sustainability, consumption of nonsustainable, novel, and relatively inexpensive fashion continues to be almost addictive.

Central to the issue of sustainable fashion lies what Black terms *the* "fashion paradox" (Black 2010: 244). Her book *Eco-chic: The Fashion Paradox* (2008) deals with the seemingly incompatible factors of environmental concerns set against personal aesthetic desires for high-end attire. Black's paradox is most evident in the phenomenon of fast fashion and is primarily applicable to the consumption practices of more affluent Western consumers. Many years before Black, Gilles Lipovetsky in his *The Empire of Fashion* (1994) outlined another paradox but here in far more cynical terms. For him ethics and the "ecological movement" are one of a number of paradoxes within the driving forces of fashion. The more the power of fashion to dominate our lives increases, the more noticeable is the concurrent ethical surge for eco-products. He explains this paradox in part by showing how marketing of values such as ethics pays, and how faddish forms of eco-purchasing are simply a new stage of fashion consumption, mixing what he calls eco-consumption and eco-business. He argues that the "newness" of fashion and the ecological movement that focuses on the future and the long-lasting are not that radically different. They are specific examples "in which the seduction of marketing annexes the 'respect for nature' niche" (Lipovetsky 1994: 248). There is now, he feels, no escape from the fashion system.

OVERVIEW OF ISSUES

The fashion industry, with its long supply chain, is extremely complex, and this has made it difficult for the question of sustainability to be given thoroughgoing research attention (Black 2010: 244). Acknowledging the complexity of the current segmented fashion market of which fast fashion is a part, there are a number of issues of present concern. An overview of writings on the subject will be a first step to set the scene. It is then important to consider the nature of fast fashion, one of the factors that stimulated the sustainable dress debate, and its place in the spectrum of the fashion consumer market. Importantly, questions of "value" will thread their way through the text as we explore what might be termed the "ethical turn," noticeable in certain socially aware Western design products over the first decade of the twenty-first century.

Second, and in association with this, questions are raised about so-called green and ecofashion.[2] Here we look briefly at localized, small-scale slow fashion (found alongside consumption of mass online or mall fashions) whose complexities Clark (2008) has carefully studied. This attire, she argues, is far more complicated than just being simply an alternative to fast fashion (428). Also canvassed are certain previously discussed paradoxical issues that arise between the desire to look attractively clothed and the issue of ethical consumption.

It is interesting to note that when attention and criticism have focused on problems of the world's clothing and textile industries, it has been largely, but not entirely, from a Eurocentric perspective. We need to acknowledge transnational aspects of a subject of this kind. In fact, there are sustainable practices taking place in many Asian countries and among diasporic communities in places like London. In India, for instance, firms like Conserve in New Delhi upcycle plastic bags to make accessories such as bags and belts (Quinn 2010: 138–39). Other enterprises like Dharam Pal Woollen Mills at Panipat, Haryana, import used Western garments and remake them into various products to sell back to discount stores in the United States and Italy.

Finally, if we take the widest definition of sustainability, we find many non-Western societies have different imperatives from the West. Sustainability in certain indigenous cultures, in parts of Asia, South America, and the South Pacific, for instance, may mean a powerful desire to prevent the loss of certain forms of customary dress, ones outside Western mainstream fashion. Reclamation or continuation of indigenous kinds of attire using age-old styles and practices of textile production (sometimes fused with new styles) is being encouraged in many places in order to maintain connections with the past (Schevill 2010: 4), thus challenging fashion's temporary nature. So the text concludes by extending the very term *sustainability* in relation to fashion and indeed dress beyond that of prevention of environmental damage. It does this by examining certain non-Western examples, as it ponders the possible future of this field of study.

EARLY CONCERNS AND APPROACHES

Aside from the "back to nature" romanticism of the hippie movement, since the 1970s a trickle of general disquiet about environmental degradation has grown exponentially, especially in the more developed areas of the world. The popular media expressed this concern, as did the probes of investigative journalists, to say nothing of academic critiques.

A sense of urgency to respond to these problems was evident as early as 1972 with *The Limits to Growth,* the first report to the Club of Rome (Meadows et al. 1972). It focused on predicaments facing the world, including problems generated by excess consumption. Greenpeace was founded in 1971. Antisweatshop, antifur (People for the Ethical Treatment of Animals [PETA] started in 1981), and antiglobalization consumer activists gathered force, increasingly drawing attention to unethical clothes-manufacturing practices and the polluting effects of textile production on ecosystems.

By the 1990s, published scientific research into textiles and sustainability plus business analyses of consumer behavior had multiplied. The term *sustainable consumption* entered common parlance by the early 1990s (Birtwistle and Moore 2007: 210). This was exactly at the time the concept of fast fashion was emerging as a commercial factor. Although somewhat belated in comparison to studies of sustainable land use, housing, and water, publications on the subject of clothing, textiles, and their degrading production methods began more frequently to offer research-based and worrying understanding about their nonbiodegradable effects (Bahorsky 1998; Kumar and Aggarwal 1994). At the same time, mass fashion and dress more generally, linked to eco-sustainability, were increasing analyzed from a wide range of research specialties, conceptual frameworks, and methodologies.

Especially since the late twentieth century, work has been done in relation to economic factors, scientific and business studies, consumer behavior, resource conservation, marketing, global manufacturing, and retailing (for example, Birtwistle and Moore 2007; Kunz and Garner 2011). By the middle of the first decade of the twenty-first century, research attention shifted to broader considerations. These focused on greater integration of sustainable fashion and dress in terms of cultural phenomena more generally (Reinach 2005: 47). About this time fast fashion came to be a topic of interest to academic researchers concerned with consumption and the industry itself. This new interest sits well with changes in the discipline of fashion and clothing studies, in particular what Lise Skov and Marie Riegels Melchior class as the production-based research approach. This method focuses on the mutual interrelationship of production and consumption, sometimes called the *fashion system.* This is in opposition to the more segmented interest in supply chains, branding, or retailing that is more the province of economic and business studies (Skov and Melchior 2010: 15).

Publication of serious, wide-ranging analyses of dress, textiles, and environmental sustainability increased fairly rapidly from the early twenty-first century. Margaret Maynard's chapter "Clothing: Is There a Responsible Choice?" in her *Dress and Globalisation* (2004), was one of the first occasions when a dress historian questioned ethical and environmental responsibility in relation to clothing, on both a personal and a corporate level. Since this publication, critical writing on the subject of fashion and social responsibility has grown significantly in academic circles and the broader print media. Sandy Black has played a leading academic role in her networked website Interrogating Fashion (2005), bringing together artists, scientists, designers, and so on to challenge existing fashion and clothing practices.[3] She also published *Developing Considerate Design,* with Claudia M. Eckert (2009), as well as an essay "Ethical Fashion and Ecofashion" in *The Berg Companion to Fashion* (2010), edited by Valerie Steele. Here too we must mention Kate Fletcher's *Sustainable Fashion and Textiles: Design Journeys* (2008), a significant work based around sustainable design and practical applications as ways to affect consumption.

In the same year an important special issue of *Fashion Theory* on ecofashion was published, edited by Regina A. Root (Root 2008a). The authors included in this issue held a generally positive view that changes toward a future in which ecofashion played a major part were a distinct possibility. According to Nathaniel Dafyyd Beard, citing consumption figures of dress products made of organic cotton, he felt it possible that 2006–2008 would be regarded as a watershed period when sustainable or ecofashion moved from being a small segment of the market to a real commercial proposition (2008: 452). Sarah Scaturro had an equally positive opinion of current and improved technologies of manufacturing, which she suggested could bring increased sustainability in production methods for textiles. She claimed there is indeed a hopeful future for what she terms *eco-tech fashion* (2008: 487). Technology and sustainability can be symbiotic in the long term. However, these views have yet to be proved and may reflect a Western bias.

Regina Root, editor of the special issue, asks two pertinent questions: when is sustainable fashion a sign of political action rather than simply a "media event" (and one could add a tokenistic gesture), and how could the "lens of sustainability" change the direction of fashion theory itself? (Root 2008b: 420). This second question is more difficult to answer than the first although it is of special interest for fashion studies, today a vigorously expanding field. Fashion wearing is a site of aesthetic pleasure for many, a locus of desire and a device for the communication of status and personal expression. To imagine that fashion and design creativity would be seriously deflected by theories of wearing entirely colored by issues of sustainability is difficult to envisage in the present global commercial environment. Yet the topic is of major concern to many in the academic community, including theorists, as well as those teaching fashion as a design subject and the nexus between material/object-based studies and the practical.

FASHION AND FAST FASHION

Before we consider specific issues related to fast fashion, it is important to explain that in the twenty-first century the term *fashion* may be used in different ways. Fashion is a process demonstrating changes over time, at its heart the endless and deliberate negation of what has come immediately before it (Riello and McNeil 2010: 1). However, fashion is now no longer univocal. The range of categories that define it brings to the field of current fashion studies considerable complexity. Until the later 1960s, the genre of haute couture, centered especially on Western women's attire, mainly sourced from Paris, was the preserve of the extremely moneyed class. It was and is a top-down design process. Its products demonstrate the relentless pursuit of individualistic style; its quality and design acumen (often conveyed via glossy fashion images) drives consumer desire. In this sense the term *fashion* describes extremely pricey and lavish one-off styles, the concept of a signature designer, realized by highly skilled artisans (with very small output and clientele). Luxury custom-made men's tailoring (the great skill we associate with London's Savile Row) is also labor-intensive, but its garments are less subject to the regular, often radical, changes seen in women's high fashion. Bespoke tailoring is expensive, but a new mood of interest in looking well dressed has emerged among professional men, with suits now considered lifelong investments if properly cared for (Meagher 2011a). In one sense men's quality clothing is the more sustainable option.

Since the 1960s, fashion has split into many categories of prêt-à-porter, mass and volume fashion, and street style, and these have greatly complicated the picture (Crane 2000: 135). This industry, of which fast fashion is a part, is vast. According to Regina Root, it employs about 26.5 million people worldwide (2008b: 419). In the previous year, it was estimated that there were about 40 million jobs in the global textile and clothing industries (Hines and Bruce 2007). Fast fashion, a form of volume product, is far different from couture or ready-to-wear attire and has its own characteristics. It is more tangential, based on demand-led business models, in tune with ever-changing styles or fads, and widely sold in slick middle-range chain stores on high streets or in malls. Trend-spotting on the catwalk and elsewhere is a key to its success. The term *massclusivity* is used of fast fashion to indicate its position as one straddling high and middle-of-the-road style (Tokatli 2008: 23). The clothes are a step up from the generic mass-produced and globalized, relatively uniform everyday clothing worn all over the world from Nepal to Peru.

What exactly is *fast fashion*? The term, especially associated with the products of the Spanish firm Zara but also others like Mango and H&M, was in use by the later 1990s (Kunz and Garner 2011: 149). Sometimes called the "quick-response" method, the facilitation of "rapid access to the latest styles" has been inextricable from innovations in communication technology. It is dependent on ever-developing interactive digital networks and rapid marketing processes (Sheridan, Moore, and Nobbs 2006). Zara, a pioneer of fast fashion principles (part of the Inditex conglomerate), and Gap are good examples of the hold so-called fast fashion has on the consumer psyche. Zara's products are fabric rather than garment led, and digitization enables the company to shrink the time taken from the initial design to volume production and the final sales point. The enhanced product design or "hot" product, which reflects the latest trends, is cunningly matched with minimal turnaround times to create maximum profit (Cachon and Swinney 2011: 778). Topshop expects its clothes to be worn no more than ten times (Birtwistle and Moore 2007: 211).

At the core of fast fashion is a fashionability where speed of making is easily applied to the high-quality intricacies of classic garments (Tokatli 2008: 22, 23). It presents the aura of exclusivity in that it offers relatively few items for sale. Immediately desirable, these soon disappear from the racks, and customers miss out on opportunities if they do not purchase the items immediately. Companies introduce new designs every six weeks (Black 2010: 252), and in the case of Zara novel styles of merchandise are in their stores, if outsourced to Spain, with a two- to three-week lead time (Kunz and Garner 2011: 149). What were biannual seasonal designs are now replaced by the introduction of merchandise more and more quickly. These firms sell globally at an ever-lowering cost. As quality is lowered and clothes can be purchased cheaper, they become more disposable (Black 2010: 252). As they become cheaper and cheaper, consumers return to the store in ever shorter time cycles.

In an interesting twist, fast fashion companies like H&M have combined with couturiers and high-end designers, in this case Donatella Versace, to refigure the very nature of exclusivity. The designer Collette Dinnegan (the first Australian to regularly show her ready-to-wear collection in Paris) has made a version of her high-class lines to sell in down-market stores as a way to engage new customers. For instance, she produced her Wild Hearts Lingerie in 2008 for Target, a medium-price chain store, following Target's contracted range from Stella McCartney in 2007. At the same time the exclusive Burberry brand is engaging a wide audience of consumers by its skillful use of the immediacy of Facebook, Twitter, and Instagram and its exceptionally popular social networking site Art of the Trench[4] (Meagher 2011b: 48).

Similar dispensers of "hot" fashions are many online marketing sites, such as that of the interactive trend-aware company ASOS, supposedly the largest online-only fashion and beauty store in the United Kingdom. The ASOS website allows consumers to see the most popular outfits over the recent past, be part of a fashion community, upload a favorite photograph of themselves, express their own fashion personality, and develop a style profile.[5] Made in the Now, a "real-time" news-based company, produces new T-shirt designs every twenty-four hours, partly based on Facebook and Twitter votes.[6] The company's designs respond to breaking media stories. They claim to offer an alternative to wasteful fast fashions by supplying only on demand. They claim their goods are both sustainable and more instantaneous than fast fashions. The relationship between the provider and the purchaser of fashion has thus shifted dramatically. Fashion expertise, once personalized and the province of expert fitters, vendeuses, and style advisors, has shifted to more emphasis on individual choice, personal taste, and now interactivity via social media sites.

These types of stylish dress are some of the most problematic products in any discussion about the nature of sustainability. In 2006 UK consumers on average purchased 77 pounds (35 kilograms) of clothing per year, with one-eighth sent to charities for reuse and the rest discarded (Allwood et al. 2006). In fact, much fast fashion goes to landfill, where synthetics don't decompose and wool produces methane as it decays (Birtwistle and Moore 2007: 212). According to the latter two authors, in the previous few years consumers had appeared little interested in the social or environmental impact of what they wore (214). Probably a major reason is that sophisticated marketing and business expertise has educated consumers to expect constant newness, and advertising has become increasingly skillful in raising desires.

Initially, Zara (with 4,300 stores in 73 countries by 2011) was held in some regard for its sole use of local European workers, but this has changed. As a number of supplier firms in countries such as Morocco, India, and Turkey have gained the competence to manufacture intricately worked high-quality garments with the required flexibility and speed, Zara has turned to sourcing from these countries. In 2008 they also employed workers in places like India to spot trends and produce designs rather than simply provide low-paid outworkers (Tokatli 2008: 27). For less complicated production, the company looks to Sri Lanka, India, Pakistan, Vietnam, and Indonesia (25, 35). While accessibility to fashion seems on the face of it to be greater than ever for many levels of consumers, this kind of practice is not benign. The swifter turnaround times put more and more pressure on low-paid clothing workers wherever they are, and as Black suggests, "Complex ethical issues are... hidden behind all fashion-purchasing decisions" (2010: 253).

Thus the question of value is extremely pertinent to fast fashion, with its use of new manufacturing technologies and ability to make replaceable clothes at greater and greater speed. Manufacturers who cut corners and embrace substantial improvements in technology (in particular digitization) and the ability to access low-paid workers in remote and underdeveloped parts of the world make this clothing both profitable and popular but of dubious social value in its widest sense. The ethical nature of fast fashion is indeed problematic, as more and more products of questionable quality and with a short life span come onto the market.

Many global brands proclaim ethical credentials, but what exactly does "ethics" mean in each case? Like the term *natural,* it is subjective and very hard to define. An interesting example of eco-ethics is found at fashion-conscious.com. This company stocks only designs that have a supposedly ethical and eco dimension—be it recycled, organic, non-toxic, fair trade, sustainable, vegan, or nonexploitative. To help the consumer determine the ethics of each item for sale in the online store, the company has created symbols that denote the specific ethical status of the designers and their products. This is a slightly puzzling concept as it appears some items are deemed more ethical than others. The problem with fast fashion is that its desirability and devotion to newness make compatibility with ethical requirements challenging, if not impossible.

STYLISH ALTERNATIVES TO THE NEW

Recently, other approaches to fashion have emerged that do not fit with the received understanding we have of high or fast fashion. These challenge fashion's preoccupation with the new as outlined by Clark (2008). Some offer remaking as an alternative, as well as recycling, use of secondhand items, and even sharing, but nevertheless have a special place within the system. Elsewhere, some small companies are endeavoring to dampen down consumption of new fashions by refashioning existing clothes that still look stylish (Scaturro 2008: 485). These products are increasingly evident in niche marketing and supposedly empowering online sites like Etsy. The latter claims to be "the world's handmade marketplace" and includes details of designers and the ways in which clothing but also other nondress products were made.[7]

It is true that many concerned designers have taken the issue of producing sustainable dress/fashion and textiles very seriously. Quinn in his chapter "Sustainability" gives detailed accounts of highly imaginative designers devising methods of recycling clothing overproduced by large companies and transforming discarded industrial fabrics into textiles (2010: 110). He points to a growing market for products that satisfy consumer interest in acquiring garments that will not harm the environment. An example offered by Clark is the Junky Styling label, located in the United Kingdom, which favors longevity: quality used garments for men and women undergo "surgery," with the input of both the designer and the customer, to "upstyle" individual garments. Their creations have penetrated high-end style as they have shown at London Fashion Week and have celebrity customers (Clark 2008: 438). "New recycled garments" are also the preserve of the TRAIDremade label (Textile Recycling for Aid and International Development) started in 2002 (439). This is a fashion label for men and women of one-off creations using secondhand textiles and clothing. It has a flagship store in London's Camden area.

A further novel way to acquire stylish clothing outside the paradigm of fast fashion is clothes swapping, called *swishing,* which is a form of collaborative consumption, not anticonsumption. Clothes can be swapped at places like The Super Swish Clothes Shop, Covent Garden, London, which combines glamour and ethics, or via swishing parties now taking place all over the world. The term is invented and means "rustling" clothes from friends. There is also the online website Swishing, where you can buy items based on credits or swap clothes, if you don't have enough credit from an item you have swapped, you can part-buy another garment, making up the difference with cash.

Vast numbers of people all over the world wear charity shop and secondhand dress by necessity. Retro or vintage dressing is also embraced by the affluent if it fits with their sense of style. Sustainability, in the case of the first, is by necessity rather than design. Both these forms of dressing are kinder to the environment than the constant use of new clothing. Appreciation for the unique quality and imaginative restyling of secondhand or vintage dress is a big factor in the latter kinds of purchases, which mark an important alternative form of consumption governed by personal rather than dictated taste. Whether this kind of clothing will ever entirely overtake the global demand for new clothing is debatable.

SUSTAINABILITY: THE BROADER PICTURE

If we take a wide definition of sustainability in relation to dress, one including environmental issues but also beyond, we find many non-Western societies have different priorities. While fast fashion is the primary focus in this essay, fashion/attire generally has different connotations in the less developed environments of the world and indeed in poverty-stricken places within metropolitan cultures everywhere. Here the constant replenishment with new products is not possible financially. In the less developed world, the cycle of dress operates in location-specific orders of temporality, for instance, in terms of types and availability of new and used clothing, and the manner in which secondhand goods are reused. In underdeveloped parts of Africa, Asia, and South America, sites are chosen for outsourcing manufacture of fast new fashions at the lowest cost. But new clothes made for a multinational company may be discarded by purchasers in the developed world and may return to the location of their making as cheap secondhand gear. It is possible for brands designed, say, in the United States to be made in Vietnam, returned to the United States, and then reexported as new or secondhand attire, perhaps to the detriment of the local textile industry.

In underdeveloped countries, bales of secondhand clothing are sourced largely from thrift shops and other charity organizations, mainly from the United States, but also the United Kingdom and Europe, and frequently marketed on the street. Sub-Saharan Africa is the world's largest secondhand clothing destination (Hansen 2010: 235). The complexity and meanings accorded this secondhand trade are extraordinary. The reuse of these commodities cuts down on consumption of new clothing, but in turn stylish dressing is reconstituted. Lead researcher Karen Tranberg Hansen has shown the complexities of how Africans create their own versions of fashionable appearances by the practice of *salaula* (in Zambia) or so-called *kaunjika* in Malawi (239). Consumers rummage among goods, then pick and choose, oftentimes altering imported secondhand Western goods to achieve a desired look (Hansen 1999, 2000).

Yet sustainability in certain indigenous cultures, in parts of Asia, South America, and the South Pacific, for instance, may mean a powerful desire to prevent the loss of certain forms of customary clothing, especially for dance performances, ceremonies, and feasts, but also more widely. In Papua New Guinea the art of *bilas* (self-decoration) especially at dance performances (Cochrane 2010: 265) is not static, nor is it cultural preservation in any rigid sense. In many instances, the intention is ongoing inventiveness and novelty but absorbed into a traditional style that sustains connections with the past. It is a form of reinstatement or reframing of local attire combining versions of age-old styles and practices of textile production, with perhaps some incorporation of modern imported materials and features. Sandra Niessen, Ann Marie Leshkowich, and Carla Jones, discussing the Asian process of reinstating previous styles as part of sustaining traditions, terms it "self-Orientalizing," where these apparent traditional styles are in fact conscious and strategic remakings of the past (2003: 31). On the other hand, garments such as the Chinese *cheongsam* or the *shalwar kamiz* are now globalized clothes that may, to some degree, find their way into the designs of fast fashion, it being important to distinguish between the various imperatives.

In New Zealand, the Māori resistance to the intrusion of Europeans and their way of life has contributed to a late twentieth- and early twenty-first-century flowering of their culture, including self-adornment. Modern synthetic materials can be used where traditional ones are unavailable, and sometimes styles are adapted to modern usage in some way. There is, for instance, the revival of authentic weaving techniques for cloaks, although weavers are unable to access all the former customary resources of flora and fauna except *harakeke* (Wallace 2010: 258). Kanaks in New Caledonia care less for

European-style metropolitan dress, except for formal occasions, than for what is termed Oceanic style, printed shirts for men and print dresses for women (Angleviel 2010: 487). Rei Matau women on the island of Yap in Micronesia still wear traditional woven *lavalava* waist wraps with no covering above the waist to signal cultural identity. Polyester is now preferred as more durable and less coarse than plant fibers (Petrosian-Husa 2010: 503). In other struggling economies in the South Pacific (Fiji, for instance), women wear Western dress for office and formal wear but often modified to local tastes, while at home for special occasions they favour *sulu jiaba,* a layered dress and underskirt (Ewins 2010: 442–43). As well, secondhand clothes are mixed with customary dress made from local materials for village life and indigenous celebrations.

CONCLUSION: A SOCIAL DILEMMA

There is little doubt that by the end of the first decade of the twenty-first century many consumers, primarily in developed parts of the world, have become increasingly aware of their social responsibilities regarding protection of environmental resources (Kunz and Garner 2011: 99). This is perhaps less so in the acquisition of fashion and dress generally. Indications are that changes to excess consumption of volume fashion, including fast fashion, did emerge in the aftermath of the 2010 global financial crisis and the second phase of financial instability during 2011. These uncertainties seem to have produced a new wave of cautious consumers, many preferring to shun mainstream retailers, reduce garment purchases, and spend online or save in other ways. It has also had a profound effect on corporate profits for retailers. The newfound reticence to spend has apparently not affected the luxury market and diffusion lines of top designers. Here growth has not been dampened. And the slump has had differential outcomes. In China the GFC seems to have caused a relatively minor down turn and a review of the textile and garment industry in 2011 shows China exported US$153.22 billion worth of garments, a growth of 18.35 percent compared to the previous year, 2010.[8]

The question is, will environmentally sound forms of dressing be embraced that will satisfy consumers preoccupied with their stylish appearances? Will public rejection of the wasteful nature of fashion ever occur, even if clothing companies highlight their supposed "green" credentials? Perhaps fast fashion, and the aesthetic sophistication of consumers, is fundamentally incompatible with ethical resource management. All corporate success is measured by turnover, growth, and expanding profits. Given continuing financial troubles in Europe and the United States, and concerns about high unemployment, it may be that scale and costs associated with sustainable solutions will not find mass industry support. One issue might be where progress toward alliances (perhaps convergence) between computing, communications, electronics, textiles, and fashion sits with environmental optimism. As Colin Gale and Jasbir Kaur note in their chapter "Future Wear," once technological innovation in clothing and textile production has begun, and manufacturers see its commercial possibilities, there is no going back (Gale and Kaur 2004: 190). But can "smart" clothing ever be environmentally neutral?

It is possible to argue that fundamental and thoroughgoing changes to the global fashion status quo may happen only in the event of a major worldwide recession and day of reckoning for the environment as a whole. That said, indigenous practices, perhaps drawn in part from locally grown materials, might prove to outlast other modern equivalents. It is also interesting to see that recently new lightweight wool fabrics are showing a significant resurgence in profitability. Wool is less harmful to the environment than artificial fibers. It is very long-lasting and is economically sustainable, although at present it is being directed primarily to premium fashion markets.

Alongside hopes for cutting other commodities, like fuel consumption, it may be some time until the fashion system will change its priorities, if it ever does. The question remains, is diversity of style in new clothing something an increasingly resource-depleted world can afford? The Sustainable Apparel Coalition, formed in 2011 with major companies onboard, including Nike, Esprit, Patagonia, Walmart, Marks & Spencer, Gap, and a host of others, may show the way forward. But perhaps the phrase *sustainable fashion* is largely rhetorical, an environmental gloss to corporate "business as usual." If so, what then might be the future of this field of study?

NOTES

1. This is vigorously demonstrated by Naomi Klein (2000) in her No Logo chapter "The Discarded Factory."
2. See the useful definition of relevant terms in Thomas (2008).
3. Sandy Black, Interrogating Fashion, 2005, http://www.interrogatingfashion.org (accessed February 3, 2012). This research was supported by the London College of Fashion, University of the Arts, London, funded by Engineering and Physical Sciences Research Council and Arts and Humanities Research Council.
4. Art of the Trench, http://www.artofthetrench.com (accessed May 8, 2013).
5. ASOS, http://www.asos.com (accessed February 4, 2012).
6. Made in the Now, http://www.madeinthenow.com (accessed May 8, 2013).
7. Etsy, http://www.etsy.com (accessed May 8, 2013).
8. "A Review of China's Textile and Garment Industry 2011," *ATA Journal for Asian Textiles and Apparel*, April 2012, http://www.adsaleata.com/Publicity/ePub/lang-eng/article-8506/asid-73/Article.aspx (accessed July 25, 2013).

BIBLIOGRAPHY

Allwood, Julian M., Søren Ellebæk Laursen, Cecilia Malvido de Rodriguez, and Nancy M. P. Bocken. 2006. *Well Dressed? The Present and Future Sustainability of Clothing and Textiles in the United Kingdom.* Cambridge: University of Cambridge Institute for Manufacturing.

Angleviel, Frédéric. 2010. "Dress in New Caledonia." In Margaret Maynard (ed.), *Berg Encyclopedia of World Dress and Fashion,* vol. 7, *Australia, New Zealand, and the Pacific Islands,* 484–87. Oxford: Berg.

Bahorsky, Michael S. 1998. "Textiles: Regulatory Aspects and Reviews." *Water Environment Research* 70 (4): 690–93.

Beard, Nathaniel Dafyyd. 2008. "The Branding of Ethical Fashion and the Consumer: A Luxury Niche or Mass-Market Reality?" *Fashion Theory: The Journal of Dress, Body and Culture* 12 (4): 447–68.

Birtwistle, Grete, and Christopher M. Moore. 2007. "Fashion Clothing—Where Does It All End Up?" *International Journal of Retail and Distribution Management* 35 (3): 210–16.

Black, Sandy. 2008. *Eco-chic: The Fashion Paradox.* London: Black Dog.

Black, Sandy. 2010. "Ethical Fashion and Ecofashion." In Valerie Steele (ed.), *The Berg Companion to Fashion,* 251–60. Oxford: Berg.

Black, Sandy, and Claudia Eckert. 2009. *Developing Considerate Design: Meeting Individual Fashion and Clothing Needs within a Framework of Sustainability.* In Frank T. Piller and Mitchell M. Tseng (eds.), *Handbook of Research in Mass Customization and Personalization,* 813–32. Hackensack, NJ and London: World Scientific Press.

Cachon, Gerard P., and Robert Swinney. 2011. "The Value of Fast Fashion: Quick Response, Enhanced Design and Strategic Consumer Behaviour." *Management Science* 57 (4): 778–95.

Clark, Hazel. 2008. "SLOW + FASHION—an Oxymoron—or a Promise for the Future...?" *Fashion Theory: The Journal of Dress, Body and Culture* 12 (4): 427–46.

Cochrane, Susan. 2010. "Festivals Pacific-Style." In Joanne B. Eicher (ed.), *Berg Encyclopedia of World Dress and Fashion,* vol. 10, *Global Perspectives,* 264–66. Oxford: Berg.

Crane, Diana. 2000. *Fashion and Its Social Agendas: Class, Gender and Identity in Clothing.* Chicago: University of Chicago Press.

Ewins, Roderick. 2010. "Fijian Dress and Body Modifications." In Margaret Maynard (ed.), *Berg Encyclopedia of World Dress and Fashion,* vol. 7, *Australia, New Zealand, and the Pacific Islands,* 435–43. Oxford: Berg.

Fletcher, Kate. 2008. *Sustainable Fashion and Textiles: Design Journeys.* Oxford: Earthscan.

Gale, Colin, and Jasbir Kaur. 2004. *Fashions and Textiles: An Overview.* Oxford: Berg.

Hansen, Karen Tranberg. 2000. "Other People's Clothes: The International Second-Hand Clothing Trade and Dress Practices in Zambia." *Fashion Theory: The Journal of Dress, Body and Culture* 4 (3): 245–74.

Hansen, Karen Tranberg. 2010. "Secondhand Clothing." In Joanne B. Eicher (ed.), *Berg Encyclopedia of World Dress and Fashion,* vol. 10, *Global Perspectives,* 232–37. Oxford: Berg.

Hines, Tony, and Margaret Bruce. 2007. *Fashion Marketing: Contemporary Issues.* Amsterdam: Butterworth-Heinemann.

Klein, Naomi. 2000. *No Logo.* London: Flamingo.

Kunz, Grace I., and Myrna B. Garner. 2011. *Going Global: The Textile and Apparel Industry.* 2nd ed. New York: Fairchild Books.

Lipovetsky, Gilles. 1994. *The Empire of Fashion: Dressing Modern Democracy.* Princeton, NJ: Princeton University Press.

Maynard, Margaret. 2004. *Dress and Globalisation.* Manchester: Manchester University Press.

Maynard, Margaret. 2010. "Globalization and Dress." In Joanne B. Eicher (ed.), *Berg Encyclopedia of World Dress and Fashion,* vol. 10, *Global Perspectives,* 252–63. Oxford: Berg.

Meadows, Donella H., Dennis L. Meadows, Jørgen Randers, and William W. Behrens III. 1972. *The Limits to Growth: A Report for the Club of Rome's Project on the Predicament of Mankind.* London: Universe Books.

Meagher, David. 2011a. "Editor's Letter." *Wish,* June 11, p. 14.

Meagher, David. 2011b. "Tweet, Tweet." *Wish,* December 11, pp. 48–50.

Niessen, Sandra, Ann Marie Leshkowich, and Carla Jones (eds.). 2003. *Re-orienting Fashion: The Globalization of Asian Dress.* Oxford: Berg.

Petrosian-Husa, Carmen C. H. 2010. "Lavalava (Cloth) of the Rei Metau." In Margaret Maynard (ed.), *Berg Encyclopedia of World Dress and Fashion,* vol. 7, *Australia, New Zealand, and the Pacific Islands,* 502–7. Oxford: Berg.

Kumar, P., and R. K. Aggarwal. 1994. "Impact of Industrial Effluents on the Soil and Water Quality of the Desert Ecosystem and Its Management." *Advances in Forestry Research in India* 11: 79–104.

Quinn, Bradley. 2010. *Textile Futures: Fashion, Design and Technology.* Oxford: Berg.

Reinach, Simona Segre. 2005. "China and Italy: Fast Fashion versus Prêt à Porter: Toward a New Culture of Fashion." *Fashion Theory: The Journal of Dress, Body and Culture* 9 (1): 43–56.

Riello, Giorgio, and Peter McNeil. 2010. "Introduction." In Giorgio Riello and Peter McNeil (eds.), *The Fashion History Reader: Global Perspectives,* 1–14. Oxford: Routledge.

Root, Regina A. (ed.). 2008a. "Ecofashion." Special issue, *Fashion Theory: The Journal of Dress, Body and Culture* 12 (4).

Root, Regina A. 2008b. "Letter from the Editor." *Fashion Theory: The Journal of Dress, Body and Culture* 12 (4): 419–25.

Scaturro, Sarah. 2008. "Eco-tech Fashion: Rationalizing Technology in Sustainable Fashion." *Fashion Theory: The Journal of Dress, Body and Culture* 12 (4): 469–88.

Schevill, Margot Blum. 2010. "Introductory Note to Latin America and the Caribbean." In Margo Schevill (ed.), *Berg Encyclopedia of World Dress and Fashion,* vol. 2, *Latin America and the Caribbean,* 3–4. Oxford: Berg.

Sheridan, Mandy, Christopher Moore, and Karinna Nobbs. 2006. "Fast Fashion Requires Fast Marketing: The Role of Category Management in Fast Fashion Positioning." *Journal of Fashion Marketing and Management* 10 (3): 301–15.

Skov, Lise, and Marie Riegels Melchior. 2010. "Research Approaches." In Joanne B. Eicher (ed.), *Berg Encyclopedia of World Dress and Fashion,* vol. 10, *Global Perspectives,* 11–16. Oxford: Berg.

Thomas, Sue. 2008. "From 'Green Blur' to Ecofashion: Fashioning an Eco-lexicon." *Fashion Theory: The Journal of Dress, Body and Culture* 12 (4): 427–46.

Tokatli, Nebahat. 2008. "Global Sourcing: Insights from the Global Clothing Industry—the Case of Zara, a Fast Fashion Retailer." *Journal of Economic Geography* 8 (1): 21–38.

Wallace, Patricia. 2010. "Introduction to Māori Dress." In Margaret Maynard (ed.), *Berg Encyclopedia of World Dress and Fashion,* vol. 7, *Australia, New Zealand, and the Pacific Islands,* 249–59. Oxford: Berg.

26

Design for Sustainability in Fashion and Textiles

KATE FLETCHER

INTRODUCTION

> In many ways, the environmental crisis is a design crisis. It is a consequence of how things are made.
>
> —Sim Van der Ryn and Stuart Cowan (1996: 9)

The direct link between products, production, their implied consumption, and ecological and social impacts has, over the last twenty years, led to a wide range of changes across the fashion supply chain, from conceptualization and design through manufacturing and distribution to waste management and recycling. Just as in the wider global debate on sustainability, where a spectrum of viewpoints coexist, there are many different fashion-sector responses to ecological and social imperatives. This chapter explores this variety through the lens of design for sustainability, an emerging field of study that uses a broad view of design to increase environmental and social quality across all sectors, including fashion.

The capacity of design to influence the sustainability profile of goods and services was acknowledged by the Brundtland Report. Best known for its popularization of the term *sustainable development,* the report also made recommendations for a new approach to design and production, setting out terms for "a production system that respects . . . the ecological base" and "a technological system that searches continuously for new solutions" (World Commission on Environment and Development 1987: 65). The particular focus on design in Brundtland is justified by the large relative effects of design decisions on the entire product life cycle: it is estimated that 80 percent of a product's environmental and economic costs are committed by the final design stage, before production begins (Graedel, Comrie, and Sekutowski 1995: 19). It follows from this that by integrating sustainability considerations into design, there is potential to bring far-reaching ecological and social benefits—benefits that flow courtesy of design's position at the beginning of the industrial chain. When sustainability considerations are built into the earliest stage of product conceptualization and design development, the effect can be to prevent impacts from occurring, so minimizing the need for remedial cleanup action further down the chain. This anticipatory potential has led to design actions being described as "the most proactive direct action one can take to achieve [impact] prevention" (Keoleian and Menerey 1994: 664), and this frames design, and those who employ design thinking, as powerful agents for change in sustainability, an agency that has profound reciprocal implications for the nature of design and the manufacturing industries (see, for example, Manzini 1994; Thorpe 2007; Walker 2006).

The two-way transformative effect of sustainability on design is perhaps not seen as widely in fashion design. Mathilda Tham explores a range of possible reasons for this, including the flippant way in which fashion is often viewed from both outside and inside the profession: "an immoral, self-indulgent industry . . . that lacks gravitas and a strong conceptual framework" (2008: 194); seen thus, fashion appears to occupy an incongruous place within the grounded, values-driven paradigm of sustainability. Sociologist Barbara Vinken (2005, in Tham 2008: 193) traces the roots of this "superficial" viewpoint and notes a strong gender bias: fashion has long had associations with femininity, idleness, social amusement, and consumption, which continue through some approaches to fashion education, emphasizing, for example, "personal creativity, crafts skills and intuition rather than analysis" (194). Indeed, design roles in the mass-market sector are largely populated by women with little formal education beyond undergraduate-level fashion design (and certainly not in environmental issues), who, according to Tham's research, place little importance in their work on critical analysis and who often lack control over their creative practice (124). Against such a context, and in the light of their limited knowledge about sustainability themes and cynicism about the industry's willingness to change (131), fashion designers' response to sustainability has been, perhaps unsurprisingly, fitful. Yet a number of strong educational projects focused on fashion design students and tutors, such as the Labour Behind the Label project Fashioning an Ethical Industry,[1] have been working to improve knowledge and skills around sustainability issues in general and, in the case of Fashioning an Ethical Industry, workers' rights in particular.

THE MAGNITUDE OF THE SUSTAINABILITY CHALLENGE

Regardless of the slow pace and irregularity of the fashion sector's uptake of sustainability ideas, the magnitude of the sustainability challenge for all sectors, including fashion, continues to underscore the urgency of change. This was highlighted most notably in recent times by the Club of Rome in its report *The Limits to Growth* (Meadows et al.

1972), in which it outlined what it named as the "global problematique": how to reconcile expanding population and consumption levels on a planet of finite limits, and the effect of not doing so ("collapse"). Almost two decades later, Paul and Anne Ehrlich helped enumerate this challenge with a simple equation, the IPAT identity (1990: 58), the product of population size, levels of consumption, and the environmental efficiency of current technologies. They argued that in order to maintain the effects of human actions at their current level, the desired size of impact reduction over the next forty years, a period in which the world population is set to double, is predicted to lie between a factor of four and a factor of twenty. In essence, it states that in order to contain pollution levels as consumption increases, the impact of products and services will have to be reduced by up to 95 percent, or to one-twentieth of today's level. It seems difficult to overstate the enormity of this task. Even today's best practices and cutting-edge techniques, as described variously in texts like *Factor Four* (Weizsäcker, Lovins, and Lovins 1997) and *World Changing* (Steffan 2008), rarely offer the promise of impact reduction at any level higher than the most conservative of the Ehrlichs' estimates. What is more, few best-practice technologies, products, or services make it into the mainstream and become widely adopted, underlining still further the gap between current behavior and demanding sustainability goals. As Stuart Walker and Ralf Nielson comment:

> The magnitude of change required by sustainability is so significant that it cannot be achieved by small incremental improvements to our current approaches. It is the "current approaches" themselves, which, in many respects are the primary obstacle, therefore small improvements to these approaches are unlikely to achieve the changes necessary for sustainability. (1998: 8)

LIFE-CYCLE THINKING

A widely shared foundational idea underpinning design for sustainability is life-cycle thinking, the goal of which is to minimize a product's combined negative effects on ecological and social systems by pursuing a globalized or holistic systems approach to design. In the last two decades the intellectual framework of life-cycle thinking has significantly shaped the sustainability work within the fashion industry. Simply, it involves directing attention not only to fiber type, material provenance, or the processing stage that a company deals with directly but also to the whole physical life cycle of the product, from raw materials to end of life. It sees garments as a mosaic of interconnected flows of materials and labor and as potential satisfiers of needs and not simply as isolated resources, processes, or sources of one-off environmental, social, and cultural impact in production.

Life-cycle thinking is inspired by the language and study of ecology and works to understand the multiple interrelationships that link material, industrial, and economic systems with nature. These connections operate at different scales and with different spheres of influence, some on a direct local level and others globally. In life-cycle thinking, openness to these relationships is a key precursor to change, reflecting the dynamic effect of each part on every other part. The goal of this global view is to optimize the sustainability of the whole product system and to have this take priority over increasing the effectiveness of individual system parts or life-cycle phases. And unlike in the past, when each life-cycle phase was the concern of discrete companies or industries (spinners, weavers, white goods manufacturers, etc.), now the success of the whole entails joint responsibility for all players to reduce impact. This makes things like waste, for example, as much a concern and focus for designers and consumers as for recyclers.

TWO DISTINCT APPROACHES

Design-for-sustainability work can be seen to cluster around two distinct approaches. The first approach, which is the more investigated, focuses on improving current products, including current processes. It is, in effect, a problem-minimizing strategy that takes the current industrial model as the starting point for improvement toward sustainability. The second approach calls for new concepts and visions on how to fulfill basic human needs, including an openness to redesigning the systems that shape design, production, and consumption: economic models, business practices, sociocultural behavior.

The existence of two distinct approaches is confirmed by Matthew Simon (1994), who differentiates between "weak" and "strong" sustainability in design and sees designers as practicing either "technocentric design" (weak sustainability) or "ecocentric design" (strong sustainability). The concepts of techno- and ecocentrism reflect differences in philosophical positions regarding conceptions of nature and the environment and ways to implement sustainable development (Pepper 1996: 37). The former believes that society will solve environmental problems through science, technology, and economics; the latter frames solutions as emerging from a perspective that sees humankind as part of a global system whose natural laws impose limits on resource consumption and growth and that emphasizes decentralized, democratic, and small-scale solutions and substantial behavioral change.

Today the majority response to the sustainability issues of the fashion sector reflects a technocentric position, which typically comprises the development of more efficient processes, innovation around fiber types, and supply-chain management and recycling initiatives (see, for example, European Commission 2003). Technocentrism promotes sustainability not as a process to transform the sector at root but as a mechanism to modify practices and minimize harm through a technology- and science-led revision of existing ways of doing business. The acceptance of current structures and logic leads to limited questioning of the causes of systemic sustainability challenges, most notably the impact of consumerist materialism. Thus a limitation of the technocentric approach is the possibility that the environmental benefit of "better" products may be lost by their overconsumption, a phenomenon described as the rebound effect. Indeed, the lack of acknowledgment of consumption's effects on sustainability within the sector's environmental and ethical response has helped lead to the framing, in some quarters, of the current state of affairs in fashion and sustainability as oxymoronic (see, for example, Black 2008; Clark 2008)—a critique given added succor by the commercial fashion sector's overt reliance on the trend-induced premature obsolescence of clothing, image, and "the new" as key mechanisms to generate new sales and foster business growth. The source of the tension is the clash between short-term commercial fashion business priorities (including those which use "green" materials and efficient supply chains) and long-term sustainability goals. For those technocentric solutions proposed by the sector are not geared toward a profoundly different order and type of change that is necessary to achieve sustainability. This has proved an enduring challenge. A decade and a half ago Victor Margolin (1998: 86) articulated it as at the crux of the problem: "the proposals for change have been all too modest, and have never come out strongly against the expansion model of economic growth." He goes on, "Design must disengage itself from consumer culture ... [and] participate in projects for the welfare of humankind both inside and outside the market economy."

Yet not all philosophical positions on sustainability are limited to selecting from existing strategies. Ecocentrism operationalizes a different epistemological position, one that involves questioning the current paradigm, system goals, and deep-rooted structures. The result for those working from this position is that systemic challenges, like consumption, are an integrated and essential part of the response of a transformed system, with commercial opportunities emerging from a sustainability-oriented sector. Here the concern is about alternative sustainability-oriented ways of doing and being, some of which already exist within our current understanding, and a raft of roving multidimensional challenges that extend far beyond the traditional boundaries of the fashion sector and include economics, psychology, resource management, and social behavior. This approach, *design for sustainability,* combines global, local, and elementary needs, and ones that address the conservation of the *quality* of natural resources, rather than their *quantity* (van Berkel, Willems, and Lafleur 1997: 64). A focus on quality, not quantity—or effectiveness, not efficiency—is also evident in William McDonough and Michael Braungart's text *Cradle to Cradle* (2002), in which they argue for a restructuring of all industrial activity around two closed loops in order to reorient human systems around sustainability goals.

For authors such as the eminent industrial ecologist John Ehrenfeld (2008), the design writer John Thackara (2005), and the highly respected Ezio Manzini (1994), this distinction is an essential one as the future shape and direction of society are grappled with, involving many systemic challenges and "systemic discontinuities." The ecocentric approach is grounded in systems thinking, where a focus on improving social and ecological quality is an implicit part of the design process and where large-scale improvements are seen to flow most often from examining the rules, goals, and defining logic of a system (Meadows 2010). I have argued elsewhere (Fletcher 2008: 60–73) that insight gained from systems thinking can aid the process of transformation toward

TABLE 26.1 SUMMARY OF DIFFERENCES BETWEEN DESIGN APPROACHES

	TECHNOCENTRIC DESIGN	ECOCENTRIC DESIGN
Starting point	Based on current model	Sees current model as part of the problem
Timeframe	Short-term	Long-term
Target	Quantity	Quality
Scale	Large scale	Small scale
Type of solution	Technological solutions	Sociocultural soutions
Focus	Product or process	Broad systems remit
Effect	Problem-minimizing	Sustainability-creating
Design goal	Redesign of what exists	Giving form to radical alternatives
Keywords	Repair, refine	Rethink, revision

sustainability in the fashion sector. It involves moving from a reductionist approach to tackling sustainability issues (i.e., looking at individual sources of pollution, problematic materials, inefficient processes) to a whole industry-as-system approach. Systems thinking can, for example, help explain why certain types of changes or design approaches are preferred—most commonly those that produce benefits quickly, are felt directly by the innovator, and are already within its sphere of influence. In addition, it shows how, somewhat counterintuitively, this most common approach to driving improvements brings the smallest promise of change:

> A focus on standards or efficiency targets tends to bring the most limited change because it involves only minor adjustments to a product or process. Adjusting numbers may change efficiency ratings, but because these improved ratings are being applied to the same fibres, processed with the same machinery, sold by the same retailers as before, the system does not change much. (Fletcher 2008: 61)

Modeling the fashion sector as a complex system offers an overarching framework for understanding the potential effectiveness of an array of different design approaches with a range of different scales, targets, and time frames. It also provides an effective platform to pull together more recent developments in design thinking from within the ecocentric design perspective: product-service-system design, social innovation for sustainability, co-design, postgrowth design (see, for example, papers from the LeNS conference, in Ceschin, Vezzoli, and Zhang 2010). Table 26.1 provides a summary of differences between the technocentric and ecocentric design approaches.

TERMINOLOGY

Against such a context, a plethora of terminology has emerged that reflects some of the complexities and aspirations of the sustainability challenge. While terms such as *green fashion, ecofashion, ethical fashion,* and *sustainable fashion* are often considered near synonyms, there are subtle differences in meaning that mark an evolution in both theory and practice in design for sustainability in fashion. *Green fashion,* for instance, has an explicitly environmental agenda and often has a single-issue and explicitly product-oriented focus (see, for example, *Green Designed Fashion* [Bierhals 2008]). *Ecofashion* also has a focus on products, though it takes a more integrated approach, working more across the product's life, as typified by Sass Brown's book *Eco Fashion* (2010). *Ethical fashion* often has a dual meaning: as a broad, general, catch-all term for activity in the sustainability arena and as a more specific focus on worker-related issues and animal rights.[2] *Sustainable fashion* or *fashion for sustainability* suggests awareness of systemic influences and complex interdependencies between material and cultural fashion components over the long term. For me, this makes possible the emergence of a working definition of fashion sustainability: that which fosters ecological integrity, social quality, and human flourishing through the products, practices of use, and relationships enabled by fashion. The term, if not this definition, is now in common usage in a wide number of texts: *Sustainable Fashion and Textiles: Design Journeys* (Fletcher 2008), *Sustainable Fashion: Why Now?* (Hethorn and Ulasewicz 2008), *Sustainable Fashion: A Handbook for Educators* (Parker and Dickson 2009), *Shaping Sustainable Fashion* (Gwilt and Rissanen 2011), and *Fashion and Sustainability: Design for Change* (Fletcher and Grose 2012).

HISTORICAL CONTEXT

While design for sustainability has taken on a particular importance at the end of the twentieth and beginning of the twenty-first centuries, it is not only a recent phenomenon. The ideas embodied in design for sustainability were, for example, evident in some of the work of William Morris (Madge 1993: 151). Further, Buckminster Fuller in the 1930s, and Victor Papanek until his death in 1999, explored numerous concepts found today. Although not a designer, Fritz Schumacher in his seminal work *Small Is Beautiful* (1973) helped shape many of the social, structural, and economic arguments that facilitate design for healthy, equitable, and autonomous living. Alistair Fuad Luke (2009: 33–52) provides a detailed survey of the development of design with regard to environmental, technological, market, and political factors from the 1750s to the beginning of the twenty-first century.

The evolution of ideas in the discipline of design for sustainability has paralleled the environmental movement more generally. In the 1970s, when there was a period of sustained focus on the environmental implications of economic growth and development, design for sustainability was similarly characterized by "concern over the consequences of modern economic development and the materialist way of life it had created, in both industrialised and developing countries" (Madge 1993: 156). This focus is perhaps most visible in Papanek's approach to design and the environment, which included elements of environmental value, needs, and equity. His seminal text, *Design for the Real World,* published in Britain in 1972, shook the design establishment with its vocal condemnation of the design world's infatuation with (as he saw it) both superficial styling and useless products. In contrast, Papanek's main remit was to design for a whole range of minority groups in society with special needs—the elderly, children, the short of stature—and together, he argued, these groups amounted to a majority. In many ways Papanek's vision anticipated the meeting of sustainable development and design in that it saw design in a broad social and global context. His last text, *The Green Imperative: Ecology and Ethics in Design and Architecture* (1995), can be seen to reflect many of these themes, such as dwelling, "spiritual" elements of design, decentralized production, and anthropological studies of indigenous peoples and many of their simple and effective design solutions.

THE ROLE OF THE DESIGNER

As described previously, the discipline of design for sustainability has enlarged its scope and field of action over the last two decades. This evolution has opened up a debate about the role of design itself, adding to already ongoing discussions about design's purpose and practices in a changing global world. Benny Banerjee (2008: 3) describes design as currently at an "inflection point," where larger ecological, sociocultural, and economic forces are causing a reexamination of both design's prevalent value systems and the places where design skills are traditionally applied. This can be identified as readily in fashion design as in any other design discipline. From a sustainability perspective, such scrutiny is leading to exploration of the potential emergence of new roles for designers—and new places to apply intuitive, expressive, creative design capacities, outside of the traditional private and product-based routes, and new ways to contribute to the public, social, and ecological good, perhaps as facilitators, intensifiers, and educators (Fletcher and Grose 2012: 154–79). Here it is design thinking, a more strategic, less overtly tactical, incremental view of design that is put forward to help tackle global challenges and that results in differences that engage and value people (Brown 2009).

INTRODUCTION TO DESIGN-FOR-SUSTAINABILITY STRATEGIES

When operating within a strategic role, sustainability can be fully embraced as a complex, multifactorial challenge, where change is leveraged in multiple ways and from many different points of departure. The following sections explore this work with reference to some working examples from the fashion industry. Some of the early work done under the rubric of design for sustainability, while well intentioned, often lacked grounding in hard environmental data in order to validate the assumptions made. Here responses were built around preconceived notions about which activities were considered to be high impact and which were considered ecosystem "friendly." Perhaps the most pervasive example of this was the simplistic assumption, now discredited, that natural fibers are "good" for the environment and synthetic ones "bad." Yet as the field has developed, so has the availability of data on the resource consumption and pollution effects of different fibers, key manufacturing processes, and life-cycle stages, with the effect that decision making is now often supported with tools and matrices based on holistic studies of resource use and pollution effects: life-cycle assessment (LCA). At the time of writing, for example, giant global brands Levi's and Nike had both recently published eco-matrices for key product areas in order to make more transparent—and, they would argue, more rigorous—current production choices from a sustainability perspective (*Eco Textile News* 2010; Nike 2011). While LCA is not an exact science and is itself based on a large number of assumptions and incomplete information (Heiskanen 2002), it has had a profound effect on design-for-sustainability work, most notably by operationalizing the philosophy of holism through the provision of defendable sets of quantitative data.

An LCA can take many forms and is often used more as a screening tool to scope out or identify areas of key impact rather than to generate a global data set for a particular product—often because of the time and cost implications of conducting a full LCA. That being said, some full LCAs have been conducted for fashion products. The earliest and most influential of these was of a polyester blouse, conducted in 1993 on behalf of the American Fiber Manufacturers' Association (a trade body representing synthetic and cellulosic fiber producers; Franklin Associates 1993). The findings show that as much as 82 percent of energy use, 66 percent of solid waste, "over half" of the emissions to air (for carbon dioxide specifically the figure is 83 percent), and "large quantities" of waterborne effluents (96 percent if measured by biological oxygen demand alone) are amassed during the consumer care phase of the blouse's life (i.e., laundering), and that impacts associated with producing the blouse (including polyester manufacture) and disposing of the blouse at the end of its life are small in comparison. At the time it was first published, the study's findings provided valuable political capital to synthetic fiber producers, who were coming under increasing pressure over their environmental performance and were keen to deflect attention away from their core business practices. Yet the study had an alternative, and arguably more constructive, legacy: that of showing that environmental issues stretch beyond the bounds of individual corporations and that the sustainability performance of a product requires joint responses from all those—farmers, producers, manufacturers, retailers, consumers, and disposal organizations—with a stake in a garment's life cycle.

Reflecting this ethos of shared responsibility, strategies have been developed that use design thinking to address impacts that arise in all life-cycle phases. Carolien van Hemel (1998: 30) provides a summary of these as part of her PhD, in which she also developed the Ecodesign Strategy Wheel, a tool to support designers in quickly identifying impacts associated with a product's life and showing the potential benefits of a redesign.

TABLE 26.2 SUMMARY OF DESIGN-FOR-SUSTAINABILITY STRATEGIES

LIFE-CYCLE PHASE	GOAL	STRATEGY
Materials selection	Choose low-impact materials	• Avoid materials that damage human health or ecological health or that deplete resources • Use minimal resources • Use renewable resources • Use waste by-products • Use recycled or reused materials
Production	Optimize manufacturing	• Minimize manufacturing waste • Minimize energy used in production • Minimize number of production methods and operations • Minimize number of components/materials
Distribution	Distribute product efficiently	• Reduce product and packaging weight • Use reusable or recyclable packaging • Use an efficient transport system • Use local production and assembly
Use	Design for low-impact use	• Reduce energy inefficiencies • Reduce water-use inefficiencies • Reduce material-use inefficiencies
	Optimize product lifetime	• Build in user's desire to care for product long term • Design for take-back programs • Build in durability • Design for maintenance and easy repair • Design for upgrades • Design for second life with a different function
End of life	Optimize end of life	• Integrate methods for product collection • Provide for ease of disassembly • Provide for recycling or downcycling • Design for reuse or "next life of product" • Provide for reuse of components • Provide ability to biodegrade • Provide for safe disposal

The *OKALA Ecodesign Guide* (White, Belletire, and St. Pierre 2007: 34) updates van Hemel's strategy wheel, listing strategies for innovation at five phases of the life cycle (see Table 26.2).

In addition to five life cycle–based categories, the Okala publication, like Carolien van Hemel, includes a further set of innovation possibilities, describing opportunities to engage with sustainability that go beyond individual products or product life cycles to include functional innovation, systems change, and redesign of consumer practices, behavior, and even lifestyles. These are listed as follows:

- Rethink how to provide the benefit
- Serve needs provided by associated products
- Anticipate technological change and build in flexibility
- Provide product as service
- Share among more users
- Design to mimic nature
- Use living organisms in product (White, Belletire, and St. Pierre 2007: 34)

The list can, however, be further expanded to include a number of emerging design-for-sustainability themes:

- Co-design
- Design for empathy
- Design for changing sociocultural norms
- Design for localism
- Design for active users
- Design of alternative economic and business models, including postgrowth models and "slow" principles and values
- Design to meet fundamental human needs

In the sections that follow, short working examples will be introduced that highlight innovation from across these themes. In many cases, these possible areas of innovation constitute future practice in this field of study, and while they are often in their embryonic stage of development and are often shaped at the fringes, their future potential is not limited to the edges of fashion-sector activity but can also apply to the mainstream.

CHOOSE LOW-IMPACT MATERIALS

Materials selection is often one of the first areas where fashion brands and designers choose to act in order to promote sustainability. For example, a key part of Esprit's pioneering E-collection in the early 1990s was low-impact materials (Grose 1994). Also starting in the 1990s, ecofashion pioneer Katherine Hamnett politicized fiber selection by releasing a press release with her (PVC-free) collection on the pollution effects caused by PVC, a key trend at the time (Bellos 1995). Since then, and with varying degrees of commitment, most fashion brands have selected low-impact materials for at least some garments in their range. For most materials, information about resource consumption and pollution effects is available, though it is still rarely in a form that allows an easy comparison between different fibers. For some brands like the tiny British label Izzy

Lane,[3] for example, fibers (specifically wool fibers) are the focus of its business model, and in particular the pursuit of ethical husbandry practices associated with raising sheep. Here the pursuit of best practice for a given fiber has led a designer to diversify into farming and producing raw material with the desired ethics and provenance. Other design brands too have reached upstream from the studio into fiber production. The Danish label Noir,[4] for example, has established an organic cotton farm in Uganda in order to supply its own fiber needs and establish a model for other fashion businesses. Within specific fiber categories, there are now quite well-established protocols of best practice, some of which includes fully certified status such as fair trade or organic (see, for example, Fletcher 2008). When selecting from a wide palette of materials, the choices are more complex, with trade-offs between key resources commonplace. For example, those fibers that are most energy-intensive (typically synthetic fibers) have low demands for water. Conversely, those fibers that draw on little energy in cultivation and extraction are often extremely water-intensive to produce (cotton being the obvious example). Brands such as the British retailer Marks & Spencer[5] respond to these challenges by drawing up commitments to use minimum volumes of preferred materials, including recycled polyester, organic wool, linen, and fair trade cotton.

OPTIMIZE MANUFACTURING

Manufacturing decisions in a global sector like fashion are notoriously difficult to control from a sustainability perspective because of the complexity of the supply chain and the disparities between processing machinery, chemical compounds, pollution-treatment facilities, labor practices, and so on at different producing factories. In an attempt to overcome these challenges, Nike, the U.S.-based global sports and footwear brand, once vilified for its unethical production practices, has been working to optimize manufacturing decisions taken by designers using the Environmental Apparel Design Tool (Nike 2011)—an updated version of its Nike Considered Index that also includes processing decisions. The tool serves as a functional calculator with the ability to measure the impact of materials and processing routes commonly used in manufacturing apparel products and adds category points together in a range from "best" to "needs improvement" in order to support design decision making. In the manufacture phase, the "best" category is reserved for those pieces with no garment treatments; "better" for those with basic wash, reduced-water wash, silicone wash, "eco ball," or enzyme wash/bio polish; "good" for items processed with bleach, lasers, ozone wash, or mechanical distress; and "needs improvement" for those garments with pumice/stone wash, resin garment treatment, enzyme wash with stones, chemical wash with stones, acid or chemical wash or spray, or potassium permanganate in stone wash or spray. Nike has published its tool on its website for review in a move that is reflective of a bigger trend toward transparency throughout the industry supply chain and is an active player in the Sustainable Apparel Coalition, which is working to develop a precompetitive common approach for measuring and evaluating fiber and fabric efficiency and improve supply-chain performance industry-wide.[6]

OPTIMIZE PRODUCT LIFETIME

Developing garments for a satisfying and long period of use is a resource-efficient design strategy of which durability—and in particular emotional durability (Chapman 2005)—is a key component. Building a nuanced understanding of the multiple, interrelated, and personal factors that trigger sustained use (rather than just storage) of fashion clothes is an ongoing challenge for work in this field, which is clearly influenced by the economic logic of fashion commerce as much as by individual behavior. In a recent eponymous project, 132 5. Issey Miyake, the pioneering Japanese fashion designer has developed a collection that responds to a number of sustainability themes including optimized lifetimes.[7] The pieces, inspired by the Japanese tradition of origami and produced in materials including recycled polyester, fold flat into geometric forms. When unfolded, they become multifaceted tubes that can be recreated in different garment configurations. This adaptability, promoted through a system of press stud attachments at key points, allows the wearer to adjust or change the shape of the garment from a cocktail dress to a long skirt, with temporary seams or darts, arguably providing the wearer more opportunities to wear the piece and so optimize the resources embodied therein. The logic is simple: a garment worn twice as often has half the environmental impact per wearing.

OPTIMIZE END OF LIFE

In a conventional model of fashion design, a designer and brand's interest in a garment stops at the shop doors of the retail space. Life-cycle thinking expands this model, and the fate of a garment during its use, at the end of its life, and in its future reuse, becomes a key part of the design strategy. It is certainly the case that some end-of-life design strategies, like recycling, are widely known and advocated within fashion-sector circles, yet this is rarely done with an integrated framework where the ease and effectiveness of eventual recycling and materials reuse are an initial design concept priority. A body of work known as design for recycling has been developed in other disciplines, notably industrial design, to establish guidelines and priorities for good practice in this area. While design for recycling principles have been translated into a fashion and textile context (see Fletcher 2008: 106), take-up appears to be limited to the outdoor sportswear segment, with most high-street and high-end fashion brands preferring to leave reuse and recycling of their clothes to third parties like charities and local authorities. This is likely for a number of reasons, not least the perceived low value of used clothes and the high volumes involved—two factors that, when combined, are rarely seen as a positive resource by these corporations. By contrast, for technical outdoor sportswear producers, which have strong brand connections to nature, and by association to natural system properties like loops and cycles, returned used garments are a visible means of "closing a loop" and gaining new (used) raw material to work into other products. The Swedish brand Klättermusen,[8] for example, facilitates its recycling program rECOver through financial incentives based on a deposit scheme, levied on all products at the point of purchase. Customers who return used products get back their deposit, ranging from €1 to €20, depending on the article. Klättermusen currently makes new pants and backpacks from heavily worn returned pieces; for those returned products that are less worn, it repairs some pieces and donates them to charity.

CO-DESIGN

Design initiatives that seek to promote sustainability through transformation of fashion industry practices work with a changed set of rules and goals shaping their activity. One example of this is co-design. For those working with ideas of co-design (design with others), the business model is shaped fundamentally by the goal of collaboratively designing products together with the people who will use them. Co-design principles of inclusiveness, cooperative processes, and participative action work to disrupt hierarchical power relations (as exemplified in most fashion brands) and offer users of clothes more control over their garments' design and production (von Busch 2008). Fundamentally, co-design contests the economic growth–driven logic of most fashion activities today and sits at the fringes of fashion activity, offering a small-scale, human, and skill-centered response to conventional fashion practice. One example is Antiform,[9] which works within the Hyde Park community in Leeds, United Kingdom, to create fashion cooperatively. Tapping into some preexisting sewing, repair, craft, and embellishment skills, and offering training where skills are in short supply, Antiform has facilitated the creation of an eight-piece collection, made by sixty-four local people (beaders, knitters, artists, seamstresses, and volunteers) sold in the local districts of Leeds. All materials for the collection are waste clothing gathered in the area from free monthly exchange events that bring an influx of materials and people into the project. The symbiotic relationship between the resulting collection and the materials exchange is key to the project's development, allowing local residents to get involved in many different levels of the project, creating a new system for local fashion.

POSTGROWTH DESIGN

Like principles of co-design, postgrowth design activities challenge at a root level the priorities and values of existing industry structure and goals. Postgrowth ideas, first developed thirty years ago in a branch of economics known as ecological economics—perhaps most notably by Herman Daly (1992)—offer an alternative to the predominant economic model, which is structurally reliant on economic growth tied to expanding resource use: on making and selling increasingly more units to improve market share, increase profit, and stay in business. The response from Daly, among others (see, for example, Jackson 2009), is to reimagine an overarching economic logic that works within planetary limits and looks for ways to add value, meet needs, and provide employment without constantly expanding material throughput. One project that is exploring these ideas is Local Wisdom,[10] an action research fashion project that explores the "craft of use" associated with garments as one mechanism to enhance people's fashion experiences within the limits of the clothes they already have. It does this by gathering images and object histories associated with tending and using clothes and transforming these into a body of design inspiration and work that cumulatively constitutes a platform of "next practice" in fashion created from a starting point of qualitative development rather than growth in material throughput (Fletcher 2011).

CONCLUSIONS

Design for sustainability has greatly enlarged its range and field of action over the last twenty years. During this time its attention has shifted from technical material, processing, and environment-based issues to a broader, more sociocultural remit—a shift that has occurred in fashion design as in other disciplines. Parallel to this change is a shift in perspectives about the role of design and the potential of design thinking, reflecting the fact that sustainability issues extend beyond strict disciplinary boundaries and draw on many other areas of study, including, among others, economics, future studies, environmental science, psychology, and ecology. This expanding role has also led to design and design thinking being employed in places and contexts far outside design's traditional territory, opening up opportunities for designers to operate not just as shapers of material goods for the traditional marketplace but also as creators of new business models, ways of behavior, and social priorities that are based on sustainability values. While many of the design-for-sustainability ideas and strategies reviewed in this chapter did not originate in fashion, the fashion sector has employed many of them to good environmental and ethical effect, with projects, companies, or individuals working in most, if not all, of the areas highlighted in these pages. The sustainability challenges for the fashion industry are arguably little different than for most other sectors: a combination of material and supply-chain issues and deeper, systemic challenges linked to the goals and priorities of the sector. These are, however, perhaps exaggerated in fashion because of the short-lived nature of many fashion products due to trend-induced perceived (not actual) obsolescence and the globalized international division of labor that has led to lowering production costs and garment prices in recent years; this, together with a rise in consumptive materialism, has led to increasing levels of consumption. Yet in spite of these difficulties, whatever the sustainability achievements that are secured in fashion, they will be disseminated widely, for the currency of fashion is global and as such fashion has significant potential to lead the transformation toward sustainability.

NOTES

1. Fashioning an Ethical Industry, http://www.fashioninganethicalindustry.org/home/ (accessed January 7, 2011).
2. Ibid.
3. Izzylane, http://www.izzylane.com/ (accessed January 7, 2011).
4. Noir, http://www.noir.dk/ (accessed May 13, 2013).
5. "Plan A: Doing the Right Thing," Marks & Spencer, http://plana.marksandspencer.com/ (accessed January 7, 2011).
6. Sustainable Apparel Coalition, http://www.apparelcoalition.org/ (accessed November 2, 2011).
7. 132 5. ISSEY MIYAKE, Issey Miyake website, 2010, http://www.isseymiyake.com/en/brands/132_5.html (accessed January 5, 2011).
8. Klättermusen, http://www.klattermusen.se/start_EN.php?lang=EN&curr=EUR (accessed January 7, 2011).
9. Antiform, http://www.antiformonline.co.uk/ (accessed January 7, 2011).
10. Local Wisdom, http://www.localwisdom.info/ (accessed January 7, 2011).

BIBLIOGRAPHY

Banerjee, Benny. 2008. "Designer as Agent of Change: A Vision for Catalyzing Rapid Change." In Carla Cipolla and Pier Paolo Peruccio (eds.), Proceedings of Changing the Change Design, Visions, Proposals and Tools Conference, July 10–12, Turin, Italy, 192–205.

Bellos, Alex. 1995. "Queen of Shock Who Makes Sure Her Designs Keep Their Street Cred." *The Guardian,* September 23, p. 5.

Bierhals, Christine Anna. 2008. *Green Designed Fashion.* Stuttgart, Germany: Fusion.

Black, Sandy. 2008. *Eco Chic: The Fashion Paradox.* London: Black Dog.

Brown, Sass. 2010. *Eco Fashion.* London: Laurence King.

Brown, Tim. 2009. *Change by Design.* New York: Harper Collins.

Ceschin, Fabrizio, Carlo Vezzoli, and Jun Zhang (eds.). 2010. *Sustainability in Design: Now! Challenges and Opportunities for Design Research, Education and Practice in the XXI Century,* LeNS conference proceedings, Bangalore India, September. Sheffield, UK: Greenleaf.

Chapman, Jonathan. 2005. *Emotionally Durable Design: Objects, Experiences, Empathy.* London: Earthscan.

Clark, Hazel. 2008. "SLOW + FASHION—an Oxymoron—or a Promise for the Future…?" *Fashion Theory: The Journal of Dress, Body and Culture* 12 (4): 427–46.

Daly, Herman. 1992. *Steady-State Economics.* 2nd ed. London: Earthscan.

EcoTextile News. 2010. "Jean Therapy." 38 (October): 26–27.

Ehrenfeld, John A. 2008. *Sustainability by Design.* New Haven, CT: Yale University Press.

Ehrlich, Paul, and Anne Ehrlich. 1990. *The Population Explosion.* London: Hutchinson.

European Commission. 2003. *Integrated Pollution Prevention and Control: Reference Document on Best Available Techniques for the Textiles Industry.* Brussels: European Commission.

Fletcher, Kate. 2008. *Sustainable Fashion and Textiles: Design Journeys.* London: Earthscan.

Fletcher, Kate. 2011. "Post Growth Fashion and the Craft of Users." In Alison Gwilt and Timo Rissannen (eds.), *Shaping Sustainable Fashion,* 165–75. London: Earthscan.

Fletcher, Kate, and Lynda Grose. 2012. *Fashion and Sustainability: Design for Change.* London: Laurence King.

Franklin Associates. 1993. *Resource and Environmental Profile Analysis of a Manufactured Apparel Product: Woman's Knit Polyester Blouse.* Washington, DC: American Fiber Manufacturers Association.

Fuad Luke, Alistair. 2009. *Design Activism.* London: Earthscan.

Graedel, T. E., P. Reaves Comrie, and J. C. Sekutowski. 1995. "Green Product Design." *AT&T Technical Journal* (November/December): 18–25.

Grose, Lynda. 1994. "Incorporating Environmental Objectives through the Design Process and through Business." In *Globalization—Technological, Economic and Environmental Imperatives, 75th World Conference of the Textile Institute, Textile Institute, Manchester,* 77–81. Manchester: Textile Institute.

Gwilt, Alison, and Timo Rissanen. 2011. *Shaping Sustainable Fashion.* London: Earthscan.

Heiskanen, Eva. 2002. "The Institutional Logic of Lifecycle Thinking." *Journal of Cleaner Production* 10: 427–37.

Hethorn, Janet, and Connie Ulasewicz. 2008. *Sustainable Fashion: Why Now? A Conversation Exploring Issues, Practices, and Possibilities.* New York: Fairchild Books.

Jackson, Tim. 2009. *Prosperity without Growth.* London: Sustainable Development Commission.

Keoleian, Gregory A., and Dan Menerey. 1994. "Sustainable Development by Design: Review of Lifecycle Design and Related Approaches." *Air and Waste* 44 (May): 645–68.

Madge, Pauline. 1993. "Design, Ecology, Technology: A Historiographical Review." *Journal of Design History* 6 (3): 149–66.

Manzini, Ezio. 1994. "Design, Environment and Social Quality: From 'Existenzminimum' to 'Quality Maximum.'" *Design Issues* 10 (1): 37–43.

Margolin, Victor. 1998. "Design for a Sustainable World." *Design Issues* 14 (2): 83–92.

McDonough, William, and Michael Braungart. 2002. *Cradle to Cradle: Remaking the Way We Make Things.* New York: North Point.

Meadows, Donella H. 2010. *Thinking in Systems: A Primer.* London: Earthscan.

Meadows, Donella H., Dennis L. Meadows, Jørgen Randers, and William Behrens. 1972. *The Limits to Growth.* London: Earth Island.

Nike. 2011. "Environmental Apparel Design Tool." http://www.nikebiz.com/responsibility/nikeenvironmentaldesigntool (accessed January 5, 2011).

Papanek, Victor. 1972. *Design for the Real World.* London: Thames and Hudson.

Papanek, Victor. 1995. *The Green Imperative: Ecology and Ethics in Design and Architecture.* London: Thames and Hudson.

Parker, Liz, and Marsha A. Dickson (eds.). 2009. *Sustainable Fashion: A Handbook for Educators.* Bristol, UK: Labour Behind the Label.

Pepper, David. 1996. *Modern Environmentalism: An Introduction.* London: Routledge.

Schumacher, Ernest F. 1972. *Small Is Beautiful.* London: Abacus.

Simon, Matthew. 1994. "Sustainable Product Design Workshop." Paper presented at Design for Environment and Implementation of Environmental Aspects in Product Design, BWI, Zurich, November.

Steffan, Alex (ed.). 2008. *World Changing: A User's Guide for the Twenty First Century.* New York: Abrams.

Thackara, John. 2005. *In the Bubble: Designing in a Complex World.* Cambridge, MA: MIT Press.

Tham, Mathilda. 2008. "Lucky People Forecast: A Systemic Futures Perspective on Fashion and Sustainability." PhD diss., Goldsmiths, University of London.
Thorpe, Ann. 2007. *The Designer's Atlas to Sustainability.* Washington, DC: Island Press.
van Berkel, Rene, Ester Willems, and Marije Lafleur. 1997. "The Relationship between Cleaner Production and Industrial Ecology." *Journal of Industrial Ecology* 1 (1): 51–65.
Van der Ryn, Sim, and Stuart Cowan. 1996. *Ecological Design.* Washington, DC: Island Press.
van Hemel, Carolien G. 1998. "Ecodesign Empirically Explored: Design for Environment in Dutch Small and Medium Sized Enterprises." PhD diss., Delft University of Technology.
Vinken, Barbara. 2005. *Fashion Zeitgeist: Trends and Cycles in the Fashion System.* Oxford: Berg.
von Busch, Otto. 2008. *FASHION-able: Hactivism and Engaged Fashion Design.* Gothenburg: Art Monitor.
Walker, Stuart. 2006. *Sustainable by Design: Explorations in Theory and Practice.* London: Earthscan.
Walker, Stuart, and Ralf Nielson. 1998. "Systemic Shift: Sustainable Development and Industrial Design Methodology." *Journal of Sustainable Product Design* 4: 7–17.
World Commission on Environment and Development (WCED). 1987. *Our Common Future.* Oxford: Oxford University Press.
Weizsäcker, Ernest, Amory B. Lovins, and L. Hunter Lovins. 1997. *Factor Four: Doubling Wealth, Halving Resources.* London: Earthscan.
White, Philip, Steve Belletire, and Louise St. Pierre. 2007. *OKALA Ecodesign Guide.* Phoenix, AZ: Industrial Designers Society of America.

27

Fashion and the Design of Prosperity: A Discussion of Alternative Business Models

SIMONETTA CARBONARO AND DAVID GOLDSMITH

INTRODUCTION

Although "business as usual," that is, business practices that prioritize short-term financial profit above long-term sustainability, is clearly still the overwhelmingly dominant mode of global operation, there are also signs that innovative business models and social initiatives are in some cases improving the way we clothe, feed, and shelter ourselves and may even indicate an evolutionary change toward more cooperative business models, more empathic social relationships, and more sustainable ways of living. Indicators of this change may be seen, for example, in the aims of the transition movement to live within local biocapacities[1] or the many thousands of grassroots groups and organizations that are springing up across the world that are devoted to improving environmental and social circumstances[2] and, within the fashion realm, the initiative of leading global brands to work together toward more sustainable production methods.[3]

The environmental and social problems caused by current mainstream fashion systems and habits are well known (Allwood et al. 2006; Cline 2012; Hoffman 2007; Ross 2004; Shell 2009; Siegle 2011). Optimists may hold the belief that humanity is already beginning to respond creatively to the profound pressures we face. If it is true that we are on the verge of transformation, it is also true that we can expect radical shifts in the way we make, wear, and assign meaning to our clothing. In fact, there may be opportunities for fashion (considered here not just a commodity for consumption but also a symbol of individual and societal values) to not only contribute to the remodeling of our world but also lead the way toward better lives of real prosperity. Fashion, or, more broadly, dress, has this opportunity because it is a universal need that, similar to food, is a constant private and public reminder and representation of individual and cultural identity. Further, fashion is a cultural and creative force that is highly competent in the areas of communication and change; it is imaginable that this intrinsic competence can be directed toward sustainable goals.

Indeed, alternative fashion practices have already been documented in books such as Sandy Black's *Eco-chic: The Fashion Paradox* (2008) and *The Sustainable Fashion Handbook* (2012), Kate Fletcher's *Sustainable Fashion and Textiles: Design Journeys* (2008), Sass Brown's *Eco-fashion* (2010), and Kate Fletcher and Lynda Grose's *Fashion and Sustainability: Design for Change* (2012). These new modes are also seen in the growing number of exhibitions of sustainably oriented fashion practices, an early example being Well Fashioned: Eco Style in the UK (Crafts Council, 2006). Another exhibition, Eco-fashion: Going Green (2010) at the Museum at the Fashion Institute of Technology in New York City, used six categorizing themes connected with environmental, social, economic, or cultural impacts.

Whether garments are made using large-scale global industrial systems or small-scale local artisanal methods is a crucial way of considering sustainability and fashion. By far the dominant means of manufacturing fashion today is the industrial globalized model. It is well described in Grace Kunz and Myrna Garner's (2011) *Going Global: The Textile and Apparel Industry* and evidenced in Pietra Rivoli's (2005) *The Travels of a T-Shirt in the Global Economy: An Economist Examines the Markets, Power and Politics of World Trade,* Rachel Snyder's (2007) *Fugitive Denim: A Moving Story of People and Pants in the Borderless World of Global Trade,* and Kelsey Timmerman's (2009) *Where Am I Wearing? A Global Tour to the Countries, Factories, and People That Make Our Clothes.* Alternatively, craft-based apparel production that is carried out at home or in small, sometimes cooperative enterprises is not nearly so well understood as the large-scale model, especially as it may relate to economic and social change (Littrell and Dickson 2010: 11). These two models are considered here in the context of two production sites in India.

This chapter diverges from standard academic format in several ways. The conversational format replicates the ongoing communication between the two authors, business consultant and design management professor Simonetta Carbonaro and textile designer and PhD candidate David Goldsmith, in ways that parallel their working methods as practitioners and social researchers, advisor and advised. They have at times written broadly, keeping in mind the etymology of the word *university* (the whole, the aggregate) and acknowledging that the issues raised here relate to the whole of human experience. Even if, after several years of collaboration connected with the Design of Prosperity initiative,[4] the authors are largely in agreement with one another, they have chosen to leave their respective voices apparent to give an indication of their different perspectives as they together explore possible solutions to the paradox (Black 2008) of "sustainable fashion."

The pages that follow start with some of the broad socioeconomic circumstances that situate the notion of sustainable fashion. Next, the role design has in creating prosperity is presented, and cases are discussed. Finally, it is proposed that fashion, a practice that has always dealt with beauty and sociocultural transformation, can lead the movement toward better lives.

MASS-MARKET VALUE CHAINS AND THE WONDERLAND ECONOMY

David Goldsmith: It is increasingly common to hear, and with good reason, that high-consumption cultures, epitomized by the United States, where the ecological footprint per capita is about fourteen times greater than in India (Global Footprint Network 2012), must transition to new ways of living if there is to be any chance of creating long-term sustainability.

The quantity of fashion offerings in the world market is staggering and has increased dramatically in terms of pace and volume over the past decades. Ethical living campaigner and journalist Lucy Siegle cites a fourfold increase since 1980 in the number of garments acquired yearly in the United Kingdom (Textrends.org, cited in Siegle 2011: 3). Swedish retailer Gina Tricot's spring 2011 advertising slogan "New Fashion Everyday" unabashedly illustrates the phenomenon that Siegle describes. Unfortunately, such "new fashion" on any given day is not meaningfully different from what it was the day before or what it will be the day after. A customer in this circumstance has what I call *faux choix*: she is free to choose between this, that, or the other cheaply produced mass-market product, none of which differs markedly from the rest. Whatever the reasons people embrace mass-market fashion (see Teri Agins's *The End of Fashion* [2000] and Yuniya Kawamura's *Fashion-ology* [2005] for the sociological and marketing-driven underpinnings of the fashion industry), this behavior now seems grotesquely out of alignment with the kind of careful and conscious consumption that would make sense given our planetary and social problems.

Simonetta Carbonaro: Indeed, Lizabeth Cohen (2004), Juliet Schor (2005), Richard Sennett (2006), Raj Patel (2009), and especially Benjamin Barber in his *Consumed: How Markets Corrupt Children, Infantilize Adults, and Swallow Citizens Whole* (2007), all contend that consumption as it exists today in the high-income saturated markets has become a kind of involuntary servitude. The flood of essentially similar cheap products, poor in design and quality but overloaded with marketing-driven "symbolic" signs and images, is one of the main reasons why some consumers in countries with historically high rates of consumption are becoming reluctant to buy. After decades of dealing with the fast fashion dynamic that pushes them toward rapidly taking up and rapidly rejecting branded fashionable products that are overcharged with equally rapidly changing status symbol values, consumers are beginning to experience a loss of appetite for shopping and partaking in excessive material consumption. Reduced consumption is embedded in many of the alternative fashion practices seen today, and specifically indicated in social expressions such as the voluntary simplicity movement, the proliferation of and second life ateliers, the swapping movement, the Church of Stop Shopping, and the one-dress-for-one-year Uniform Project.[5] Conforming to the fast fashion rhythm has become not only a financially challenge in times of economic downturn but also a fatiguing, frustrating, and time-consuming process (Carbonaro and Votava 2009, 2010). This is part of the reason why, for example, in the United States, expenditures on apparel have fallen over the past decades, from 7 percent of consumers' overall spending in the 1970s to 3.3 percent in 2011 (Apparel Strategist 2011).

This puts the system of industrial mass consumption in trouble because when supply overcomes demand, as has been happening especially in the oversaturated markets, the industrial system paradoxically transforms itself into a tremendously inefficient and therefore unsustainable system. When offer exceeds demand, each one of the actors of such a growth-based economic system—brands, suppliers, retailers, consumers—try to countermeasure the deficit (in sales or real income) by raising their own efficiency. This drives the vicious cycle of price erosion and reduction of unit costs evident in the fast fashion sector. It also forces industry to consolidate in order to generate even larger-scale impacts through more and more standardization and the development of a constant flow of always "new" product variants, as promoted by the Gina Tricot advertising slogan mentioned previously, to counterbalance the general price decline. This dynamic also fosters the development of myriad novelties dependent on what could be called *marketing-driven design,* whose purpose is merely to cosmetically embellish so-called new products so that they in turn can serve as mere vehicles for extravagant investments in marketing (Carbonaro and Votava 2010). In a system that is reliant on hyperconsumption of short-lived products, there is a low quota of products of real innovation. Furthermore, consumers have little chance to perceive the intrinsic material quality of the thousands and thousands of new products, nor to realize what might be true differences in products. If differences still exist, they are lost in an avalanche of marketing-driven design and messages, which load products with persuasive emotional narratives rather than with any truly design-driven "meaning" (Verganti 2008). As a result, consumers just go for the cheapest offer. By doing so, prices are kept low, which keeps consumption, the prime enemy of sustainability, high (Cline 2012; Shell 2009; Siegle 2011). As a business consultant and professor of design management and humanistic marketing, I advise my clients and students to respond to current ethical (and therefore aesthetic and economic) imperatives (Guillet de Monthoux 2004). This means shifting to consumption models that reduce the volume of products loaded with marketing-driven added values and instead increase the percentage of products with real value and meanings linked to the "aesth-ethics" of more sustainable ways of life.

DG: This growth-based consumption economy, which you call the "Wonderland Economy" (Carbonaro 2013) because the material abundance it produces leads to a sense of wonderment (if not intoxication), has developed over two centuries of industrial and technological revolutions and socioeconomic shifts. It is the reason that so many people have such an unprecedented abundance of material possessions or, as eminent anthropologist Daniel Miller (2010) calls it, "stuff." But this form of living seems to be losing relevance as humanity begins to deal with unprecedented phenomena such as the trespassing of the "Planetary Boundaries" (Rockström and Klum 2012), and the compression of time and space that are part of the impending social conditions that Manfred Steger (2009) calls "globality."[6] A long list of economists and social scientists, including Ernst Friedrich Schumacher (1973), Herman Daly (1991), Richard Sennett (2006), Joseph Stiglitz, Amartya Sen, and Jean-Paul Fitoussi (2009), Tim Jackson (2009), Dan O'Neill, Rob Dietz, and Nigel Jones (2010), and Paul Hawken (2010), Serge Latouche (2010), have proposed slow-growing, more locally oriented economic systems as alternatives to the current model. They argue that the global growth-based system is failing because it recklessly exploits the limited resources and biodiversity of earth that allow us to live yet does not do a good enough job of providing adequate human-centered benefits, such as health, education, political voice, or a flourishing natural environment. In the fashion realm, Kate Fletcher, in "Slow Fashion: An Invitation to Systems Change" (2010), conceptualizes how a slow fashion system, as compared to the growth-based fashion industry, would be based on a more holistic human-centered evaluation of costs and benefits.

SC: Slowing down our systems is essential. Time and physical space are two dimensions that ought to occupy a central position in our thinking about sustainability because they are also nonrenewable resources. They should thus be handled with care and be integral components of deliberations on our economic, environmental, social, and especially *cultural* growth. Even if, on a purely theoretical basis, the unlimited growth model could, with the help of "silver bullet" technologies (of which there are none on the horizon), create a "cradle-to-cradle" (McDonough and Braungart 2002) eco-efficient sustainable goods industry, this would reveal itself as an empty myth (Welford 1997). The concept of today's eco-modernism is based on a simplistic principle of "producing more with less" (Schmidheiny 1992), with little regard for the need to design an ecology of the mind and spirit that would cultivate the ability to see alternatives to the Wonderland Economy. According to the findings of Nobel laureate psychologist Daniel Kahneman, we are currently in transition from an economy of material wealth to an economy in search of happiness (Kahneman, Deiner, and Schwarz 2003; Kahneman and Krueger 2006). In such a real-world economy, high value is assigned to those immaterial "goods" that cannot be exchanged, reproduced, or replaced—for example, security, peace, friendship, forthrightness, culture, knowledge, or simply time. Similarly, environmental scholar John Ehrenfeld (2008), building on eminent psychologist Erich Fromm's work, talks about two modes of human experience: having and being. What counts in the being model is that which is physically intangible: our convictions and values. Today there is more validity than ever in the early twentieth-century social scientist Max Weber's insight ([1914] 1978) that consumption is a process of life *choices*—not just life*styles*—linked to one's own values system. A paradigm shift from a society of having to one of being would mean a cultural and social transformation that would necessarily also transform, with luck, the basis of our economy.

THE DESIGN OF PROSPERITY

DG: Since industrialization began, there have been arguments against orienting society around industrial efficiency (Jevons 1866; Polimeni et al. 2009; Sale 1995). In 1933 the influential economist John Maynard Keynes wrote,

> The decadent international but individualistic capitalism, in the hands of which we found ourselves after the war, is not a success. It is not intelligent, it is not beautiful, it is not just, it is not virtuous—and it doesn't deliver the goods. In short we dislike it, and we are beginning to despise it. But when we wonder what to put in its place, we are extremely perplexed. (1933: 755–69)

Even if the perplexity continues to this day, urgent calls are being heard for the reconstruction of our economic foundations so that they assume the limits and value of natural capital, expect wealth equity, and integrate human development (Bello 2004; Berry 2010; Meadows, Randers, and Meadows 2004; O'Neill Dietz, and Jones 2010; Singer 2004). In the design world there has been a tremendous wave of awareness and interest in using design as a tool for improving life on earth. David Wann (1996); Victor Papanek (2005); Cameron Sinclair, Kate Stohr, and Cynthia Barton (2006); John Thackara (2006); Cynthia Smith (2007); Tim Brown (2009); Clive Dilnot (2009); Roberto Verganti (2009); and Carlo Arnaldo Vezzoli and Ezio Manzini (2010) are some of the leaders of the discourse asserting that design that ignores the conservation of natural resources and human well-being cannot any longer be properly thought of as design. Looking back over the past century, it might be useful to consider three design dictums. "Form follows function," attributed to the early twentieth-century architect Louis Sullivan and embraced by numerous modernist designers (Woodham 1997), described a design ethos in which the revelation of the practical use of industrially produced goods was paramount. A postmodernist adage, "form follows fiction," is associated with the sort of whimsical products, such as home products company Alessi's corkscrews, that embed a narrative, cartoon-like dimension in their physical form. I have proposed "form follows faction," which names the existing design ethos (Papanek 2005; Pilloton 2009; Sinclair, Stohr, and Barton 2006; Smith 2007) that is founded on a sociopolitical commitment and seeks to create products, services, and systems that above all else aim to improve the quality of life on our planet.

SC: Surely, the most important task for designers today is to prefigure ways of thinking, ways of living, and ways to express this, both materially and immaterially, that help humanity achieve the growth of culture, that is, the human dimensions of education, the arts, science, knowledge, craftsmanship, experience, and, last but not least, wisdom. As far as this concerns the fashion industry, it will mean a fundamental reorientation from an industry that (like others) has situated the environment and human needs within its economic structure, to one that instead situates its economic structure within the realm of planetary resiliency and human needs. By understanding and recognizing ecological biophysical and the *immanent* and *intrinsic* value of these matters, capitalism, along with fashion as a component of the market, could transcend itself (Ruffolo 2008). By decoupling capitalism from its dependence on so-called *added value* (the trickery that keeps the consumption machine cycling), we may be able to find a way out of the perplexity of capitalism that Keynes describes. If so, capitalism, in a more reasonable form, could probably exist for many centuries more, because it would enter a phase based not primarily on consumption but on real human needs and culture. Such a culture-based economy is the only kind of economy that could allow for unlimited growth and prosperity. In short, the main role of design today is not to help with the consumption of material goods but to create a viable—and beautiful—future. That is the core idea behind the Design of Prosperity initiative.

FASHION DESIGN AS RADICAL ACTION

DG: What the Design of Prosperity proposes in some ways seems like a far-fetched vision.

SC: It is a radical vision, but one that is shared by many people in all kinds of enterprises, academic disciplines, and research institutes. For example, the Swedish Foundation for Environmental Research (MISTRA) in 2010 awarded a €4.5 million grant for interdisciplinary research that aims to position fashion as an agent for leading society toward a more sustainable future (Cato 2010: 5). It is already clear that fashion designers can simultaneously be sensitive seismographs of cultural activity, accelerators of long-term social trends, and drivers of cultural transformation. The task in hand is to harness the creative power of fashion to nudge society, as it has done in the past, in a new direction. Take, for example, the impacts made by Vivienne Westwood's rebellious sartorial stand against the British bourgeoisie (Bolton and Koda 2007; Wilcox 2005) or Giorgio Armani's provision of a strong new silhouette for women to participate in the male-dominated working world (Celant and Koda 2000; Whiteside and White 2002).

DG: One could reach farther back in time to Gandhi's celebrated calls in the 1930s and 1940s (see Joshi 2002: 3) for Indians to produce their own homespun, handwoven cloth, or *khadi*. It was a successful campaign in terms of symbolism, and together with a boycott of British textile goods, it gave economic leverage to India's fight for national independence (Bean 1989; McGowan 2009; Ramagundam 2008; Roy 1993).

SC: These kinds of careful reconsideration of meaning and modes of production are also being embraced by many contemporary fashion designers working to move beyond "business as usual" and standardized aesthetics. We see this, for example, in labels like Sweden's Dream and Awake by Amanda Ericsson and the UK-based Junky Styling (Figure 27.1), a label founded by self-taught designers Annika Sanders and Kerry Seager in 1997. Both brands play with the symbolic and material

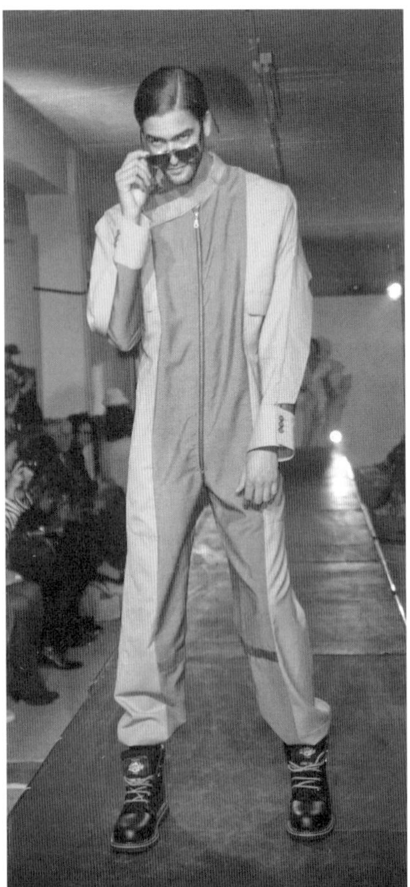

FIGURE 27.1 Junky Styling jumpsuit from the 2012 Junky Air collection inspired by air and the notion of elevation. Repurposed from two men's suits.
Credit: Photograph by Ben James.

value of recycled clothing and share an aesthetic playfulness with experimental designer Martin Margiela, who has created intellectually provocative fashion such as

> skirts made out of the kind of scarves that can be collected at a flea market; clothes made out of old clothes which have been taken apart and then put back together again; pullovers made out of old stockings, in which the heels model the breasts and the elbows. (Vinken 2005: 143)

DG: In the United States, Alabama Chanin, the fashion and home furnishings cottage industry started by fashion designer Natalie Chanin in the small city of Florence, Alabama, utilizes the quilting and embroidery skills of "former factory workers, retired teachers, widows, housewives, and secretaries" living in the area (Fletcher 2008: 144). These relatively expensive garments, all of which are hand-stitched and some of which are hand-dyed using locally grown indigo, have been widely admired, and the business model is looked at as an example of an alternative way to create compelling, therefore more sustainable, fashion (Clark 2008; Reiley and DeLong 2011; Figure 27.2).

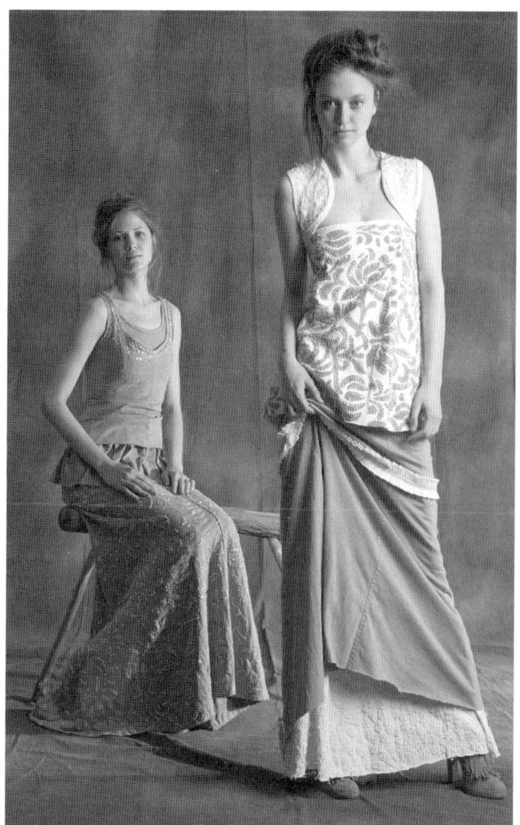

FIGURE 27.2 Alabama Chanin garments, hand-appliquéd and embroidered by women living in the vicinity of Florence, Alabama, United States, 2012.
Credit: Photograph by Peter Stanglmayr.

SC: Small handcraft-based fashion labels have the freedom to create aesthetically extreme and emotionally provocatively experimental garments, and are critical catalysts for change, but we should not forget that the large-scale industrial structure of the fashion sector has a profound capacity for encouraging widespread transformation. Large-scale impacts are achievable through large-scale industrial processes, such as the recycling of polyester or the creation of global scientific safety standards. Let us now discuss two polar opposite cases that we are familiar with and that happen to be within a short geographic distance of one another in central India.

VESTO COME PENSO AND GUDI MUDI

SC: The first case is the apparel collection designed by sustainable fashion pioneer Katherine Hamnett for Coop Italia, called Vesto Come Penso, "I Dress as I Think," launched in spring 2012. Coop (the Italian abbreviation for a consumers' cooperative model of business) is a retailing chain established in 1854 in Turin. It is owned by its approximately 7.9 million member-consumers, a community that pushed Coop's top management for the development of a new ethical fashion collection of clothing. Coop member-consumers wanted Coop, as the number-one distribution company in Italy with more than €13 billion in sales annually (Coop Italia 2013), to develop new ecological and fair trade apparel. Coop, although primarily known as a supermarket and hypermarket chain, was in fact a pioneer of ethical clothing in Italy, launching its first organic and fair trade apparel collection in 1994. However, in more recent years, the development and assortment of their fair trade and organic offering were declining—as were sales in this category. Coop management took their members' requests seriously and took the opportunity to revive their previous role as innovators. Maura Latini, vice president of Coop Italia, has formulated the parameters for what the collection ought to embody:

> When we think about fashion, we don't only think about colors, styles and all those elements that are always changing, ephemeral and that follow the seasons and cycles of the fast fashion system. We think instead that the substance of fashion is made of the same matter as our ideas and our values: first of all the respect for and right to work. One of the ways that we do that is by joining in solidarity with the farmers and suppliers of the southern parts of the world by paying a fair trade premium that is not linked to market oscillations and which finances initiatives and services in the workers' communities.[7]

With Vesto Come Penso, Coop aimed to link the dignity of human labor with respect for the environment, and manifest that with Hamnett's women's, men's, and children's collection of dresses and pants, and her iconographic T-shirts with

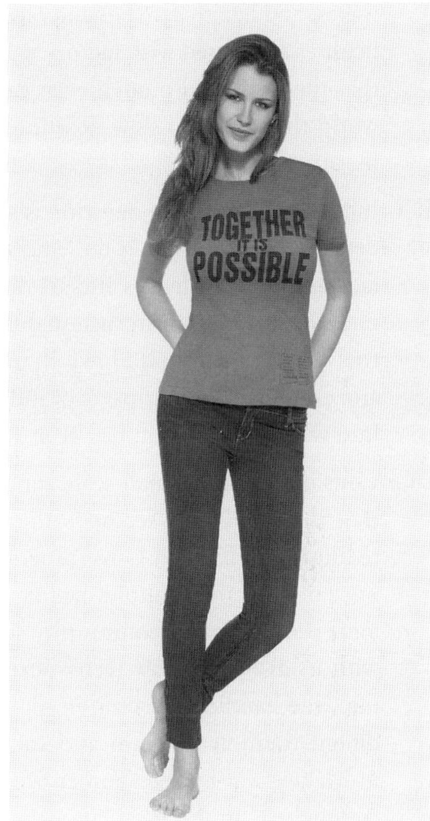

FIGURE 27.3 Katherine Hamnett organic cotton fair trade slogan T-shirt for the Vesto Come Penso line of clothing by Coop Italia, Italy, 2012. *Credit*: © Coop Italia.

slogans such as "Save the Future," "Stop and Think," and "Together It Is Possible" (Figure 27.3).

DG: With this "new and improved" mass-market offer, Coop is attempting to mitigate the inequity of wealth distribution on our planet. One of the suppliers of Coop Italia's fair trade and organic collection is Pratibha Syntex Limited, a huge producer of knitwear in Pithampur, in the state of Madhya Pradesh, India. Pratibha turns out—utilizing its state-of-the-art machinery, up-to-date environmental practices, and more than 7,000 employees—some 55 million garments per year.[8] Their production campuses, which I visited while they were producing the Hamnett line for Coop Italia, are located in a predominantly rural region that is seriously impoverished, with nearly 40 percent of the population below the poverty line (Ray et al. 2009: 225). There are several million people in this state, according to the Indian government, who lack adequate food, clean water, fuel, and hygienic facilities. Pratibha's social efforts include subsidizing schools and providing financial support and guarantees to 28,000 farmers who produce organic cotton for their business under the international certifying organization FLO-CERT's fair trade standards. In this situation, a job at Pratibha, which offers training, above-average wages, and health care benefits, seems to be—even with the tedium, noise, and difficulties associated with factory work—a means to a better life. But I am concerned that the industrial model, even such a relatively "nice" one, is inappropriate for a world that needs to slow down, reduce consumption, and at the same time create meaningful work.

SC: Indeed, whenever the question is about sustainability, the answer always begins, "It depends on . . ." There is no "one-size-fits-all" solution. As a global community, we face multiple challenges and are only starting to understand the interdependent dimensions of long-term sustainability. But we know that developed or "postindustrial" parts of the world have an urgent requirement to mitigate the harmful social and environmental impacts of industrial mass manufacturing within the countries into which production has been relocated.

DG: Considering now small-scale modes of production, it might be a surprising fact that the handloom sector is the second-largest source of employment in India (Ministry of Textiles, Government of India n.d.: 135). In Maheshwar, a small city not far from the Pratibha factory, handloom weaving has been a key part of the local economy and community identity since the seventeenth century. Together with its associated low-tech vocations (yarn spinning, bobbin winding, and dyeing), the handloom sector employs about 35 percent of the workforce.[9] The handloom training program and social business Gudi Mudi was launched in 2009 in Maheshwar by the WomenWeave Charitable Trust. Gudi Mudi (which means "scrunched" in the local language and references the puckered texture of some of their fabrics) initially relied on private and government grants but is now largely self-supporting through sales, both domestic and international, of its handloomed fabrics.[10] Much of their production is done with yarn hand-spun on-site from organic cotton, and is colored with either natural or lower-impact synthetic dyes. Their current products, mostly plain-weave striped and checked scarves and yardage, are woven on simple looms by economically and socially marginalized women (and a few men).

WomenWeave's mission, in part, is "to provide weavers a creative, practical and multi-disciplinary learning experience thereby enabling them to ethically and equitably engage in the global marketplace" (Murphy 2012). As a small-scale artisanal producer of fabrics, Gudi Mudi faces significant challenges and opportunities, many of which I have observed during my field research there. Among the issues are gaining finance and developing infrastructure for training and product development; finding customers for slowly made, variable products in a fashion market that usually expects quickly made, invariable products; developing a business model that takes advantage of the "long-tail" Internet-enabled economy (Anderson 2008); educating customers on the intrinsic value of artisan-made objects; and negotiating the complex issue of fair trade.[11] On the other hand, there are important benefits of this small-scale model that should be considered in relationship to long-term sustainability. First, in terms of social welfare, the trainees have a good amount of freedom to set their own hours, which allows them to balance their personal and family responsibilities with their desire for economic gain. The site is within walking distance of almost all who work there, which, following historical principles of fair trade (Littrell and Dickson 2010), helps the holistic development of the community. There are also signs, such as increases in environmental awareness and higher levels of self-confidence, that those involved in this program and social businesses are part of the global movement toward sustainability that we have discussed. Importantly, if one way to reach sustainability is by consuming fewer but more meaningful items, handmade textiles, by being scarce and intrinsically embedded with emotional resonance, have a unique contribution to make. Ironically, one difficulty Gudi Mudi faces with regard to making the most special products they can, is procuring locally grown organic cotton, which is efficiently commandeered by large-scale manufacturers such as Pratibha!

SC: Competition for resources is one example of the "it depends" dilemma connected with systemic thinking about sustainability, and it points to the need to think beyond the technical aspects of sustainability, such as measuring environmental impacts, and the necessity of work that provides human dignity. Products must also serve the *aesthetic* dimensions of human needs. Otherwise, just mitigation of the mechanical systems will be achieved. We should understand and act on the knowledge that aesthetics and ethics belong to the same nature—tools that satisfy the human need for uniqueness and originality, and for changing the ecology of the mind.

The strength and relevance of a project like Coop Italia are based on this critical point. By creating a very strong aesthetic that simultaneously shines a spotlight on the cleaner and more ethical value chain that produced it, and by choosing an iconic activist and radical fashion designer such as Hamnett, Coop Italia is bringing to many people the message that choosing what to buy and what to wear can be a gesture embodying potentially radical economic and social activism.

DG: The Vesto Come Penso project shows the power of a globally dispersed initiative (designed in the United Kingdom, branded and sold in Italy, manufactured in India) to foster change through careful planning and clear messaging. At the other end of the spectrum, the aspect of human touch and uniqueness that is evident in small-scale, local, or artisanal production of apparel could also help reorient consumers toward more "nutritious" ways of dressing. Rahul Mishra is one fashion designer who believes so. In his case, by using handloomed fabrics (Figure 27.4), he aims "not to grow rich and famous but to make the people around [him] prosperous."[12] Eschewing industrial perfection, he says, "Though ancient, handloom is as contemporary as my vision. The problems we encounter with it, as in other areas of modern life, are often the most beautiful things that happen to us."[13]

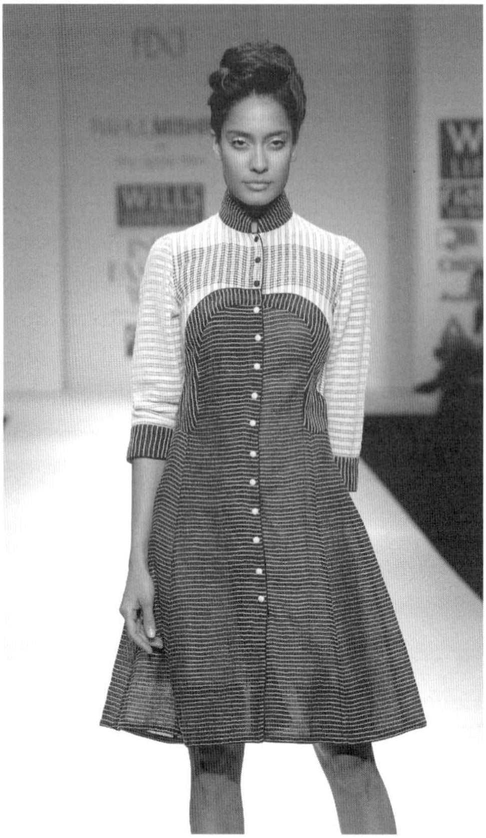

FIGURE 27.4 Rahul Mishra dress, 2010, made with handloomed fabrics from Women-Weave's Gudi Mudi social enterprise, India. *Credit*: © Rahul Mishra.

FASHION AND THE DESIGN OF PROSPERITY

SC: At this point in societal transformation, there are a number of ways that designers could engage with the production of fashion. One route would be to enter into the still-growing luxury product market, which, thanks to the sudden wealth of China, Russia, Brazil, and other rapidly developing countries, is richer than ever. Take the example of PPR Group. In 2011 their luxury brands, Gucci, Bottega Veneta, and Yves Saint Laurent, had a sales growth of almost 23 percent to €4.9 billion (*Pambianco News* 2012). This "business as usual" road has been financially rewarding, but for how long that will continue remains to be seen. Alternatively, designers and fashion stakeholders can take on more entrepreneurial roles by confronting humanity's pressing evolutionary challenges and embracing a humanistic ethos that celebrates the designing of a new economy of significance and meaningfulness. Although we have focused on the large scale and the small scale, the recognition of global interdependence remains the key to a sustainable future, regardless of the production model. Both large scale and small scale, industrial and artisanal—in fact, hybrid approaches for a vast variety of circumstances around the world—should be pursued and investigated through practice as well as academic research. In my view, the best-case scenario would be one in which fashion designers, artisans, entrepreneurs, and marketers come to think of themselves, not only as creators of products, artifacts, sales, and profits, but as the propellers of a new postindustrial economy and the creators not only of garments of style but of styles of thought. As mentioned at the beginning of this dialogue, fashion, because of its ubiquity, its communicative capacity, and its physiological and psychological importance, has a unique opportunity to stimulate new and better habits (from Latin *habitus,* meaning ways of being and not only appearing). Today, a good number of individuals and communities of practice are taking action to restore a future we thought we had lost. They are working on the design of a new notion of prosperity that, unlike the conventional notion of progress, does not allow us to scorch the earth and plunder its riches. Imagine we have two visions of the future standing on either side of us. On one side is the notion of *design,* with its embedded meaning "to draw and plan" (from Old French *dessein*) but also "to choose and designate" (from Latin *designare*) and, by implication, "to look forward." On the other side is *prosperity,* a concept that harbors the ancient Indo-European word *spara,* "to save." It is a word that, like *freedom, brotherhood,* or *equality,* has deeper meanings than the simple sentiment we might associate with the wealthy conformist who, in the golden dusk of a setting sun, enjoys "tranquility" despite the ailments and afflictions that are spreading around the world. The two words, put together in the phrase the Design of Prosperity, become an optimistic notion—but one that requires a vehicle for it to materialize. When fashion embodies this forward-looking notion of the design of prosperity, we would then see fashion and society heading together in a truly meaningful and sustainable direction.

NOTES

1. For the transition movement, see http://www.transitionnetwork.org.
2. See, for example, http://www.wiser.org.
3. See, for example, the Sustainable Apparel Coalition, http://www.apparelcoalition.org.
4. The Design of Prosperity (thedesignofprosperity.com) is an initiative spearheaded by Professor Carbonaro, begun in 2005 at the Swedish School of Textiles at the University of Borås. It is distinguished by cooperation between the academic, cultural, and business communities, with the aim of exploring through conferences and workshops how change and innovation can give rise to new concepts and patterns of prosperity. While not exclusively focused on textiles or fashion, as are the United Kingdom's annual RITE conferences (Reducing the Impact of Textiles on the Environment) or the social and environmental projects of NICE (Nordic Initiative, Clean and Ethical), the Design of Prosperity shares similar goals.
5. For an example of the voluntary simplicity movement, see the Simplicity Institute, http://simplicityinstitute.org. For the Church of Stop Shopping, see http://www.revbilly.com, and for the Uniform Project, visit http://www.theuniformproject.com.

6. Manfred Steger, professor of global studies and director of the Globalism Research Centre at RMIT University, uses the term *globality* to "signify a *social condition* characterized by tight global economic, political, cultural, and environmental interconnections and flows that make most of the currently existing borders and boundaries irrelevant" (Steger 2009: 8; emphasis original).
7. Maura Latini, personal communication with Simonetta Carbonaro, December 2011.
8. Atul Mittal, personal communication with David Goldsmith, January 2012.
9. Ganesh Verma, personal communication with David Goldsmith, January 2012.
10. Hemendra Sharma, personal communication with David Goldsmith, February 2012.
11. For a thorough explanation of fair trade certification and its relationship to artisanal enterprises, see Mary Littrell and Marsha Dickson's *Artisans and Fair Trade: Crafting Development* (2010).
12. Jasmeen Dugal, "Rahul Mishra," ExplosiveFashion, http://www.explosivefashion.in/know_your_designers.php?id=8 (accessed June 10, 2012).
13. Rahul Mishra, personal communication with David Goldsmith, March 31, 2012.

BIBLIOGRAPHY

Agins, Teri. 2000. *The End of Fashion: How Marketing Changed the Clothing Business Forever.* New York: Harper Paperbacks.

Allwood, Julian M., Søren Ellebæk Laursen, Cecilia Malvido de Rodríguez, and Nancy M. P. Bocken. 2006. *Well Dressed? The Present and Future Sustainability of Clothing and Textiles in the United Kingdom.* Cambridge: Cambridge University Institute for Manufacturing.

Anderson, Chris. 2008. *The Longer Long Tail: The Revised and Updated Edition: Why the Future of Business Is Selling Less of More.* New York: Hyperion.

Apparel Strategist. 2011. "Apparel Spending Continues to Outperform in October." Apparel-Strategist.com, November 26. http://apparelstrategist.com/childrens-apparel-spending-continues-to-underperform-in-october (accessed July 10, 2012).

Barber, Benjamin R. 2007. *Consumed: How Markets Corrupt Children, Infantilize Adults, and Swallow Citizens Whole.* New York: Norton.

Bean, Susan S. 1989. "Gandhi and Khadi: The Fabric of Indian Independence." In Annette B. Weiner and Jane Schneider (eds.), *Cloth and Human Experience,* 355–76. Washington, DC: Smithsonian Institution Press.

Bello, Walden. 2004. *Deglobalization: Ideas for a New World Economy.* London: Zed Books.

Berry, Wendell. 2010. *What Matters? Economics for a Renewed Commonwealth.* Berkeley, CA: Counterpoint.

Black, Sandy. 2008. *Eco-chic: The Fashion Paradox.* London: Black Dog.

Black, Sandy. 2012. *The Sustainable Fashion Handbook.* London: Thames and Hudson.

Bolton, Andrew, and Harold Koda. 2007. *AngloMania: Tradition and Transgression in British Fashion.* New York: Metropolitan Museum of Art.

Brown, Sass. 2010. *Eco-fashion.* London: Laurence King.

Brown, Tim. 2009. *Change by Design: How Design Thinking Transforms Organizations and Inspires Innovation.* New York: HarperBusiness.

Carbonaro, Simonetta. 2009. "Ein Interview mit Simonetta Carbonaro: Radikales Umdenken erforderlich oder das Design eines neuen Wohlstandes." In Martina Fineder, Robert Temel, and Christian Dögl (eds.), *Irresistibly Responsible: Focus Design: Innovations for Man and Society in Flux,* 43–45. Vienna: departure wirtschaft, kunst und kultur.

Carbonaro, Simonetta. 2013. "Fashion and Resilience: The Design of a New Prosperity." Keynote speech at Crafting the Future, The European Academy of Design conference, Gothenburg, Sweden, April 17.

Carbonaro, Simonetta, and Christian Votava. 2009. "The Function of Fashion? The Design of New Styles of… Thought." *Nordic Textile Journal* 9 (1): 31–45.

Carbonaro, Simonetta, and Christian Votava. 2010. "Form Follows Sense: New Innovation and Design Strategies for Crisis-Ridden Times." In Michael Sahmiyeh (ed.), *Creating Desired Futures: How Design Thinking Innovates Business,* 51–68. Boston: Birkhäuser.

Cato, Martina (ed.). 2010. *Mistra Future Fashion Research Program: Background Paper.* Stockholm: Mistra (the Swedish Foundation for Strategic Environmental Research).

Celant, Germano, and Harold Koda. 2000. *Giorgio Armani.* New York: Guggenheim Museum.

Clark, Hazel. 2008. "SLOW + FASHION—an Oxymoron—or a Promise for the Future…?" *Fashion Theory: The Journal of Dress, Body, and Culture* 12 (4): 427–46.

Cline, Elizabeth L. 2012. *Overdressed: The Shockingly High Cost of Cheap Fashion.* New York: Portfolio/Penguin.

Cohen, Lizabeth. 2004. *A Consumers' Republic: The Politics of Mass Consumption in Postwar America.* New York: Vintage Books.

Coop Italia. 2013. "Rapporto di Sostenibilità e Valori 2012." Coop Italia, Casalecchio di Reno, Bologna, Italy.

Daly, Herman. 1991. *Steady-State Economics.* Washington, DC: Island Press.

Dilnot, Clive. 2009. "Ethics in Design: 10 Questions." In Hazel Clark and David Brody (eds.), *Design Studies: A Reader,* 180–90. Oxford: Berg.

Ehrenfeld, John R. 2008. *Sustainability by Design: A Subversive Strategy for Transforming Our Consumer Culture.* New Haven, CT: Yale University Press.

Fletcher, Kate. 2008. *Sustainable Fashion and Textiles: Design Journeys.* London: Earthscan.

Fletcher, Kate. 2010. "Slow Fashion: An Invitation to Systems Change." *Fashion Practice: The Journal of Design, Creative Process and the Fashion Industry* 2 (2): 259–66.

Fletcher, Kate, and Lynda Grose. 2012. *Fashion and Sustainability: Design for Change.* London: Laurence King.

Global Footprint Network. 2012. *Country Factsheets.* Oakland, CA: Global Footprint Network. http://www.footprintnetwork.org (accessed May 7, 2012).

Guillet de Monthoux, Pierre. 2004. *The Art Firm: Aesthetic Management and Metaphysical Marketing.* Stanford, CA: Stanford Business Books.

Hawken, Paul. 2010. *The Ecology of Commerce.* Rev. ed. New York: First Harper Business.

Hoffman, Leslie (ed.). 2007. *Future Fashion White Papers.* New York: Earth Pledge.

Jackson, Tim. 2009. *Prosperity without Growth: Economics for a Finite Planet.* London: Earthscan.

Jevons, William Stanley. 1866. *The Coal Question: An Inquiry Concerning the Progress of the Nation, and the Probable Exhaustion of Our Coal Mines.* London: Library of Economics and Liberty.

Joshi, Divya. 2002. *Ghandhiji on Khadi: Selected and Compiled with an Introduction.* Mumbai: Gandhi Book Centre.

Kahneman, Daniel, Edward Deiner, and Norbert Schwarz (eds.). 2003. *Well-Being: Foundations of Hedonic Psychology.* New York: Russell Sage Foundation.

Kahneman, Daniel, and Alan B. Krueger. 2006. "Developments in the Measurements of Subjective Well-Being." *Journal of Economic Perspectives* 20 (1): 3–24.

Kawamura, Yuniya. 2005. *Fashion-ology: An Introduction to Fashion Studies.* Oxford: Berg.

Keynes, John Maynard. 1933. "National Self-Sufficiency." *The Yale Review* 22 (4): 755–69.

Kunz, Grace I., and Myrna B. Garner. 2011. *Going Global: The Textile and Apparel Industry.* New York: Fairchild Books.

Latouche, Serge. 2010. *Farewell to Growth.* Cambridge, UK: Polity.

Littrell, Mary A., and Marsha A. Dickson. 2010. *Artisans and Fair Trade: Crafting Development.* Sterling, VA: Kumarian.

McDonough, William, and Michael Braungart. 2002. *Cradle to Cradle: Remaking the Way We Make Things.* New York: North Point.

McGowan, Abigail. 2009. *Crafting the Nation in Colonial India.* New York: Palgrave Macmillan.

Meadows, Donella, Jorgen Randers, and Dennis Meadows. 2004. *Limits to Growth: The 30-Year Update.* White River Junction, VT: Chelsea Green.

Miller, Daniel. 2010. *Stuff.* Cambridge, UK: Polity.

Ministry of Textiles, Government of India. n.d. *Annual Report 2010–2011.* http://texmin.nic.in/annualrep/ar_10_11_english.pdf (accessed May 12, 2013).

Murphy, Marilyn. 2012. "We Have Gold in Our Hands." *Clothroads: A Global Textile Market,* February 7. http://www.clothroads.com/we-have-gold-in-our-hands/ (accessed May 12, 2013).

O'Neill, Dan W., Rob Dietz, and Nigel Jones. 2010. *Enough Is Enough: Ideas for a Sustainable Economy in a World of Finite Resources.* Leeds, UK: Center for the Advancement of the Steady State Economy.

Pambianco News. 2012. "Il fascino del lusso traina i conti di PPR che supera i 12 miliardi." http://www.pambianconews.com/il-fascino-del-lusso-traina-i-conti-di-ppr-che-supera-i-12-miliardi/ (accessed February 17, 2012).

Papanek, Victor. 2005. *Design for the Real World: Human Ecology and Social Change.* Chicago: Academy Chicago.

Patel, Raj. 2009. *The Value of Nothing: How to Reshape Market Society and Redefine Democracy.* New York: Picador.

Pilloton, Emily. 2009. *Design Revolution: 100 Products That Empower People.* New York: Metropolis Books.

Polimeni, J. M., Kozo Mayumi, Mario Giampietro, and Blake Alcott. 2009. *The Myth of Resource Efficiency: The Jevons Paradox.* London: Routledge.

Ramagundam, Rahul. 2008. *Gandhi's Khadi: A History of Contention and Conciliation.* New Delhi: Orient Longman.

Ray, Shovan, Amita Shah, Alok R. Chaurasia, and Rahul Banerjee. 2009. *Poverty Reduction Strategy for Madhya Pradesh.* Mumbai: Indira Gandhi Institute.

Reiley, Kathryn, and Marilyn DeLong. 2011. "A Consumer Vision for Sustainable Fashion Practice." *Fashion Practice: The Journal of Design, Creative Process and the Fashion Industry* 3 (1): 63–84.

Rivoli, Pietra. 2005. *The Travels of a T-Shirt in the Global Economy: An Economist Examines the Markets, Power and Politics of World Trade.* Hoboken, NJ: Wiley.

Rockstöm, Johan, and Mattias Klum. 2012. *The Human Quest: Prospering within Planetary Boundaries.* Stockholm: Stockholm Text Publishing.

Ross, Robert J. S. 2004. *Slaves to Fashion: Poverty and Abuse in the New Sweatshops.* Ann Arbor: University of Michigan Press.
Roy, Tirthankar. 1993. *Artisans and Industrialization: Indian Weaving in the Twentieth Century.* Oxford: Oxford University Press.
Ruffolo, Giorgio. 2008. *Il capitalismo ha i secoli contati.* Turin, Italy: Einaudi.
Sale, Kirkpatrick. 1995. *Rebels against the Future: The Luddites and Their War on the Industrial Revolution: Lessons for the Computer Age.* Cambridge, MA: Perseus.
Schmidheiny, Stephan. 1992. *Changing Course: A Global Business Perspective on Development and the Environment.* Geneva: World Business Council for Sustainable Development.
Schor, Juliet B. 2005. *Born to Buy: The Commercialized Child and the New Consumer Culture.* New York: Scribner.
Schumacher, E. F. 1973. *Small Is Beautiful: Economics as If People Mattered.* New York: Harper.
Sennett, Richard. 2006. *The Culture of the New Capitalism.* New Haven, CT: Yale University Press.
Shell, Ellen Ruppel. 2009. *Cheap: The High Cost of Discount Culture.* New York: Penguin.
Siegle, Lucy. 2011. *To Die For: Is Fashion Wearing Out the World?* London: Fourth Estate.
Sinclair, Cameron, Kate Stohr, and Cynthia Barton (eds.). 2006. *Design Like You Give a Damn: Architectural Responses to the Humanitarian Crises.* New York: Metropolis Books.
Singer, Peter. 2004. *One World: The Ethics of Globalization.* New Haven, CT: Yale University Press.
Smith, Cynthia E. (ed.). 2007. *Design for the Other 90 Percent.* New York: Cooper-Hewitt National Design Museum, Smithsonian Institute.
Snyder, Rachel Louise. 2007. *Fugitive Denim: A Moving Story of People and Pants in the Borderless World of Global Trade.* New York: Norton.
Steger, Manfred B. 2009. *Globalization: A Very Short Introduction.* Oxford: Oxford University Press.
Stiglitz, Joseph, Amartya Sen, and Jean-Paul Fitoussi. 2009. *Report by the Commission on the Measurement of Economic Performance and Social Progress.* Paris: Government of France.
Thackara, John. 2006. *In the Bubble: Designing in a Complex World.* Cambridge, MA: MIT Press.
Timmerman, Kelsey. 2009. *Where Am I Wearing? A Global Tour to the Countries, Factories, and People That Make Our Clothes.* Hoboken, NJ: Wiley.
Verganti, Roberto. 2008. "Design, Meanings, and Radical Innovation: A Metamodel and a Research Agenda." *Journal of Produce Innovation Management* 25 (5): 436–56.
Verganti, Roberto. 2009. *Design-Driven Innovation: Changing the Rules of Competition by Radically Innovating What Things Mean.* Boston: Harvard Business Press.
Vezzoli, Carlo Arnaldo, and Ezio Manzini. 2010. *Design for Environmental Sustainability.* London: Springer.
Vinken, Barbara. 2005. *Fashion Zeitgeist: Trends and Cycles in the Fashion System.* Oxford: Berg.
Wann, David. 1996. *Deep Design: Pathways to a Livable Future.* Washington, DC: Island Press.
Weber, Max. [1914] 1978. *Economy and Society.* Berkeley: University of California Press.
Welford, Richard. 1997. *Hijacking Environmentalism: Corporate Responses to Sustainable Development.* London: Earthscan.
Whiteside, Patricia, and Nicola White. 2002. *Giorgio Armani.* London: Carlton.
Wilcox, Claire. 2005. *Vivienne Westwood.* London: Victoria and Albert Museum.
Woodham, Jonathan M. 1997. *Twentieth-Century Design.* New York: Oxford University Press.

RESOURCES BIBLIOGRAPHY

SECTION I: FASHION/DRESS AND TIME

Bauman, Zygmunt. 2000. *Liquid Modernity.* Cambridge, UK: Polity.
Clark, Judith. 2005. *Spectres: When Fashion Turns Back.* London: V&A Publishing.
Taylor, Lou. 2004. *Establishing Dress History.* Manchester: Manchester University Press.
Twigg, Julia. 2013. *Fashion and Age: Dress, the Body and Later Life.* London: Bloomsbury.
Wilson, Elizabeth. 1985. *Adorned in Dreams: Fashion and Modernity.* London: Virago.

SECTION II: FASHION, IDENTITY, AND DIFFERENCE

Entwistle, Joanne. 2000. "Fashioning the Career Woman: Power Dressing as a Strategy of Consumption." In Mary R. Andrews and Mary Margaret Talbot (eds.), *All the World and Her Husband: Women, Consumption and Power,* 224–38. London: Continuum International.
Entwistle, Joanne, and Elizabeth Wilson (eds.). 2001. *Body Dressing.* Oxford: Berg.
Hebdige, Dick. 1979. *Subculture: The Meaning of Style.* London: Methuen.
Paulicelli, Eugenia, and Hazel Clark (eds.). 2009. *The Fabric of Cultures: Fashion, Identity, Globalization.* Oxford: Taylor and Francis.

SECTION III: SPACES OF FASHION

Goffman, Erving. 1990. *The Presentation of the Self in Everyday Life.* London: Penguin.
Lefebvre, Henri. 1991. *The Production of Space.* Oxford: Blackwell.
Massey, Doreen. 2005. *For Space.* London: Sage.
Potvin, John. (ed.). 2009. *The Places and Spaces of Fashion, 1800–2007.* London: Routledge.

SECTION IV: FASHION AND MATERIALITY

de la Haye, Amy. 2008. "One Object, Multiple Interpretations." *Fashion Theory: The Journal of Dress, Body and Culture* 12 (2): 137–58.

Pearce, Susan M. 1992. *Museums, Objects and Collections: A Cultural Study.* Washington, DC: Smithsonian Institution Press.

Taylor, Lou. 2004. *Establishing Dress History.* Manchester: Manchester University Press.

Woodward, Ian. 2007. *Understanding Material Culture.* Los Angeles: Sage.

SECTION V: FASHION, AGENCY, AND POLICY

Craik, Jennifer. 1993. *The Face of Fashion.* London: Routledge.

Hansen, Karen Tranberg. 2004. "The World in Dress: Anthropological Perspectives on Clothing, Fashion, and Culture." *Annual Review of Anthropology* 22: 369–92.

Maynard, Margaret. 2004. *Dress and Globalisation.* Manchester: Manchester University Press.

Root, Regina A. 2010. *Couture and Consensus: Fashion and Politics in Postcolonial Argentina.* Minneapolis: University of Minnesota Press.

SECTION VI: SCIENCE, TECHNOLOGY, AND NEW FASHION

Beylerian, George M., and Andrew Dent. 2007. *Ultra Materials: How Materials Innovation Is Changing the World.* Ed. Bradley Quinn. London: Thames and Hudson.

Braddock Clarke, Sarah E., and Jane Harris. 2012. *Digital Visions for Fashion and Textiles.* London: Thames and Hudson.

Philips Electronics. 2000. *New Nomads: An Exploration of Wearable Electronics by Philips.* Rotterdam: 010 Publishers.

Seymour, Sabine. 2008. *Fashionable Technology: The Intersection of Design, Fashion, Science and Technology.* Vienna: Springer.

SECTION VII: SUSTAINABLE FASHION IN A GLOBALIZED WORLD

Allwood, Julian M., Søren Ellebæk Laursen, Cecilia Malvido de Rodríguez, and Nancy M. P. Bocken. 2006. *Well Dressed? The Present and Future Sustainability of Clothing and Textiles in the United Kingdom.* Cambridge: University of Cambridge Institute for Manufacturing.

Black, Sandy. 2012. *The Sustainable Fashion Handbook.* London: Thames and Hudson.

Dickson, Marsha A., Suzanne Loker, and Molly Eckman. 2009. *Social Responsibility in the Global Apparel Industry.* New York: Fairchild Books.

Ehrenfeld, John A. 2008. *Sustainability by Design: A Subversive Strategy for Transforming Our Consumer Culture.* New Haven, CT: Yale University Press.

Fletcher, Kate, and Lynda Grose. 2012. *Fashion and Sustainability: Design for Change.* London: Laurence King.

Hethorn, Janet, and Connie Ulasewicz (eds.). 2008. *Sustainable Fashion: Why Now? A Conversation Exploring Issues, Practices, and Possibilities.* New York: Fairchild Books.

INDEX